Iatrogenic Neurology

Iatrogenic Neurology

José Biller, M.D., F.A.C.P.

Professor and Chairman, Department of Neurology, Indiana University School of Medicine; Chief, Neurology Services, Department of Neurology, Indiana University Medical Center, Indianapolis

Butterworth–Heinemann

Boston Oxford Johannesburg Melbourne New Delhi Singapore

Every effort has been made to ensure that the drug dosage schedules within this text are accurate and conform to standards accepted at time of publication. However, as treatment recommendations vary in the light of continuing research and clinical experience, the reader is advised to verify drug dosage schedules herein with information found on product information sheets. This is especially true in cases of new or infrequently used drugs.

Recognizing the importance of preserving what has been written, Butterworth–Heinemann prints its books on acid-free paper whenever possible.

Butterworth–Heinemann supports the efforts of American Forests and the Global ReLeaf program in its campaign for the betterment of trees, forests, and our environment.

Library of Congress Cataloging-in-Publication Data

Iatrogenic neurology / [edited by] Jose Biller.
p. cm.
Includes bibliographical references and index.
ISBN 0-7506-9840-3
1. Neurotoxicology. 2. Drug--Side effects. 3. Therapeutics--Complications 4. Iatrogenic diseases. I. Biller, Jose.
[DNLM: 1. Iatrogenic Disease. 2. Neurologic Manifestations. QZ 42 I1144 1998]
RC347.5.I28 1998
616.8--dc21
DNLM/DLC
for Library of Congress 97-39911
CIP

British Library Cataloguing-in-Publication Data
A catalogue record for this book is available from the British Library.

The publisher offers special discounts on bulk orders of this book.
For information, please contact:

Manager of Special Sales
Butterworth–Heinemann
225 Wildwood Avenue
Woburn, MA 01801-2041
Tel: 781-904-2500
Fax: 781-904-2620

For information on all Butterworth–Heinemann publications available, contact our World Wide Web home page at: http://www.bh.com

10 9 8 7 6 5 4 3 2 1

Printed in the United States of America

To our patients

Contents

Contributing Authors

Marie Di Nome Acierno, M.D.
Assistant Professor of Ophthalmology and Neurology, University of Mississippi Medical Center, Jackson

Harold P. Adams, Jr., M.D.
Professor of Neurology and Director, Division of Cerebrovascular Diseases, University of Iowa College of Medicine, Iowa City

John C. Andrefsky, M.D.
Assistant Director, Neuromedical/Neurosurgical Intensive Care Unit, The Cleveland Clinic Foundation

José Biller, M.D., F.A.C.P.
Professor and Chairman, Department of Neurology, Indiana University School of Medicine; Chief, Neurology Services, Department of Neurology, Indiana University Medical Center, Indianapolis

Rajesh K. Bindal, M.D.
Resident, Section of Neurological Surgery, Indiana University School of Medicine, Indianapolis

Allison Brashear, M.D.
Assistant Professor, Department of Neurology, Indiana University School of Medicine, Indianapolis

Karen S. Caldemeyer, M.D.
Assistant Professor, Section of Neuroradiology, Department of Radiology, Indiana University School of Medicine, Indianapolis

James J. Corbett, M.D.
McCarty Professor and Chairman, Department of Neurology, and Professor, Department of Ophthalmology, University of Mississippi Medical Center, Jackson

David S. Currier, M.D.
Assistant Clinical Professor of Anesthesiology, Indiana University School of Medicine, Indianapolis

Andrew J. DeNardo, M.D.
Clinical Assistant Professor of Radiology, Indiana University School of Medicine; Staff Neuroradiologist, Methodist Hospital of Indiana, Indianapolis

Edward J. Dropcho, M.D.
Professor, Department of Neurology, Indiana University School of Medicine; Chief, Neurology Service, Richard Roudebush Veterans Affairs Medical Center; Director, Neuro-Oncology Program, Indiana University Cancer Center, Indianapolis

David W. Dunn, M.D.
Associate Professor, Departments of Neurology and Psychiatry, Indiana University School of Medicine; Child Neurologist and Child Psychiatrist, James Whitcomb Riley Hospital for Children, Indianapolis

Martin R. Farlow, M.D.
Professor and Vice-Chairman of Research, Department of Neurology, Indiana University School of Medicine, Indianapolis

Jeffrey I. Frank, M.D.
Director, Neuromedical/Neurosurgical Intensive Care Program, The Cleveland Clinic Foundation

Bhuwan P. Garg, M.D.
Professor, Department of Neurology, Indiana University School of Medicine; Director, Section of Pediatric Neurology, James Whitcomb Riley Hospital for Children, Indianapolis

Stacy L. Greenspan, D.O.
Neuroradiology Fellow and Instructor, Section of Neuroradiology, Department of Radiology, Indiana University School of Medicine, Indianapolis

Ann Marie Hake, M.D.
Neurodegenerative Disease Research Fellow, Department of Neurology, Indiana University School of Medicine, Indianapolis

Kylene K.H. Huler, M.D.
Chief Resident, Department of Neurology, Indiana University School of Medicine, Indianapolis

Robert Jay Huler, M.D.
Assistant Professor, Department of Orthopedic Surgery, Indiana University School of Medicine; Spinal Surgeon, Indiana University Hospitals; Director of the Scoliosis and Spinal Deformity Clinics, James Whitcomb Riley Hospital for Children; Orthopedic Consultant, Indiana Comprehensive Hemophilia Center, Indianapolis

John C. Kincaid, M.D.
Associate Professor, Department of Neurology, and Director of Electromyography Laboratory, Indiana University School of Medicine, Indianapolis

Margaret A. Laycock, M.D.
Clinical Assistant Professor, Department of Neurology, Indiana University School of Medicine, Indianapolis

Marc D. Malkoff, M.D.
Associate Professor, Department of Neurology, Indiana University School of Medicine; Director, Neuroscience Critical Care Unit, Indiana University Hospital, Indianapolis

James F. Meschia, M.D.
Senior Associate Consultant in Neurology, Mayo Clinic Jacksonville, Florida

Paul B. Nelson, M.D.
Professor and Chairman, Section of Neurosurgery, Indiana University School of Medicine; Chief of Neurosurgery, Indiana University Hospital, Indianapolis

Nina A. Paleologos, M.D.
Assistant Professor of Neurology, Northwestern University Medical School, Chicago; Co-Director, Neuro-Oncology Program, Evanston Hospital, Evanston, Illinois

Robert M. Pascuzzi, M.D.
Professor and Vice-Chairman, Department of Neurology, Indiana University School of Medicine, Indianapolis

Hema Patel, M.D.
Clinical Assistant Professor, Department of Neurology, Section of Pediatric Neurology, Indiana University School of Medicine, Indianapolis

John P. Phillips, M.D.
Clinical Assistant Professor, Department of Neurology, Section of Pediatric Neurology, Indiana University School of Medicine, Indianapolis

Karen L. Roos, M.D.
Professor, Department of Neurology, Indiana University School of Medicine, Indianapolis

Charles E. Schultz, M.D.
Neuromuscular Disease Fellow, Department of Neurology, Indiana University School of Medicine, Indianapolis

John A. Scott, M.D.
Clinical Associate Professor of Radiology, Indiana University School of Medicine; Interventional Neuroradiologist, Methodist Hospital of Indiana, Indianapolis

Michael A. Sloan, M.D.
Department of Neuroscience, Harbin Clinic, Rome, Georgia

B. Todd Troost, M.D.
Professor and Chairman, Department of Neurology, Wake Forest University School of Medicine, Winston-Salem, North Carolina

Melissa A. Waller, M.S., CCC-A
Clinical Audiologist, Department of Otolaryngology, University of Texas Southwestern Medical Center, Dallas

Kelda Harris Walsh, M.D.
Clinical Assistant Professor of Psychiatry, Child Psychiatry Section, Indiana University School of Medicine; Medical Director of Psychiatry, Adolescent Unit, LaRue Carter Hospital, Indianapolis

Linda S. Williams, M.D.
Clinical Assistant Professor, Department of Neurology, Indiana University School of Medicine, Indianapolis

Joanne Wojcieszek, M.D.
Clinical Assistant Professor, Department of Neurology, Indiana University School of Medicine, Indianapolis

Preface

Exalted G-d, before beginning my sacred task to bring healing to Your mortal creatures, I beg You grant me the courage and strength to faithfully execute my duties. Guard me from the blindness of avarice and the thirst for glory and honor. Endow me with the strength to equally serve the rich and the poor, the good and the wicked, friend and enemy—to simply see in each, a fellow human being in pain. Inspire me with the desire to learn from more learned physicians, for the art of medicine, to which I have dedicated myself, is infinite. Protect me, however, from the scorn and ridicule of those who are older or more respected. Let the truth alone guide me, for any professional compromise can bring only illness and tragedy to Your mortal creatures. Oh most compassionate and merciful L-rd, strengthen me both in body and soul and implant within me a spirit of wholesomeness.

The Physician's Prayer
Rabbi Moses ben Maimon (Maimónides 1135–1204)

Primum non nocere

Better science and recent medical progress have brought dramatic advances in methods of diagnosis and treatment; however, reports of adverse reactions have accompanied these advances. The incidence of iatrogenic illness is probably underestimated, and iatrogenic illness accounts for a considerable number of all hospital admissions. *Iatrogenesis* refers to the consequences of medical actions and results from errors of omission or of commission. Although iatrogenesis has a long history, it represents a considerable part of the complexity of modern medicine and dictates the need for rapid dissemination and exchange of medical information. In light of the expansive use of technology, the incidence of iatrogenic illness increases in hospitalized patients, especially the elderly as well as neonates, and with the increasing use of polypharmacy.

Awareness of iatrogenic illness and its consequences, as well as understanding of the basic mechanisms underlying its manifestations, avoids delays in diagnosis and treatment. Physicians should consider iatrogenic disease in every differential diagnosis and always weigh the probable benefit of each test or treatment against its possible risks. Side effects usually occur soon after a drug is started, but unpredictable hazardous events occur not uncommonly with considerable delay and further experience. Risk factors that contribute to iatrogenic neurologic disorders are multifactorial. Neurologic sequelae can range from minor transient disturbances to severe deficits or even death.

This book reviews some of the more frequent undesirable neurologic events that may result from the use of commonly prescribed drugs and certain diagnostic or therapeutic procedures, as well as strategies to prevent their occurrence. Astute and vigilant care and careful monitoring for untoward events are needed to prevent unnecessary distress and morbidity and to reduce the risks of iatrogenic neurologic illness.

It remains only to thank my wife, Célika, and my children, Sofía, Gabriel, and Rebecca, for their patience, encouragement, and love, and Susan Pioli, Director of Medical Publishing, and Jana Friedman, Assistant Editor, of Butterworth–Heinemann for their support and advice. Finally, I wish to express my gratitude to Dana Tackett, Production Editor, and the staff of Silverchair Science + Communications for their helpful suggestions.

J.B.

Chapter 1

Complications of Lumbar Puncture and Myelography

Stacy L. Greenspan and Karen S. Caldemeyer

Objectives

- To recognize that lumbar puncture and myelography are invasive procedures and may occasionally be associated with serious complications
- To learn that there are indications for myelography despite the widespread use of magnetic resonance imaging (MRI)
- To increase familiarity with the common complications associated with lumbar puncture and the most common etiologies for their cause
- To appreciate the importance of the history of contrast agents used for myelography and why the search for new agents continues
- To recognize some of the more common radiographic findings associated with lumbar puncture and myelography complications
- To understand that the cause of spinal headaches is multifactorial and difficult to assess objectively

Myelography, a procedure once commonly performed to evaluate extradural and intradural pathology as well as intramedullary processes, has been almost completely replaced by MRI. Residents today often wonder whether they need to learn how to perform myelography, since MRI is the study of choice in most instances of spine and spinal cord pathology. However, myelography is not obsolete and remains the method of choice because of its easy availability for the majority of the world population where MRI is less available.[1] Myelography has a role in the evaluation of the spine when MRI is contraindicated, as in patients with pacemakers and other implantable electronic devices, as well as in patients with aneurysm clips. Myelography may also be useful in patients with previous surgical fixation, where computed tomography (CT) and MRI may be degraded by significant metal artifact. The evolution of myelography is interesting, and although a relatively simple procedure to perform, it is not without risks. Fortunately, in the 1990s, the complications are relatively minor and infrequent.

History of Myelography and Contrast Agents

Evaluation of spine and spinal cord pathology via myelography is performed by injecting a contrast agent into the subarachnoid space, either in the mid to lower lumbar region or upper cervical region (C1–C2 puncture). In the early 1920s, several researchers injected air into the subarachnoid space and were able to successfully localize spinal cord tumors.[2] In 1922, poppy seed oil was accidentally introduced into the subarachnoid space by Sicard and Forrestier while performing an extradural injection to treat sciatica.[3] They observed how easily visualized and how freely mobile this agent was within the subarachnoid space. Because of its high viscosity and nonmiscibility with the spinal fluid, however, the oil was difficult to remove and often irritated the pia-arachnoid lining. Diodrast (Per-Abrodil) was used in the early 1930s, but it too was difficult to remove and caused meningeal irritation. Some long-term disabilities were also reported with the use of this agent.[2] In the early 1930s, sodium methiodal (Abrodil) was introduced as the first water-soluble organic iodine compound to be used for myelography. However, studies with this compound were halted during World War II.[3] In the late 1930s and early 1940s, Thorotrast was recommended for myelography. Thorotrast emits alpha radiation with a half-life of 1.4×10^{10} years. The use of Thorotrast was associated with severe systemic reactions, intense arachnoiditis, and delayed development of malignancies.[3] In the late 1940s, Abrodil grew in popularity in Scandinavian countries, but not in the United States, due to its irritating effects on the spinal cord and meninges.[3] In 1940, the University of Rochester introduced iophendylate (Pantopaque), another oily medium that was less viscid and irritating than poppy seed oil (Lipiodol) (Figures 1.1A and B).[3] Pantopaque formed oily globules within the cerebrospinal fluid (CSF) but was more readily removed than Lipiodol. As a result of its immiscibility and insolubility with CSF, Pantopaque did not demonstrate significant neurotoxicity. However, its prolonged exposure to CSF was implicated as a cause for arachnoiditis.[2] Meglumine iothalamate (Conray-60) and meglumine iocarmate (Dimer-X), two water-soluble ionic agents, were introduced in the 1960s and 1970s, but these, too, did not gain widespread acceptance due to their neurotoxic effects.[3] In the late 1970s and early 1980s the first nonionic medium, metrizamide (Amipaque) was introduced, dramatically changing the picture. In the mid to late 1980s newer nonionic water-soluble contrast media such as iohexol (Omnipaque) and iopamidol (Isovue) were introduced (Figures 1.1C and D). Today, water-soluble ionic contrast media are contraindicated for intrathecal use and have been replaced with newer nonionic, low-osmolar agents. Research continues to find new nonionic agents with an even greater margin of safety.

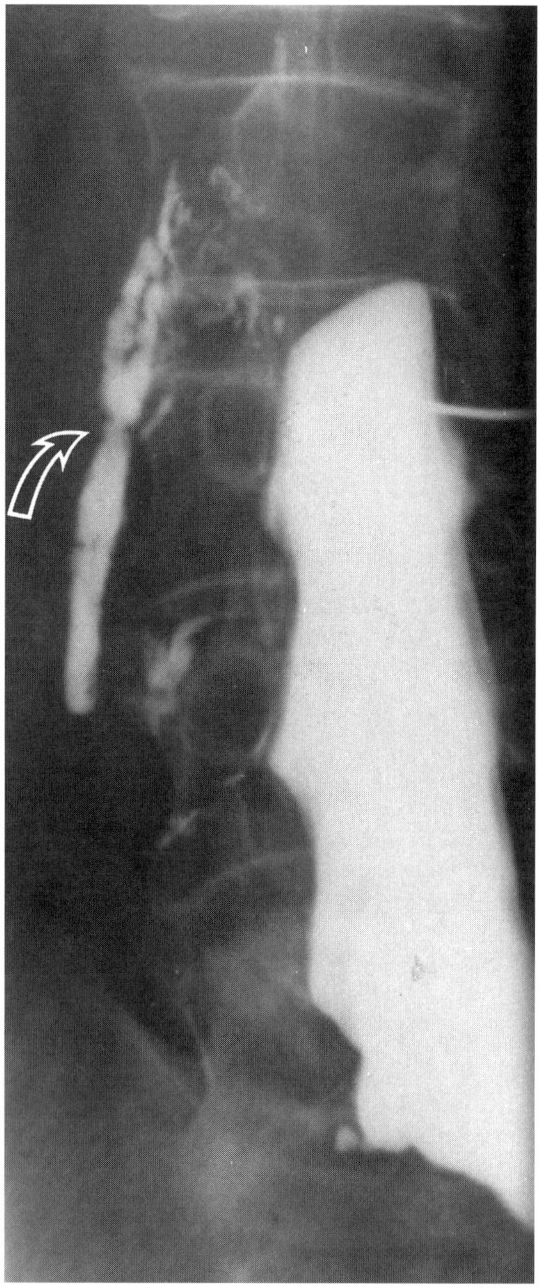

A

Figure 1.1. Pantopaque myelogram. Oblique lumbar (A) and lateral cervical views (B) of a Pantopaque myelogram demonstrate the dense contrast in the subarachnoid space. Note how difficult it is to identify the filling defect of discrete nerve roots or the spinal cord due to the dense opacification. Also, note the extra-arachnoid globules of oily Pantopaque dissecting along the planes of the psoas muscles (open arrow) as well as the intracranial extension (solid arrow).

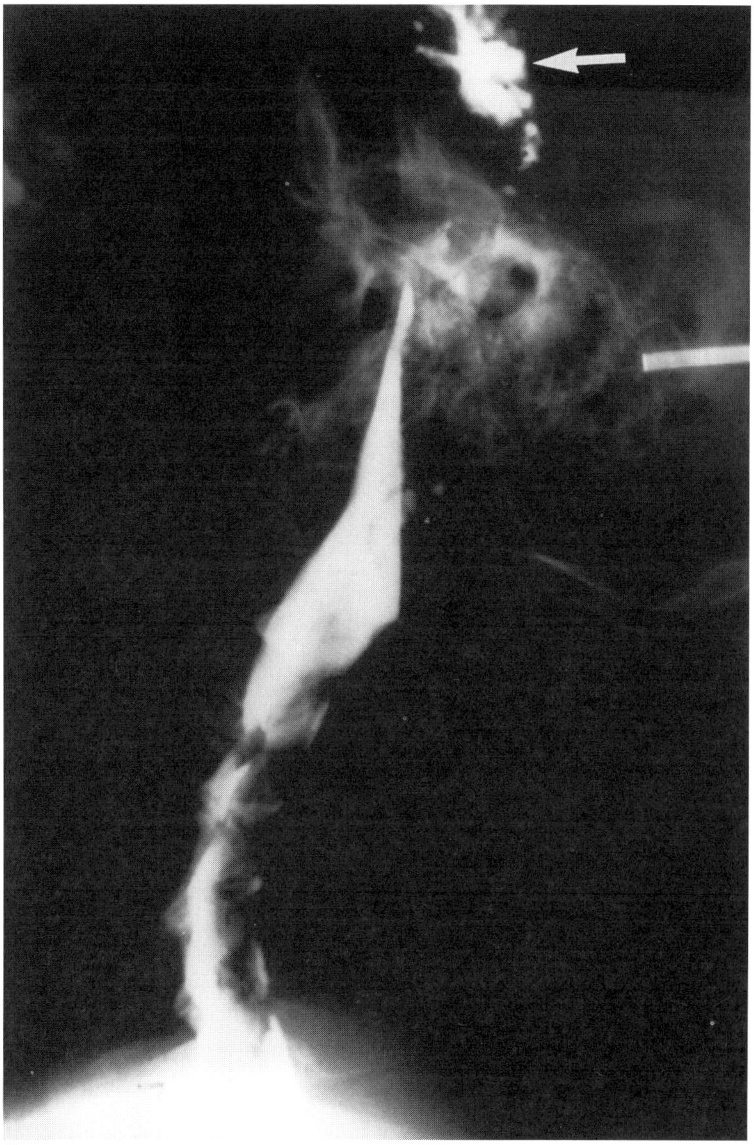

B

Complications

Before myelography is performed, it is essential to obtain a medical history from the patient and inform the individual of the potential risks of the procedure. Currently, the risks associated with myelography are minor and infrequent, but certain adverse effects occur more commonly than others, and in some instances, can result in debilitating outcomes. Spinal headache is by far the most frequent complication after myelography.[4] Infection is a potential serious complication and can be related to the technique and experience of the person performing the procedure. Arachnoiditis is another potential serious complication and can result from the irritating effects of the contrast agent on the meninges. Seizures were more common in the past with the more neurotoxic, low-osmolar, water-soluble, nonionic compounds (e.g., metrizamide) but are still seen occasionally in patients with epilepsy or taking medications that lower the seizure threshold (e.g., phenothiazines, tricyclic antidepressants, and monoamine oxidase inhibitors). Injury to the spinal cord, a nerve root, or the intervertebral disk is extremely uncommon but can result in permanent neurologic deficits. Worsening of brain herniation or spinal cord compression may occur with lumbar puncture and withdrawal of spinal fluid in patients with unrecognized increased intracranial pressure or spinal block.[5] Puncture-induced hemorrhage is most commonly encountered in patients with an underlying bleeding diathesis. Epidermoid tumors, venous intravasation, and cardiac or respiratory failure are additional potential complications of myelography, but with careful technique and adequate patient history, these adverse effects should be kept to a minimum.

Spinal Headache

The most common complication after myelography is a spinal headache.[4] A spinal headache is characterized by its positional nature in which the headache is aggravated by sitting, standing, coughing, or straining and relieved in the recumbent position. The headache may be accompanied by neck stiffness, nausea, vomiting, visual disturbance, tinnitus, or deafness.[4] Approximately 90% of headaches begin within 3 days after puncture and typically last 3–5 days.[4] Headache has been reported to occur after myelography in 4–60% of patients.[6] Several theories have been proposed for the etiology of spinal headaches. Persistent leakage of CSF from the dural puncture site is the most common proposed mechanism. The dura mater, composed of dense connective tissue, may not seal after needle puncture. In the upright position, a pressure gradient from the subarachnoid to epidural space of 40–50 cm of water exists.[4] Raskin's theory is that the sudden decrease in CSF pressure activates adenosine receptors, producing venous and arterial vasodilatation that subsequently results in a spinal headache.[6] Others believe that the decrease in CSF volume in the closed volume central nervous system (CNS) results in a compensatory increase in blood volume through vasodilatation of the pain-sensitive cerebral veins.[4] Support of these theories includes the successful treatment of headaches with vasoconstrictors such as caffeine and theophylline. August Bier, in the late 1800s,

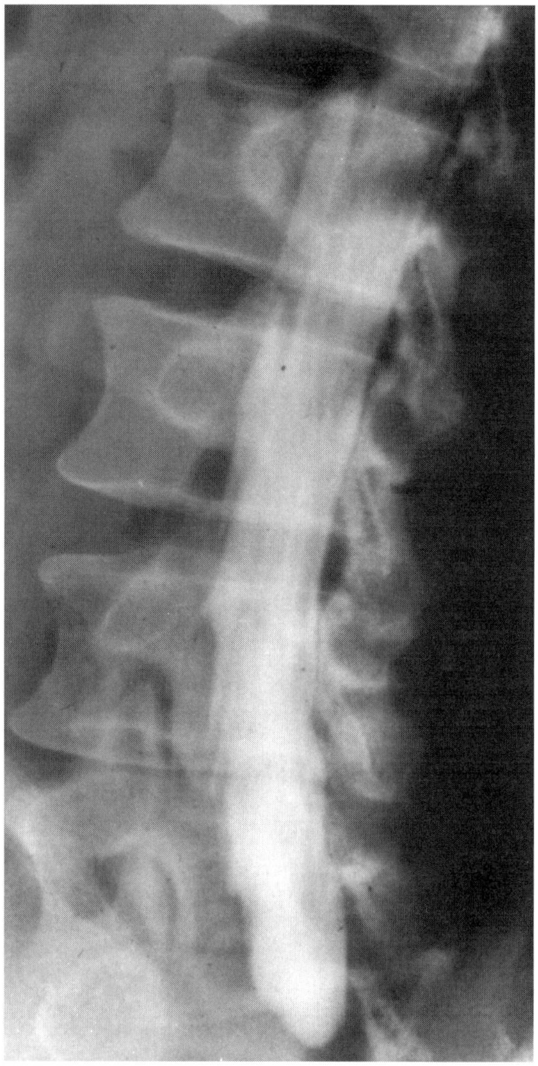

C

Figure 1.1. *continued.* Oblique lumbar view of a water-soluble contrast myelogram (C) and anteroposterior cervical view (D) show less dense opacification of the subarachnoid space. Individual nerve roots and the spinal cord can be easily identified.

proposed that the loss of CSF hydraulic cushioning due to CSF leakage may lead to sagging of intracranial contents and tension on the brain's anchoring devices when the patient stands upright. His theory surfaced when he experienced a headache after attempting to perform a lumbar puncture on himself for spinal anesthesia.[7] Traction on cranial and upper cervical nerves may be the cause of the audi-

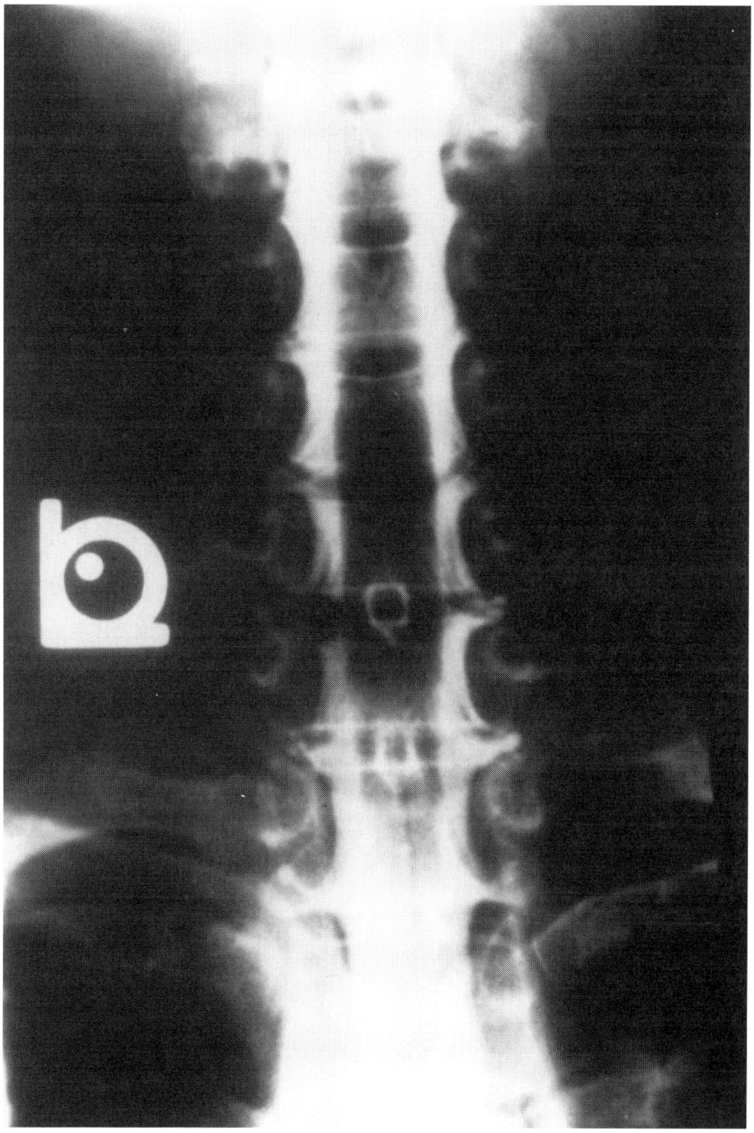

D

tory and vestibular symptoms, nausea, and neck stiffness.[5] Others believe that headache is related to a direct neurotoxic effect of the contrast agent used.

Needle Size

Varying needle sizes and configurations have been correlated with the incidence of headache after dural puncture. Rolfe and Maguire studied the incidence of postlumbar puncture headache (PPH) that occurred after lumbar injections with 18-, 19-, and 22-gauge needles.[8] They found no significant difference between the varying needle sizes. However, Tourtellotte et al.[9] and Wilkinson and Sellar[10] found conflicting results when they compared the incidence of PPH using 22- versus 26-gauge spinal needles. Tourtellotte et al. found that not only were headaches more frequent after myelography with 22-gauge needles (36% versus 12%), but they were also more severe (44% versus 0%). Wilkinson and Sellar found no significant increased incidence of PPH using 22-gauge needles. However, smaller-gauge needles may be impractical for lumbar puncture for fluid withdrawal or myelography where contrast is injected or in postsurgical patients with significant scar tissue. Some authors believe that the size of the dural perforation appears to be less important than factors relating to age, sex, type of myelogram, and experience of the individual myelographer.[7, 8]

Tapered Versus Beveled Needles

Tapered, pencil-point tip needles have been compared with the traditional beveled cutting edge needles (Figure 1.2). In the study by Prager et al., it was found that patients had a lower incidence of spinal headaches after myelography when the pencil-point tip needles were used versus the beveled needles.[6] Jones et al. found similar results with the atraumatic, conical tip needle.[11] The theory is that the tapered, blunter, pencil-point tip needles produce less damage to the dural fibers by pushing them apart rather than cutting them as with beveled edge needles. Thus, healing of the dural fibers is more rapid, resulting in less CSF leakage and ultimately fewer spinal headaches.[6] The pencil-point tip needles, however, have a side hole rather than an end hole, which increases the risk of an extra-arachnoid injection, whereas the beveled cutting edge needles have only an end hole, decreasing the risk of an extra-arachnoid injection (Figure 1.3). Also, the tapered pencil-point needles used in the studies by Prager et al.[6] and by Jones et al.[11] were considerably more expensive. Orientation of the needle bevel parallel to rather than perpendicular to the spine has been reported to decrease PPH in some studies but not others.[4]

Positioning (Bed Rest Versus Early Ambulation)

Positioning of the patient after myelographic procedures has been shown by Skalpe and Nakstad[12] to play a significant role in the incidence of PPH, whereas others believe that in well-hydrated patients positioning has no significant effect on the incidence of PPH.[13–15] Skalpe and Nakstad found the lowest frequency of spinal headaches in patients who were placed in the prone position for 1 hour after myelography and recommend this precaution for all patients.[12] Also, in their study, the highest frequency of headache occurred in patients who were ambulant after the procedure. Kuuliala and Goransson found no significant difference in postprocedural headaches when patients chose early ambulation or bed rest after iohexol (Omnipaque) myelography.[15] Guiati et al. also found no difference in the incidence of headaches between patients who were ambulatory and those who were kept at bed rest.[14] Postacchini and Massobrio found no significant difference in the incidence of side effects when they compared outpatients with inpatients following iopamidol myelography.[16]

C1–C2 Puncture Versus Runup Myelography

Another variable studied is puncture site. Skalpe and Nakstad found a higher incidence of spinal headache in patients after cervical myelography with a lumbar puncture technique than cervical myelography with a C1–C2 puncture technique.[12] This may be due to the head-down tilting necessary to move the contrast medium up to the cervical spine when a lumbar approach is used, increasing the chance for contrast to extend intracranially.[12, 17] Macpherson et al. found no significant difference in the incidence of headache in patients undergoing direct C1–C2 puncture versus runup myelography from the lumbar route.[18]

Age, Sex, Normal Myelogram Results, Body Mass, Physician Experience, Paramedian Approach, and Cerebrospinal Fluid Removal

It is clear that there may be many causes of the postmyelographic headache. The type of intrathecal contrast currently available is limited to the new low-osmolar, nonionic agents that significantly reduce the possibility of a chemical-related neurotoxic effect. In 1993, Harrison concluded that the incidence of headache following myelography and diagnostic lumbar puncture is relatively equal.[7] Thus, the postmyelographic headache is thought to be related to a dural fistula rather than a direct effect of contrast medium toxicity.

Certain variables such as age and gender cannot be altered. Studies have found a significantly increased incidence of PPH in young adults.[4, 6] Patients ages 20–40 years are most likely to develop PPH; the elderly and patients younger than 20 years are at less risk.[4] Although no scientific basis can be attributed to the higher incidence in this group of patients, younger patients are more likely to become active more quickly after a myelographic proce-

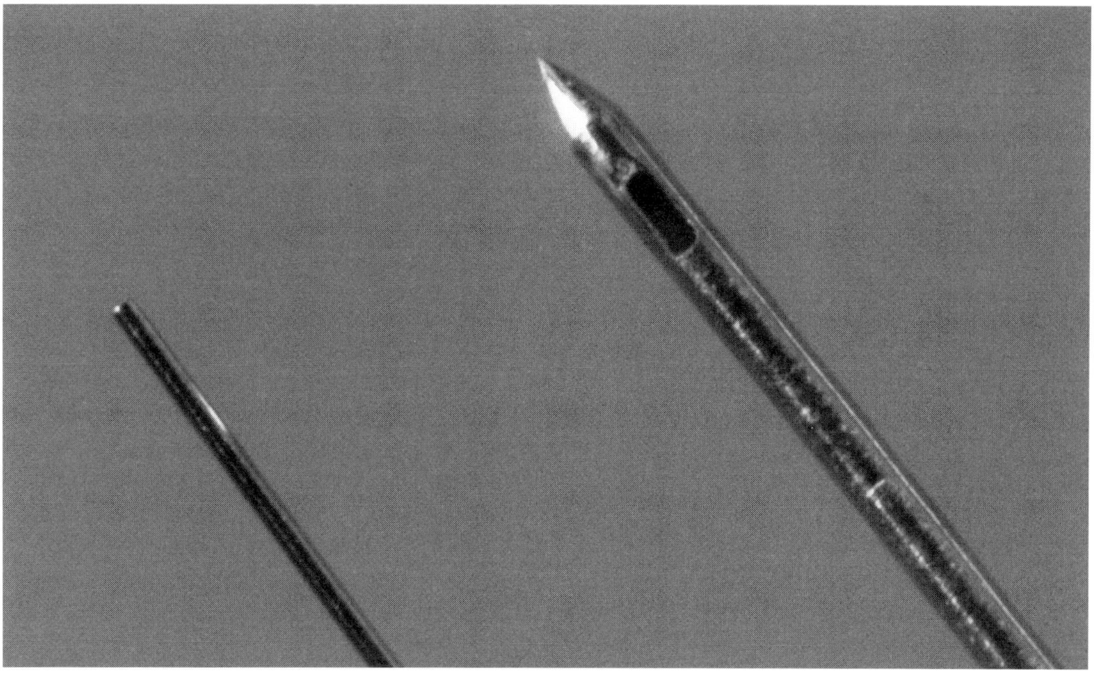

A

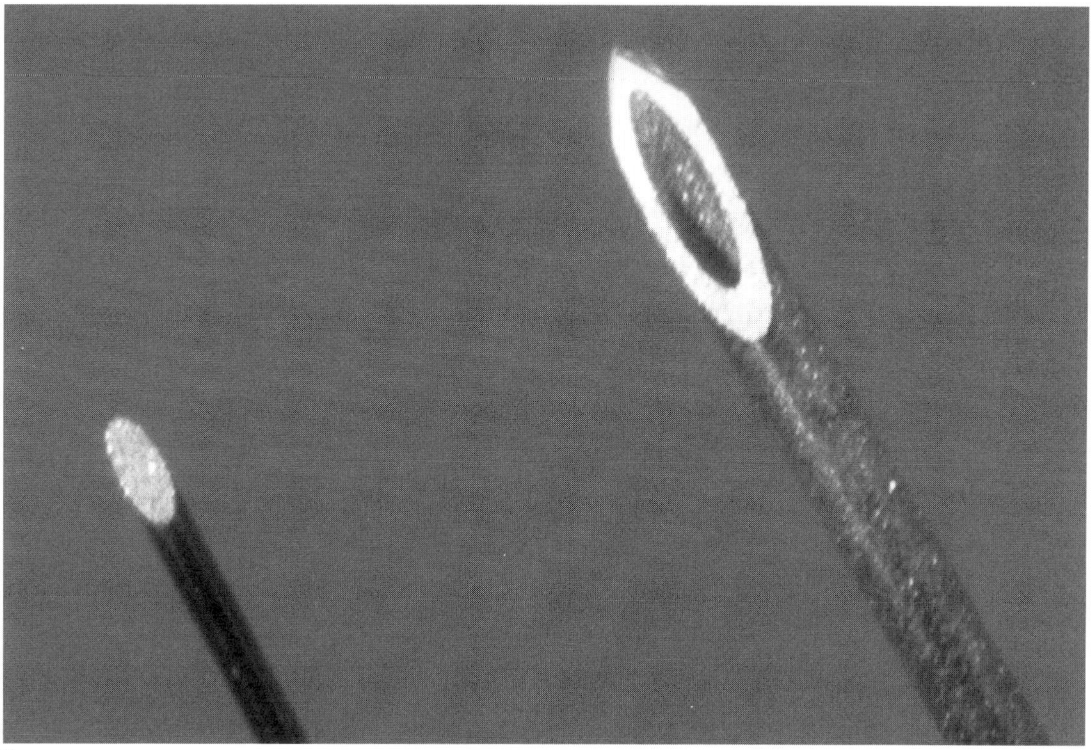

B

Figure 1.2. Tapered versus beveled needles. (A) Tapered, pencil-point tip needles have a blunt tip with a side hole that increases the risk of extra-arachnoid injections. (B) Beveled needles have a sharper tip with an end hole, decreasing the risk of extra-arachnoid injection.

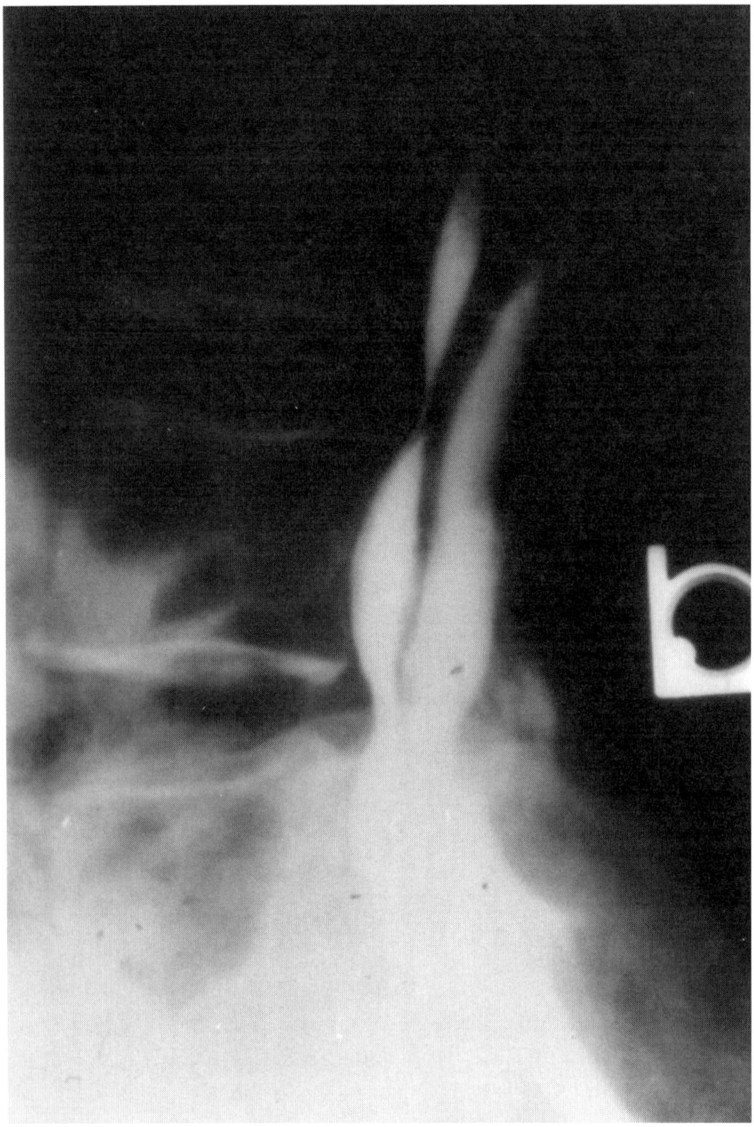

A

Figure 1.3. Subdural injection. Lateral (A) and oblique (B) views of a lumbar myelogram demonstrate a mixed injection with contrast present both in the subarachnoid and subdural spaces.

dure, increasing their risks for postmyelographic headache. Other studies have reported a higher incidence of PPH in women.[4, 7, 9, 11, 16, 19, 20] Although both psychological and endocrinologic factors have been postulated as explanations, no direct correlation has been documented in women. Patients with migraines or other types of headaches more commonly report PPH.[4, 13] Women suffer from migraines more commonly than men, and the abnormal cerebral vasoreactivity experienced after a myelographic procedure may have a greater adverse effect on women. Interestingly, the incidence of headaches after myelography has been reported to be higher in patients with normal examinations versus those with abnormal findings.[4, 11, 13, 20] The cause for this incidence remains unclear but may be attributed to a higher pain threshold in patients with chronic pain[9] or possibly to the increased secretion of endorphins caused by the underlying disease.[13] Others have hypothesized that patients with normal myelography results may be more likely to develop headache because they are angry that the study did not reveal the cause of their complaints.[4] Wilkinson and Sellar[9] and Wagner et al.[21] did not find a significant correlation between increased incidence of PPH and normal myelographic findings. Low body

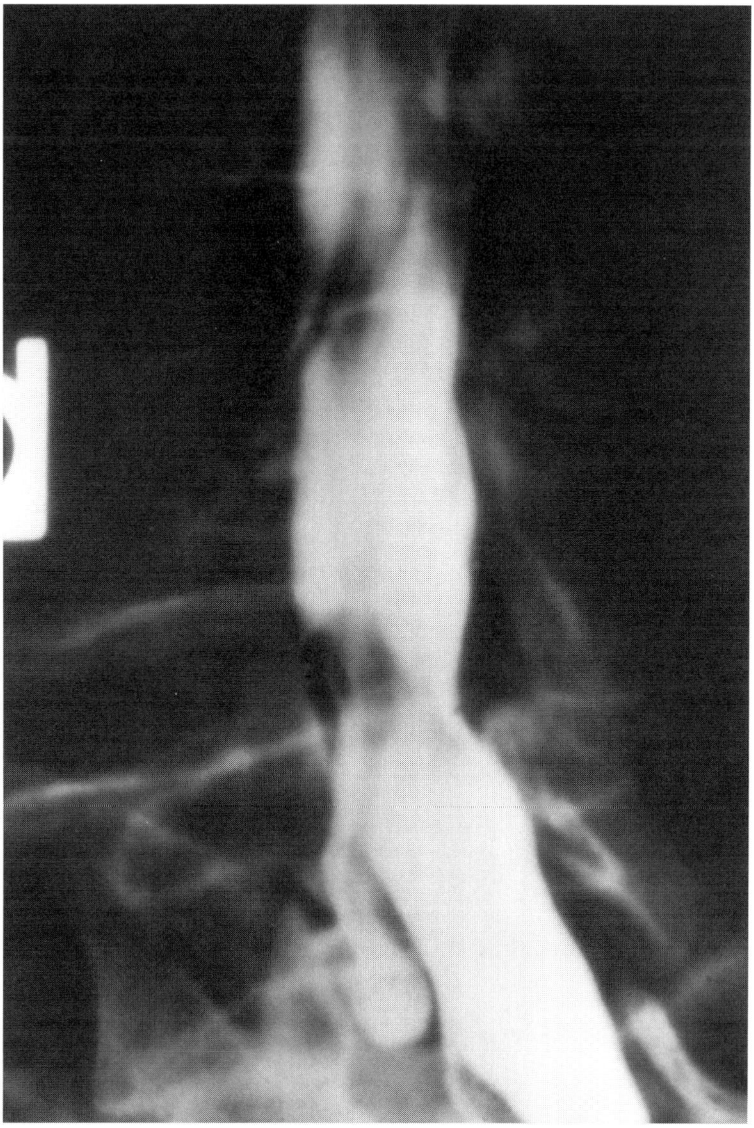

B

mass index has been reported to be associated with a greater risk of PPH.[4] A paramedian approach and an experienced physician are both associated with lower PPH rates in some studies.[4] Hypovolemia and removal of CSF have been inconsistently associated with a higher incidence of PPH.[4]

As long as those who perform myelography adhere to careful technique using needle gauges of 20 or less and restrict patients to bed rest for several hours after the procedure, complications of postmyelographic headache should be minimized. Management of PPH includes bed rest, hydration, analgesics, antiemetics, and methylxanthines. If conservative measures fail, PPH can be rapidly treated with an epidural blood patch of autologous blood, which presumably results in fibrinous sealing of the dural tear.[4, 5]

Arachnoiditis

Spinal arachnoiditis can result from a variety of causes, including infection, intrathecal hemorrhage, trauma, and space-occupying lesions such as disk prolapse, as well as agents injected into the subarachnoid space from either spinal anesthesia or myelography. Myelography with Pantopaque and water-soluble contrast media, both ionic and nonionic, has been shown to produce a meningeal inflammatory reaction in animals (Figures 1.4 and 1.5).[22] In humans, however, although histologic changes of arachnoiditis have been reported after intrathecal injection of these agents, the changes are often accompanied by absent or minimal clinical findings. The introduction of the new nonionic water-soluble contrast agents (e.g., iohexol) has been shown to produce even less meningeal irritation and subsequently reduced leptomeningeal adhesions.

In humans reabsorption of water-soluble contrast media by spinal villi and granulations has been shown to commence almost immediately after lumbar injection.[23] The rate of reabsorption is increased if the patient is maintained in the supine position because the contrast is mixed throughout the subarachnoid space, allowing for contact with a greater surface area of arachnoid granulations throughout the spinal canal.[23] If the patient is maintained in an upright position, there is less mixing of contrast with the CSF and hence delayed reabsorption. This results in an increased duration of contact of the contrast medium with the arachnoid in the caudal sac. The increased volume and concentration of contrast media collecting in the caudal subarachnoid space in an erect patient may result in arachnoiditis. If a patient is dehydrated, it may further slow the reabsorption of contrast media, increasing the risk for arachnoiditis.[23] If during the procedure, more CSF is withdrawn than the amount of contrast media injected, the CSF pressure may drop enough to slow or stop CSF absorption.

Pantopaque, despite being withdrawn from the subarachnoid space after myelography, results in residual oily droplets that collect in the caudal sac. Unabsorbed Pantopaque is responsible for delayed arachnoiditis in some cases. Some of these cases result in severe, acute symptomatology, whereas other patients develop a more chronic arachnoiditis with more insidious symptomatology months or years after the original insult.[2] Patients with arachnoiditis typically complain of pain involving one or more roots and paresthesias in an irregular distribution. Similar complications are seen with the use of metrizamide, which is soluble in CSF. This complication is rarely seen today due to the introduction of the newer generation of low-osmolar, nonionic, water-soluble contrast agents.

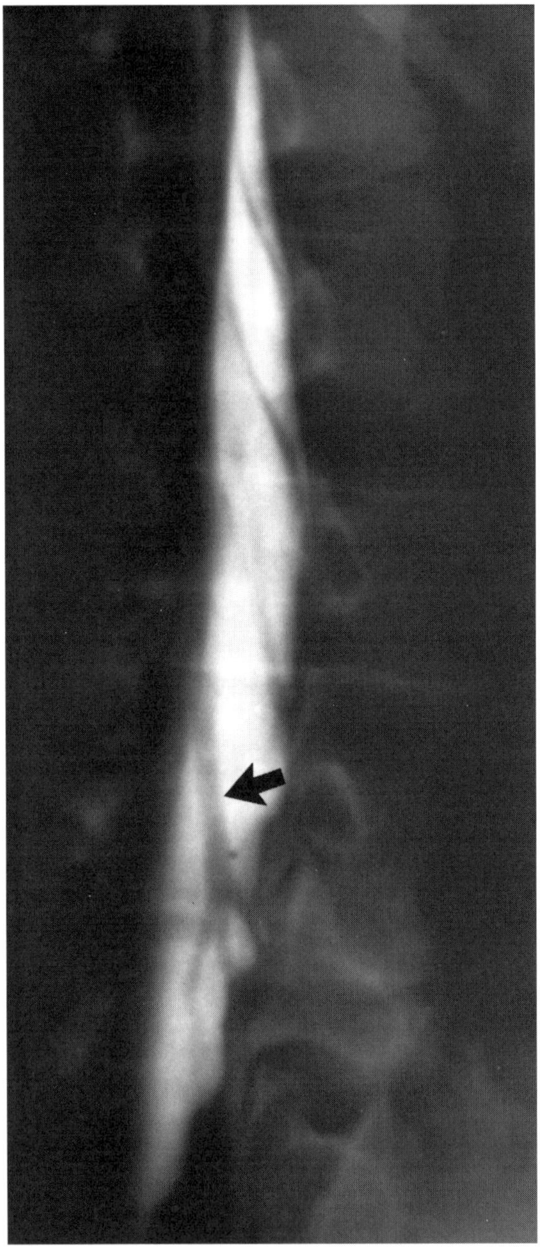

A

Figure 1.4. Arachnoiditis. (A) This water-soluble contrast myelogram shows marked thickening of the caudal nerve roots (arrow). Compare these nerve roots with the normal, thin nerve roots shown in Figure 1.1C. (B) Axial postmyelogram computed tomographic scan demonstrates contrast in the subarachnoid space with a few round filling defects representing thickened, clumped nerve roots.

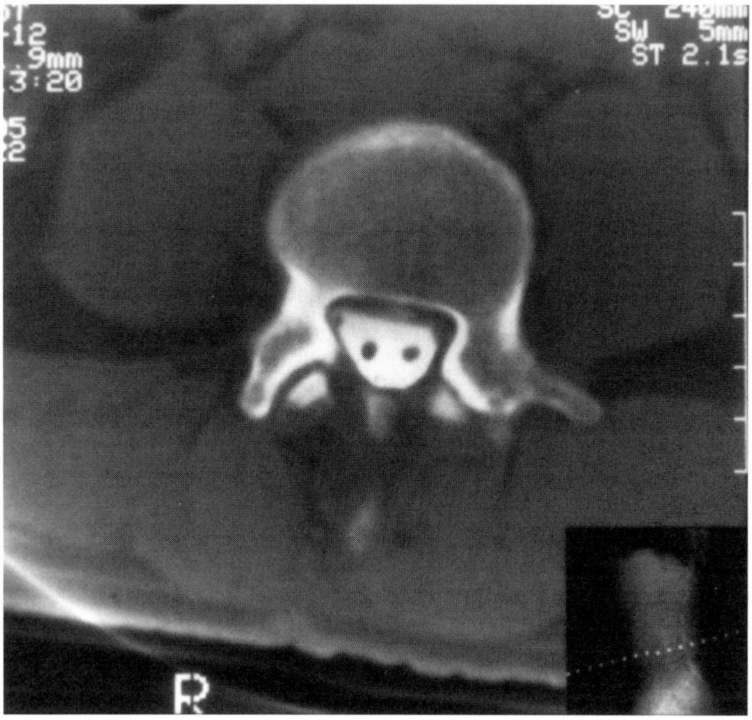

B

Seizures

Intrathecal iodinated contrast media infrequently cause neurotoxic side effects such as urticaria, facial edema, nausea, vomiting, hallucinations, or seizures. In the 1970s, the introduction of meglumine iothalamate (Conray 280) was the outcome of a search for a water-soluble contrast medium.[24] Despite the manufacturer's warnings not to inject meglumine into the subarachnoid space, many Indian radiologists resorted to using meglumine because iophendylate (Pantopaque) was frequently not available. Bagchi reports a case of a middle-aged man with a 2-year history of left-sided sciatica who underwent myelography with Conray.[24] His procedure resulted in violent convulsions, subarachnoid hemorrhage, and death. Praestholm and Lester also reported serious complications, including tonic-clonic muscle spasms in numerous patients after meglumine myelography.[25] Taminiau and Slooff[26] and Morrey and O'Brien[27] reported three cases of severe myoclonic seizures after meglumine myelography that resulted in bilateral femoral neck fractures. Haase et al. reported several cases of vertebral body fracture after meglumine myelography secondary to severe tonic-clonic muscle spasms.[28] Thus, Conray and its water-soluble ionic counterparts were demonstrated to be unsafe for intrathecal injection, as stated in the manufacturer's warning.

Water-soluble ionic contrast media, once used for lumbar myelography, is associated with an increased incidence of toxicity and irritating effects resulting in spasmodic muscle contractions as well as a slight decrease in blood pressure. The intensity of the contractions sometimes leads to dreadful, untoward effects such as vertebral body fracture, femoral neck fractures, and ilium and pubis fractures.[26–28] Other seizure-related complications included intracerebral and subarachnoid hemorrhage with temporary or permanent neurologic sequelae.[24] Since the introduction of nonionic contrast media, the use of intrathecal ionic contrast agents has been abandoned. Metrizamide, although nonionic, was the agent most commonly used in the early 1980s and was associated with generalized motor seizures. Risk factors identified for causing an increased incidence of seizures included the coadministration of other medications such as phenothiazines, thioxanthenes, tricyclic antidepressants, monoamine oxidase inhibitors, CNS stimu-

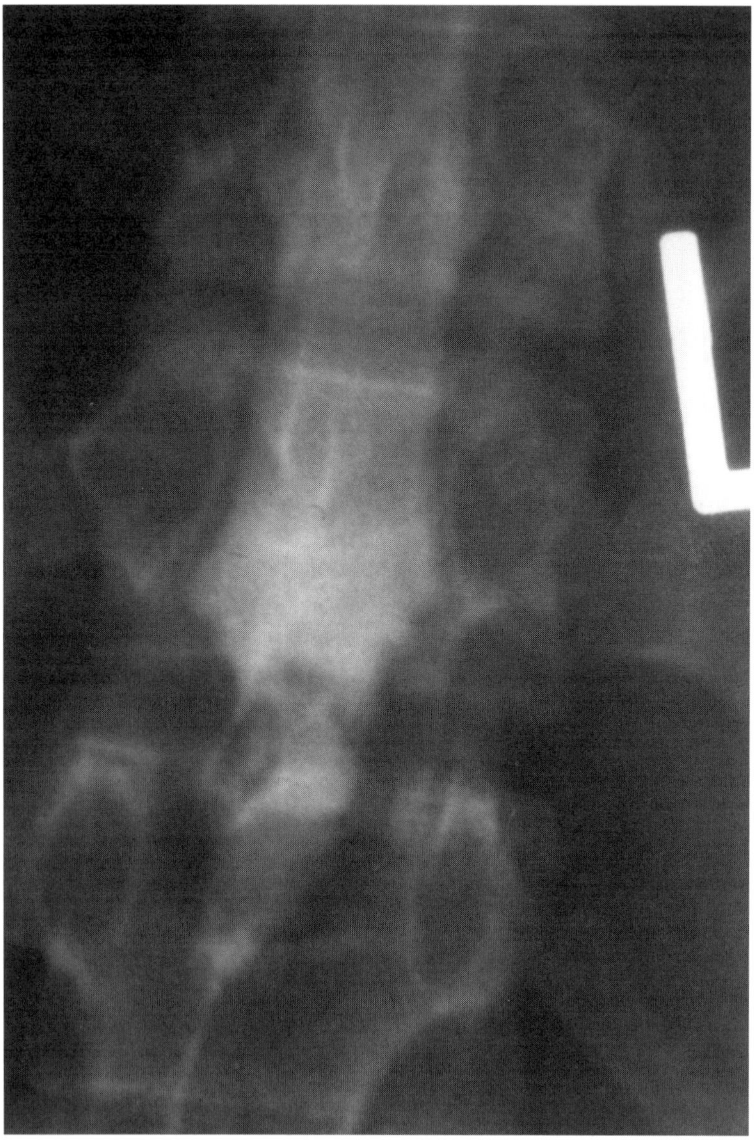

C

Figure 1.4. *continued.* (C) An anteroposterior myelogram showing a featureless sac with scarring and contraction of nerve root sleeves and distal thecal sac.

lants, and miscellaneous medications such as meperidine (Demerol) and metoclopramide (Reglan), which have the effect of lowering a patient's seizure threshold. Also, patients with a history of seizure or who were administered high concentrations and large volumes of contrast, especially if dehydrated, had an increased risk of seizure. Phenobarbital, but not diazepam, may possibly be effective as a prophylactic drug in patients at risk for a seizure who are undergoing myelography. This prophylactic procedure was found to be effective in rabbits.[17] Although the onset of activity of diazepam is rapid, its duration of action is short. Thus, diazepam rapidly penetrates into and redistributes out of the brain, whereas phenobarbital has a much longer duration of activity.

Electroencephalographic (EEG) abnormalities, as an expression of toxic encephalopathy, have been shown after both metrizamide and iohexol myelography.[29] Transient EEG abnormalities with metrizamide are well documented in the literature.[30] Drory et al.[29] detected EEG abnormalities in 10–75% of patients after administering metrizamide; Ekholm and Fischer[30] recorded EEG

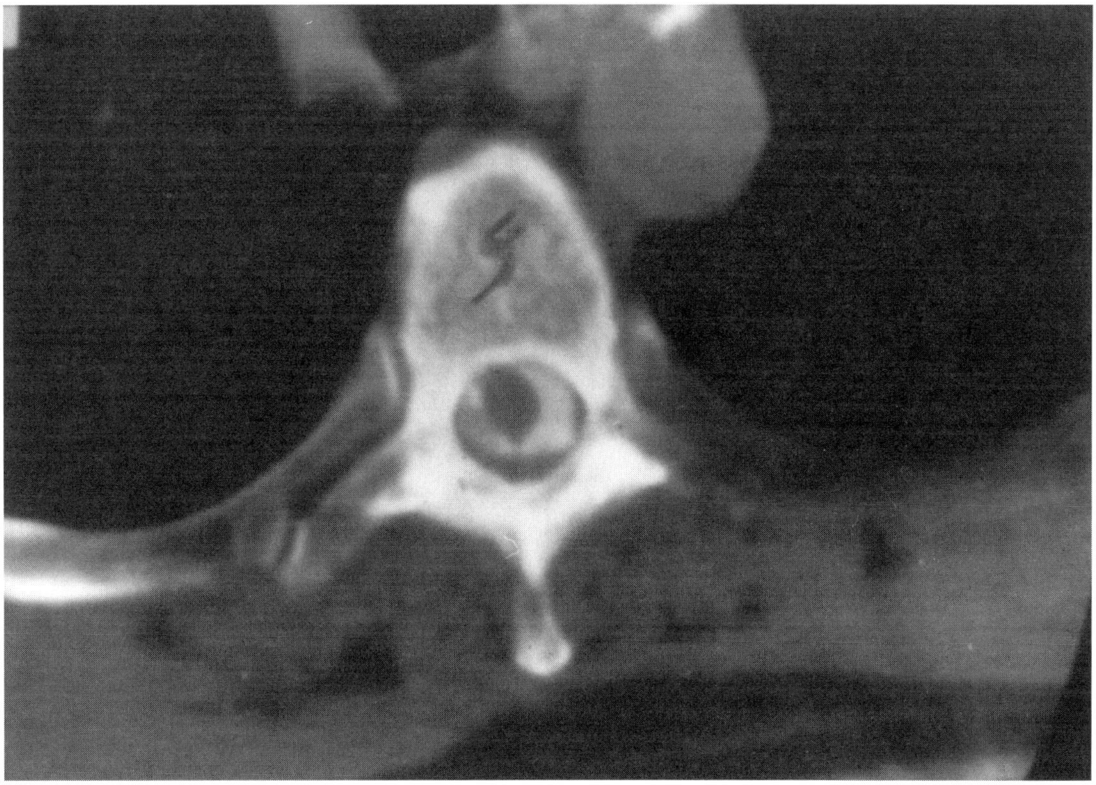

Figure 1.5. Arachnoiditis. Postmyelogram computed tomographic scan showing the spinal cord adherent to the right posterior margin of the vertebral body. Also, the cord has lost its normal rounded configuration.

abnormalities in 16–35% of patients following metrizamide injection. Maximal EEG changes were noted by 24 hours postinjection due to delayed diffusion of contrast medium into the intracellular space. EEG changes were infrequently noted before 2 hours but were frequently seen after 5 hours.[23] EEG changes typically disappeared after 24 hours, although Drory et al. reported EEG changes up to 5 days after metrizamide myelography. Most of the changes were described as an increase in slow activity, though rarely paroxysmal activity was recorded.[29] Drory et al. also studied the EEG abnormalities after iohexol myelography and reported these to be less frequent (2–24% of patients) and less severe than metrizamide myelography.[29] In addition, side effects of iohexol are less severe than metrizamide, consisting of mostly mild headache or nausea, but never seizures or significant behavioral changes according to Drory et al.[29] The differences between iohexol and metrizamide appear to be related more to their variations in chemical structure.[30]

Both metrizamide and iohexol, being water-soluble agents, are reabsorbed through the arachnoid granulations within the spinal canal, into the blood, and finally excreted by the kidney. Studies have shown metrizamide to be associated with a higher incidence of severe adverse effects such as behavioral changes and seizures.[30] This difference in neurotoxicity is attributed to the presence of a glucosamine side chain on the metrizamide molecule. This glucosamine side chain acts as a glucose analogue within the brain parenchyma. The result is competitive inhibition of hexokinase, the specific membrane glucose carrier, with a decrease in intracellular glucose and hence impaired cerebral neuron metabolism. Researchers were able to demonstrate a decrease in carbon dioxide production in hippocampal tissue slices from rats when metrizamide was added, indicating that normal metabolism was interrupted.[30, 31] Iohexol does not have this glucosamide side chain in its chemical structure and has not been shown to influence normal brain functioning. Thus, iohexol has replaced its predecessor metrizamide due to its more desirable margin of safety.

Convulsions with iohexol have not been reported, confirming that iohexol is less epileptogenic than metrizamide.

Intraspinal Epidermoid

Epidermoid tumors make up less than 2% of CNS tumors and rarely occur in the spinal canal.[32] When epidermoid tumors occur in the spinal canal, they may be acquired or congenital in origin. Congenital tumors are thought to arise from displaced ectodermal elements during embryogenesis and are associated with congenital dermal sinuses.[32] Acquired epidermoid tumors are thought to result from the implantation of epidermal elements into the subarachnoid space after a lumbar puncture with a nonstylet needle or failing to reinsert the stylet during removal of the needle from the subarachnoid space (Figure 1.6). This theory accounts for the increased incidence of spinal epidermoid tumors in the lumbar region. A small piece of epidermis has been shown to be removed from inserted needles in more than 60% of punctures in a study by Gibson and Norris.[33] The incubation period can vary from 2 to 23 years as the epidermal elements grow. These tumors are typically pearly in appearance and range from a few millimeters to several centimeters and may be single or multiple.[34]

Injury to the Cord, Nerve Root, or Disk

The C1–C2 puncture technique carries a slightly increased risk of complications due to the location of the puncture site. Inadvertent injection of contrast into the cervical spinal cord can occur (Figure 1.7). Johansen et al. reported a case where 3 ml of metrizamide was accidentally injected into the spinal cord of a 45-year-old woman who suffered immediate left-sided paralysis as well as head and back pain.[35] Eight months after the procedure she still had a residual paresis of her left upper extremity. Additional reports of inadvertent injection of metrizamide into the spinal cord via a C1–C2 puncture resulted in no permanent sequelae.[35] Nakstad and Kjartansson in 1988 reported a case of accidental spinal cord injection of approximately 2 ml of iohexol during a C1–C2 puncture.[36] The patient had no complaints during or after the injection. Both Nakstad and Kjartansson thought that the lower toxicity of iohexol was responsible for the lack of neurologic findings in their patient.

Young and Burney reported a complication of a transected nerve root in a 41-year-old woman.[37] The woman underwent Pantopaque myelography for low back and leg pain. The procedure was uneventful, and all but 2 ml of Pantopaque were successfully withdrawn. When no further contrast could be removed, the patient began experiencing radiating left hip pain. At that point, the needle stylet was replaced, and the needle was removed, producing severe unremitting radiating pain. The needle was examined on removal and disclosed a 7-cm nerve filament within its end. Presumably, the nerve filament became trapped within the needle's side hold, and as the stylet was replaced, it wedged the nerve root against the inner wall of the needle. When the needle was withdrawn the nerve filament snapped. Similar cases were experienced by Kennedy and Steinfeld[38] and Hungerford and Powers[39] when they performed Pantopaque myelography using the Cuatico (multi-side hole) needle and by Brody et al.[40] when they used the Chynn aspiration cannula. All of these cases have a common factor: The needles used in these procedures are designed with at least one side hole with or without an end hole. These cases demonstrate a few important points that were especially important during the days of Pantopaque myelography. First, the needle should not be withdrawn while applying negative pressure. Second, suction should be gentle and should be halted at the first sign of pain. Finally, the water-soluble contrast agents available today do not need to be aspirated from the spinal canal; however, before removal of the needle, the stylet should be replaced, and both needle and stylet should be withdrawn as a unit slowly.[39] Improper technique may also cause traumatic perforation of the annulus fibrosus with resultant prolapse of disk material (Figure 1.8).[3] Inadvertent injury or contrast injection into the spinal cord may also occur in patients with an unrecognized tethered cord or syrinx (Figure 1.9).

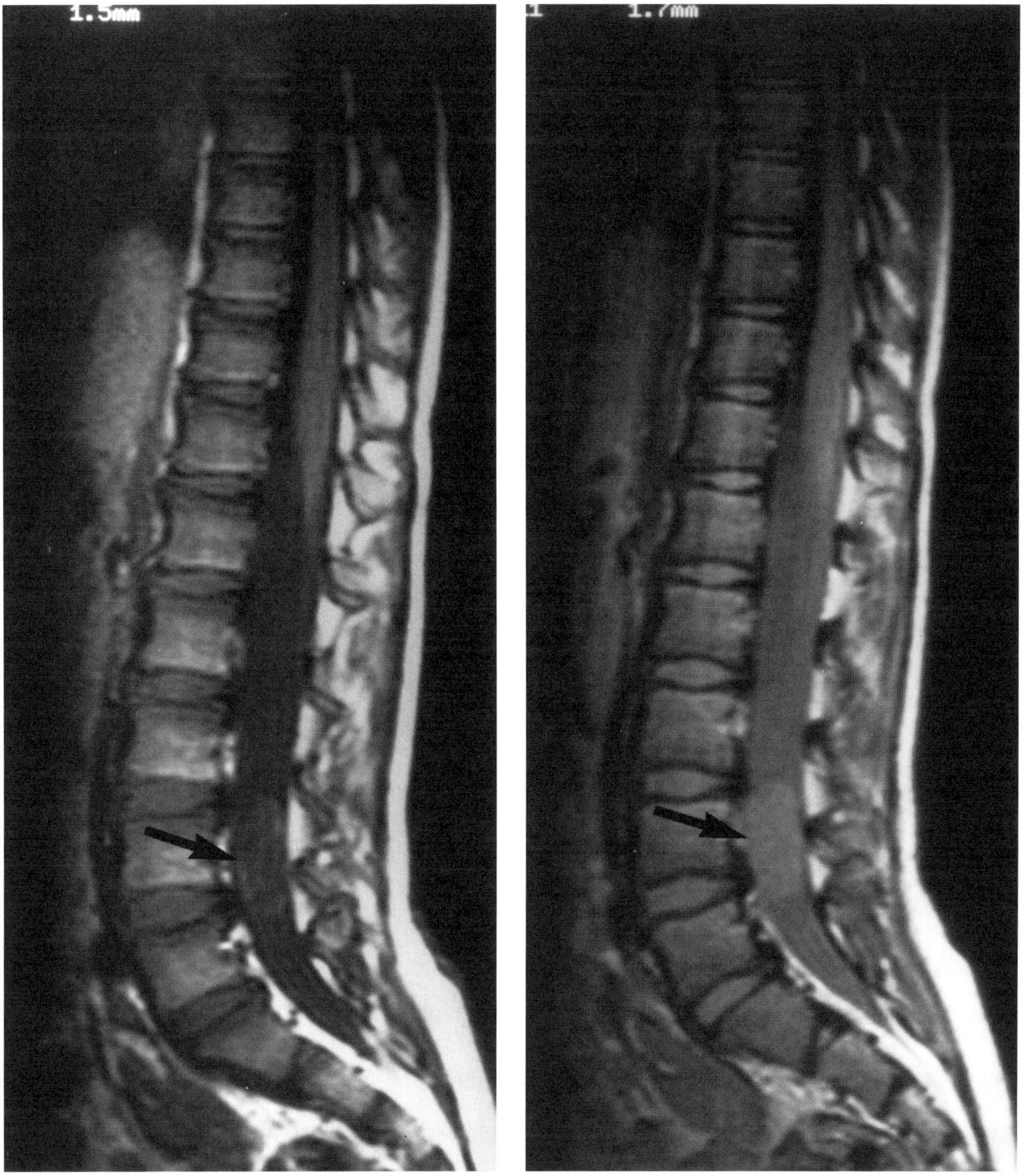

A B

Figure 1.6. Acquired epidermoid tumor in a 5-year-old boy with severe back pain and history of lumbar puncture as young infant. Sagittal T1-weighted precontrast (A) and proton density (B) images show an oval intrathecal mass that is slightly hyperintense to cerebrospinal fluid (arrows).

Infection

Observing meticulous aseptic technique is of utmost importance when performing myelography because the subarachnoid space has a relatively low resistance to infection. Failure to do so may result in the introduction of organisms into the subarachnoid space and regional soft tissues, increasing the risk of subsequent meningitis, osteomyelitis, septic arthritis, and soft tissue or epidural abscess (Figures

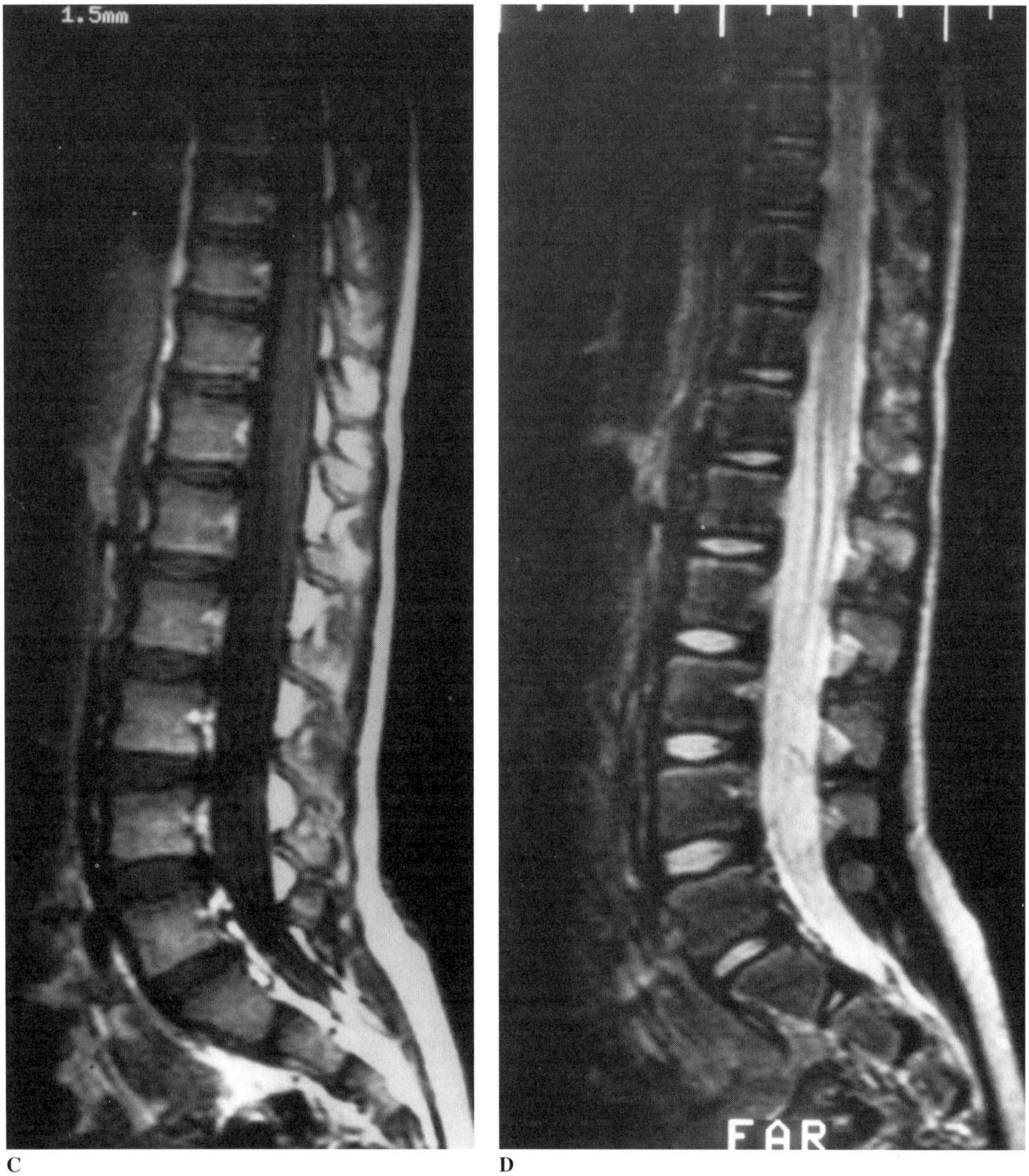

C D

Figure 1.6. *continued.* (C) Sagittal T1-weighted postcontrast image shows no enhancement. (D) On the T2-weighted sagittal image, the mass is difficult to differentiate from cerebrospinal fluid due to similar signal intensity.

1.10 and 1.11).[3] Broad-spectrum antibiotics should be administered for at least 5–7 days should there be a break in aseptic technique. Lumbar puncture is contraindicated if infection is present in the skin overlying the spine.[6]

Venous Intravasation

Venous intravasation is not considered problematic today due to the use of water-soluble nonionic agents that are commonly injected intravenously for

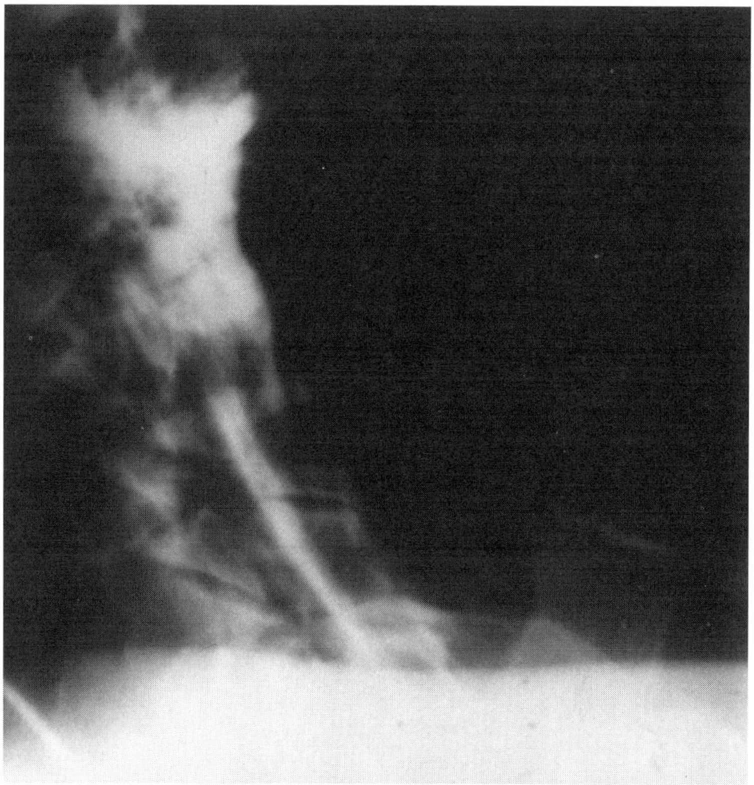

A

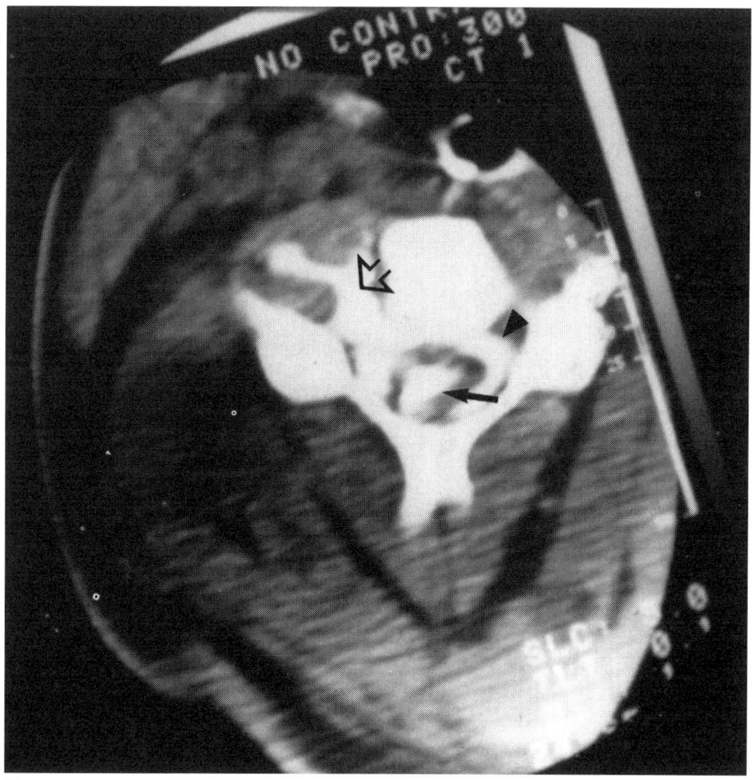

B

Figure 1.7. Intramedullary injection of contrast media. (A) Cervical myelogram shows a multicompartmental injection of contrast in the epidural, subdural, subarachnoid, and intramedullary spaces. (B) Contrast is seen in the epidural (open arrow) and subdural spaces, as well as within the spinal cord (solid arrow). Some contrast is also present in the subarachnoid space (arrowhead).

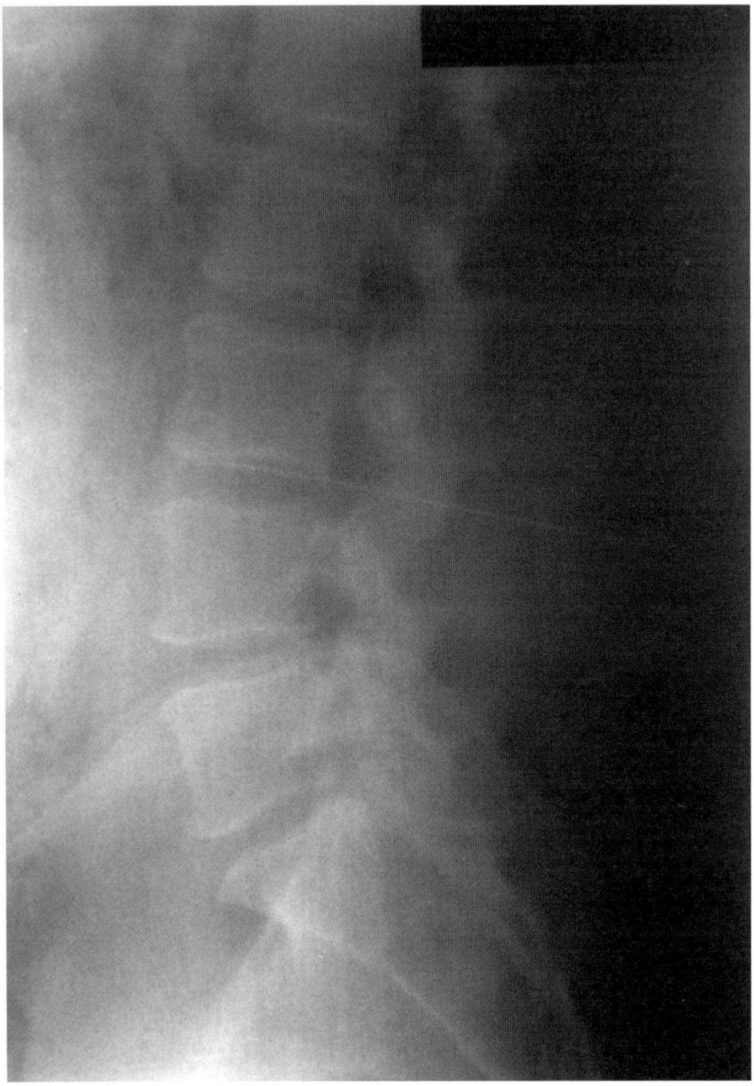

Figure 1.8. Inadvertent injury to disk. After placement of the spinal needle, fluoroscopy revealed that the needle had advanced too deeply into the intervertebral disk, which may result in traumatic disk herniation.

various studies. However, in the past, injection of Pantopaque into the vertebral vein system could result in tiny pulmonary oil emboli.

Cardiac or Respiratory Arrest

During myelography, patients are usually prone and may be poorly monitored. Therefore, cardiac or respiratory distress may not be immediately recognized. A single case report by Cooper in 1964 described a young, relatively healthy man who suffered a cardiac arrest after myelography.[3] A 43-year-old man who was apprehensive, but otherwise healthy, with low back pain and left sciatica underwent routine myelography on an x-ray tilt table. The patient fainted as the table was raised approximately 35 degrees toward the feet. The table was returned to a Trendelenburg position and the patient promptly regained consciousness. The procedure was attempted again after medication was administered to prevent orthostatic hypotension.

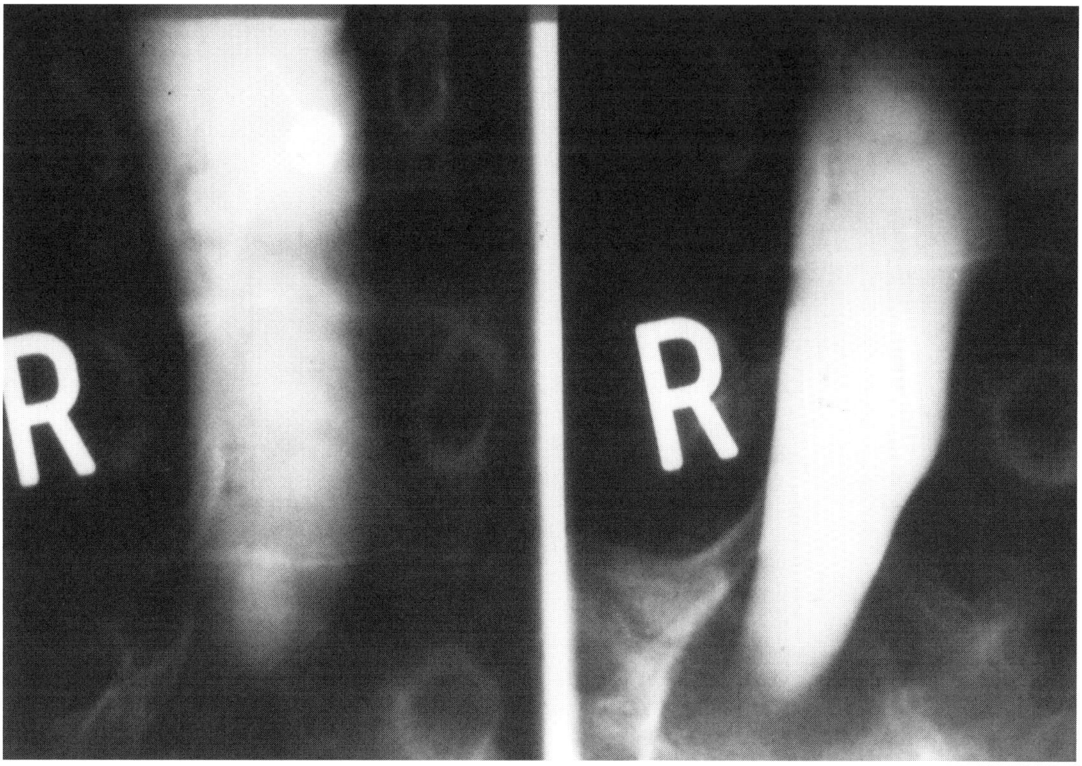

A

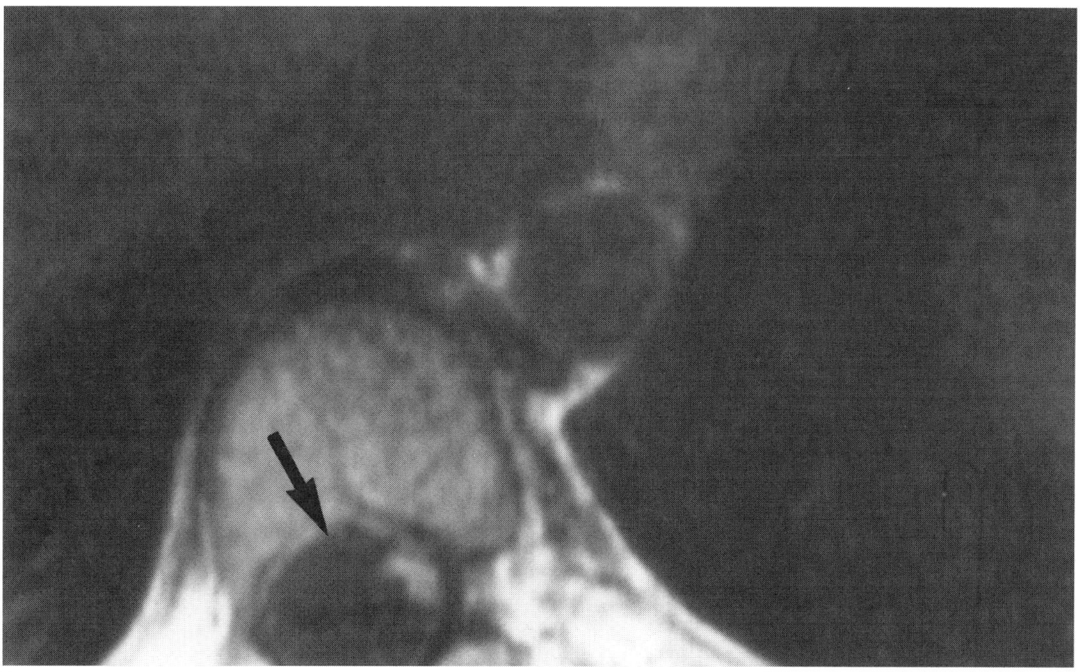

B

Figure 1.9. Inadvertent injection into a syrinx cavity. (A) Lumbar myelogram shows an amorphous appearance of the contrast without visualized nerve roots. (B) Spinal magnetic resonance imaging shows the patient has an unrecognized syrinx (arrow). Injection into the syrinx cavity was the cause of the appearance on myelography.

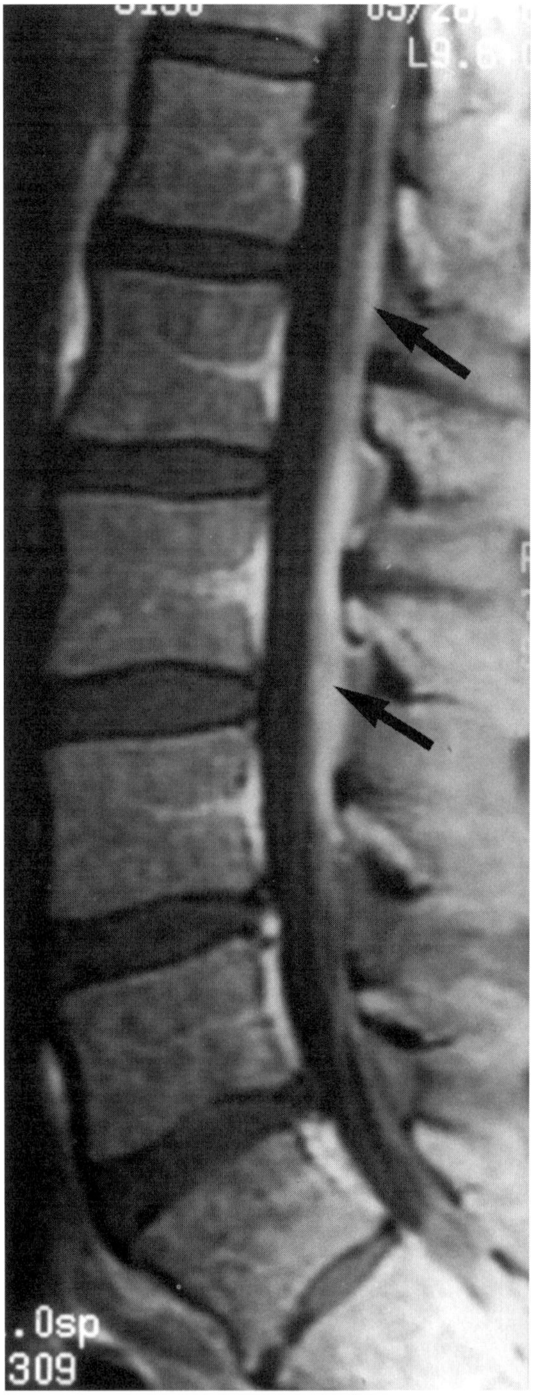

Figure 1.10. Subarachnoid infection. Postcontrast sagittal T1-weighted magnetic resonance imaging of the lumbar spine reveals linear enhancement along the conus medullaris and cauda equina (arrows). This represented intrathecal infection due to contamination of the subarachnoid space during lumbar puncture.

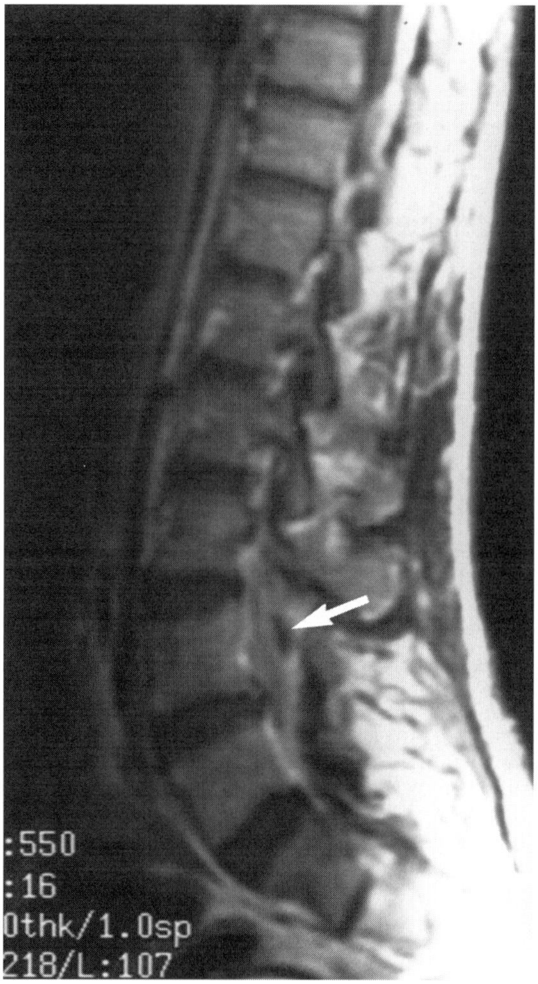

A

Figure 1.11. Epidural abscess. Sagittal (A) and axial T1-weighted (B) images postcontrast show a small epidural abscess (arrow) as a complication of dural puncture.

The patient fainted again as the table was tilted up, but did not regain consciousness as the table was lowered. The patient required cardiopulmonary resuscitation, but recovered. This case illustrates that apprehension can produce increased vagal tone, and a patient with an unusually labile circulatory system may experience syncope and even cardiac arrest.

It is not uncommon to witness mild symptoms of orthostatic hypotension such as dizziness, sweating, lightheadedness, and nausea. In any patient with a history of orthostatic hypotension or severe

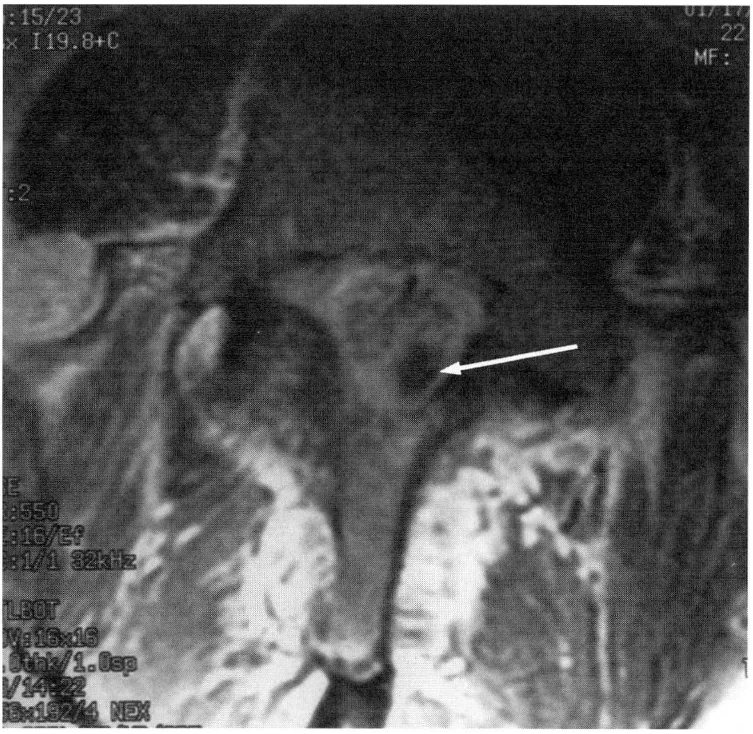

B

anxiety, it may be wise to obtain a blood pressure measurement before performing the examination, both in the supine and upright positions.

In 1976, Benedict and Janower[41] reported a case of respiratory arrest that occurred in a 55-year-old woman undergoing Pantopaque myelography. The woman had a history of metastatic carcinoma of the breast with infiltration of her phrenic nerves, which was not known before performing the procedure. During the procedure she was placed prone in the head-down position in order to move the contrast agent into the lower cervical region. A few minutes later, she became apneic and cyanotic, and resuscitative measures failed as she died 3 weeks later. Although this example is rare, it exemplifies the point that attention should be paid to the patient's respiratory function. In this case, tumor infiltration of the phrenic nerves resulted in diaphragm paralysis when the patient was placed in the prone position, and the head-down position probably further impaired respiration. In patients with muscular or neuromuscular disorders, the potential exists for respiratory compromise while undergoing myelography.

Epidural, Subdural, and Subarachnoid Hemorrhage

Thrombocytopenia or other bleeding diathesis or systemic heparin or warfarin administration increases the risk of puncture-induced hemorrhage (Figure 1.12). Lumbar puncture is not performed at our institution, except for urgent clinical indications, in patients with platelet count of less than 50,000 per μl.

Worsening of Neurologic Deficits

Herniation may occur in patients with unrecognized increased intracranial pressure. All patients should be carefully evaluated for papilledema or signs of increased intracranial pressure before lumbar puncture and a head CT performed in questionable cases. With the availability of CT, this complication should be infrequently seen. Withdrawal of fluid may cause worsening of neurologic dysfunction in patients with a severe spinal stenosis and convert an incomplete spinal block into a complete spinal block.

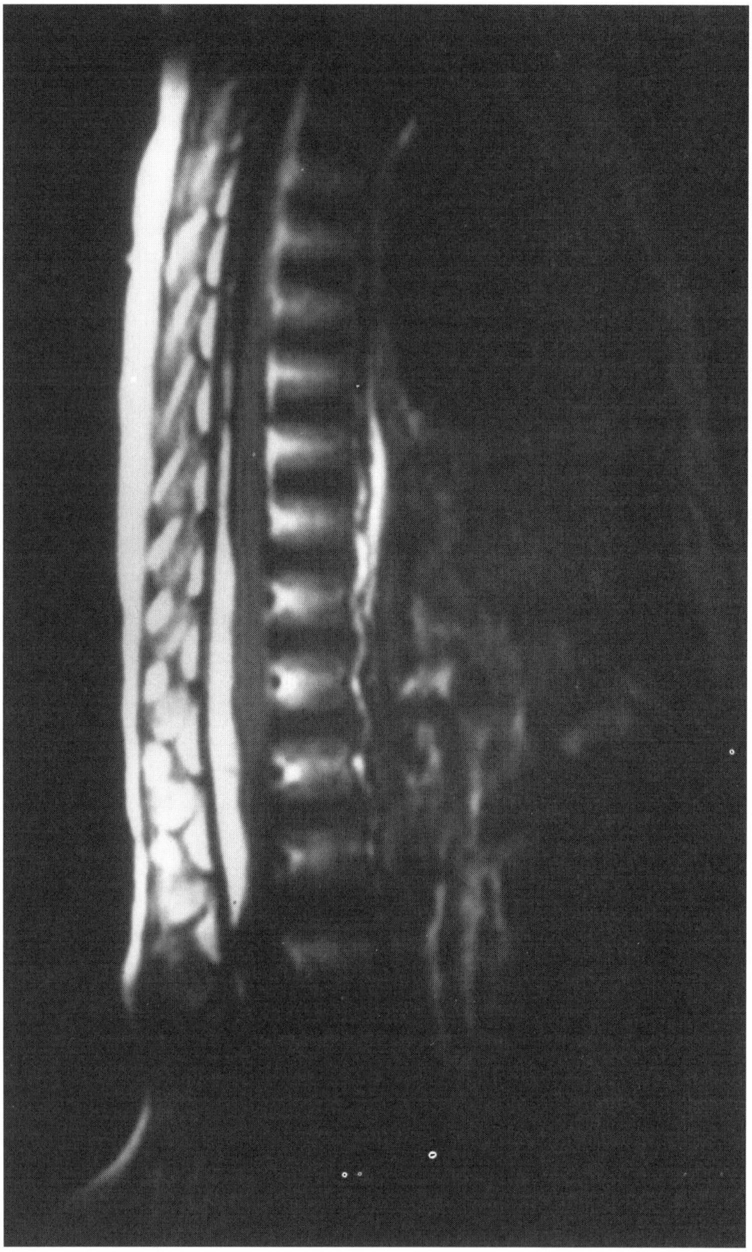

A

Figure 1.12. Lumbar puncture-induced subdural hematoma. Sagittal (A) and axial (B) noncontrasted T1-weighted images show a fusiform area of bright signal posterior to the cord and thecal sac. This represents methemoglobin within a subdural hematoma.

Conclusion

Lumbar puncture is a frequently performed procedure in patients suspected of CNS pathology. Myelography, on the other hand, is infrequently requested due to the widespread availability of MRI. However, in patients with contraindications for MRI, myelography followed by CT is the study of choice. Both lumbar puncture and myelography are invasive procedures, and although relatively simple to perform, can be associated with both immediate and delayed complications. With careful aseptic technique and patient screening, these complications can be minimized.

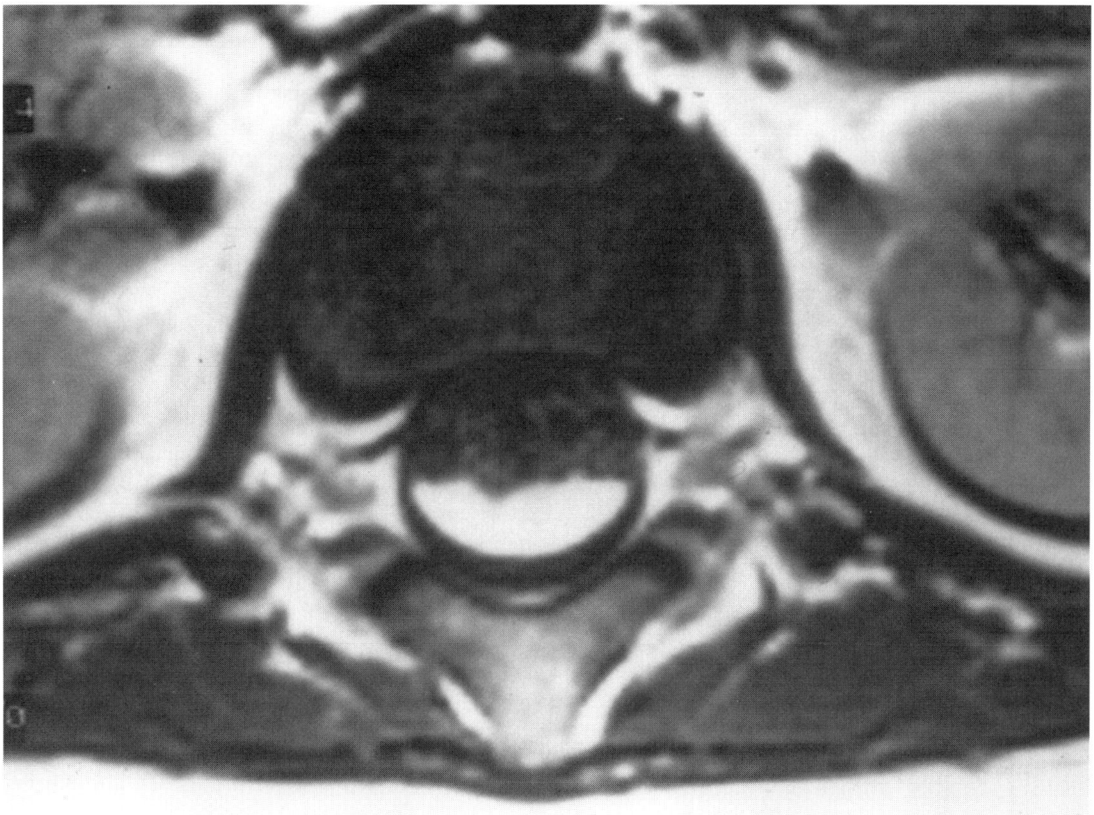

B

References

1. Maly P, Sundgren P, Baath L, et al. Adverse reactions in myelography. Correlation between animal research and clinical practice. Acta Radiol Suppl 1995;399:230.
2. Peterson HO. The hazards of myelography. Radiology 1975;115:237.
3. Shapiro R. Myelography (4th ed). Chicago: Year Book Medical, 1984.
4. Peterman SB. Postmyelography headache: a review. Radiology 1996;200:765.
5. Rowland LP. Merritt's Textbook of Neurology (9th ed). Baltimore: Williams & Wilkins, 1995.
6. Prager JM, Roychowdhury S, Gorey MT, et al. Spinal headaches after myelograms: comparison of needle types. AJR Am J Roentgenol 1996;167:1289.
7. Harrison PB. The contribution of needle size and other factors to headache following myelography. Neuroradiology 1993;35:487.
8. Rolfe EB, Maguire PD. The incidence of headache following various techniques of metrizamide myelography. Br J Radiol 1980;53:840.
9. Wilkinson AG, Sellar RJ. The influence of needle size and other factors on the incidence of adverse effects caused by myelography. Clin Radiol 1991;44:338.
10. Tourtellotte WW, Henderson WG, Tucker RP, et al. A randomized, double-blind clinical trial comparing the 22 versus 26 gauge needle in the production of the post-lumbar puncture syndrome in normal individuals. Headache 1972;12:73.
11. Jones MJ, Selby IR, Gwinnutt CL. Technical note: the influence of using an atraumatic needle on the incidence of post-myelography headache. Br J Radiol 1994;67:396.
12. Skalpe IO, Nakstad P. Myelography with iohexol (Omnipaque): a clinical report with special reference to the adverse effects. Neuroradiology 1988;30:169.
13. Hallam DM, Sonne NM, Jensen GS, et al. Headache after lumbar iohexol myelography: the influence of a history of headaches and early ambulation. Neuroradiology 1993;35:319.
14. Guiati AN, Guadagnoll DA, Quigley JM. Relationship of side effects to patient position during and after metrizamide lumbar myelography. Radiology 1981; 141:113.
15. Kuuliala IK, Goransson HJ. Adverse reactions after iohexol lumbar myelography: influence of postprocedural positioning. AJR Am J Roentgenol 1987;149:389.
16. Postacchini F, Massobrio M. Outpatient lumbar myelography. Analysis of complications after myelography

comparing outpatients with inpatients. Spine 1985; 10:567.
17. Saltiel E, Adelman DC, Ellis JC, et al. Generalized motor seizure following metrizamide cisternography. Drug Intelligence Clin Pharm 1984;18:894.
18. Macpherson P, Teasdale E, McGeorge AP. Direct puncture versus run up cervical myelography with iopamidol: comparison of side effects, EEG changes and radiographic quality. J Neurol Neurosurg Psychiatry 1983;46:959.
19. Skalpe IO. Adhesive arachnoiditis following lumbar radiculography with water-soluble contrast agents. Radiology 1976;121:647.
20. Sand T, Stovner LJ, Dale L, et al. Side effects after diagnostic lumbar puncture and lumbar iohexol myelography. Neuroradiology 1987;29:385.
21. Wagner A, Jensen C, Saebye A, et al. A prospective comparison of iotrolan and iohexol in lumbar myelography. Acta Radiol 1994;35:182.
22. Haughton VM. Intrathecal toxicity of iohexol vs. metrizamide. Survey and current state. Invest Radiol 1985;20:S14.
23. Sage MR. Kinetics of water-soluble contrast media in the central nervous system. AJR Am J Roentgenol 1983;141:815.
24. Bagchi AK. Convulsions, subarachnoid haemorrhage and death following myelography with meglumine iothalamate 280. Surg Neurol 1976;5:285.
25. Praestholm J, Lester J. Water-soluble contrast lumbar myelography with meglumine iothalamate (Conray). Br J Radiol 1970;43:303.
26. Taminiau AHM, Slooff TJJH. Bilateral femoral neck fractures as a complication of myelography. Acta Orthop Scand 1980;51:621.
27. Morrey BF, O'Brien ET. Femoral neck fractures following water-soluble myelography induced spinal seizures. J Bone Joint Surg Am 1977;59:1099.
28. Haase J, Jepsen BV, Bech H, et al. Spinal fracture following radiculography using meglumine iothalamate (Conray). Neuroradiology 1973;6:65.
29. Drory VE, Avrahami E, Neufeld MY, et al. EEG recordings following intrathecal iohexol administration. Clin Neuropharmacol 1990;13:318.
30. Ekholm S, Fischer H. Neurotoxicity of metrizamide. Arch Neurol 1985;42:24.
31. Morris TW, Ekholm SE, Simon JH, et al. In vitro models for testing the metabolic effects of myelographic contrast media. Invest Radiol 1988;23:S213.
32. Baba H, Wada M, Tanaka Y, et al. Intraspinal epidermoid after lumbar puncture. Int Orthop 1994;18:116.
33. Gibson T, Norris W. Skin fragments removed by injection needles. Lancet 1958;2:983.
34. Pear BL. Iatrogenic intraspinal epidermoid sequestration cysts. Radiology 1969;92:251.
35. Johansen JG, Orrison WW, Amundsen P. Lateral C1–2 puncture for cervical myelography. Report of a complication. Radiology 1983;146:391.
36. Nakstad PH, Kjartansson O. Accidental spinal cord injection of contrast material during cervical myelography with lateral C1–C2 puncture. AJNR Am J Neuroradiol 1988;9:410.
37. Young DA, Burney RE. Complication of myelography—transection and withdrawal of a nerve filament by the needle. N Engl J Med 1971;285:156.
38. Kennedy TF, Steinfeld JR. Nerve rootlet avulsion as a complication of myelography with the Cuatico needle. Radiology 1976;119:389.
39. Hungerford GD, Powers JM. Avulsion of nerve rootlets with the Cuatico needle during removal after myelography. AJR Am J Roentgenol 1977;129:485.
40. Brody PA, London SS, Sung MA. Nerve root avulsion. A complication of myelography using the Chynn needle. Radiology 1977;125:734.
41. Benedict KT, Janower ML. Respiratory arrest—a fatal complication of myelography. Radiology 1977;122: 729.

Chapter 2

Complications of Cerebral and Spinal Angiography

Andrew J. DeNardo and John A. Scott

Objectives

- To understand that cerebral and spinal angiography carry inherent risks that need to be considered when contemplating their use in the diagnosis of a given patient
- To appreciate the level of risk to the patient when undergoing these diagnostic procedures
- To understand the factors that may put a patient at higher risk, and interventions or techniques that may be used to reduce risk
- To recognize complications that may need immediate action and others that may be observed or treated conservatively
- To stratify the risk of angiography against the natural history of the diseases these tests are most useful in diagnosing
- To understand that complications occur without warning in the best of hands, and that there are both acceptable as well as unacceptable levels of risk that need to be addressed at all levels of practice

Historical Perspective

The evaluation of the vascular tree with radiography and contrast injection developed soon after the discovery of x-rays. However, it took the advent of rapid film changers; biocompatible contrast agents; and the ingenuity of Seldinger, Dotter, and Moniz before cerebral angiography became a viable diagnostic tool.[1–3] Before the development of diagnostic angiographic catheters and transfemoral angiography, standard techniques for delivering contrast involved direct puncture of the cerebral vessels and retrograde injection of the brachial arteries to assess the vertebral arteries. With the advent of digital subtraction technology, it became possible to rapidly perform angiography.

Before the widespread use of computed tomography (CT), angiography provided information about intracranial masses by evaluating vascular displacement and neovascularity. In the early 1970s, CT became the primary diagnostic tool for evaluating masses, and angiography was relegated primarily to the diagnosis of cerebrovascular diseases.

Technological advancements improved safety and comfort as well as the accuracy of diagnosis. Advancements have been made steadily in angiographic equipment, angiographic catheters and wires, and contrast materials. The most important advancement in the equipment was digital subtraction technology, which allows rapid image acquisition and viewing. Increased transmission of torque and thin-wall catheters have made angiography faster and safer. Important progress has also been made in radiographic contrast agents. The earliest agent, Thorotrast, was not only a contrast agent but also a beta-emitting isotope that resulted not only in delayed soft-tissue sarcomas but also chronic granulomas when extravasation occurred.[4, 5] Water-soluble contrast agents replaced Thorotrast, and more recently nonionic and low-osmolar agents have resulted in better patient tolerance.

Cerebral Angiography: Introduction

The diagnostic algorithms addressing cerebral vascular pathology are changing. Improvements in magnetic resonance angiography, CT angiography, and ultrasound and Doppler studies have reduced the need for cerebral angiography in many disease states. Indeed, the number of cerebral angiograms performed at most institutions has decreased significantly over the last several years.[6, 7] These less invasive diagnostic tools, however, have not fully replaced diagnostic angiography due to the better spatial resolution and temporal information seen with angiography. Detecting aneurysms, arteriovenous malformations, vasculitis, and especially carotid stenosis can all be accomplished with noninvasive imaging. In each case, however, therapeutic intervention may be altered significantly by information available only with contrast angiography.

Complications that occur as a result of cerebral angiography may be a result of vascular access, arterial contrast injection (general or specific to the central nervous system [CNS]), or selective catheterization and injection. Minimizing the risk while obtaining maximal useful information should be the goal of these procedures. All procedures should be tailored to the specific signs and symptoms, with additional information being sought only when there is clinical relevance. Complications occur at a certain acceptable rate at every institution. No complication that occurs during a study performed without indication is acceptable.

Certain factors affect the level of risk at any individual institution. As with most procedures, skill level has a significant impact on the complication rate. Acceptable levels of proficiency or expertise are difficult to determine. How many angiograms does it take to become proficient or expert? How many procedures per year does it take to maintain proficiency? The involvement of trainees has been shown to result in an increased complication rate.[8–10] This does not mean that we should not provide this training, but training should be limited to individuals who demonstrate earnest interest and the requisite skills. As the use of cerebral angiography continues to decrease, it may be beneficial to develop centers of excellence where complications can be monitored and kept to acceptably low levels.

General and Neurologic Risk

The risk of permanent neurologic deficit is the most important complication to consider when assessing the role of cerebral angiography in the diagnostic algorithm. One might also consider addressing the severity of the deficits in terms of disability. Many studies have addressed the former issue and the larger series report an average risk of approximately 0.3% or less for permanent deficit. The risk may be as low as 0.1% in good hands. The risk of transient neurologic deficit is approximately 0.5–2.0%.[8–19]

Mani et al. reported in a three-part series the risk and factors affecting the overall risk found in an analysis of 5,000 cerebral angiograms.[8, 13, 14] They found no difference in the rate of complications related to the specific vessel injected, number of vessels evaluated, or type of contrast used. There was a positive correlation between length of the procedure or age of the patient and frequency of complications. They found that complication rates were significantly higher when the procedure lasted more than 80 minutes or the patient was older than age 40 years. Procedures were performed in significantly less time at nontraining institutions. The survey was taken from two training and two nontraining institutions. Overall, neurologic complication rates were considerably higher at training (3.9%) versus nontraining (0.9%) institutions, yet permanent deficits after cerebral angiography were equal (0.1%). In a separate analysis, the risk of neurologic complications was found to be higher (1.2–1.9%) in patients with atherosclerotic cerebrovascular disease, in postoperative and post-traumatic states, and with subarachnoid hemorrhage. Patients evaluated for headache, tumor, or seizure and those with normal angiogram results had lower neurologic complication rates (0.2–0.5%).[8, 13, 14]

Further series have addressed overall and neurologic complication rates of cerebral angiography. Waugh and Sacharias in their series of 939 patients found a rate of 0.3% for permanent neurologic deficits.[11] Systemic complications were seen in 1.8%, with no cases of renal failure.

Heiserman et al., in a more recently reported series, noted a 1% incidence of all neurologic events and 0.5% incidence of permanent deficit.[12] In their series, the risk of neurologic deficit strongly correlated with history of stroke and transient ischemic attack or carotid bruit. Faught et al., in a later but much smaller series of 147 patients, confirmed increased risk in patients with atherosclerotic disease and stenosis, as well as the number of previous transient ischemic attacks.[15] Their overall rate of neurologic complications was much higher (total, 12.2%; permanent, 5.2%) than reported in other series. It is unclear why their risk of stroke was so high, but the sample size is the smallest of the reported series, and incidence of neurologic complications the highest. In one of the few prospective series, McIvor et al. analyzed 230 examinations and found little difference in complication rates based on some of the same variables addressed by Mani et al.[9] McIvor et al. also noted lower neurologic complication rates when the procedure was performed by an experienced radiologist. The mean time of examination was 18 minutes shorter when performed by an experienced radiologist. They found no difference in morbidity between the use of ionic versus nonionic contrast. In probably the best analyzed prospective series, Dion et al. evaluated the neurologic event rate after cerebral angiography in 1,002 procedures both at 24 and 72 hours.[16] The rate of stroke at 24 hours was 1.3% (0.1% permanent) and between 24 and 72 hours was 1.8% (0.3%) permanent. Their non-neurologic complication rate (consisting mostly of local groin hematoma) was 7.2%. Although their study reliably compiled information about postangiographic events beyond 24 hours, they believed that angiography could not unequivocally be causally related to these events. Earnest et al. found similar complication rates in a series of 1,517 angiograms.[17] They noted an overall rate of 8.2%, with a neurologic event rate of 2.6% (0.33% permanent). The permanent neurologic event rate was increased in patients evaluated for cerebrovascular disease (0.62%). They also found an increased complication risk with advanced age, elevated creatinine level, and number of catheters used, likely reflecting the difficulty of examination. Gasparini et al., in a small series of 218 patients, found a 6.9% neurologic event rate with a 0.4% rate of permanent deficit.[18] Procedure time and difficulty of examination were the major factors associated with neurologic complication. Eisenberg et al., in a study of 301 patients, reported a 1.3% neurologic event rate without any permanent deficits.[19] This series again supports a relatively low neurologic morbidity. A series of 1,095 patients by Grzyska et al. noted a 0.45% neurologic event rate, with 0.09% of these events being permanent.[10] They thought that there was benefit to newer technical advances, primarily nonionic contrast and digital subtraction technique. Perhaps the gains were the result of decreased examination times associated with these advances. They also emphasized the need for close supervision of trainees and proposed catheter manipulation time limits for trainees to reduce risk imposed to patients.

A summary of the major series reporting complications indicates a relatively low rate of permanent neurologic morbidity. The factors most commonly implicated in the complication rates are duration of examination and operator experience. The complexity of the examination in terms of difficulty of selection of the brachiocephalic vessels is likely the primary underlying factor. Patients with tortuous brachiocephalic vessels and uncoiled aortic arches can pose a significant challenge to the best angiographers and may require multiple catheter exchanges. Patient age is also another easily measured factor reflecting the same process. The number of catheter exchanges may be the best measure of the technical difficulty of an examination.

Contrast-Related Complications

Injection of iodinated contrast agents directly into the vascular system carries a risk of both systemic and local complications. The choice of radiographic contrast agents has multiplied. Nonionic agents do not offer clearly significant improved safety in terms of reduction of potential neurotoxicity, but patient comfort and less frequent nausea make many procedures quicker and thereby indirectly safer. There is some experimental and clinical evidence to suggest lower neurotoxicity of the nonionic contrast agents.

Many factors go into choosing contrast agent, including cost, tolerance, and anticoagulant effect. Most physicians choose the agent perceived to be the safest; however, among the commonly used contrast agents real differences in neurologic complication rates related solely on the specific contrast chosen have not been clearly demonstrated.

Neurotoxicity

Nakagawa et al. evaluated nonionic contrast agents in order to identify factors that may account for neurotoxicity.[20] Electroencephalographic (EEG) changes and behavior were evaluated with respect to the specific contrast agents administered to mice. They noted abnormal EEG changes with ionic contrast media, as well as iopromide, iosimide, and metrizamide. They concluded that the nonionic contrast agents iohexol, iopamidol, iotrolan, and iocibidol were well tolerated with respect to EEG, and the ionic contrast and nonionic agents metrizamide and iopromide were not. Nonionic contrast agents were also better tolerated in terms of general behavior.

Skalpe et al. performed a clinical comparison of ionic (meglumine metrizoate) and nonionic (metrizamide) agents for cerebral angiography and found changes on EEG more frequently with ionic than with the nonionic contrast agents.[21] Bradycardia was seen more frequently with the ionic agent.

Idiosyncratic Reactions

There are many sporadic reports of poorly understood neurologic events associated with cerebral angiography in the medical literature.[20, 22–36] Most of these events are not easily explained by single emboli and are transient in nature. The most commonly reported of these events is transient global amnesia. Some authors have implied a relationship to the volume of contrast injected,[23] whereas others have implicated the type of contrast.[29] These events have been reported with both ionic and nonionic contrast agents. These events are too infrequent to make any strong statements about causation except to state that they can be seen during or shortly after cerebral angiography and, in fact, have been reported in association with noncerebral angiography.[37] Other transient neurologic events in this category include cortical blindness[22–28] and encephalopathy.[29] Once again, the nature of these events is likely related to the direct injection of contrast material into the cerebral vessels and may be the manifestation of a direct toxic effect on the neurons and glia. Alternatively, cerebral dysfunction may be secondary to induction of focal seizures.

Transient Global Amnesia. Transient global amnesia is not a syndrome unique to cerebral angiography, yet there are many reports of an association with angiography. The exact mechanisms underlying this relationship are unknown. It is unlikely that all of the events reported are caused by emboli. The typical event occurs in the periangiography period and almost always resolves within 24 hours. The syndrome has been reported both with ionic and nonionic contrast agents. Advanced age seems to be associated with a higher risk of developing this syndrome.

Giang et al. reported two cases of transient global amnesia that occurred after cerebral angiography with nonionic contrast (iopamidol).[30] Two similar cases were reported with iohexol by Brady et al.[31] Pexman et al. reviewed 12 cases of amnesia seen with a 0.8% incidence after cerebral angiography.[32] Nine of their patients (all older than age 40 years) had typical transient global amnesia; however, three younger patients were thought to have exacerbation of temporal lobe epilepsy as a cause of their amnesia. Eight of their patients experienced similar episodes before angiography. Pexman et al. believed embolic events were to blame in the majority of their cases, whereas contrast toxicity was a cause in the minority (three cases). Schamschula and Soo reported two cases of transient global amnesia using nonionic contrast that resolved within 24 hours.[33] Cochran et al. reported seven cases of transient global amnesia that occurred after cerebral angiography.[34] All patients recovered within 24 hours. Vertebral artery spasm was noted in one patient.

Haley has reported encephalopathy that occurred after cerebral angiography in three elderly men.[29] All three received ionic contrast media (meglumine iothalamate). Two patients became stuporous, yet all recovered within several days. Contrast toxicity was blamed for the events.

Transient Cortical Blindness. Several reports of cortical blindness following cerebral angiography are present in the literature.[22–28] One report describes contrast enhancement of the occipital cortex present on CT during the episode of blindness, providing evidence for blood-brain barrier breakdown.[23] This particular patient also had diminished renal function. It is unclear whether these findings are direct or indirect effects of the contrast. It may also be possible that these clinical syndromes seen in rare association with cerebral angiography are related to undetected embolic events.

Studdard et al. reported a case of transient cortical blindness in which there was contrast enhancement of the occipital cortex present on several CT scans after angiography.[23] They concluded that the event was a direct toxic effect of the contrast agent. Their patient had renal impairment, which probably contributed to persistent cortical enhancement. Focal seizures were also implicated. Shyn and Bell reported an additional case of transient cortical blindness in which evidence of blood-brain barrier breakdown with occipital cortical enhancement was noted postangiogram.[27] They postulated disruption of the blood-brain barrier resulting from the contrast and subsequent contrast neurotoxicity. Kermode et al. reported transient cortical blindness in six patients, with both low-osmolar ionic and nonionic contrast media.[24] Persistent cortical blindness has also been reported to occur after cerebral angiography. In these cases hypercoagulability secondary to the contrast injection was implicated.[26] Vasospasm has also been noted in association with the syndrome of transient cortical blindness in one of six cases reported by Ritter et al.[28] They postulated contrast stasis and direct contrast toxicity as alternative causes.

Cranial Nerve Deficit

Lapresle et al. reported a single case of transient VII, IX, X, and XII, nerve palsy following cerebral angiography.[35] The authors explained this unique deficit by the expected pattern of vascular supply. It remains unclear whether the event resulted from thromboembolism, vasospasm, or direct contrast toxicity. The patient was a 28-year-old woman being evaluated for transient ischemic attack, perhaps reflecting an underlying hypercoagulable state. An unusual cause of third nerve palsy has also been reported in association with posterior communicating artery aneurysm thrombosis following angiography.[38]

Transverse Myelopathy

Transverse myelopathy has also been reported following cerebral angiography. Seitz and Hintze described two patients who suffered incomplete transverse myelopathy after vertebral angiography in one patient and thyrocervical angiography in the second.[39] They postulated that the events were related to contrast in one case and may have been due to contralateral vertebral artery hypoplasia in the other. Ramirez-Lassepas et al. reported three cases of cervical myelopathy following angiography.[40] Only one of these patients had undergone cervical angiography, and the authors also concluded that the events were a result of arterial contrast injection reaching the spinal vascular supply. Ionic contrast was used in all of their cases.

Anaphylactoid Reactions

Anaphylactoid reactions to radiographic contrast injection are uncommon. These may be severe and life threatening or more commonly mild. Mild reactions cause itching and hives, whereas severe reactions may induce life-threatening hypotension, bradycardia, and angioedema. The exact nature of these reactions is not known. The role of complement and IgE-mediated events seems to be a rare occurrence, and the release of histamine from mast cells is more likely a direct toxic effect.[41, 42] Vik et al. studied the effect of nonionic and low-osmolar ionic agents on complement activation in the serum of nonallergic individuals and found no evidence of complement activation with iodixanol and no evidence of histamine release with the addition of other contrast agents.[41] They concluded that anaphylactoid reactions are probably not mediated by complement.

Anaphylactoid reactions can occur in individuals with no prior exposure and can be severe. Fortunately, most reactions are mild, and itching or hives can be handled with simple measures. The incidence of severe reactions is low and appears to be less common in association with arterial than with venous injections.[43]

Numerous pretreatment regimens have been proposed for patients who have had prior systemic reactions to administration of iodinated contrast. Almost all of these include corticosteroid administration 12, 4, and 1 hours before the planned procedure. The addition of diphenhydramine decreases the risk of reaction to some extent. The benefit of H_2 blockers is less clear. Lower osmolar and nonionic agents may have an additional benefit in reducing the risk of minor and severe reactions.[43,44] Some researchers have recommended the addition of a beta agonist to a pretreatment regimen, again without much supporting evidence.

Prior history of contrast reaction is the major predisposing factor when considering risk. Other factors such as history of asthma or use of beta-blockers have also been implicated as increasing the risk of a reaction.[45–47] Women may also be at slightly greater risk.[48]

Lasser et al., in a survey of contrast-related reactions, found that the incidence of anaphylactoid reactions during contrast examinations was significantly less with nonionic contrast agents (44.4 per million) than with either ionic low- or high-osmolar agents (193.8 per million).[49] Severe reactions were also lower with nonionic agents (10.5 per million) versus ionic agents (37.4 per million). Fatal reactions, however, were slightly higher with nonionic contrast media (6.4 per million) versus ionic agents (3.9 per million).[44] The only proven strategy for protection from severe and minor anaphylactoid reactions in susceptible individuals is the preprocedure administration of corticosteroids.[45, 49]

Lasser et al. noted a significant protective effect of a two-dose (12 and 2 hours before examination) over a single-dose (2 hours prior) corticosteroid administration before contrast administration in reducing the incidence of anaphylactoid reaction.[49] Pretreatment does not guarantee that severe and even life-threatening reactions will not occur.[50]

Other risk-reducing regimens are not as clearly beneficial. Greenberger et al., in a prospective series of patients with prior reaction to contrast, found no benefit to the addition of either an H_1-blocker (cimetidine) or beta-antagonist (ephedrine).[51]

Renal Toxicity

Renal toxicity with intravascular use of contrast agents is well documented. Acute renal failure, although rare, has been documented following cerebral arteriography.[52] Acute tubular necrosis associated with contrast is usually reversible. Factors implicated in increasing risk are diminished creatinine clearance, hyperproteinemia, and dehydration. A newer hypoglycemic agent metformin has been implicated in potentiating the deleterious effects of contrast on renal function. Intravascular contrast should not be administered to dehydrated patients, and if emergent angiography needs to be performed, every effort at rehydration should be made. The risk of producing irreversible renal injury in a well-hydrated patient even with marked renal insufficiency appears to be quite low. Diabetic nephropathy has been stated to be a more specific risk factor for developing contrast-induced tubular necrosis. Total contrast dose has also been implicated as a causative factor leading to nephrotoxicity.[53, 54] Weinrauch et al. suggest an increased risk of nephrotoxicity in patients with diabetic nephropathy and an association with increased contrast doses.[55] They recommend keeping azotemic patients well hydrated periprocedurally and using no more than 50 ml per m^2 body surface. In the face of renal insufficiency, injection volumes should be kept to a minimum and test injections should be used only as needed. Biplane digital subtraction capability is a great advantage and allows orthogonal imaging with improved contrast visualization. This combination provides the maximal diagnostic information with minimal contrast injection.

The incidence of renal failure from contrast examinations is very low (1–2 per million). The risk associated with ionic contrast media appears to be only slightly higher (1.22 per million) than with the nonionic agents (1.08 per million). The relative incidence of renal failure as a percentage of all reported reactions, however, was higher with nonionic contrast, reflecting the even greater reduction in anaphylactoid reactions.[44] The use of nonionic instead of ionic contrast in terms of nephrotoxicity is also supported by experimental data. Khoury et al. found decreased toxicity of nonionic contrast as measured by elevations in urinary protein following arterial contrast examinations.[53] Cavaliere et al. evaluated the excretion of certain protein markers of tubular injury and found nonionic (iopamidol) contrast media to be less toxic to the renal tubules than ionic (diatrizoate) contrast media.[56]

Other risk-reducing strategies have been investigated and are worthy of note. In a prospective series of azotemic patients, a calcium channel blocker (nitrendipine) was shown to help preserve glomerular filtration rate in patients receiving iodinated contrast material.[57] Erley et al. found similar results in patients given theophylline before contrast. The patients were also protected from the deleterious effects measured by less reduction in glomerular filtration rate compared with controls.[58]

Seizures

Rare reports of seizures following cerebral angiography are present in the literature. An EEG demonstrated continuous epileptiform activity, and the diagnosis of nonconvulsive status epilepticus was made in a patient with altered consciousness after cerebral arteriography with iothalamate meglumine.[59]

Pituitary Apoplexy

An interesting case of pituitary apoplexy was reported following cerebral angiography. The patient had regression of acromegaly and pituitary insufficiency after this event.[60] Another patient with this event was studied with an ionic contrast agent (ioxaglic acid).[61] The patient complained of headache 6 hours after examination. It is unclear whether the cause was increased intra-arterial pressure, thrombosis, or infarction related to contrast with subsequent hemorrhage.

Hemiballismus

Five cases of transient involuntary leg movements during cerebral arteriography have been reported. The movements were contralateral to the side of injection. The etiology is obscure.[36]

Cardiac Effects

Hayakawa et al. noted heart rate changes of greater than 20% in patients undergoing cerebral arteriography.[62] They found tachycardia in 14.9% and bradycardia in 7.1% (including two patients with asystole, 0.5%). Bradycardia was noted much more frequently in younger patients who were not premedicated with atropine and in patients with subarachnoid hemorrhage or arteriovenous malformation. Patients with neoplastic diseases and those with an initial sinus bradycardia were most likely to suffer tachycardia. In another study the incidence of bradycardia was higher with ionic than nonionic contrast.[21]

Local Complications

Local complications of cerebral angiography occur at the site of arterial puncture. This may be femoral, axillary, or brachial. Direct puncture techniques are not considered here. Most of these complications are related to hemorrhage but vessel injury with occlusion, distal embolization,[63, 64] nerve injury due to access attempts, or compression are to be considered.

AbuRahma et al. reported an analysis of complications in 707 arteriograms.[65] Local complication rates for the femoral approach were 9% versus 27% for the axillary approach. Brachial plexus injury was 13% in patients undergoing the axillary approach. They found a higher incidence of complications with selective versus nonselective cerebral arteriography, but both methods had similar neurologic complication rates. Postarteriographic contrast renal failure was associated with a higher contrast load. Overall complication rates were also related to catheterization time, amount of contrast used, and number of vessels punctured. Uchino, in a series of 333 patients using a transbrachial approach with a 4-French catheter system, found local complication rates of 2.1%, but noted that complication rates were significantly higher in women than in men.[66] Lilly et al. retrospectively reviewed 10,589 arteriograms for the factors that determined risk of transfemoral arteriography.[67] Severe local complications (requiring surgical repair) occurred in 47 patients (0.4%). The strongest factor associated with local bleeding was puncture site outside the common femoral artery. Minor risk factors included older age and female gender. Obesity and postprocedure anticoagulation were not associated with increased local complications as might have been expected. Gritter et al. catalogued complications associated with transbrachial arteriography using a pigtail catheter for nonselective digital subtraction angiography of the brachiocephalic vessels.[68] In 660 cases, only two (0.3%) major local complications occurred. Minor complications consisted of local arm pain (17.5%), transient parerethises (7.3%), and hematoma formation (9.5%). From these data, we can conclude that, if possible, femoral access should be used. Brachial access is a reasonable alternative, and axillary access is used as a last resort.

Serious life-threatening hemorrhage can result from femoral puncture, particularly if common femoral puncture is not performed. Low puncture can lead to difficulty in applying pressure to the puncture site and large hemorrhages into the thigh.

High puncture can result in retroperitoneal hemorrhage with disastrous results.[69]

Hemorrhagic complications may not always be avoided. The utility of obtaining routine coagulation parameters prior to angiography is in question. Darcy et al. prospectively studied 1,000 patients to asses the utility of pretest coagulation parameters in relation to the risk of bleeding.[70] They found that hematomas developed in 8.1% of patients with abnormal coagulation parameters and in 9.7% of patients with normal profiles. Increased bleeding complications were seen in patients with a low platelet count ($<100 \times 10^9$ per liter). Physiologic factors may also impose a greater risk to some patients. Extreme caution is advised when contemplating angiography in a patient with connective tissue disorders, especially Ehlers-Danlos syndrome because of the risk of severe vascular injury due to the friable vascular wall in these patients, especially in type I and IV patients.[71]

Inadvertent Thrombus or Plaque Embolization

Embolic material may arise from the catheterized vessel or from the catheter or guidewire placed into the vessel. Embolic material can be a thrombus dislodged from the catheter or blood vessel, a plaque from the vessel wall, catheter or wire fragments, or air. Embolic events likely account for the temporary and permanent neurologic complications. Many emboli that develop during angiography lyse spontaneously and cause only temporary neurologic deficits. Ginsberg et al. reported two cases of embolic events demonstrated during angiography with angiographic resolution of the emboli and clinical resolution of the accompanying symptoms.[72] Mamon et al. performed in vitro studies evaluating potential factors that could lead to thromboembolic events during angiography.[73] They found increased activation of coagulation factors with nonionic (iohexol) contrast as opposed to ionic (diatrizoate, ioxaglate) contrast agents. Their findings suggested an inhibition of thrombin with ionic contrast and a lack of inhibition with nonionic contrast. They also noted increased thrombin formation in glass versus plastic tubes. Gawel et al. demonstrated platelet aggregation after angiography in five patients, as measured by elevations in serum beta thromboglobulin levels.[74] They suggested a trial of antithrombotic therapy during cerebral arteriography.

Inadvertent Air Embolism

Despite careful catheter hygiene, some air microemboli move into the cerebral circulation. Information has been carefully obtained concerning the significance and avoidance of air microemboli. Markus et al. used transcranial Doppler (TCD) to assess the occurrence of air microemboli during angiography and to find ways to reduce the frequency of air emboli that may contribute to morbidity of cerebral angiography.[75] They found that air was introduced at the time the contrast or saline was drawn up into a syringe and during injection into the catheter. Allowing the filled syringe to stand several minutes before injection markedly reduced the number of air emboli insonated by TCD. Slower injections reduced the number of air emboli that may form as a result of cavitation associated with rapid injection. The cavitation effect was seen more prominently with saline and low-viscosity contrast agent injection. Care should also be taken to flush catheters slowly with saline. Ginsberg et al. evaluated the risk of air emboli with relation to the type of syringe used for injection.[76] They found no significant difference between glass and plastic syringes with respect to air emboli. Gerraty et al. correlated microembolic events seen in 24 patients by TCD with clinical and magnetic resonance imaging (MRI) findings.[77] Microemboli demonstrated by TCD during angiography had signal characteristics of air. The number of emboli seen (average, 51 per procedure per vessel) increased with the injection volume. No correlation with clinical events or MRI changes could be made.

Foreign Particle Emboli

Foreign particles, most likely introduced during angiography, have been demonstrated in resected arteriovenous malformations and have refractile properties. These foreign particles were not evaluated for chemical structure and may arise from catheters or guidewires or as imperceptible particles within injected materials. It is common practice to wipe guidewires with saline-soaked cotton sponges, and this could also be a rich source of embolic material. It is unclear to what extent these foreign particles might contribute to neurologic events during cerebral angiography.[78]

Embolic Complications in Children

Pettersson et al. reported a rate of 0.4% embolic complications in children in a series of 3,731 cerebral angiograms.[79] None had permanent sequelae, and only one demonstrated transient neurologic deficit. The investigators concluded that embolic events in children have a much lower risk of inducing neurologic deficit for reasons that are not clear. Possibilities proposed were the use of general anesthesia in most of their patients, different response to ischemia in children, or different types of emboli in children. An additional possibility is the better potential for collateral supply in children. It is not clear whether this protective effect is isolated to young children as in their series or if perhaps this is a gradually disappearing effect as one ages.

Intimal Dissection

An exact incidence of intimal dissection is not known. The guidewire or catheter and forceful injection can result in intimal injury. As with spontaneous dissection of the carotid or vertebral arteries, these iatrogenic lesions frequently heal without sequelae. However, dissection can proceed to vessel occlusion, vessel stenosis, or pseudoaneurysm.[80] As with spontaneous dissection, the lesion can act as an embolic source and treatment should be aimed at reducing this risk.

Aneurysm Rupture

Aneurysm rupture during cerebral angiography is a frightening event. There are numerous reports of contrast extravasation demonstrated in the literature during angiography.[81–87] It is difficult, however, to glean how much cause and effect can be attributed to the events. Almost all of the patients reported were being evaluated for acute subarachnoid hemorrhage and are clearly at risk for early rebleeding. There is some evidence of slight increases in arterial flow during cerebral arteriography that might account for some increased risk of rehemorrhage during angiography.[81] However, this risk needs to be placed in perspective with the importance of adequate diagnostic imaging in cases of acute subarachnoid hemorrhage. There may be some increased risk of rupture in female subjects.[83, 84]

Koenig et al. summarized 10 cases of aneurysm rupture during angiography and reported that there is no increased risk associated with internal carotid injection over common carotid injection, and delayed arteriography was not justified.[88] Aoyagi and Hayakawa, however, analyzed the reported cases along with six of their own and concluded that there may be increased risk of rerupture from cerebral arteriography if the procedure is done within 3 hours of initial hemorrhage.[82] They also noted that these patients had a much worse outcome compared with patients with early rerupture not associated with angiography.

Periangiographic aneurysmal hemorrhage likely carries a higher morbidity and mortality than expected with spontaneous rebleeding. Murray and Wortzman, in analysis of three cases and the literature, concluded that the morbidity and mortality of aneurysm rupture during angiography was higher than expected with rerupture alone.[85]

Postangiography Headache

Some patients experience a headache with cerebral angiography. Ramadan et al. evaluated 45 consecutive patients after cerebral angiograms with regard to headache.[89] They found a 33% incidence of headache, with unilateral headaches more common (60%) than bilateral (40%). Onset after angiography was typically delayed, with a mean interval of 125 minutes (±99 minutes). Associated symptoms included nausea (20%), vomiting (7%), photophobia (33%), and phonophobia (20%). The headaches had the characteristics associated with vascular origin without aura. Prior history of headache in postangiography headaches was seen in 53% versus 23% in the nonpostangiography group. The authors postulated contrast- or catheter-induced release of vasoactive substances such as serotonin or nitric oxide.

Shuaib and Hachinski reported clinical analysis of 142 patients who received 149 cerebral angiograms.[90] They found that there was no increased risk of neurologic complications in these patients as had been previously suggested in the literature. They recorded a neurologic event rate of 2.6% as compared with 2.8% seen in 1,002 nonmigraine patients. They concluded that cerebral angiography is safe in patients with a history of migraine, even during an acute headache.

Radiation Risk

Radiation effects from a single or even multiple diagnostic cerebral arteriography are difficult to measure in terms of morbidity. Casselden measured ocular lens doses received during both digital subtraction and conventional film screen cerebral angiography.[37] He found that using the digital subtraction technique the patient dose was a fraction of a centigray (0.327), whereas the dose during film screen angiography was considerably higher. In either case, the doses are not large enough to cause some of the early deleterious effects such as alopecia or skin burns that have been reported with interventional procedures. The long-term effects, such as radiation induction of tumor, are only theoretical at these doses. Extrapolation of larger doses known to cause induction of tumors with a long lag time to the lower doses has been proposed; therefore, any reduction in dose may be considered beneficial. Due to the long time between radiation exposure and the development of tumors (15–20 years), dose reduction is particularly important in younger patients who may live long enough to develop a radiation-induced tumor.

Radiation reduction can be accomplished in several ways. The choice of digital subtraction technique as noted previously is an important consideration. Appropriate shielding of nonimaged areas and collimation of the primary beam to reduce scatter is important. Doses delivered by newer angiographic equipment are lowered with improved beam filtration (reducing unwanted lower energy photons) and pulsed fluoroscopy (diminishing actual radiation time with the same visualization time). Minimizing fluoroscopy time and the number of angiographic runs should be the primary strategy for radiation reduction.

Spinal Angiography

Angiography of the supply to the spinal cord carries similar risks to those of cerebral angiography. Direct toxic effects of the contrast agent, embolic events, and vessel injury are potential hazards during spinal angiography. One must consider that in a complete spinal angiography performed for evaluation of potential vascular malformation, the number of vessels evaluated may be as many as 30–35 and may require multiple catheter exchanges. These factors alone can be important in determining risk, both neurologic and non-neurologic.

Forbes et al. found that the incidence of complications during spinal angiography was similar to that of cerebral angiography.[91] In a series of 96 patients, they found an incidence of permanent neurologic event of 0.7%, with all neurologic events at 2.2%. Systemic events of 3.7% and local puncture complications of 8.2% were reported. Inadvertent emboli and vessel injury, particularly to the anterior spinal arteries, are the most likely causes of permanent injury to the cord. Care must be taken when injecting contrast or flushing the catheter while the catheter is within a spinal artery that gives rise to anterior spinal supply. A case of extravasation of contrast during spinal angiography has also been reported; this patient suffered paraplegia as a result.[92]

Conclusion

Many of the risks of cerebral or spinal angiography are related to the difficulty of the technique and to the experience and skill of the angiographer. Some complications, however, are a result of contrast reactions that are rarely foreseen. The risk of neurologic complications (particularly permanent) using current techniques should be very low. Some of the complications reported temporally associated with cerebral angiography, such as aneurysm rupture or pituitary apoplexy, are too uncommon to adequately address in a risk-reduction approach.

References

1. Doby T. Cerebral angiography and Egas Moniz. AJR Am J Roentgenol 1992;159:364.
2. Schierhorn H. [Egas Moniz, Wilhelm Lohr and cerebral angiography. An expedition into the discovery of the cerebral vessels]. [German] J Hirnforsch 1981;22:491.
3. Crisan V. [Egas Moniz (1874–1955), creator of cerebral angiography and prefrontal leukotomy]. [Romanian] Rev Med Interna Neurol Psihiatr Neurochir Dermatovenerol Neurol Psihiatr Neurochir 1979;24:71.
4. Isner JM, Sazama KJ, Roberts WC. Vascular complications of thorium dioxide. Am J Med 1978;64:1069.
5. Johnson PK, Babb RR. Cholangiocarcinoma in a patient previously given thorotrast. Am J Dig Dis 1975;20:384.
6. Wagner WH, Treiman RL, Cossman DV, et al. The

diminishing role of diagnostic arteriography in carotid artery disease: duplex scanning as definitive preoperative study. Ann Vasc Surg 1991;5:105.
7. Larson EB, Oomenn GS, Margolis MT, Loop JW. Impact of computed tomography on utilization of cerebral angiograms. AJR Am J Roentgenol 1977;129:1.
8. Mani RL, Eisenberg RL. Complications of catheter cerebral arteriography: analysis of 5,000 procedures. III. Assessment of arteries injected, contrast medium used, duration of procedure, and age of patient. AJR Am J Roentgenol 1978;131:871.
9. McIvor J, Steiner TJ, Perkin GD, et al. Neurologic morbidity of arch and carotid arteriography in cerebrovascular disease. The influence of contrast medium and radiologist. Br J Radiol 1987;60:117.
10. Grzyska U, Freitag J, Zeumer H. Selective cerebral intraarterial DSA. Complication rate and control of risk factors. Neuroradiology 1990;32:296.
11. Waugh JR, Sacharias N. Arteriographic complications in the DSA era. Radiology 1992;182:243.
12. Heiserman JE, Dean BL, Hodak JA, et al. Neurologic complications of cerebral angiography. AJNR Am J Neuroradiol 1994;15:1401; discussion 1408.
13. Mani RL, Eisenberg RL. Complications of catheter cerebral arteriography: analysis of 5,000 procedures. II. Relation of complication rates to clinical and arteriographic diagnoses. AJR Am J Roentgenol 1978;131: 867.
14. Mani RL, Eisenberg RL, McDonald EJ Jr, et al. Complications of catheter cerebral arteriography: analysis of 5,000 procedures. I. Criteria and incidence. AJR Am J Roentgenol 1978;131:861.
15. Faught E, Trader SD, Hanna GR. Cerebral complications of angiography for transient ischemia and stroke: prediction of risk. Neurology 1979;29:4.
16. Dion J, Gates P, Fox AJ, et al. Clinical events following neuroangiography. A prospective study. Acta Radiol Suppl 1986;369:29.
17. Earnest F IV, Forbes G, Sandok BA, et al. Complications of cerebral angiography: prospective assessment of risk. AJR Am J Roentgenol 1984;142:247.
18. Gasparini M, Arosio M, Galbiati N, et al. Neurologic complications of cerebral angiography. Ital J Neurol Sci 1986;7:353.
19. Eisenberg RL, Bank WO, Hedgcock MW. Neurologic complications of angiography for cerebrovascular disease. Neurology 1980;30:895.
20. Nakagawa H, Arita S, Kobayashi S, et al. [Neurotropic effects of nonionic contrast media]. [Japanese] Nippon Yakurigaku Zasshi 1989;93:187.
21. Skalpe IO, Lundervold A, Tjorstad K. Cerebral angiography with nonionic (metrizamide) and ionic (meglumine metrizoate) water soluble contrast media. A comparative study with double blind technique. Neuroradiology 1977;14:15.
22. Helsley JD. Cortical blindness following cerebral angiography. W Va Med J 1995;91:324.
23. Studdard WE, Davis DO, Young SW. Cortical blindness after cerebral angiography. Case report. J Neurosurg 1981;54:240.
24. Kermode AG, Chakera T, Mastaglia FL. Low osmolar and nonionic x-ray contrast media and cortical blindness. Clin Exp Neurol 1992;29:272.
25. Stevens JM, Barter S, Kerslake R, et al. [Transient cortical blindness after cerebral angiography: report of a case]. [Portuguese] Arq Neuropsiquiatr 1984;42:298.
26. Hansen PE, Stenbjerg S. Possible increased tendency to thrombosis after cerebral angiography. Acta Neurol Scand 1979;59:148.
27. Shyn PB, Bell KA. Transient cortical blindness following cerebral angiography. J La State Med Soc 1989; 141:35.
28. Ritter G, Busse K, Rittmeier K. [Cortical blindness following arteria vertebralis angiography]. [German] Radiologe 1976;16:424.
29. Haley EC Jr. Encephalopathy following arteriography: a possible toxic effect of contrast agents. Ann Neurol 1984;15:100.
30. Giang DW, Kido DK. Transient global amnesia associated with cerebral angiography performed with use of iopamidol. Radiology 1989;172:195.
31. Brady AP, Hough DM, Lo R, Gill G. Transient global amnesia after cerebral angiography with iohexol. Can Assoc Radiol J 1993;44:450.
32. Pexman JH, Coates RK. Amnesia after femorocerebral angiography. AJNR Am J Neuroradiol 1983;4:979.
33. Schamschula RG, Soo MY. Transient global amnesia following cerebral angiography with non-ionic contrast medium. Australas Radiol 1994;38:196.
34. Cochran JW, Morrell F, Huckman MS, Cochran EJ. Transient global amnesia after cerebral angiography. Report of seven cases. Arch Neurol 1982;39:593.
35. Lapresle J, Lasjaunias P, Thevenier D. [Transitory paralysis of cranial nerves IX, X and XII as well as the left VII after angiography. Contribution to the ischemic pathology of the cranial nerves]. [French] Rev Neurol (Paris) 1980;136:787.
36. Komiyama M, Yasui T, Izumi T. Transient involuntary movement of the leg (monoballismus) during cerebral angiography. AJNR Am J Neuroradiol 1995;16:1942.
37. Casselden PA.Ocular lens dose in cerebral vascular imaging. Br J Radiol 1988;61:202.
38. Griffiths PD, Gholkar A, Sengupta RP. Oculomotor nerve palsy due to thrombosis of a posterior communicating artery aneurysm following diagnostic angiography. Neuroradiology 1994;36:614.
39. Seitz D, Hintze A. [Myelomalacia following vertebral angiography with a femoral catheter]. [German] ROFO Fortschr Geb Rontgenstr Nuklearmed 1976;125:59.
40. Ramirez-Lassepas M, McClelland RR, Snyder BD, Marsh DG. Cervical myelopathy complicating cerebral angiography. Report of a case and review of the literature. Neurology 1977;27:834.
41. Vik H, Froysa A, Sonstevold A, et al. Complement acti-

vation and histamine release following administration of roentgen contrast media. Acta Radiol Suppl 1995; 399:83.
42. Baxter AB, Lazarus SC, Brasch RC. In vitro histamine release induced by magnetic resonance imaging and iodinated contrast media. Invest Radiol 1993;28:308.
43. Bush WH, Swanson DP. Acute reactions to intravascular contrast media: types, risk, factors, recognition and specific treatment. AJR Am J Roentgenol 1991;157:1153.
44. Lasser EC, Lyon SG, Berry CC. Reports on contrast media reactions: analysis of data from reports to the U.S. Food and Drug Administration. Radiology 1997;203:605.
45. Porri F, Vervloet D. [Reactions to iodinated contrast media. (review)]. [French] Allerg Immunol (Paris) 1994;26:374.
46. Laxenaire MC, Torrens J, Moneret-Vautrin DA. [Fatal anaphylactic shock in a patient treated with beta-blockers]. [French] Ann Fr Anesth Reanim 1984;3:453.
47. Lang DM, Alpern MB, Visintainer PF, Smith ST. Elevated risk of anaphylactoid reaction from radiographic contrast media is associated with both beta-blocker exposure and cardiovascular disorders. Arch Intern Med 1993;153:2033.
48. Lang DM, Alpern MB, Visintainer PF, Smith ST. Gender risk for anaphylactoid reaction to radiographic contrast media. J Allergy Clin Immunol 1995;95:813.
49. Lasser EC, Berry CC, Talner LB, et al. Protective effects of corticosteroids in contrast material anaphylaxis. Invest Radiol 1988;23(Suppl 1):S193.
50. Madowitz JS, Schweiger MJ. Severe anaphylactoid reaction to radiographic contrast media. Recurrences despite premedication with diphenhydramine and prednisone. JAMA 1979;241:2813.
51. Greenberger PA, Patterson R, Tapio CM. Prophylaxis against repeated radiocontrast media reactions in 57 cases. Adverse experience with cimetidine and safety of beta-adrenergic antagonists. Arch Intern Med 1985;145:2197.
52. Adornato B, Winestock D. Acute renal failure. A complication of cerebral angiography. Arch Neurol 1976;33:687.
53. Khoury GA, Hopper JC, Varghese Z, et al. Nephrotoxicity of ionic and nonionic contrast material in digital vascular imaging and selective renal arteriography. Br J Radiol 1983;56:631.
54. Robinson JS, Arzola DD, Moody RA. Acute renal failure following cerebral angiography and infusion computerized tomography. Case report. J Neurosurg 1980;52:111.
55. Weinrauch LA, Friedberg SR, Elia JA. Acute renal failure after cerebral arteriography in a diabetic patient. Neuroradiology 1977;12:197.
56. Cavaliere G, Arrigo G, D'Amico G, et al. Tubular nephrotoxicity after intravenous urography with ionic high-osmolal and nonionic low-osmolal contrast media in patients with chronic renal insufficiency. Nephron 1987;46:128.
57. Neumayer HH, Junge W, Kufner A, Wenning A. Prevention of radiocontrast-media-induced nephrotoxicity by the calcium channel blocker nitrendipine: a prospective randomised clinical trial. Nephrol Dial Transplant 1989;4:1030.
58. Erley CM, Duda SH, Schlepckow S, et al. Adenosine antagonist theophylline prevents the reduction of glomerular filtration rate after contrast media application. Kidney Int 1994;45:1425.
59. Vickrey BG, Bahls FH. Nonconvulsive status epilepticus following cerebral angiography. Ann Neurol 1989;25:199.
60. Louwerens M, de Herder WW, Postema PT, et al. Pituitary insufficiency and regression of acromegaly caused by pituitary apoplexy following cerebral angiography. Eur J Endocrinol 1996;134:737.
61. Suga T, Kagawa S, Goto H, et al. [A case of pituitary adenoma progressing to pituitary apoplexy on the occasion of cerebral angiography]. [Japanese] No Shinkei Geka 1996;24:475.
62. Hayakawa K, Nishimura Y, Yoshida M, et al. ECG changes during cerebral angiography. An analysis of 334 patients—942 cerebral angiographies. Neuroradiology 1984;26:369.
63. Gaspar MR, Yellin AE. Femoral artery occlusion caused by percutaneous angiography: mechanisms and management. Acta Chir Belg 1977;76:323.
64. Jacobsson B, Paulin S, Schlossman D. Thromboembolism of leg following percutaneous catheterisation of femoral artery for angiography. Symptoms and signs. Acta Radiol Diagn (Stockh) 1969;8:97.
65. AbuRahma AF, Robinson PA, Boland JP, et al. Complications of arteriography in a recent series of 707 cases: factors affecting outcome. Ann Vasc Surg 1993;7:122.
66. Uchino A. Local complications in transbrachial cerebral angiography using the 4-F catheter. So Neurol Med Chir (Tokyo) 1991;31:647.
67. Lilly MP, Reichman W, Sarazen AA Jr, Carney WI Jr. Anatomic and clinical factors associated with complications of transfemoral arteriography. Ann Vasc Surg 1990;4:264.
68. Gritter KJ, Laidlaw WW, Peterson NT. Complications of outpatient transbrachial intraarterial digital subtraction angiography. Work in progress. Radiology 1987; 162(1 Pt 1):125.
69. Kaufman JL. Pelvic hemorrhage after percutaneous femoral angiography. AJR Am J Roentgenol 1984; 143:335.
70. Darcy MD, Kanterman RY, Kleinhoffer MA, et al. Evaluation of coagulation tests as predictors of angiographic bleeding complications. Radiology 1996;198: 741.
71. Slingenberg EJ. Complications during intravascular diagnostic manipulations in the Ehlers-Danlos syndrome. Neth J Surg 1980;32:56.
72. Ginsberg LE, Stump DA, King JC, et al. Transient neurologic deficits due to embolic occlusion and immedi-

ate reopening of the cerebral arteries. Stroke 1985; 16:522.
73. Mamon JF, Hoppensteadt D, Fareed J, Moncada R. Biochemical evidence for a relative lack of inhibition of thrombin formation by nonionic contrast media. Radiology 1991;179:399.
74. Gawel M, Burkett M, Rose FC. Platelet activation following cerebral angiography. Acta Neurol Scand 1980;61:240.
75. Markus H, Loh A, Israel D, et al. Microscopic air embolism during cerebral angiography and strategies for its avoidance [see comments]. Lancet 1993;341: 784.
76. Ginsberg LE, Stump DA, King JC, et al. Air embolus risk with glass versus plastic syringes: in vitro study and implications for neuroangiography. Radiology 1994;191:813.
77. Gerraty RP, Bowser DN, Infeld B, et al. Microemboli during carotid angiography. Association with stroke risk factors or subsequent magnetic resonance imaging changes? Stroke 1996;27:1543.
78. Vinters HV, Kaufmann JC, Drake CG. "Foreign" particles in encephalic vascular malformations. Arch Neurol 1983;40:221.
79. Pettersson H, Fitz CR, Harwood-Nash DC, et al. Iatrogenic embolization: complication of pediatric cerebral angiography. AJNR Am J Neuroradiol 1981;2:357.
80. Golabek R, Karwowski B. [Radiological image of aneurysm of the internal carotid artery as a complication of angiography]. [Polish] Wiad Lek 1989; 42:263.
81. Nornes H. Internal carotid artery blood flow during cerebral angiography. Neuroradiology 1977;12:219.
82. Aoyagi N, Hayakawa I. Rerupture of intracranial aneurysms during angiography. Acta Neurochir (Wien) 1989;98:141.
83. Dublin AB, French BN. Cerebral aneurysmal rupture during angiography with confirmation by computed tomography: a review of intra-angiographic aneurysmal rupture. Surg Neurol 1980;13:19.
84. Nascimento SH. [Rupture of intracranial aneurysm during angiography. Report of a case and review of the literature]. [Spanish] Acta Neurol Latinoam 1976;22:189.
85. Murray JB, Wortzman G. Contrast medium extravasation from aneurysmal rupture during cerebral angiography. Clin Radiol 1977;28:277.
86. Hayakawa I, Watanabe T, Tsuchida T, Sasaki A. Perangiographic rupture of intracranial aneurysms. Neuroradiology 1978;16:293.
87. Liliequist B, Lindqvist M, Probst F. Rupture of intracranial aneurysm during carotid angiography. Neuroradiology 1976;11:185.
88. Koenig GH, Marshall WH Jr, Poole GJ, Kramer RA. Rupture of intracranial aneurysms during cerebral angiography: report of ten cases and review of the literature. Neurosurgery 1979;5:314.
89. Ramadan NM, Gilkey SJ, Mitchell M, et al. Postangiography headache. Headache 1995;35:21.
90. Shuaib A, Hachinski VC. Migraine and the risks from angiography. Arch Neurol 1988;45:911.
91. Forbes G, Nichols DA, Jack CR Jr, et al. Complications of spinal cord arteriography: prospective assessment of risk for diagnostic procedures. Radiology 1988;169:479.
92. Mosely IF, Tress BM. Extravasation of contrast medium during spinal angiography: a case of paraplegia. Neuroradiology 1977;13:55.

Chapter 3

Complications of Interventional Neuroradiology

John A. Scott and Andrew J. DeNardo

Objectives

- To understand the complications common to all embolization procedures involving the extracranial circulation and means of their avoidance
- To understand the complications common to all embolization procedures involving the intracranial circulation and means of their avoidance
- To become familiar with the various embolic agents, indications for their use, and associated potential complications
- To understand that the venous anatomy of dural arteriovenous fistulas (DAVFs) predict the clinical behavior, prognosis, therapeutic options, and hence potential complications
- To recognize the complications associated with the treatment of inoperable cerebral aneurysms using endovascular techniques
- To appreciate the broad spectrum of interventional neuroradiologic procedures, the complexity of the vascular anatomy of the head and neck, and the need for proper training to safely perform these procedures

Since the 1970s, endovascular treatments and the specialty of interventional neuroradiology has undergone tremendous growth and change. Most of this growth has been in the evolution of embolization procedures for vascular lesions of the brain, spine, spinal cord, head, and neck. This chapter concentrates on the complications associated with these procedures. Advances have also been made in the endovascular treatment of acute stroke and balloon dilation of cerebrovascular atherosclerotic lesions. The techniques and complications associated with these techniques are beyond the scope of this chapter and are not discussed.

The safe performance of interventional neuroradiologic procedures requires a cooperative multidisciplinary team composed of interventional neuroradiologists, neurosurgeons, neurologists, plastic surgeons, otorhinolaryngologists, neuroanesthesiologists, intensive care physicians, x-ray technicians, and radiologic nurses. This team must discuss and agree on the treatment plan and its goals. The patient and family should be active in this discussion. They should be informed about the disease to be treated, its natural history, and the treatment options and their respective risks and benefits. The discussion should occur well in advance of the planned procedure so that there is sufficient time for the patient to assimilate the information presented and have the opportunity to have all questions answered.

Improvements in radiographic equipment, angiographic devices, radiographic contrast agents, and neuroanesthesia, together with advances in the knowledge of vascular anatomy and pathology, have diminished the morbidity of neurointerventional procedures. Endovascular embolization procedures are performed using fluoroscopic guidance; therefore, high-quality angiographic equipment is imperative for safety. High-resolution, biplane, digital radiographic imaging with road mapping capabilities and live, subtracted fluoroscopy are necessary to adequately visualize the microcatheters and embolic agents that are currently used.

The development of and continued refinements in variable stiffness microcatheters, microguidewires, flow-directed microcatheters, and embolic devices have allowed more selective catheterization and improved treatment outcomes. Nonionic contrast agents, although more expensive, have less neurotoxicity and are better tolerated by patients.

Neuroanesthesia is also important for patient safety during embolization procedures. Most procedures are performed on an awake, but sedated patient, which allows for close neurologic monitoring. Fentanyl and midazolam are commonly used for analgesia and sedation. It is essential that the patient be motionless during the procedure for adequate imaging; thus, general anesthesia may be necessary in uncooperative patients. If using electrophysiologic monitoring during the procedure, one must remember that certain anesthetic agents may alter their readings.

It must be emphasized that the possession of these tools is not a substitute for proper training in their use and in the understanding of the complex vascular anatomy of the head and neck that is necessary to allow for safe performance of neurointerventional procedures.

This chapter attempts to introduce the complications associated with the wide spectrum of interventional neuroradiologic embolization procedures. Complications that are common to the vascular anatomic area treated, regardless of disease (i.e., head and neck tumors, intracranial disease), are covered in the first part of the chapter. This discussion is followed by complications specific to the disease entity treated. Means to avoid these complications and their treatment are discussed.

Arterial Embolization of Vascular Lesions of the Head, Neck, and Dura

Vascular lesions of the head, neck, and dura share a common arterial supply (branches of the external carotid artery); therefore, the techniques of transarterial endovascular treatment and the associated complications are similar. Lesions in this anatomic region that are amenable to embolization include vascular neoplasms of the head and neck (paraganglioma, juvenile nasopharyngeal angiofibroma, hemangioma, extracranial arteriovenous malformation [AVM], arteriovenous fistula), vascular lesions of the dura (meningioma, hemangiopericytoma, DAVF), and intractable epistaxis.

Because of the rich collateral vascular network of the head and neck, proximal embolization or surgical ligation of feeding arteries is not effective in devascularizing these lesions. Distal catheterization with microcatheters and embolization of the lesion nidus with particulate or liquid embolic material has proven more effective.[1, 2]

A thorough understanding of the functional microvascular anatomy of the head and neck (Table 3.1), the anastomoses to the intracranial circulation, and the blood supply to the cranial nerves is important to avoid cranial nerve palsies, blindness, and stroke.[3]

Provocative testing of vessels that may have cranial nerve supply can be performed by the superselective arterial injection of 50 mg of lidocaine (Xylocaine) followed by appropriate testing of that cranial nerve. If transient palsy results, the vessel should not be embolized with small particulate or liquid embolic agents.[4]

Embolic agents that are in current use may be broadly divided into particulate and liquid agents. The choice of embolic agent depends on multiple factors, including lesion histology, presence and size of arteriovenous shunting, catheter position, potential anastomoses, and desired permanence of vascular occlusion. Polyvinyl alcohol (PVA) particles are the most widely used particulate agent. PVA is available in sizes ranging from 50 to 1,000 mm. Although PVA is a permanent embolic agent, the particles are irregular in shape, and embolized vessels may recanalize through the interstices between the particles. PVA is usually reserved for preoperative or palliative embolization. Smaller particles (less than 150 microns in length) are more likely to pass through vascular anastomoses and should be used with caution in this situation. Small particles may also pass through arteriovenous shunts if the shunts are larger than the particle size.[5]

N-butyl-2-cyanoacrylate (NBCA), a tissue adhesive, is the most commonly used liquid embolic agent. It is used when a permanent embolic agent is necessary, such as in lesions in which embolization

Table 3.1. External Carotid Artery Branches, Major Anastomoses, and Potential Complications

Artery and Branches	Anastomosis	Complication
Internal maxillary artery		
Anterior deep temporal artery	Ophthalmic artery	Blindness
Infraorbital artery	Ophthalmic artery	Blindness
Sphenopalatine artery	Ophthalmic artery	Blindness
Artery of foramen rotundum	Inferolateral trunk (ICA)	ICA stroke Blindness
Middle meningeal artery	Inferolateral trunk	ICA stroke Blindness
Petrosal branch		CN VII, VIII palsy
Cavernous branch		CN III, IV, V, VI palsy
Accessory meningeal artery	Inferolateral trunk	ICA stroke Blindness CN III, IV, V, VI palsy
Occipital artery		
Stylomastoid branch		CN VII, VIII palsy
C1 and C2 branches	Vertebral artery	Posterior circulation stroke
Facial artery	Ophthalmic artery	Blindness
Ascending pharyngeal artery		
Neuromeningeal branch		CN IX, X, XI, XII palsy
Clival branches	Meningohypophyseal trunk	ICA stroke Blindness

ICA = internal carotid artery; CN = cranial nerve.

is planned as the sole means of treatment (e.g., inoperable AVMs). This agent polymerizes into a solid cast when it contacts ionic solutions, such as saline or plasma. The polymerization time may be prolonged by mixing the agent with iophendylate, ethiodol, or acetic acid,[6] allowing the agent to reach the nidus of the lesion before polymerization. Tantalum or tungsten powder is also added to the embolic mixture to render it radiopaque. NBCA in its liquid state has low viscosity, which allows it to be injected through microcatheters and penetrate deep into the nidus of a lesion. These properties also allow for passage through small vascular anastomoses, and its use carries a higher risk of stroke and cranial nerve palsy.[1] The catheter must be quickly removed after the injection of NBCA to prevent it from being glued within the vessel.

Paragangliomas

Paragangliomas are vascular tumors of neural crest origin and most commonly occur in the jugular bulb, middle ear, and carotid body. These tumors may secrete epinephrine, norepinephrine, or both in 5% of cases. Preoperative angiography and embolization may provoke secretion of these substances and precipitate a hypertensive crisis. Patients suspected of having a secretory tumor should be premedicated for 1 week with phentolamine or phenoxybenzamine and volume expansion.[7] Hypertensive crises that occur during embolization may be treated with phentolamine, labetalol, propranolol, or sodium nitroprusside.[7]

Embolization of carotid body paragangliomas may cause carotid sinus syndrome in rare cases.[8] Atropine and ephedrine are the drugs of choice to treat this condition, but may be ineffective. In these cases, immediate surgical resection of the mass or transection of the glossopharyngeal nerve and superior roots of the vagus nerve may be necessary.[8] Meperidine should be given for pain control rather than morphine because the former drug is vagolytic and the latter is vagotonic.[9]

Meningioma

Preoperative embolization of the dural arterial blood supply of meningiomas decreases intraopera-

Table 3.2. Classification of Dural Arteriovenous Fistulas According to Location

Location	Sinus Outflow	Retrograde Outflow	Common Symptoms
Cavernous sinus	Common	Rare	Bruit, orbital symptoms (proptosis, chemosis, conjunctival edema, cranial nerve palsy, decreased visual acuity)
Transverse/sigmoid sinus	Common	May occur	Bruit, headache If retrograde outflow, neurologic deficit, seizures, hemorrhage
Tentorium	Rare	Common	Neurologic deficit, seizures, hemorrhage
Anterior fossa	Rare	Common	Hemorrhage, seizure, neurologic deficit
Foramen magnum	Rare	Common (perimedullary)	Myelopathy

Table 3.3. Classification of Dural Arteriovenous Fistulas According to Venous Outflow

Type	Venous Outflow
I	Normal antegrade sinus outflow
IIa	Insufficient antegrade sinus outflow with retrograde reflux into sinus
IIb	Insufficient antegrade sinus outflow with retrograde reflux into cortical veins
IIa+b	Insufficient antegrade sinus outflow with retrograde reflux into both sinus and cortical veins
III	Outflow directly into cortical vein
IV	Outflow directly into cortical vein with associated venous ectasia
V	Outflow into spinal perimedullary veins

Source: Reprinted with permission from C Cognard, YP Gobin, L Pierot, et al. Cerebral dural arteriovenous fistulas: clinical and angiographic correlation with a revised classification of venous drainage. Radiology 1995;194:671.

tive blood loss, thereby facilitating surgical resection and reducing postoperative complications.[10, 11] Postembolization peritumoral and subarachnoid hemorrhage has been reported, presumably secondary to tumor necrosis.[12] Hemorrhage or increased mass effect due to tumor edema may necessitate emergent resection.[13]

Dural Arteriovenous Fistula

DAVFs, also referred to as dural AVMs, are acquired arteriovenous communications within the dura of the walls of a venous sinus or cortical venous tributary. The transverse sigmoid and cavernous sinuses are most commonly involved. DAVFs are classified according to their anatomic location and anatomy of the venous outflow—features that predict presenting symptoms and clinical course (Tables 3.2 and 3.3). Higher-grade lesions are characterized by retrograde cortical venous outflow and are more likely to present with aggressive symptoms (e.g., neurologic deficit, seizures, hemorrhage, increased intracranial pressure, and myelopathy).[14] Treatment options vary and are dictated by symptomatology and angiographic features. Those lesions that are low risk based on angiography may be treated conservatively, provided the symptoms are tolerated by the patient. Conversely, those that demonstrate cortical venous outflow or present with hemorrhage require complete obliteration of the fistula.

Carotid Jugular and Occipital Artery Compression

DAVFs of the lateral or cavernous sinuses may be treated by manual arterial self-compression, a technique first described by Halbach, in which complete thrombosis can be achieved in nearly one-third of cases.[15, 16] This therapy is reserved for low-risk fistulas; whereas complete obliteration of the fistula by more aggressive therapy is indicated for high-risk lesions or those that present with hemorrhage. Potential complications of compression therapy include cerebral ischemia, bradycardia, and hypotension due to carotid occlusion and carotid sinus stimulation. Therefore, initial compressions should be observed by a physician to ensure that the treatment will be tolerated by the patient.[15, 16]

Transarterial Embolization

Superselective catheterization and embolization of the external carotid dural arterial supply to DAVFs is effective in diminishing the arteriovenous shunts and may result in complete thrombosis of the lesion. The incidence of obliteration is lower than that achieved with transvenous embolization[17]; therefore, we reserve this treatment as a palliative procedure in patients with low-risk DAVFs or for preoperative devascularization.

In addition to the potential complications common to all external carotid arterial embolizations, the arteriovenous communications encountered with DAVFs pose other hazards. Liquid embolic material may pass through the shunts and occlude venous outflow, resulting in venous infarction and hemorrhage.[18]

Transvenous Embolization

Complete occlusion of DAVFs can be achieved with a high rate of angiographic and clinical cure by packing the involved sinus with embolic material introduced via a transvenous or direct surgical approach.[17, 19, 20] High-risk DAVFs that involve the cavernous sinus and lateral sinus lesions are the most common lesions treated in this manner. The inferior petrosal sinus or superior ophthalmic vein is catheterized to reach DAVFs involving the cavernous sinus. Lateral sinus lesions are accessed via either jugular vein. Stainless steel or platinum fiber coils and platinum detachable coils are the most widely used embolic material, although transvenous embolization has also been performed with liquid embolic agents.

It must be emphasized that this treatment should be performed only for high-risk DAVFs in which the involved sinus is not functioning as a pathway for normal cerebral venous outflow. Embolization and occlusion of the sinus in this situation carry great risk for venous infarction and intracerebral hemorrhage. The venous phase of the diagnostic arteriography should be carefully examined for evidence of cerebral venous drainage toward the involved sinus. Lesions that demonstrate this finding should be excluded from transvenous therapy.

Vascular perforations of the sinus or venous access, although unusual, may occur and require prompt management.[21] Anticoagulation should be immediately reversed, and the perforation or involved vascular compartment should be closed with coils or other appropriate embolic device.[21] Perforation of the superior ophthalmic vein results in intraorbital hematoma and may necessitate emergent surgical evacuation.[22]

All attempts should be made to occlude the sinus at the point of the fistula(s). Deposition of coils or other embolic devices in other locations in the sinus or in the venous outflow conduits may result in cortical venous rerouting, venous occlusion, infarction, and hemorrhage.[20, 23]

Intracranial Embolization

The development of microcatheters, microguidewires, and flow-guided microcatheters has made superselective catheterization of cerebral arteries possible and has allowed for safe embolization of vascular lesions and intracerebral arterial infusion of drugs and chemotherapeutic agents.

The methods of catheterization, devices employed, and certain complications are common to all intracerebral lesions treated by endovascular techniques. Ischemic complications may be due to catheter-induced vascular injury causing vasospasm or dissection. Thrombi may form on catheters and guidewires or between catheters when using coaxial catheter systems. To minimize the incidence of thromboembolic complications, intracerebral embolization procedures are usually performed under full heparinization. Heparinized saline is used to flush catheters and to perfuse the dead space between catheters in coaxial systems.

Catheter or guidewire vascular perforations are usually the cause of hemorrhagic complications. Prompt fluoroscopic recognition of contrast extravasation, reversal of anticoagulation, and closure of the vessel or perforation are necessary to reduce morbidity and mortality.[21]

Cerebral Arteriovenous Malformations

Embolization has become an accepted therapy for cerebral AVMs with the following treatment goals: (1) preoperative embolization of large AVMs to

Table 3.4. Hemorrhagic Complications in 403 Patients

Cause	Incidence and Location	Outcome
Perforation, 8 (2%)	Subarachnoid, 8 (2%)	Mild deficit, 1 (0.25%)
Nidal aneurysm, 3 (0.74%)	Parenchymal, 9 (2.2%)	Severe deficit, 4 (1%)
Venous occlusion, 4 (1%)	Intraventricular, 2 (0.5%)	Death, 4 (1%)
Undetermined, 4 (1%)	—	—

Source: Reprinted with permission from C Cognard, YP Gobin, L Pierot, et al. Cerebral dural arteriovenous fistulas: clinical and angiographic correlation with a revised classification of venous drainage. Radiology 1995;194:671.

decrease surgical and postoperative morbidity, (2) pre-stereotaxic radiation to decrease nidus size, (3) palliative embolization for patients with intractable seizures or progressive neurologic deficit, and (4) the sole means of therapy in small lesions in which total occlusion may be achieved.[24]

Complications associated with brain AVM embolization may be categorized into hemorrhagic or ischemic events that occur during the procedure or in the postoperative period. Intracerebral hemorrhage may result with microcatheter arterial perforation or secondary to occlusion of the lesion venous outflow with embolic material. The use of soft, flow-guided microcatheters with NBCA as the embolic agent has reduced the incidence of vascular perforation. Prompt recognition and appropriate treatment should be instituted to reduce the associated morbidity.[21] Hemorrhage may occur acutely if embolic material passes through the arteriovenous shunts and occludes draining veins. Proper adjustment of acrylate polymerization time appropriate for the shunt to be embolized minimizes the incidence of this untoward event. Delayed venous occlusion and hemorrhage also may be seen secondary to a low-flow state in a recently embolized AVM.[25] A course of anticoagulation in the immediate postembolization period may be warranted with those lesions thought to be at risk for this occurrence.[25] The incidence and outcomes of the hemorrhagic complications in one retrospective series are outlined in Table 3.4.[24]

Ischemic complications occur secondary to occlusion of normal cerebral vessels with embolic material. Normal vessels may arise from the pedicle to be embolized distal to the catheter tip and may not be recognized on pre-embolization superselective angiography, or they may arise proximal to the catheter tip and become occluded if there is reflux of embolic material. Cerebral ischemia may also result if there is retrograde thrombosis of the embolized feeding vessel proximal to the point of occlusion.[25] Superselective amobarbital sodium (Amytal) testing has been shown to diminish ischemic complications due to retrograde thrombosis of a feeding pedicle or due to occlusion of unrecognized normal cortical vessels arising from the feeding pedicle.[24, 26] This test consists of injecting 35–50 mg of amobarbital sodium through the microcatheter before embolization. A neurologic examination is then performed appropriate to the territory tested. This test may be augmented by the concomitant use of electroencephalographic or somatosensory evoked potential monitoring.

Pulmonary embolization with embolic material, although infrequent, has also been described.[27]

Cerebral Aneurysm

The current treatment of choice for cerebral aneurysms is surgical clip ligation. In the late 1980s, a new embolic device consisting of electrical detachable coils was developed (Guglielmi Detachable Coil [GDC], Target Therapeutics, Fremont, CA) and was recently approved by the Food and Drug Administration for the treatment of cerebral aneurysms. This device was designed as a less invasive, nonsurgical means of occluding cerebral aneurysms in those patients who are not surgical candidates or in whom surgery failed. To treat an aneurysm using this technique, the tip of a microcatheter is guided into the aneurysm lumen. A GDC coil soldered to a microguidewire is passed through the microcatheter into the aneurysm. The solder attachment to the guidewire firmly attaches the coil to the wire and allows the coil to be repositioned or withdrawn. Once the coil is properly positioned within the aneurysm, a 1-mA direct current is applied to the proximal end of the microguidewire. Within a few minutes, this current detaches the coil by electrolytically dissolving the guidewire just proximal to the solder junction.

Technical complications associated with GDC embolization include cerebral ischemia and hemorrhage. Cerebral ischemia may result when coils or thrombus at the aneurysm neck protrude into the parent artery, resulting in stenosis or occlusion. Appropriate treatment with thrombolysis, balloon angioplasty, or surgical removal may be necessary.[28] A thrombus may form in an aneurysm neck remnant that remains postembolization and embolize into the distal cerebral circulation. Current recommendations include a short (48-hour) course of heparinization followed by long-term aspirin therapy.[28] Hemorrhagic complications may occur with aneurysm perforation by the guidewire, catheter, or coils. Prompt closure of the aneurysm and reversal of anticoagulation may save the patient from this life-threatening complication.

Table 3.5 summarizes a report of the complications encountered in 403 patients with acute aneurysmal hemorrhage treated with GDC embolization. Thirty-seven technical complications (9.18%) occurred, resulting in death in seven patients (1.74%).[28]

Table 3.5. Guglielmi Detachable Coil Technical Complications in 403 Patients

Technical Complication	Number of Patients
Aneurysm perforation	11 (2.7%), 6 deaths
Arterial vasospasm	2 (0.5%)
Parent artery occlusion	12 (3%)
Cerebral embolization	10 (2.5%)
Coil migration	2 (0.5%)

Source: Reprinted with permission from F Viñuela, G Duckwiler, M Mawad. Guglielmi detachable coil embolization of acute intracranial aneurysm: perioperative anatomic and clinical outcome in 403 patients. J Neurosurg 1997;86:475.

Intracranial Angioplasty and Papaverine Infusion for Subarachnoid Hemorrhage Vasospasm

Clinically significant vasospasm can occur in up to one-third of patients who initially survive aneurysmal subarachnoid hemorrhage. Intracerebral angioplasty and intra-arterial papaverine infusion have been shown to improve the caliber of affected vessels and reverse neurologic deficits in those patients who do not respond to medical management,[29, 30] provided it is performed soon after the onset of neurologic deficits. Current guidelines for patient selection include (1) acute onset of neurologic deficit after subarachnoid hemorrhage that cannot be attributed to other causes, (2) deficit does not improve with medical therapy, (3) lack of infarct on computed tomography, and (4) angiographic vasospasm in a vascular distribution consistent with the deficit.[31]

To minimize the risk of vessel rupture, balloon angioplasty is performed with a soft, low-pressure, silicone balloon permanently attached to a microcatheter. The balloon diameter is 3 mm when inflated; therefore, vessels beyond the M1, P1, and A1 segments are not dilated.

Papaverine is an opium alkaloid that acts on smooth muscle to cause vasodilatation of cerebral arteries. To dilate vasospasm in vessels distal to those amenable to angioplasty, a dose of 300 mg per vessel may be infused over 30–40 minutes through a microcatheter that is positioned as close as possible to the affected vessels. The vasodilatory effect lasts only 24–48 hours; therefore, repeat treatments may be necessary.

Vessel rupture may occur when the balloon is overinflated or if balloon dilation is performed on vessels beyond the M1, A1, or P1 segments. In one reported series, this complication occurred in two of 60 patients.[31]

Transitory neurologic deficits have been reported in patients with vasospasm treated with papaverine.[32] These symptoms include cranial nerve palsies, obtundation, and respiratory arrest and may be more common when the vertebrobasilar circulation is infused.[32] The mechanism of action is uncertain, but may be due to direct effect on the central nervous system[32] or secondary to precipitation of the drug and microembolization in a low-flow state.[33] Mydriasis commonly occurs when papaverine is infused below or at the origin of the ophthalmic artery.

Temporary Balloon Test Occlusion of the Internal Carotid Artery

Balloon test occlusion of the internal carotid artery is performed before permanent occlusion by surgical or endovascular techniques when carotid artery sacrifice is necessary for treatment of aneurysms or skull base tumors. The internal carotid to be tested is catheterized with a nondetachable balloon catheter. After systemic anticoagulation, the balloon is inflated just to the point of vessel occlusion, and the patient is observed for 20–30 minutes with repeated neurologic testing. The balloon is immediately deflated in the event of neurologic change. This test is often combined with concomitant brain blood flow imaging (e.g., hexamethylpropyleneamine oxine [HMPAO] radionuclide single-proton emission computed tomography brain scan, stable xenon computed tomographic scan) or electroencephalographic monitoring, in an attempt to identify patients who are at risk for delayed stroke.

One large series reported an overall complication rate of 3.2% associated with this test.[34] In 500 patients, there were eight asymptomatic complications (six carotid dissections, one carotid pseudoaneurysm, and one middle cerebral artery embolus). Eight patients experienced neurologic deficits, of which six were transitory and two permanent.

Other reported complications include transitory ocular ischemia (visual loss, periorbital pain), which may result when heparinized saline is perfused distal to the occlusion balloon at a rate that completely replaces oxygenated blood.[35] Symptoms are reversible when the perfusion is slowed or stopped.

Permanent Balloon Occlusion of the Internal Carotid Artery

Permanent occlusion of the internal carotid artery is used as a treatment for aneurysms of the upper cervical, petrous, or cavernous internal carotid artery that are not amenable to surgery and as a preoperative adjunct for skull base tumors when carotid artery sacrifice is anticipated. Cerebral ischemia may be the result of emboli that may propagate from the carotid stump beyond the occlusion or from diminished perfusion of the ipsilateral cerebral hemisphere.

Before the development of temporary balloon occlusion testing, abrupt carotid occlusion resulted in a stroke rate of 26% and a 12% mortality.[36] A review of reported cases in the literature showed a 4.7% rate for stroke and no mortality in patients who underwent permanent balloon occlusion of the internal carotid artery after a negative balloon test occlusion.

Carotid Cavernous Fistula

The dural attachments of the internal carotid artery at its exit from the carotid canal and at the anterior clinoid process make it susceptible to shear injuries resulting from blunt head trauma. Lacerations of the cavernous internal carotid artery may result in an arteriovenous fistula with the surrounding cavernous sinus. Penetrating injuries, spontaneous fistulas secondary to angiodysplasias (e.g., Ehlers-Danlos syndrome), or rupture of a cavernous carotid aneurysm are less common etiologies.

The resultant hypertension and flow reversal in the cavernous sinus and its venous tributaries commonly cause orbital symptoms. These symptoms may include proptosis, chemosis, orbital bruit, cranial nerve palsy, and increased intraocular pressure. If the fistula is left untreated, approximately 40–50% of patients will have visual impairment.[37, 38] Other symptoms include cerebral ischemia, acute visual loss, cerebral hemorrhage, and epistaxis. These less common manifestations portend a more ominous course and indicate emergent treatment.[39]

Before the development of detachable balloons, carotid cavernous fistulas (CCFs) were treated surgically with nondetachable balloons[40] or autologous muscle emboli.[41] In 1974, Serbinenko described the simple, but elegant method to treat CCFs using detachable balloons.[42] Despite improvements in balloons and delivery catheters, this technique is essentially unchanged and remains the treatment of choice for this lesion. The balloons, made of latex or silicone, are attached to the end of a microcatheter with varying degrees of strength of attachment. A latex ligature tied around the neck of the balloon or a self-sealing valve incorporated into the neck of the balloon prevents balloon deflation when it is detached from the catheter. The balloon is negotiated through the fistula, progressively inflated (usually with isotonic contrast) in the cavernous sinus, occluding the fistula with preservation of the internal carotid artery lumen, and detached from the microcatheter. Satisfactory closure of the fistula with preservation of the internal carotid artery is achieved in approximately 80% of cases.[43, 44] In the remaining cases, it may be necessary to occlude the internal carotid artery at the site of the carotid laceration in order to close the fistula. This may be necessary in those lesions in which there is a large laceration or complete transection of the internal carotid artery or when the balloon protrudes significantly into the carotid lumen. CCFs may recur acutely in up to 8% of cases due to balloons shifting in position or prematurely deflating.[1, 43]

Potential complications in the treatment of CCFs from the transarterial route include thromboembolism, premature balloon detachment with intracranial embolization, cerebral ischemia in cases of carotid occlusion, and cranial nerve palsies. These complications may result in permanent neurologic deficit in 2–4%.[1, 43] Transient ischemic deficits have been reported in 3%.[43] Cranial nerve III and VI palsies may occur after embolization, but are permanent in only rare cases. These deficits resolve in the weeks after the procedure, possibly due to slow deflation of the balloon.[1, 44] Patients are anticoagulated during the procedure to minimize the risk of thromboembolism. Premature balloon detachment, an unusual complication, is avoided by careful manipulation of the balloon catheter system in the carotid lumen, avoidance of unnecessary balloon inflation in the carotid lumen, and the use of balloons that have stronger attachments to the microcatheter. Surgical retrieval of a balloon that embolized into the distal intracranial circulation has been reported.[45] If carotid occlusion is necessary to occlude a CCF, a carotid occlusion test should be performed first to minimize the risk of cerebral ischemia (see the previous discussion on temporary balloon test occlusion of the internal carotid artery).

CCFs that have been unsuccessfully treated from a transarterial route may be treated from a transvenous approach. This technique consists of catheterizing the inferior petrosal sinus via the femoral or jugular vein or the superior ophthalmic vein by direct surgical exposure. The catheter system is then advanced into the cavernous sinus, and detachable balloons or coils are used to close the fistula. Venous perforation or partial occlusion of cavernous sinus venous outflow with venous rerouting into the cerebral veins or ophthalmic venous system may occur. These procedural complications may result in intracerebral or intraorbital hemorrhage.[43]

Conclusion

Advances in radiographic equipment, endovascular devices, and in the understanding of cerebrovascular anatomy have allowed treatment of many neurologic lesions with interventional neuroradiologic techniques. As has been discussed, these new techniques have associated morbidities. A thorough understanding of the disease processes and means of endovascular therapy that comes with proper training is necessary for the safest performance of these procedures.

References

1. Lasjaunias P, Berenstein A. Surgical Neuroangiography (Vol 2). Endovascular Treatment of Craniofacial Lesions. Berlin: Springer-Verlag, 1987.
2. Kagetsu NJ, Berenstein A, Choi IS. Interventional radiology of the head and neck. Cardiovasc Intervent Radiol 1991;14:325.
3. Lasjaunias P, Berenstein A. Surgical Neuroangiography (Vol 1). Functional Anatomy of Craniofacial Arteries. Berlin: Springer-Verlag, 1987.
4. Horton JA, Kerber CW. Lidocaine injection into external carotid branches: provocative test to preserve cranial nerve function in therapeutic embolization. AJNR Am J Neuroradiol 1986;7:105.
5. Repa I, Moradian GP, Dehner LP, et al. Mortalities associated with use of a commercial suspension of polyvinyl alcohol. Radiology 1989;170:395.
6. Brothers MF, Kaufmann JCE, Fox AJ, Deveikis JP. N-butyl-2-cyanoacrylate—substitute for IBCA in interventional neuroradiology: histopathologic and polymerization time studies. AJNR Am J Neuroradiol 1989;10:777.
7. Halbach VV, Hieshima GB, Higashida RT, David CF. Endovascular Therapy of Head and Neck Tumors. In F Viñuela, VV Halbach, JE Dion (eds), Interventional Neuroradiology. Endovascular Therapy of the Central Nervous System. New York: Raven, 1992;17.
8. Eskridge JM, Harris AB, Finch L, Alotis MA. Carotid sinus syndrome and embolization procedures. AJNR Am J Neuroradiol 1993;14:818.
9. Eskridge JM. Interventional neuroradiology. Radiology 1989;172:991.

10. Macpherson P. The value of preoperative embolisation of meningioma estimated subjectively and objectively. Neuroradiology 1991;33:334.
11. Dean BL, Flom RA, Wallace RC, et al. Efficacy of endovascular treatment of meningiomas: evaluation with matched samples. AJNR Am J Neuroradiol 1994; 15:1675.
12. Suyama T, Tamaki N, Fujiwara K, et al. Peritumoral and intratumoral hemorrhage after gelatin sponge embolization of malignant meningioma: case report. Neurosurgery 1987;21:944.
13. Nelson PK, Setton A, Choi IS, et al. Current status of interventional neuroradiology in the management of meningiomas. Neurosurg Clin North Am 1994;5:235.
14. Cognard C, Gobin YP, Pierot L, et al. Cerebral dural arteriovenous fistulas: clinical and angiographic correlation with a revised classification of venous drainage. Radiology 1995;194:671.
15. Halbach VV, Higashida RT, Hieshima GB, et al. Dural fistulas involving the cavernous sinus: results of treatment in 30 patients. Radiology 1987;163:437.
16. Halbach VV, Higashida RT, Hieshima GB, et al. Dural fistulas involving the transverse and sigmoid sinuses: results of treatment in 28 patients. Radiology 1987; 163:443.
17. Halbach VV, Higashida RT, Larsen DW, et al. Treatment of Dural Arteriovenous Fistulas. In RJ Maciunas (ed), Endovascular Neurological Intervention. Neurosurgical Topics. Park Ridge: American Association of Neurological Surgeons, 1995;217.
18. Lownie SP. Clinical and technical complications of endovascular therapy in the central nervous system. Semin Intervent Radiol 1993;10:243.
19. Halbach VV, Higashida RT, Hieshima GB, et al. Transvenous embolization of dural fistulas involving the cavernous sinus. AJNR Am J Neuroradiol 1989;10:377.
20. Halbach VV, Higashida RT, Hieshima GB, et al. Transvenous embolization of dural fistulas involving the transverse and sigmoid sinuses. AJNR Am J Neuroradiol 1989;10:385.
21. Halbach VV, Higashida RT, Dowd CF, et al. Management of vascular perforations that occur during neurointerventional procedures. AJNR Am J Neuroradiol 1991;12:319.
22. Teng MMH, Guo WY, Huang CI, et al. Occlusion of arteriovenous malformations of the cavernous sinus via the superior ophthalmic vein. AJNR Am J Neuroradiol 1988;9:539.
23. Lownie SP. Intracranial dural arteriovenous fistulas: endovascular therapy. Neurosurg Clin North Am 1994;5:449.
24. Viñuela F, Duckwiler G, Guglielmi G. Intravascular Embolization of Brain Arteriovenous Malformations. In RJ Maciunas (ed), Endovascular Neurological Intervention. Neurosurgical Topics. Park Ridge: American Association of Neurological Surgeons, 1995;189.
25. Duckwiler GR, Dion JE, Viñuela F, Reichman A. Delayed venous occlusion following embolotherapy of vascular malformations in the brain. AJNR Am J Neuroradiol 1992;13:1571.
26. Rauch RA, Viñuela F, Dion J, et al. Preembolization functional evaluation in brain arteriovenous malformations: the ability of superselective Amytal test to predict neurologic dysfunction before embolization. AJNR Am J Neuroradiol 1992;13:309.
27. Pelz DM, Lownie SP, Fox AJ, Hutton LC. Symptomatic pulmonary complications from liquid acrylate embolization of brain arteriovenous malformations. AJNR Am J Neuroradiol 1995;16:19.
28. Viñuela F, Duckwiler G, Mawad M. Guglielmi detachable coil embolization of acute intracranial aneurysm: perioperative anatomic and clinical outcome in 403 patients. J Neurosurg 1997;86:475.
29. Kassell NF, Helm G, Simmons N, et al. Treatment of cerebral vasospasm with intra-arterial papavarine. J Neurosurg 1992;77:848.
30. Higashida RT, Halbach VV, Cahan LD, et al. Transluminal angioplasty for treatment of intracranial arterial vasospasm. J Neurosurg 1989;71:648.
31. Eskridge JM, Newell DW, Winn HR. Endovascular treatment of vasospasm. Neurosurg Clin North Am 1994;5:437.
32. Mathis JM, DeNardo A, Jensen ME, et al. Transient neurologic events associated with intraarterial papaverine infusion for subarachnoid hemorrhage-induced vasospasm. AJNR Am J Neuroradiol 1994;15:1671.
33. Mathis JM, DeNardo AJ, Thibault L, et al. In vitro evaluation of papaverine hydrochloride incompatibilities: a simulation of intaarterial infusion for cerebral vasospasm. AJNR Am J Neuroradiol 1994;15:1665.
34. Mathis JM, Barr JD, Jungreis CA, et al. Temporary balloon test occlusion of the internal carotid artery: experience in 500 cases. AJNR Am J Neuroradiol 1995; 16:749.
35. Russell EJ, Goldberg K, Oskin J, et al. Ocular ischemic syndrome during carotid balloon occlusion testing. AJNR Am J Neuroradiol 1994;15:258.
36. Linskey ME, Jungreis CA, Yonas H, et al. Stroke risk after abrupt internal carotid artery sacrifice: accuracy of preoperative assessment with balloon test occlusion and stable xenon-enhanced CT. AJNR Am J Neuroradiol 1994;15:829.
37. Hamby WB. Carotid Cavernous Fistula. Springfield, IL: Charles C Thomas, 1966.
38. Kupersmith MJ, Berenstein A, Flamm E, Ransohoff J. Neuroophthalmologic abnormalities and intravascular therapy of traumatic carotid cavernous fistulas. Ophthalmology 1986;93:906.
39. Halbach VV, Hieshima GB, Higashida RT, Reicher M. Carotid cavernous fistulae: indications for urgent treatment. AJNR Am J Neuroradiol 1987;8:627.
40. Prolo DJ, Hanbery JW. Intraluminal occlusion of a

carotid-cavernous sinus fistula with a balloon catheter. Technical note. J Neurosurg 1971;35:237.

41. Black P, Uematsu S, Perovic M, Walker AE. Carotid-cavernous fistula: a controlled embolus technique for occlusion of fistula with preservation of carotid blood flow. Technical note. J Neurosurg 1973;38:113.
42. Serbinenko FA. Balloon catheterization and occlusion of major cerebral vessels. J Neurosurg 1974;41:125.
43. Lewis AI, Tomsick TA, Tew JM. Management of 100 consecutive direct carotid-cavernous fistulas: results of treatment with detachable balloons. Neurosurgery 1995;36:239.
44. Debrun G. Management of Traumatic Carotid-Cavernous Fistulas. In F Viñuela, VV Halbach, JE Dion (eds), Interventional Neuroradiology Endovascular Therapy of the Central Nervous System. New York: Raven, 1992;107.
45. Chalif DJ, Flamm ES, Berenstein A, Choi IS. Microsurgical removal of a balloon embolus to the internal carotid artery. Case report. J Neurosurg 1983;58:112.

Chapter 4

Neurologic Complications of Cardiovascular Procedures

Harold P. Adams, Jr.

Objectives

- To appreciate the relatively high frequency of neurologic sequelae of major cardiovascular procedures
- To note that stroke and encephalopathies are the most common central nervous system (CNS) complications of major cardiovascular operations
- To appreciate the importance of extensive atherosclerosis of the aorta as a risk factor for stroke after cardiac operations
- To understand that neurologic complications are relatively uncommon among persons having cardiac catheterization or coronary artery angiography
- To be aware that spinal cord ischemia is a potential complication of placement of an intra-aortic balloon pump
- To appreciate that stroke is the primary early neurologic complication of cardiac transplantation while CNS infections predominate at later intervals
- To appreciate that stroke after coronary artery bypass graft surgery is secondary to a number of events that can be independent of the presence of a severe stenosis of the extracranial internal carotid artery

Invasive cardiovascular procedures are used to treat individuals with severe heart diseases, including congenital anomalies, abnormal valves, intracardiac masses, or stenoses of the coronary arteries. Many major operations depend on the use of cardiopulmonary bypass. Other interventions control cardiac arrhythmias or assist or improve cardiac output. New, invasive diagnostic tests expedite evaluation of complex cardiac diseases. These innovations represent real advances in care (Table 4.1). Patients, who in the past would have died from heart disease, now are treated and cured. These procedures reduce disability and improve the quality of life. These procedures, however, also carry risks. Although local arterial, cardiac, or thoracic adverse experiences can be severe, neurologic events are highly feared sequelae. A recent report from a large multicenter study of coronary artery bypass grafting (CABG) emphasizes the problem.[1] Approximately 6% of those having operations at large medical centers developed prominent neurologic complications; one-half had strokes, and the remainder had cognitive impairments or seizures. Health care costs were increased among these patients, and a sizable proportion of these persons required long-term care. In such instances, the benefits of operation were outweighed by serious neurologic events. Roach

Table 4.1. Cardiovascular Procedures that Can Be Accompanied by Neurologic Complications

Cardiac catheterization
Coronary arteriography
Coronary artery angioplasty
Cardiac electrophysiologic studies
Cardioversion
Cardiac pacemaker
Ventricular endomyocardial biopsy
Cardiac reconstruction
Balloon valvuloplasty
Cardiac valve replacement
Coronary artery bypass grafting
Intra-aortic balloon pump
Cardiac transplantation

et al.[1] concluded that new strategies are needed to lessen the likelihood of neurologic complications. Although neurologic complications involve peripheral nerves, cranial nerves, or spinal cord, the most serious sequelae involve the brain (Table 4.2). Because of the strong relationship between heart disease and cerebrovascular disease, stroke is the most frequent complication. Heart disease and stroke have joint risk factors, including hypertension, smoking, diabetes mellitus, and hypercholesterolemia. Cerebrovascular disease is common among those with heart disease. Stroke is an important adverse reaction to heart diseases, such as atrial fibrillation, recent myocardial infarction, or rheumatic heart disease.

Table 4.2. Neurologic Complications of Cardiovascular Procedures

- Ischemic stroke
  - Embolism
    - Thromboembolism
    - Air
    - Fat
    - Foreign materials
    - Cholesterol debris
    - Microemboli
  - Hypoperfusion and hypotension
  - Arterial dissection or injury
- Retinal infarction
- Spinal cord infarction
- Intracranial hemorrhage
- Migraine
- Encephalopathy
- Depression
- Psychosis
- Seizure
- Tremor
- Limb ischemia
- Brachial plexopathy
- Mononeuropathy of any of the following nerves
  - Phrenic nerve
  - Posterior interosseus nerve
  - Recurrent laryngeal nerve
  - Suprascapular nerve
  - Anterior tibial nerve
  - Axillary nerve
  - Lateral cutaneous nerve of forearm
  - Ulnar nerve
  - Radial nerve
  - Saphenous nerve
  - Facial nerve

Frequency of Neurologic Complications for Specific Cardiac Procedures

Cardiac Catheterization or Coronary Arteriography

Neurologic events complicate approximately 0.03–1.00% of cardiac catheterizations and coronary arteriograms. Dawson and Fischer reported 10 neurologic complications in a series of 1,000 cardiac catheterizations[2]; nine were embolic events, and five involved symptoms in the vertebrobasilar circulation. Because the procedure involved insertion of the catheter via the brachial artery, local trauma to the subclavian artery was the presumed source of the symptoms. Kosmorsky et al. reported 10 patients with neuro-ophthalmologic adverse reactions in a series of 30,000 procedures.[3] Most occurred immediately after the procedure and were attributed to embolism. Another series noted visual disturbances or confusion that lasted less than 24 hours in approximately 1% of those who had cardiac catheterization.[4] The neurologic events are attributed to embolism from pieces of atherosclerotic plaque, thrombi from the catheter tip, arterial vasospasm, or hypotension.[4, 5] Migraine also can occur. Kinn and Breisblatt suggested that transient cortical blindness can result from the contrast agent, leading to an osmotic disruption of the blood-brain barrier.[6] Nonionic contrast media may improve the safety of cardiac catheterization.[7]

Coronary Artery Angioplasty, Cardiac Electrophysiologic Procedures, or Percutaneous Valvuloplasty

Galbreath et al. reported neurologic complications in approximately 2% of those who had coronary artery angioplasty; all were ischemic events.[8] A collaborative study tested the usefulness of emergent angioplasty in the management of patients with acute coronary artery occlusions.[9] No major neurologic complications were noted, and the risk was less with angioplasty than with treatment by the combination of thrombolytic therapy and anticoagulants. Overall, the risk of stroke or other major neurologic sequelae is lower with angioplasty than with CABG. Thromboembolism also complicates cardiac electrophysiologic procedures. DiMarco et al. reported adverse experiences in approximately 1.5% of cases.[10] Embolization is a rare complication of percutaneous balloon valvuloplasty.[11, 12]

Intra-Aortic Balloon Pump

Intra-aortic balloon pumps are inserted to maintain adequate perfusion in patients with severe left ventricular failure or cardiogenic shock. The apparatus is placed in the midthoracic aorta; as a result, paraparesis secondary to spinal cord ischemia is a most dreadful complication.[13–17] Symptoms occur in approximately 3% of patients.[16] Spinal cord infarction, most commonly in the lumbar or sacral regions, results from local thromboembolism, arterial dissection, fracture of an atherosclerotic plaque in the aorta, or local hypoperfusion. In addition, ischemia to nerves in the lower extremities secondary to occlusion of distal arteries, such as the femoral artery, can lead to a footdrop or distal neuropathy. Eidelman et al. reviewed the cerebrovascular complications of the use of circulatory pumps or prosthetic ventricles.[18] They noted that strokes could be secondary to decreased blood flow, increased viscosity, increased fibrinogen, increased red blood cell rigidity, and infection.

Electrical Cardioversion

Electrical cardioversion often is used to treat atrial fibrillation. Zeiler et al. reported that embolism occurs in approximately 1.3% of patients.[19] Those at the highest risk are those older than 55 years or who have coronary artery disease or cardiomyopathy.[20] A history of a previous stroke, an enlarged left atrium, diabetes mellitus, or hypertension does not predict embolism.[19] Although stroke can complicate cardioversion in individuals with a normal transesophageal echocardiographic result, Ewy,[21] Manning et al.,[22] and Klein et al.[23] concluded that if there is transesophageal echocardiographic evidence of a thrombus, the cardioversion should be postponed. Anticoagulation before and after cardioversion lowers the risk of embolization.[20–22] Emergent electrical cardioversion without anticoagulation sometimes is done for persons with recent onset atrial fibrillation and a normal transesophageal echocardiographic result. Still, some physicians prefer delaying cardioversion until the patient has received anticoagulants for at least 4 weeks.[24]

Table 4.3. Neurologic Complications in Those Having Cardiac Transplantation

Ischemic stroke
Disseminated intravascular coagulation
Infective endocarditis
Complication of biopsy
Hemorrhagic stroke
Central nervous system lymphoma
Cyclosporine toxicity
Muromonab CD3 (OKT3) toxicity
Metabolic encephalopathy
Seizures
Peripheral nerve injury
Infections
Encephalitis
Meningitis
Abscess

Cardiac Transplantation

Up to one-half of patients who have cardiac transplantation develop neurologic events, including hemorrhagic or ischemic strokes, infectious or neoplastic complications of chronic immunosuppression, and side effects from medications (Table 4.3).[25–33] Although ischemic strokes tend to appear in the perioperative period, infective complications tend to occur weeks or months later. Strokes occurring months after operation may be secondary to a local fungal arteritis secondary to *Aspergillus* or *Candida* species or as the result of infective endocarditis or disseminated intravascular coagulation.[33] Neurotoxic effects of cyclosporine include seizures, coma, encephalopathy, tremor, hallucinations, intracranial hemorrhage, and visual disturbances.[34, 35] Muromonab CD3 (OKT3) also can cause neurotoxicity.[36]

In 1965, Gilman reported neurologic deficits, most commonly cognitive impairments, in 12 of 35 people who had open-heart surgery.[37] Subsequent reports highlight the importance of postoperative neurologic abnormalities (see Table 4.2).[1, 38–63] The severity of deficits varies, and, in many cases, side effects resolve before discharge.[48] Strokes are less common than neuropsychological disturbances, which include encephalopathies, delirium, bizarre behavior, depression, memory loss, and disorientation.[46, 49, 51, 55, 56] Visual disturbances are prominent.[43, 52, 59] Blindness, monocular or binocular decreases in visual acuity, visual field defects, and visual scotomas are secondary to brain or ocular ischemia. Visual impairments also include complex visuospatial and behavioral syndromes secondary to infarctions in the occipital-parietal lobes in the border zone between the posterior and middle cerebral arteries. Neurologic complications are attributed to thromboembolism; thrombosis of intracranial arteries; embolization of fat, air, debris, or pieces of atherosclerotic plaque; hypotension; hypoperfusion; hypoxia; or metabolic disturbances.[39, 41, 42, 47, 49–52, 57–59, 61, 63] The likelihood of an increased risk of CNS complications is associated with age older than 60, hypotension, a prolonged time on cardiopulmonary bypass, or a history of stroke.[38, 45, 46, 60, 64] The frequency of strokes is highest among those who have valve replacements.

CABG is the most common major cardiovascular operation. Several groups also underscore the importance of neurologic adverse experiences of CABG.[1, 65–80] Turnipseed et al. noted eight strokes among 170 patients having CABG but found no relationship with the presence of a carotid bruit or severe carotid disease.[65] Breuer et al. reported postoperative strokes in 5.2% and prolonged encephalopathies in another 11.6% of those having surgery and noted neurologic complications were as common among persons having CABG as among those having other cardiac operations.[67] Coffey et al. reported that mortality among persons having serious neurologic complications after CABG is 29%.[68] In a series of papers, Shaw et al. reported high rates of early neurologic complications.[71, 74, 75] Signs were found in 191 of 312 patients; 5% of the cohort had strokes and 25.6% of patients had ophthalmologic complications, including retinal infarctions and emboli, decreased visual acuity, and visual field defects. Functional disability was seen only in the patients who had visual field deficits. On detailed neuropsychological assessments after surgery, deficits were noted in a majority of persons. Hse et al. reported 30 strokes complicating 2,029 operations; the patterns of the infarctions were consistent with border zone perfusion failure in two individuals and thromboembolic infarctions in the others.[77]

Mononeuropathies or brachial plexus lesions also complicate open-heart surgery.[81–84] Phrenic nerve palsies were reported in 32 cases among a series of 1,891 operations; most were in children who had a Blalock-Taussig procedure.[82] Chandler et al. reported bilateral diaphragmatic paralyses in five patients who had CABG under intense local hypothermia.[84] Lederman et al. noted peripheral nervous system complications in 63 of 421 patients having CABG; 23 involved injuries to the brachial plexus.[83] Most of the peripheral nerve complications are mild and transient. The injuries are attributed to local trauma, including cannulation of the jugular vein and compression or stretching of the nerves during positioning and surgery.

Risk Factors for Neurologic Complications of Major Cardiovascular Operations

Several factors identify those who have the greatest risk for serious neurologic sequelae after major cardiovascular operations. Events are common among older individuals.[1, 69, 79, 85] Because the average age of patients having major operations is increasing, the relationship between advanced age and serious neurologic sequelae, in particular stroke, is important.[85] The risk for stroke is associated with the high prevalence of extracranial or intracranial cerebrovascular disease, extensive aortic arch atherosclerosis, and other medical disorders that make older individuals vulnerable. Older persons also may require more extensive and complex operations.[69, 85]

Hypertension, diabetes mellitus, hypercholesterolemia, lung disease, cigarette smoking, and obesity are present frequently among those who are undergoing cardiac surgery. Diabetes mellitus does predict an increased likelihood of serious neurologic complications.[69, 85] Although the other conditions have not been correlated with an increased risk of stroke, they probably do influence the severity of the underlying heart disease or increase the likelihood of medical complications of the operation.

Those with three-vessel coronary artery disease, a left ventricular mural thrombus, left ventricular dysfunction, or atrial fibrillation have a high risk of neurologic complications.[69, 85–87] These correlations represent the severity of the underlying heart disease and reflect the difficulty and length of a cardiac operation. In addition, those having a second operation or a valve replacement have a high risk of neurologic sequelae.

Data are mixed about the influence of a history of a previous stroke or transient ischemic attack (TIA) on the frequency of serious complications after cardiovascular operations. Beall et al. evaluated the potential for recurrent stroke during CABG among 43 patients who had a stroke but no extracranial carotid artery disease; only one patient had a second stroke.[88] Conversely, Ricotta et al. concluded that a history of stroke forecasted a new neurologic event.[87] Taylor et al. found postoperative strokes after CABG in only 0.78% of patients who had a history of stroke, TIA, or atrial fibrillation, but the figure increased to 20% among those who had prior neurologic symptoms.[86] Similarly, Rorick and Furlan found new strokes after surgery in 13.4% of 126 persons who had a history of stroke.[89] Signs worsened in patients with a recent stroke, whereas signs suggestive of a new stroke were detected among patients with a remote stroke. Intraoperative hypotension can lead to hemodynamic instability and increased brain ischemia among people with recent strokes.

Overall, data suggest that a history of a TIA or stroke marks a patient as being at increased risk for serious neurologic sequelae of cardiac operations. Factors such as extracranial or intracranial arterial disease or increased vulnerability of the brain may be important. In addition, the danger of surgery may be augmented because of severe heart disease and aortic atherosclerosis among persons with previous neurologic symptoms. Although a history of either a stroke or TIA does not preclude heart surgery, the patient and family should be appraised of the high risk of complications. Whenever possible, elective cardiac surgery should be delayed for at least a few weeks after a stroke to allow the brain to recover from the ischemic event.

Finding severe atherosclerotic disease in both the coronary and cerebrovascular circulations is not a surprise because risk factors for advanced coronary artery disease are the same for premature, complex lesions of the carotid arteries. The presence of severe arterial disease in circulations other than the coronary vessels predicts an increased risk for neurologic complications, especially stroke.[72] The magnitude of the increase in risk is unclear, however, because data are conflicting.

Ropper et al. examined chances of stroke among those with carotid bruits who had elective operations.[90] Although they found little increase in the risk of stroke among patients having vascular operations, they also concluded that treatment of the carotid arteries might be needed for a patient having CABG. This opinion was bolstered by the experience of Brener et al. who noted neurologic events in 1.9% of approximately 2,000 patients who did not have carotid artery disease and 14.9% of 47 patients who had either a severe stenosis or occlusion of the internal carotid artery.[91] A subsequent series found a 15.6% rate of stroke and increased mortality among individuals with an occluded internal carotid artery.[92] Hertzer et al. found severe carotid artery disease in 275 of 9,714 patients undergoing CABG.[93] They noted a high rate of stroke when the cardiac operation was not preceded or accompanied by carotid endarterectomy (CEA). Another series found stenoses of the internal carotid arteries of more than 75% in approximately 9% of those having CABG.[94] The figure increased to 11% among those older than 60. A recent study used a preoperative oculoplethysmographic assessment of the extracranial carotid circulation and found reduced pressures in 122 of 2,312 screened patients.[95] Mortality and stroke were increased among those with a positive oculoplethysmographic result. Twenty-three patients with a positive oculoplethysmographic result had CABG without CEA, and five had major complications (21.7%). Lynn et al. reported similar results.[79]

On the other hand, Barnes et al.[96] and Barnes and Marszalek[97] could not correlate perioperative stroke with either an asymptomatic carotid bruit or carotid stenosis. Based on the low risk of stroke with CABG, Breslau et al. concluded that noninvasive screening of the carotid arteries in asymptomatic persons was not necessary before CABG.[98] Other reviews could not correlate either a bruit or stenosis of the carotid artery with the risk of perioperative stroke, largely because of the multiple mechanisms that lead to brain ischemia during heart surgery.[99, 100] Furlan and Craciun found that an asymptomatic unilateral carotid artery stenosis of less than 90% did not increase the neurologic risk of CABG.[70] Rorick and Furlan could not correlate new neurologic symptoms after operation with the severity of extracranial carotid artery disease among persons who have a history of stroke.[89] Based on a series of 5,915 people having CABG, Reed et al. concluded that the risk of stroke after heart surgery was similar to that which accompanies CEA and that prophylactic CEA might not be needed.[76] Although Ricotta et al. associated an increased risk of stroke among those with a stenosis of more than 50%, the location of the ischemic events was not related to the site of the stenotic lesion.[87]

In 1985, two reports highlighted the importance of severe atherosclerotic disease of the aorta as a cause of neurologic morbidity following cardiac surgery.[69, 101] Manipulation of a brittle, severely atherosclerotic and calcified ascending aorta can cause pieces of debris to be released. In particular, severe plaques can be fractured by clamping of the aorta. Barbut and Gold concluded that mobile atherosclerotic plaques in the ascending aorta might be the single most important factor predicting embolic complications after cardiac surgery.[102] This opinion is bolstered by the observation that five of eight strokes that occurred after surgery in one series were due to calcific emboli or atherosclerotic debris.[101]

A grading system of the severity of aortic atherosclerosis by manual examination during the operation can guide placement of an aortic clamp.[103] Those with a soft aorta or a localized atherosclerotic plaque may need only minor modifications in the surgical procedure. Individuals with advanced aortic disease, including aneurysms, are at high risk for complications, and clamping may be difficult or contraindicated. Radiologic evidence of aortic calcification forecasts an increased risk of sequelae.[79] Wareing et al. screened the ascending aorta in 1,200 patients ages 50 years or older with intraoperative ultrasonographic scanning; strokes occurred in 6.3% of 111 patients who had moderate to severe disease of the ascending aorta and who had only minor interventions.[104] Using intraoperative transesophageal echocardiography, another group found that aortic plaques that were 5 mm thick or greater or that were mobile predicted a high risk for stroke.[105] These aortic changes are most common among individuals older than 70.

The presence of severe aortic atherosclerosis partially explains the high risk of neurologic events among older persons who have cardiac operations. The aortic lesion may be the source of atherosclerotic debris (cholesterol emboli) or thrombi that go to the brain, viscera, or limbs. The presence of a brittle, hard, and friable aorta makes the surgery more difficult and alters operative strategies. In particular, clamping of the aorta is dangerous in individuals with extensive disease. Severe aortic atherosclerosis appears to be a relative contraindication for surgery. Severe disease of the ascending aorta may mandate replacement of the vessel during the heart surgery.[104] Further research on the presence, extent, and types of atherosclerotic lesions of the aorta and their associated risks for serious neurologic sequelae is needed to further lower the risk of stroke after CABG, especially in the elderly.

Prolonged cardiopulmonary bypass is a predictor of neurologic complications.[69] In part, a prolonged pump time is a surrogate for a complex cardiac lesion that necessitates a longer, more difficult operation. However, the prolonged bypass time increases the length of anesthesia, the possibility of hypotensive events, or the chances of embolization of thrombi, air, or debris.

Manipulation of the heart or chest can lead to air or fat microemboli.[61] Embolization can occur during the filling of an empty beating heart or during the redistribution of blood from the cardiopulmonary bypass machine.[63] Severe intraoperative or perioperative hypotension is a potential cause of brain ischemia with infarctions located in a border zone pattern.[69]

Recently, Mathew et al. noted that postoperative atrial fibrillation occurs in approximately one-fourth of those who have CABG.[106] Both major and minor neurologic injuries are more common and the length of hospitalization is increased among persons who had atrial fibrillation after operation. Older individuals, men, and those with a past history of atrial fibrillation or congestive heart failure have the greatest risk of atrial fibrillation.[106, 107] Atrial fibrillation also is associated with a longer clamp time and cardiopulmonary bypass.

Monitoring for Neurologic Complications During Cardiovascular Procedures and Cardiac Operations

Because general anesthesia is used during major cardiovascular procedures, intraoperative clinical monitoring for neurologic changes is not possible. Transcranial Doppler ultrasound can be used to detect microemboli in the cerebral arteries.[12, 108] The number of emboli has been associated with the likelihood of neurologic events. Electroencephalography and evoked potentials can give information about changes in perfusion during the operation; the usual findings are slowed rhythm and a decrease in voltage.[109, 110] Disturbances in the brain's electrical activity can prompt corrective responses such as increasing pump flow or the mean arterial blood pressure. Still, the usefulness of neurologic monitoring during cardiac operations is not established and its use is not as widespread as for carotid surgery.

Strategies to Lessen the Risk of Neurologic Complications During Cardiac Operations

Several groups, in observational studies, examined the potential utility of CEA in lowering the risk of stroke after CABG. Brener et al. noted one stroke among four patients with severe carotid diseases who did not have CEA and one stroke among 18 patients who had both CABG and CEA.[91] Hertzer et al. examined staging of operations for coronary and carotid disease.[93] Neurologic complications developed in 4.2% of patients who had CEA first and in 7.8% of patients who had simultaneous CABG and CEA or CABG before carotid surgery. Fillinger et al. reported one stroke ipsilateral to CEA and four deaths among 52 patients who had combined coronary and carotid operations.[111] Events were more frequent among patients who had either the coronary or carotid operation alone, although differences between the patient populations make direct comparisons difficult.

The usefulness of combining or staging CEA to protect the brain among individuals undergoing open-heart surgery is not established. Because ischemic neurologic deficits result from a number of etiologies that are independent of the presence of severe stenosis of the carotid artery, CEA does not make a major impact in reducing the risk of stroke after cardiac operation. In addition, those undergoing open-heart surgery have severe cardiac lesions that often are life threatening. The safety and utility of delaying a cardiac operation in order to do a CEA is not known, especially in those who have no neurologic symptoms. The utility of delaying cardiac surgery while the patient has CEA should be weighed against the neurologic risks of the cardiac operation. Similarly, the value of a combined CEA and CABG operation also needs to be determined.

Operative techniques have improved during the last 30 years. Surgeons have more experience. Skilled teams of anesthesiologists, operating room personnel, cardiopulmonary bypass technicians, and modern intensive care units have lowered the mortality and morbidity of cardiac operations. New equipment, especially modern heart-lung machines, have an effect. Problems such as massive air embolism can be avoided by strategies such as retrograde drainage, close attention to reservoir levels in the heart-lung machine, and high-flow suction.[47] In general, despite expanding the indications for major heart surgery to a group of individuals that may be at high risk, the likelihood of major neurologic complications has not increased; rather, the rate has declined. The absence of an increase in the rate of major sequelae reflects advances in the performance of cardiac procedures. Surgical adjuncts such as arterial line filtration or adjustments in body temperature may improve the safety of cardiac surgery.[58, 112, 113] Cardiac anesthesiologists have tested tactics to protect the brain during surgery.[114]

Anticoagulation is an important component of the ancillary care of patients having open-heart surgery, and it is particularly important for those with a mechanical valve or atrial fibrillation. Although anticoagulants are recommended strongly for the long-term prophylaxis against thromboembolism in individuals with severe heart disease, data are not clear about the optimal time of starting the medication.[115] The benefit in preventing thromboembolism must be weighed against the possibility of potentiating postoperative bleeding. Early administration of antiplatelet agents is one component of treatment of persons who have had CABG. Anticoagulants and antiplatelet agents are adjuncts of procedures such as coronary artery angioplasty.[116] These agents might be helpful in preventing embolism to the brain.

Prophylactic administration of drugs that lessen the consequences of brain ischemia might be useful among those having cardiac operations. The drugs could be started preoperatively and continued throughout the operation and after surgery. Neuroprotective drugs could have a potentially positive effect regardless of the cause of the ischemia.[117] These drugs might be effective in a setting such as heart surgery when they are not effective in persons with acute ischemic stroke because they are given before the ischemic process begins.[118] Nimodipine recently was tested in a small clinical trial that was stopped prematurely because of a lack of evidence of benefit and because of a possible prohemorrhagic effect of the drug.[119] Although this trial result was negative, other neuroprotective drugs might be useful. Additional research on the role of neuroprotective drugs in preventing brain ischemia during major cardiovascular operations is needed.

Conclusion

Brain injury is the most common serious noncardiac complication of major cardiovascular procedures, especially open-heart surgery. The brain is particularly vulnerable to embolism, hypoxia, hemorrhagic diatheses, and hypotension, all of which are potential problems during a cardiac operation. Current data demonstrate a continued high rate of major neurologic morbidity after cardiac procedures despite advances in anesthesia, operative technique, and ancillary care. One of the reasons for the high level of neurologic morbidity may be the expansion in the number of operations being performed in elderly persons who have a high risk for cerebrovascular disease and stroke. Continued efforts to lower the risk of brain injury after heart operations are needed. The human and economic consequences of severe neurologic sequelae after heart surgery remain unacceptably high.

References

1. Roach GW, Kanchuger M, Mangano CM, et al. for the Multicenter Study of Perioperative Ischemia Research Group and the Ischemia Research and Education Foundation Investigators. Adverse outcomes after cononary bypass surgery. N Engl J Med 1996;335:1857.
2. Dawson DM, Fischer EG. Neurologic complications of cardiac catheterization. Neurology 1977;27:496.
3. Kosmorsky G, Hanson MR, Tomsak RL. Neuro-ophthalmologic complications of cardiac catheterization. Neurology 1988;38:483.
4. Vik-Mo H, Todnem K, Folling M, Rosland GA. Transient visual disturbance during cardiac catheterization with angiography. Cath Cardiovasc Diag 1986;12:1.
5. Colt HG, Begg RL, Saporito JJ, et al. Cholesterol emboli after cardiac catheterization. Eight cases and a review of the literature. Medicine 1988;67:389.
6. Kinn RM, Breisblatt WM. Cortical blindness after coronary angiography. A rare but reversible complication. Cath Cardiovasc Diag 1991;22:177.
7. Davidson CJ, Mark BD, Pieper KS, et al. Thrombotic and cardiovascular complications related to nonionic contrast media during cardiac catheterization. Analysis of 8,517 patients. Am J Cardiol 1990;65:1481.
8. Galbreath C, Salgado ED, Furlan AJ, Hollman J. Central nervous system complications of percutaneous transluminal coronary angioplasty. Stroke 1985;17:616.
9. Grines CL, Browne KF, Marco J, et al. for the Primary Angioplasty in Myocardial Infarction Study Group. A comparison of immediate angioplasty with thrombolytic therapy for acute myocardial infarction. N Engl J Med 1993;328:673.
10. DiMarco JP, Garan H, Ruskin JN. Complications in patients undergoing cardiac electrophysiologic procedures. Ann Intern Med 1982;97:490.
11. Davidson CJ, Skelton TN, Kisslo KB, et al. The risk for systemic embolization associated with percutaneous balloon valvuloplasty in adults. Ann Intern Med 1988;108:557.
12. Karnik R, Valentin A, Bonner G, et al. Transcranial Doppler monitoring during percutaneous transluminal aortic valvuloplasty. Angiology 1990;41:106.
13. Honet JC, Wajszczuk WJ, Rubenfire M, et al. Neurologic abnormalities in the leg(s) after use of intraaortic balloon pump. Report of six cases. Arch Phys Med Rehabil 1975;56:346.
14. Rose DM, Jacobwitz IJ, Acinapora AJ, Cunningham JN Jr. Paraplegia following percutaneous insertion of an intra-aortic balloon. J Thorac Cardiovasc Surg 1984; 87:788.
15. Scott IR, Goiti JJ. Late paraplegia as a consequence of intra-aortic balloon pump support. Ann Thorac Surg 1985;40:300.
16. Kantrowitz A, Wasfie T, Freed PS, et al. Intra-aortic balloon pump 1967 through 1982. Analysis of complications in 733 patients. Am J Cardiol 1986;57:976.

17. Harris RE, Reimer KA, Crain BJ, et al. Spinal cord infarction following intraaortic balloon support. Ann Thorac Surg 1986;42:206.
18. Eidelman BH, Obrist WD, Wagner WR, et al. Cerebrovascular complications associated with use of circulatory support services. Neurol Clin 1993;11:463.
19. Zeiler AA, Mick MJ, Mazurek RP, et al. Role of prophylactic anticoagulation for direct current cardioversion in patients with atrial fibrillation or atrial flutter. J Am Coll Cardiol 1992;19:851.
20. Weinberg DM, Mancini J. Anticoagulation for cardioversion of atrial fibrillation. Am J Cardiol 1989;63:745.
21. Ewy GA. Optimal technique for electrical cardioversion of atrial fibrillation. Circulation 1992;86:1645.
22. Manning WJ, Silverman DI, Gordon SPF, et al. Cardioversion from atrial fibrillation without prolonged anticoagulation with use of transesophageal echocardiography to exclude the presence of atrial thrombi. N Engl J Med 1993;328:750.
23. Klein AL, Grimm RA, Black IW, et al. for the ACUTE Investigators. Cardioversion guided by transesophageal echocardiography. The ACUTE Pilot Study. A randomized, controlled trial. Ann Intern Med 1997;126:200.
24. Prystowsky EN. Management of atrial fibrillation. Simplicity surrounded by controversy. Ann Intern Med 1997;126:244.
25. Hotson JR, Pedley TA. The neurologic complications of cardiac transplantation. Brain 1976;99:673.
26. Britt RH, Enzmann DR, Remington JS. Intracranial infection in cardiac transplant recipients. Ann Neurol 1981;9:107.
27. Sila CA. Spectrum of neurologic events following cardiac transplantation. Stroke 1989;20:1586.
28. Ang LC, Gillett JM, Kaufmann JCE. Neuropathology of heart transplantation. Can J Neurol Sci 1989;16:291.
29. Andrews BT, Hershon JJ, Calanchini P, et al. Neurologic complications of cardiac transplantation. West J Med 1990;153:146.
30. Adair JC, Woodley SL, O'Connell JB, et al. Aseptic meningitis following cardiac transplantation. Neurology 1991;41:249.
31. Adair JC, Call GK, O'Connell JB. Cerebral ischemia. A complication of right ventricular endomyocardial biopsy. Cath Cardiovasc Diag 1991;21:32.
32. Fromenbaum MA, Jarcho JA, Schoen FJ. Progressive multifocal leukoencephalopathy fifty seven months after heart transplantation. J Heart Lung Transplant 1991;10:888.
33. Adair JC, Call GK, O'Connell JB, Baringer JR. Cerebrovascular syndromes following cardiac transplantation. Neurology 1992;42:819.
34. Lane RJM, Roche SW, Leung AAW, et al. Cyclosporin neurotoxicity in cardiac transplant recipients. J Neurol Neurosurg Psychiatry 1988;51:1434.
35. Vasques de Prada JA, Martin-Duran R, Garcia-Monco C, et al. Cyclosporine neurotoxicity in heart transplantation. J Heart Lung Transplant 1990;9:581.
36. Wijkicks EFM. Neurologic complications in critically ill patients. Anesth Analg 1996;83:411.
37. Gilman S. Cerebral disorders after open-heart operations. N Engl J Med 1965;272:489.
38. Javid H, Tufo HM, Najafi H, et al. Neurologic abnormalities following open-heart surgery. J Thorac Cardiovasc Surg 1969;58:502.
39. Hill JD, Aguilar MJ, Baranco A, et al. Neuropathological manifestations of cardiac surgery. Ann Thorac Surg 1969;7:409.
40. Branthwaite MA. Neurologic damage related to open-heart surgery. Thorax 1972;27:748.
41. Branthwaite MA. Cerebral blood flow and metabolism during open-heart surgery. Thorax 1974;29:633.
42. Branthwaite MA. Prevention of neurologic damage during open-heart surgery. Thorax 1975;30:258.
43. Taugher PJ. Visual loss after cardiopulmonary bypass. Am J Ophthalmol 1976;81:280.
44. Salerno TA, Lince DP, White DN, et al. Monitoring of electroencephalogram during open-heart surgery. J Thorac Cardiovasc Surg 1978;76:97.
45. Sotaniemi KA. Brain damage and neurologic outcome after open heart surgery. J Neurol Neurosurg Psychiatry 1980;43:127.
46. Kolkka R, Hilberman M. Neurologic dysfunction following cardiac operation with low-flow, low-pressure cardiopulmonary bypass. J Thorac Cardiovasc Surg 1980;79:432.
47. Mills NL, Ochsner JL. Massive air embolism during cardiopulmonary bypass. Causes, prevention, and management. J Thorac Cardiovasc Surg 1980;80:708.
48. Savageau JA, Stanton BA, Jenkins CD, Klein MD. Neuropsychological dysfunction following elective cardiac operation. I. Early assessment. J Thorac Cardiovasc Surg 1982;84:585.
49. Savageau JA, Stanton BA, Jenkins CD. Neuropsychological dysfuntion following elective cardiac operation. II. A six-month assessment. J Thorac Cardiovasc Surg 1982;84:595.
50. Taylor KM. Brain damage during open-heart surgery. Thorax 1982;37:873.
51. Furlan AJ, Breuer AC. Central nervous system complications of open heart surgery. 1984;15:912.
52. Sweeney PJ, Breuer AC, Selhorst JB, et al. Ischemic optic neuropathy. A complication of cardiopulmonary bypass surgery. Neurology 1982;32:560.
53. Aberg T, Ronquist G, Tyden H, et al. Adverse effects on the brain in cardiac operations as assessed by biochemical, psychometric, and radiologic methods. J Thorac Cardiovasc Surg 1984;87:99.
54. Sotaniemi KA, Mononen H, Hokkanen TE. Long-term cerebral outcome after open-heart surgery. A five-year neuropsychological follow-up study. Stroke 1986;17:410.
55. Moses H III, Kaden I. Neurologic consultations in a general hospital. Spectrum of iatrogenic disease. Am J Med 1986;81:955.
56. Nussmeier NA, Arlund C, Slogoff S. Neuropsychiatric

complications after cardiopulmonary bypass. Cerebral protection by a barbiturate. Anesthesiology 1986;64:165.
57. Jensen ME, Lipper MH. CT in iatrogenic cerebral air embolism. AJNR Am J Neuroradiol 1986;7:823.
58. Henriksen L, Hjelms E. Cerebral blood flow during cardiopulmonary bypass in man. Effect of arterial filtration. Thorax 1986;41:386.
59. Shahian DM, Speert PK. Symptomatic visual deficits after open heart operations. Ann Thorac Surg 1989; 48:275.
60. Aron KV, Cohen DE, Strobl FT. Effect of intraoperative intervention on neurologic outcome based on electroencephalographic monitoring during cardiopulmonary bypass. Ann Thorac Surg 1989;48:476.
61. Moody DM, Bell MA, Challa VR, et al. Brain microemboli during cardiac surgery or aortography. Ann Neurol 1990;28:477.
62. Pugsley W, Klinger L, Paschalis C, et al. Microemboli and cerebral impairment during cardiac surgery. Vasc Surg 1990;24:34.
63. van der Linden J, Casimir-Ahn H. When do cerebral emboli appear during open heart operations? A transcranial Doppler study. Ann Thorac Surg 1991;51:237.
64. Libman RB, Wirkowski E, Neystat M, et al. Stroke associated with cardiac surgery. Determinants, timing, and stroke subtypes. Arch Neurol 1997;54:83.
65. Turnipseed WD, Berkoff HA, Belzer FO. Postoperative stroke in cardiac and peripheral vascular disease. Ann Surg 1980;192:365.
66. Gonzalez-Scarano F, Hurtig HI. Neurologic complications of coronary artery bypass grafting. Case-control study. Neurology 1981;31:1032.
67. Breuer AC, Furlan AC, Hanson MR, et al. Central nervous system complications of coronary artery bypass graft surgery. Prospective analysis of 421 patients. Stroke 1983;14:682.
68. Coffey CE, Massey EW, Roberts KB, et al. Natural history of cerebral complications of coronary artery bypass graft surgery. Neurology 1983;33:1416.
69. Gardner TJ, Horneffer PJ, Manolio TA, et al. Stroke following coronary artery bypass grafting. A ten-year study. Ann Thorac Surg 1985;40:574.
70. Furlan AJ, Craciun AR. Risk of stroke during coronary artery bypass graft surgery in patients with internal carotid artery disease documented by angiography. Stroke 1985;16:797.
71. Shaw PJ, Bates D, Cartlidge NEF, et al. Early neurologic complications of coronary artery bypass surgery. BMJ 1985;291:1384.
72. Smith PLC, Treasure T, Newman SP, et al. Cerebral consequences of cardiopulmonary bypass. Lancet 1986;1:823.
73. Calabrese JR, Skewerer RG, Gulledge AD, et al. Incidence of postoperative delirium following myocardial revascularization. A prospective study. Cleve Clin J Med 1987;54:29.
74. Shaw PJ, Bates D, Cartlidge NEF, et al. Neuro-ophthalmological complications of coronary artery bypass graft surgery. Acta Neurol Scand 1987;76:1.
75. Shaw PJ, Bates D, Cartlidge NEF, et al. Neurologic and neuropsychological morbidity following major surgery. Comparison of coronary artery bypass and peripheral vascular surgery. Stroke 1987;18:700.
76. Reed GL III, Singer DE, Picard EH, DeSanctis RW. Stroke following coronary-artery bypass surgery. A case-control estimate of the risk from carotid bruits. N Engl J Med 1988;319:1246.
77. Hise JH, Nipper ML, Schnitker JC. Stroke associated with coronary artery bypass surgery. AJNR Am J Neuroradiol 1991;12:811.
78. Tuman KJ, McCarthy RJ, Najafi H, Ivanokovich AD. Differential effects of advanced age on neurologic and cardiac risk of coronary artery operations. J Thorac Cardiovasc Surg 1992;104:1510.
79. Lynn GM, Stefanko K, Reed JF III, et al. Risk factors for stroke after coronary artery bypass. J Thorac Cardiovasc Surg 1992;104:1518.
80. Brillman J. Central nervous system complications in coronary artery bypass graft surgery. Neurol Clin 1993;11:475.
81. Keates JRW, Innocenti DM, Ross DN. Mononeuritis multiplex. A complication of open-heart surgery. J Thorac Cardiovasc Surg 1975;69:816.
82. Mickell JJ, Oh KS, Siewers RD, Galuis AG, et al. Clinical implications of postoperative unilateral phrenic nerve paralysis. J Thorac Cardiovasc Surg 1978;76:297.
83. Lederman RJ, Breuer AC, Hanson MR, et al. Peripheral nervous system complications of coronary artery bypass graft surgery. Ann Neurol 1982;12:297.
84. Chandler KW, Rozas CJ, Kory RC, Goldman AL. Bilateral diaphragmatic paralysis complicating local cardiac hypothermia during open heart surgery. Am J Med 1984;77:243.
85. Jones EL, Weintraub WS, Craver JM, et al. Coronary bypass surgery. Is the operation different today? J Thorac Cardiovasc Surg 1991;101:108.
86. Taylor GJ, Malik SA, Colliver JA, et al. Usefulness of atrial fibrillation as a predictor of stroke after isolated coronary artery bypass grafting. Am J Cardiol 1987; 60:905.
87. Ricotta JJ, Faggioli GL, Castilone A, Hassett JM for the Buffalo Cardiac Cerebral Study Group. Risk factors for stroke after cardiac surgery. Buffalo Cardiac Cerebral Study Group. J Vasc Surg 1995;21:359.
88. Beall AC Jr, Jones JW, Guinn GA, et al. Cardiopulmonary bypass in patients with previously completed stroke. Ann Thorac Surg 1993;55:1383.
89. Rorick MB, Furlan AJ. Risk of cardiac surgery in patients with prior stroke. Neurology 1990;40:835.
90. Ropper AH, Wechsler LR, Wilson LS. Carotid bruit and the risk of stroke in elective surgery. N Engl J Med 1983;307:1388.
91. Brener BJ, Brief DK, Alpert J, et al. A four-year experience with preoperative noninvasive carotid evaluation

of two thousand twenty-six patients undergoing cardiac surgery. J Vasc Surg 1984;1:326.
92. Brener BJ, Brief DK, Alpert J, et al. The risk of stroke in patients with asymptomatic carotid stenosis undergoing cardiac surgery. A follow-up study. J Vasc Surg 1987;5:269.
93. Hertzer NR, Loop FD, Beven EG, et al. Surgical staging for simultaneous coronary and carotid disease. A study including prospective randomization. J Vasc Surg 1989;9:455.
94. Faggioli GL, Curl GR, Ricotta JJ. The role of carotid screening before coronary artery bypass. J Vasc Surg 1990;12:724.
95. Pillai L, Gutierrez IZ, Curl GR, et al. Evaluation and treatment of carotid stenosis in open-heart surgery patients. J Surg Res 1994;57:312.
96. Barnes RW, Liebman PR, Marszalek PB, et al. The natural history of asymptomatic carotid disease in patients undergoing cardiovascular surgery. Surgery 1981;90: 1075.
97. Barnes RW, Marszalek PB. Asymptomatic carotid disease in the cardiovascular surgical patient. Is prophylactic endarterectomy necessary? Stroke 1981;12:497.
98. Breslau PJ, Fell G, Ivey TD, et al. Carotid arterial disease in patients undergoing coronary artery bypass operations. J Thorac Cardiovasc Surg 1981;82:765.
99. Hart RG, Easton JD. Management of cervical bruits and carotid stenosis in preoperative patients. Stroke 1983;14:290.
100. Ivey TD, Strandness DE, Williams DB, et al. Management of patients with carotid bruit underlying cardiopulmonary bypass. J Thorac Cardiovasc Surg 1984;87:183.
101. Parker FB Jr, Marvasti MA, Bove EL. Neurologic complications following coronary artery bypass. The role of atherosclerotic emboli. Thorac Cardiovasc Surg 1985;33:207.
102. Barbut D, Gold JP. Aortic atheromatosis and risks of cerebral embolization. J Cardiothorac Vasc Anesth 1996;10:24.
103. Bar-El Y, Goor DA. Clamping of the atherosclerotic ascending aorta during coronary artery bypass operations. J Thorac Cardiovasc Surg 1992;104:469.
104. Wareing TH, Davila-Roman VG, Daily BB, et al. Strategy for the reduction of stroke incidence in cardiac surgical patients. Ann Thorac Surg 1993;55:1400.
105. Marschall K, Kanchuger M, Kessler K, et al. Superiority of transesophageal echocardiography in detecting aortic arch atheromatous disease. Identification of patients at increased risk of stroke during cardiac surgery. J Cardiothorac Vasc Anesth 1994;8:5.
106. Mathew JP, Parks R, Savino JS, et al. for the Multicenter Study of Perioperative Ischemia Research Group. Atrial fibrillation following coronary artery bypass graft surgery. Predictors, outcomes, and resource utilization. JAMA 1996;276:300.
107. Crosby LH, Pifalo WB, Woll KR, Burkholder JA. Risk factors for atrial fibrillation after coronary artery bypass grafting. Am J Cardiol 1990;66:1520.
108. Clark RE, Brillman J, Davis DA, et al. Microemboli during coronary artery bypass grafting. Genesis and effect on outcome. J Thorac Cardiovasc Surg 1995; 109:249.
109. Aren C, Badr G, Feddersen K, Radegran K. Somatosensory evoked potentials and cerebral metabolism during cardiopulmonary bypass with special reference to hypotension induced by prostacyclin infusion. J Thorac Cardiovasc Surg 1985;90:73.
110. Aron KV, Cohen DE, Strobl FT. Effect of intraoperative intervention on neurologic outcome based on electroencephalographic monitoring during cardiopulmonary bypass. Ann Thorac Surg 1989;48:476.
111. Fillinger MF, Rosenberg JM, Semel L, et al. Combined carotid endarterectomy and coronary artery bypass in a community hospital. Cardiovasc Surg 1993;1:7.
112. Aris A, Solanes H, Camara ML, et al. Arterial line filtration during cardiopulmonary bypass. J Thorac Cardiovasc Surg 1986;91:526.
113. Christakis GT, Koch JP, Deemar KA, et al. A randomized study of the systemic effects of warm heart surgery. Ann Thorac Surg 1992;54:449.
114. Zaidan JR, Klochany A, Martin WM, et al. Effect of thiopental on neurologic outcome following coronary artery bypass grafting. Anesthesiology 1991;74:406.
115. Stein PD, Alpert JS, Copeland J, et al. Antithrombotic therapy in patients with mechanical and biologic prosthetic heart valves. Chest 1995;108(suppl):371S.
116. Topol EJ, Califf RM, Weisman HF, Ellis SG, on behalf of the EPIC investigators. Randomised trial of coronary intervention with antibody against platelet IIb/IIIa integrin for reduction of clinical restenosis: results at six months. Lancet 1994;343:881.
117. Fisher M, Jonas S, Sacco RL. Prophylactic neuroprotection for cerebral ischemia. Stroke 1994;25:1075.
118. Trust Study Group. Randomised, double-blind, placebo-controlled trial of nimodipine in acute stroke. Lancet 1990:336:1205.
119. Legault C, Furberg CD, Wagenknecht LE, et al. Nimodipine neuroprotection in cardiac valve replacement. Report of an early terminated trial. Stroke 1996;27:593.

Chapter 5

Neurologic Complications of Anesthesia

David S. Currier and Bhuwan P. Garg

Objectives

- To know that neurologic complications are associated with general and regional anesthesia
- To become familiar with the types of neurologic complications that may occur
- To learn the manifestations of central nervous system (CNS) and peripheral nervous system complications
- To learn the etiologies of these complications
- To understand how to prevent and minimize these complications
- To know how to manage neurologic complications associated with anesthesia

Central Nervous System Dysfunction and Anesthesia

Postoperative Delirium

Delirium may occur in the immediate postoperative period or present days or even weeks later. Symptoms of postoperative delirium often fluctuate in intensity and include clouded consciousness, memory impairment, disorientation, perceptual difficulties, altered psychomotor activity, and hallucinations. Although an average incidence of 37% (range, 0–73%) has been reported,[1] the incidence depends on many factors, including patient's age, type of surgery, and anesthesia used. A 9% incidence after noncardiac surgery,[2–4] 23% after orthopedic surgery (hip fracture repair),[5] and 12–57%[6] after cardiopulmonary bypass (CPB) in the elderly has been reported. Duration of delirium is usually short, but may persist for up to 6 weeks.[7] Patients who develop delirium have longer hospital stays, higher rates of major complications, and higher rates of discharge to long-term facilities.[3, 7]

The etiology of delirium is multifactorial, with preoperative, operative, and postoperative factors contributing to its presentation. Although anesthetic concentrations may persist at low levels for several days postoperatively, this is a rare cause. Preoperative brain damage, preexisting cognitive disorder, history of seizures, age greater than 70 years, depression, addiction to drugs and alcohol, preeclampsia, and history of porphyria appear to increase the likelihood of postoperative delirium. Diabetic ketoacidosis, hypothyroidism or hyperthyroidism, and hepatic and pulmonary insufficiency can also cause delirium.

The type of anesthesia may contribute to postoperative delirium. Inhalational agents accumulate in fat tissue, especially during prolonged surgery. CNS impairment may persist for up to 6–8 days after 7 hours of isoflurane or halothane anesthesia. With shorter-acting intravenous agents such as sodium thiopental, methohexital, and propofol, the duration of cognitive impairment is considerably less, but it may extend for up to 12 hours postoperatively.[8] Ketamine is notorious for emergence delirium characterized by hallucinations, hyperexcitability, vivid dreams, and disorientation.[2] Scopolamine and atropine cross the blood-brain barrier, and the delirium is highly correlated to serum levels of these anticholinergics.[9] Narcotics, especially meperidine, and long-acting benzodiazepines, such as diazepam, chlordiazepoxide, and flurazepam, are other potential causes of delirium. High doses of corticosteroids (30 mg per kg of methylprednisolone) may produce acute psychotic reactions, depression, mania, delirium, confusion, and seizures.[10] The incidence of corticosteroid-induced delirium is 10% and appears to be dose dependent.[11] Other drugs resulting in cognitive dysfunction include phenothiazines, antihistamines, butyrophenones, cimetidine, antihypertensives, antiparkinsonian drugs, psychotropics, and cardiac drugs.[7] Withdrawal from alcohol, narcotics, and benzodiazepines also may result in delirium.

The type of surgery is important because oncologic, hip, eye, and coronary artery bypass surgery predispose to delirium. Coronary artery bypass with extended pump runs and mean perfusion pressures of less than 50 mm Hg is frequently associated with postoperative delirium.[2] Intraoperative events such as hypoxia, acidosis, hypoventilation, hypoperfusion, and anemia are common correctable causes for postoperative delirium. Hyperventilation to an arterial partial pressure of carbon dioxide ($PaCO_2$) of less than 25 mm Hg can cause cerebral vasoconstriction resulting in cerebral ischemia and confusion.

Fever, hypothermia, sepsis, pneumonia, and fat emboli can alter a patient's sensorium acutely. Metabolic abnormalities, including hypoglycemia or hyperglycemia, uremia, hyponatremia, and hyperammonemia, are potentiators for delirium. Patients undergoing transurethral resection of the prostate (TURP) are candidates for dilutional hyponatremia and subsequent confusion (TURP syndrome). Alteration in CNS neurotransmitters may play a role in the exacerbation of delirium because decreased tryptophan and acetylcholine levels and elevated cortisol levels with the stress of surgery have been associated with postoperative confusional states.[7, 9, 12]

Evaluation of patients emerging from anesthesia should be tempered by the recognition that certain neurologic abnormalities are commonly found in the postoperative period. Absence of pupillary and lid reflexes occur in 40% of neurologically intact patients.[8] Similarly, hyperreflexia and clonus can be present without an underlying neurologic condition. Reflex changes seen during emergence from anesthesia are usually bilateral; unilateral reflex changes may require further neurologic investigation.

Management of postoperative delirium depends on the potential etiology. The most readily treatable causes such as poor oxygenation, impaired ventilation, or inadequate perfusion should be considered first and treated appropriately because these are the most common causes of delirium in the postanesthesia care unit. Correction of hypothermia, hypotension, and cardiac arrhythmias may be necessary. Appropriate investigations including measurements of arterial blood gases, electrolytes, hemoglobin, and hematocrit; neuroimaging studies including cranial computed tomography, magnetic resonance imaging (MRI), as well as lumbar puncture and electroencephalography (EEG) may be indicated.

Specific pharmacologic interventions may be diagnostic and sometimes therapeutic. For instance, physostigmine may reverse the symptoms in a delirious patient suffering from central anticholinergic syndrome secondary to atropine or scopolamine. Naloxone may improve the cognitive abilities of an overnarcotized patient, and flumazenil may improve the CNS dysfunction in patients receiving excess benzodiazepines. Droperidol or benzodiazepines may lessen the severity of the delirium, especially when ketamine is administered. Oral haloperidol in small doses has been advocated for the treatment of delirium.[7] If the etiology of delirium remains elusive, supportive care and reassurance are in order, with behavior and environmental support available as needed. Ambulatory surgery and early discharge to a familiar environment may be helpful in lessening delirium and improving sleep-wake cycles. A decreased incidence of delirium occurs when high-risk patients undergo preoperative counseling.[1] The incidence may be lowered when a geriatric anesthesiologic intervention program is implemented including deep vein thrombosis prophylaxis, oxygen therapy, and preoperative and postoperative geriatric assessments.[7]

Perioperative Stroke

Perioperative stroke is a rare complication of anesthesia with a variable incidence depending on the type of surgery. The incidence of stroke is 0.37–

3.5% in general and in vascular surgery patients[13, 14]; carotid endarterectomy (CEA), open-heart surgery, and thoracoabdominal aortic surgeries place patients at a greater risk of perioperative CNS injury. Fatal cerebral damage occurs in 2% of patients undergoing cardiac procedures,[6, 8, 15] and the incidence of neurologic deficits varies from 2% to 61%.[8] When detailed neuropsychological evaluation is performed, cognitive function may be impaired in approximately 80% of patients.[8] The high morbidity and mortality in these patients are alarming, and one-half of the survivors require placement in long-term facilities.[13]

Factors placing patients at greater risk of stroke include a history of hypertension, heart disease, diabetes mellitus, smoking, obesity, preeclampsia, hypercoagulable states, and prior cerebral ischemia. Hypoxemia is rarely a cause of focal neurologic deficits. Patients with a history of transient ischemic attacks have a 21-fold greater risk of perioperative stroke compared with asymptomatic patients when undergoing peripheral vascular surgery.[16] Perioperative strokes are more likely to result from an embolic source as opposed to decreased cerebral blood flow. Cardiogenic emboli accounted for 42% of perioperative strokes in a retrospective review, whereas only 8% were attributed to arterial hypotension.[14] Most strokes do not occur intraoperatively but in the first 2–10 days postoperatively.[14, 16, 17] After CEA, 60% of strokes were found to be due to postoperative factors, whereas only 6% were identified as intraoperatively related.[18] Hypercoagulability associated with pregnancy, thrombocytosis, malignancies, and oral contraceptives increases the risk of perioperative stroke. Neurologic deficits have occurred in parturients secondary to intracranial aneurysm rupture, arteriovenous malformations, and eclampsia.[19] Vertebral artery dissection may occur with sudden neck movement, chiropractic manipulation, abrupt change in head position, laryngoscopy, and abnormal neck position under anesthesia.[19]

Physical examination may identify patients at greater risk of developing cerebral ischemia because head rotation to either side or hyperextension of the head (commonly performed for intubation) may precipitate vertebrobasilar ischemia. A controversial area concerns the advisability of performing CEA on patients with asymptomatic carotid bruits undergoing further elective surgical procedures. The presence of an asymptomatic carotid bruit is not indicative of increased perioperative stroke. The risk of perioperative stroke in patients with asymptomatic carotid bruits is 1% compared with less than 0.5% in the general population. Conversely, the risk of stroke after CEA is 2–7%.[20] Thus, prophylactic CEA may be riskier than the planned procedure.[6, 8, 17]

Certain surgical procedures are associated with a greater risk of perioperative stroke. CEA has a 2–7% incidence of stroke; however, the incidence of this complication is lower in centers of excellence.[20] Perioperative strokes that occur after CEA may be caused by embolization, hypoperfusion, improper patient selection, or associated intracranial lesions. Patients undergoing CPB also are at high risk for CNS dysfunction that resolves in the majority of patients over a period of months, with 11–35% having residual deficits up to 1 year later. Hypoperfusion during CPB may result from low flow, loss of pulsatile blood flow, hypotension, or incorrect placement of the aortic cannula. Embolism may be due to macroembolic or microembolic particles consisting of fat, air, plastic, and silicone aggregates. Longer periods of CPB and procedures that involve opening of the cardiac chambers have increased CNS complications. Warm heart surgery has a myocardial protective effect but an increased neurologic threat. Patients who remain in a comatose state after CPB have a poor prognosis, with a mortality in excess of 80%.[15]

Attention to $PaCO_2$ levels is important during anesthesia because hypercarbia vasodilates normal cerebral vessels and may lead to a stealing of blood flow from ischemic regions already maximally dilated. Lowering the $PaCO_2$ with hyperventilation may theoretically be beneficial by producing an inverse-steal, or "Robin Hood effect." However, in patients with moyamoya disease, normocapnia and normotension should be maintained because these patients experience chronic cerebral ischemia and have impaired cerebral vascular responsiveness of moyamoya vessels to hypotension and arterial carbon dioxide tensions.[21] A neutral head position with avoidance of hyperextension, excessive rotation, or flexion of the cervical spine may prevent vertebrobasilar ischemia. Ensuring normoglycemia and preventing hyperglycemia may lessen neurologic injury due to cerebral lactic acidosis during ischemia. Cerebral protection with hypothermia or a barbiturate-induced burst suppression may be used if ischemic injury is anticipated.[8]

Perioperative Seizures

Perioperative seizures may be idiopathic or related to fever, toxic metabolic encephalopathies, or structural CNS pathology. Postoperative seizures occur within 1 week in 3% of patients with impaired cerebral circulation and are often accompanied by hypertensive episodes associated with headaches.[22]

Many anesthetics are capable of altering seizure threshold. Seizures have been reported to occur several days after an enflurane anesthetic. Enflurane-induced epileptiform EEG activity is maximal at concentrations of 2–3%.[8] At any enflurane concentration, hyperventilation increases the likelihood of seizure activity and hypoventilation minimizes it. Etomidate lowers the seizure threshold and induces myoclonic movements, which may persist into the recovery period. Seizure activity is common in epileptic patients anesthetized with etomidate. Ketamine also lowers the seizure threshold, increasing the risk of postoperative seizures. Methohexital commonly produces myoclonic movements but has not consistently produced EEG epileptiform activity.[8]

A metabolite of meperidine (normeperidine) may produce myoclonus, CNS hyperexcitability, and seizures. High serum levels of local anesthetics may precipitate seizures, with an incidence of seizures during regional anesthesia varying from 1–4 per 1,000 procedures.[23] Seizures are commonly associated with narcotic, alcohol, or benzodiazepine withdrawal. Immunosuppressant drug toxicity and antibiotics such as imipenem, norfloxacin, ciprofloxacin, and penicillin derivatives may be associated with seizures.[24]

Seizures in neonates and young infants may be subtle and difficult to detect. Rarely are seizures responsible for delayed awakening from anesthesia. Hypothermic circulatory arrest for more than 60 minutes increases the incidence of seizures to 15%.[25] Metabolic abnormalities such as hyponatremia (TURP syndrome), hypoglycemia, and hypocalcemia may be associated with postoperative seizures. Patients with a history of seizures who undergo prolonged surgery can develop postoperative seizures if their antiepileptic drug levels become subtherapeutic. Administration of antiepileptic drugs on the morning of surgery is helpful. If patients are unable to take these medicines in the immediate postoperative period, parenteral supplementation is warranted.

Peripheral Nervous System and Neurologic Complications Associated with Anesthesia

Brachial Plexus Injury and Upper Extremity Nerve Injury

Peripheral nervous system injuries may arise from improper patient positioning, misadventures of regional anesthesia, or failure to maintain ventilation and circulation. Among the most frequent legal claims against anesthesiologists are peripheral nerve injuries, which account for 15% of total claims.[26] Most peripheral nerve injuries are identified immediately on recovery or within 3 days after anesthesia.[27] More claims are filed by men (69%) after administration of general anesthesia (61%) as opposed to regional anesthesia (36%).[26] The incidence of perioperative nerve injury is 0.1% after general anesthesia.[28] In axillary brachial plexus anesthesia, nerve lesions are apparent in 2.8% of patients when a paresthesia technique (intentional seeking of paresthesias) is used, as opposed to a 0.8% incidence of nerve lesions when a transarterial approach is performed.[29]

Peripheral nerve injuries result from a combination of factors including stretch, compression, comorbid conditions, preexisting nerve injuries, and administration of drugs and toxins. Stretch injuries occur from elongation of nerves, with elevation of intraneural pressure resulting in decreased blood flow and nerve ischemia. Compression can cause nerve injury by damaging surrounding vascular structures and leading to ischemia. Nerves close to bone or ligamentous structures and those nerves traveling through rigid anatomic tunnels have a greater likelihood of injury. During surgeries with excessive third spacing or patients developing tissue edema (preeclampsia), compressional nerve injury may occur. General anesthesia, longer surgeries (longer than 6 hours), and muscle relaxation increase joint laxity, predisposing to nerve injury.[27] Another factor is the "double crush syndrome."[30] Coexisting diseases (e.g., diabetes) may be the initiating injury, which then is compounded by poor intraoperative arm positioning and results, for example, in an ulnar neuropathy. Diabetes mellitus, uremia, liver disease, hypothyroidism, vitamin deficiencies, and vascular disease are other factors that promote neuronal injury.[28, 30] Specific drugs that have been found to cause peripheral nerve damage are cisplatin, vincristine, hydralazine, amiodarone, thallium, lead, and phenytoin (see Chapter 15 for discussion).

Other mechanisms for nerve injury include retractor-induced nerve injury, instrumental vaginal deliveries, direct surgical nerve injury, tourniquets, needle-induced traumatic injury, and occasionally compression injury by noninvasive blood pressure cuffs. Occasionally, hematoma formation after arterial cannulation may place nearby nerves at risk for ischemic insults. Needle-induced neurologic sequelae are rare after brachial plexus regional anesthesia. When neurologic injury occurs, it is frequently attributed to intraneural injection. A short-beveled (45-degree) needle inserted parallel to the nerve fibers may reduce the incidence of nerve injury.[31]

Ulnar nerve injuries account for 34% of the American Society of Anesthesiologists' closed claims involving peripheral nerve injuries.[31] Factors associated with ulnar nerve injury are male sex, prolonged hospitalization, body habitus, and diabetes. The ulnar nerve is highly susceptible to intraoperative injury and compressional injury. Also, when the elbow is fully flexed, the ulnar nerve is stretched within the cubital tunnel, increasing its susceptibility to ischemia. Current recommendations to avoid intraoperative ulnar neuropathy are appropriate padding and avoiding cubital tunnel pressure. When the arm is abducted, this is accomplished by supination of the forearm, thereby shifting the pressure from the cubital tunnel to the olecranon. Others believe that supination increases the stretching on the brachial plexus and advise pronation rather than supination.[32] If the forearm is fully pronated, the medial epicondyle presses against the armboard, and the ulnar groove with the ulnar nerve faces posteriorly and is free of pressure.[32] Other possible factors for ulnar nerve injury range from elbow flexion, ulnar nerve dislocation, intravenous lines, monitoring cables, poorly positioned padding, and automatic noninvasive blood pressure cuffs.[30, 33] Ulnar neuropathies have been reported after kidney transplants in which both arms were adducted.[34] It has been hypothesized that ulnar nerve injury was secondary to compression and that uremia was an important predisposing factor to ulnar nerve damage.[34] Interestingly, many patients who undergo nerve conduction studies are found to have preexisting abnormalities.[35] Postoperative ulnar nerve palsy can also occur without any apparent cause, despite careful attention to patient positioning and padding.[36]

The next most common injury involves the brachial plexus. The overall incidence of brachial plexus injury is 0.02%, but after median sternotomy it approaches 5–19%.[6, 30, 37] Injury to the brachial plexus results from arm hyperabduction (of more than 90 degrees), use of shoulder braces, and median sternotomy.[38] Other possibilities include compression or stretch injuries,[6, 37] traumatic injuries from central line placement or first rib fractures,[39] and use of anticoagulants. Also, depression of the shoulder girdle with the patient supported by wrist straps or braces in a steep Trendelenburg's position can stretch the upper roots of the brachial plexus, resulting in injury.[38] Retraction of the sternum during median sternotomy forces the clavicle into the retroclavicular space and causes the first rib to rotate superiorly, thereby increasing the distance between points of fixation of the plexus, resulting in stretch injury.[40] High-risk points of contact include the point where the brachial plexus traverses the clavicle and first rib and where the plexus emerges from the interscalene groove. The lower roots of the brachial plexus (C8–T1) are vulnerable with arm abduction and median sternotomy, whereas shoulder braces tend to injure the upper roots.[38] Hypothermia may predispose to the development of a neuropathy,[27] as may ischemia from CPB and damage to the vasonervorum.[6] Injuries are detected shortly after awakening and most recover within a 3-month period.[37, 40] Surgical exploration is not indicated for brachial plexopathies secondary to positional injury.

The radial nerve can also be damaged intraoperatively. The radial nerve can be compressed by orthopedic tourniquets, external pressure, ether screens, noninvasive blood pressure cuffs,[41] and improper arm positioning in a lateral decubitus position. Other possible causes are injection injuries, crutch palsy, Saturday night palsy, and obstetric palsy.[28] The median nerve is infrequently injured, but may be compressed in the antecubital fossa or in the carpal tunnel. This can occur with a surgeon's leaning or circumferential securing of the arm.

Recommendations to minimize brachial plexus injuries are to limit arm abduction to less than 90 degrees; avoid rotation and flexion of the neck to the opposite side; and avoid simultaneous abduction, external rotation, and extension of the upper extremity. Also, careful positioning of shoulder braces at the acromioclavicular joint to limit caudal pressure on the joint and avoiding surgical arm positions over the head may decrease brachial plexus injury. While positioning a patient, the physician should ask if that particular position would be comfortable for himself or herself. Aborting injections when paresthesias or lancinating pain are present and avoiding nerve blocks in individuals who are unable to report such paresthesias may lessen nerve injury. For many patients, the prognosis is good, with complete recovery in more than 90% of cases[27]; however, patients with diabetes and a history of alcoholism may be expected to have a more protracted recovery.

Lumbosacral Plexus Injury and Lower Extremity Nerve Injury

Lumbosacral nerve injuries are the third most common nerve injuries reported in the American Society of Anesthesiologists' closed claims database and account for 20% of the claims for postoperative nerve injury.[26, 30] Injuries are more frequent in women (72%), and 90% are associated with regional anesthesia.[26, 30] Spinal and epidural needles may injure the specific nerve roots, but this rarely occurs, with an incidence of less than 0.1%.[42] Procedures associated with lumbosacral plexus injury include childbirth, lithotomy position, and retractor-induced injury. The most likely causes for nerve injury are similar to those for brachial plexus injuries and include stretching and compression with resulting nerve ischemia.[43] The lumbosacral plexus is relatively well protected in the psoas muscle and traction injury is rare.[28] At the ala of the sacrum, the trunk of the lumbar plexus is in direct contact with bone and has an increased susceptibility for compression.

Patient positioning is a critical factor in the etiology of postoperative lumbosacral plexus injury because 1 in 3,600 patients in the lithotomy position develop a lower extremity neuropathy.[43] Risk factors include prolonged lithotomy position (of more than 4 hours), thin body habitus (body mass index of less than 20), and a history of smoking.[43] Diabetes and vascular disease are significant coexisting diseases for the precipitation of peripheral nerve injuries. The most commonly involved nerves are the common peroneal, sciatic, and femoral nerves.[43] Prognosis is dependent on the nerve injured. One-half of the patients with injuries of the common peroneal nerve or femoral nerve regain function within the first year. Injuries to the sciatic nerve have a more dismal prognosis; these patients may require lower extremity support, crutches, or prostheses for ambulatory assistance.

The peroneal nerve is fixed at the sciatic notch and the fibular neck, increasing its susceptibility to stretch injury. Also, due to its superficial location and close proximity to the fibular neck, external compression potentiates nerve ischemia. Improper positioning in stirrups, excessively tight casting, and leg dependency in a lateral decubitus position have been described as potential etiologies of peroneal nerve injury.[38] Patients undergoing knee arthroplasties may be at a higher risk for peroneal nerve injury, especially in a difficult arthroplasty with extensive soft tissue dissection.[37] The deep peroneal nerve and the tibial nerve may be injured in the popliteal fossa by inadequate padding.[38]

The superficial peroneal nerve may be injured as the nerve crosses the dorsal aspects of the foot just below the ankle. Patients who cross their legs for extended periods of times place the dependent superficial peroneal nerve at risk of injury. This position also places the nondependent extremity's sural nerve at risk. Injury to the lumbosacral plexus may occur with forceps-assisted vaginal delivery and even in normal vaginal deliveries when the fetal head is in an occipitoposterior position.[44]

The sciatic nerve becomes superficial as it passes beneath the lower border of the gluteus maximus, placing the nerve at risk for compression injury even when a patient is seated on a firm surface for extended periods of time.[28] Flexion of the hip stretches the sciatic nerve as it curves around the ischial tuberosity and the greater trochanter, placing the nerve in jeopardy during hip and femur surgeries. A lateral decubitus position may squeeze the sciatic nerve under the piriform muscle, especially in thin individuals.[32] The lithotomy position can injure the sciatic nerve if the thighs and legs are externally rotated or if the knees are extended.[32, 45] Postoperative hematoma, manipulation of the hip joint, leakage of methylmethacrylate, and direct injection injury as a complication of deep intramuscular injections may also injure the sciatic nerve.[38, 46]

The femoral nerve may be injured from a femoral hematoma as a result of arterial cannulation, retraction during pelvic surgery, and subsequent compression injury. Also, extensive flexion, abduction, and external rotation of the thigh can compress the femoral nerve.[28] The lateral femoral cutaneous nerve can be compressed when a prone jackknife position is used. Lateral femoral cutaneous neuropathy often occurs during pregnancy but is rarely disabling. Injury can also result from iliac bone harvesting, seat-belt injury, corsets, appendectomy, or lower intra-abdominal tumors. As the lateral femoral cutaneous nerve traverses beneath the inguinal ligament near the anterior iliac spine, inadequate attention to patient positioning and padding may result in nerve injury.

Recommendation to possibly minimize lower extremity neuropathies include proper patient selection for surgeries requiring a lithotomy position, limiting the duration of procedures that require a lithotomy position, and vigilant positioning of the lower extremities. This includes avoidance of leg crossing and careful attention to leg position during lithotomy, leg flexion, and dependent lateral decubitus positions. It is also imperative to ensure that the neurologic manifestations are not secondary to more severe and devastating processes, especially if regional anesthesia has been administered. Under these circumstances, other etiologies that should be considered, among others, include cauda equina syndrome, toxicity of medications, lumbar spinal canal stenosis, epidural hematoma or abscess, spinal cord infarction, and meningitis.

Neuraxial Iatrogenic Complications in Anesthesia

Complications Associated with Epidural Anesthesia

Local Anesthetic Toxicity

Local anesthetics may be associated with allergic or hypersensitivity reactions as well as systemic toxicity. It is important to differentiate systemic toxicity from an allergic reaction in the perioperative period, especially in patients who are receiving continuous epidural or subarachnoid infusions containing local anesthetic for analgesia. Systemic toxicity of local anesthetics may present with CNS dysfunction, including seizures and coma.

True allergic reactions are infrequent; however, they may be serious and life threatening. Allergic reactions to aminoamide local anesthetics are exceedingly rare; allergic reactions to aminoester local anesthetics secondary to para-aminobenzoic acid are more common. Many patients labeled as having allergies to local anesthetic agents are probably not allergic but have manifested an adverse systemic toxicity. Skin testing may be used to identify true allergic reactions. Systemic toxicity from a local anesthetic agent may result from tissue absorption, intravenous administration of excessive dose, or direct intraneural injection. Clinical effects depend on the serum level of the local anesthetic; high toxic levels may occur from accidental intravenous injections or excessive doses administered topically. CNS toxicity may be seen early, with subsequent progression to cardiac toxicity as blood levels of the local anesthetic increase.

CNS effects of lidocaine are dependent on its serum concentration. Perioral and tongue numbness, lightheadedness, visual disturbances, tinnitus, and an altered sense of well-being occur with lidocaine blood levels between 5 and 10 μg per ml. Muscular twitching, convulsions, and unconsciousness develop with blood levels of 10–13 μg per ml. Coma ensues at 15 μg per ml, and respiratory and cardiovascular depression occur at levels of 20–25 μg per ml. Factors increasing the sensitivity to local anesthetic toxicity include acidosis, hypercarbia, and use of cimetidine. Local anesthetic toxicity appears additive when combinations of esters with amides or amides with amides are administered. Unintentional intra-arterial injection during regional nerve blocks can result in CNS toxicity. Depending on the injection site, small amounts of local anesthetic may produce convulsions. For example, only 2.5 mg of bupivacaine injected into the vertebral artery during a stellate ganglion nerve block may result in convulsions. Barbiturates, benzodiazepines, and inhalational anesthetics decrease the CNS toxicity of local anesthetics.

Cardiovascular toxicity typically follows CNS symptomatology. At low doses, local anesthetics are antiarrhythmics; with increasing blood levels, myocardial depression and dysrhythmias occur. Some anesthetics such as bupivacaine and etidocaine are more cardiotoxic, and cardiovascular depression can occur without CNS manifestations. Bupivacaine has more avidity for cardiac sodium channels, and this combined with a very slow dissociation from these channels results in selective cardiotoxicity. The cardiovascular toxicity is enhanced in pregnancy, neonates, acidosis, hypoxemia, hyperkalemia, and with the addition of epinephrine.

Topical administration of local anesthetics is less likely to produce systemic toxicity unless excessive amounts are used. Eutectic mixture of local anesthetic (EMLA) cream, a mixture of lidocaine and prilocaine, is a new topical cream used for topical anesthesia prior to intravenous access and lumbar puncture in children.[47] There have been reports of prilocaine toxicity resulting in methemoglobinemia when excessive doses have been applied.[48] Usually, a dose of prilocaine of more than 500 mg is required for the development of methemoglobinemia.

Peak blood levels also depend on the site of local anesthetic application. For example, intercostal nerve blocks result in higher blood levels of local anesthetic than a caudal, epidural, or brachial plexus nerve block. The total dose administered is important; safe levels are with doses of less than 200 mg for bupivacaine, of less than 550 mg for lidocaine, of less than 500 mg for prilocaine, and of less than 500 mg for mepivacaine. Epinephrine may be used as an adjuvant with the local anesthetic to slow systemic absorption and decrease blood levels. Epinephrine may be added to the local anesthetic to assist in the diagnosis of intravascular injection by inducing tachycardia.

Management of local anesthetic toxicity requires immediate identification and appropriate emergent airway management. Oxygen and assisted ventilation may be all that is necessary. Patients who have convulsions develop hypoxia, acidosis, and hypercarbia rapidly, and anticonvulsant therapy should be initiated when appropriate. Airway control can be facilitated with succinylcholine, keeping in mind that this abolishes only the muscular activity and not the neuronal seizure activity. Some anticonvulsants such as sodium thiopental may result in cardiorespiratory depression, and inotropic support may be necessary. Cardiac arrhythmias may require cardioversion and drugs such as bretylium.

Nerve Root Injury

Nerve root injury is a rare complication of epidural or spinal anesthesia. Nerve damage may occur by several mechanisms, including direct needle trauma, intraneural injection, toxicity of the injectate, and vasospasm of the nutrient artery.[49] Needle trauma to a nerve root may be diminished by orienting the needle parallel to the neurovascular bundle.[31] Intraneural injections raise the intrafascicular pressure and create a compressive and ischemic injury to the nerve. Blunt-tipped needles may lessen the likelihood of neuronal damage as compared with sharp-beveled needles.[29, 31] Local anesthetics alone may be neurotoxic and result in altered endoneural transport, axonal death, and perineural edema (see following discussion of cauda equina and transient radicular irritation [TRI]).

Postoperatively, if a radiculopathy develops, the discomfort may be similar to the paresthesias encountered with needle placement or anesthetic injection. Paresthesias may be encountered 13% of the time with "single shot spinals," and 30% of the time with continuous spinal anesthesia.[49] These injuries usually present with minor deficits in unilateral dermatomal distribution and resolve in a few days.[44]

The most common cause of weakness, numbness, and lower extremity pain after a surgical procedure is a compressive neuropathy rather than a needle-induced traumatic injury.[44] Differentiating between these two conditions is sometimes challenging and may require the assistance of electrodiagnostic studies.[44] Other potential etiologies of postoperative neurologic deficits must be considered. These include epidural abscess and hematoma, toxicity from epidural medications, ischemia, spinal stenosis, and exacerbation of previous neurologic disease.

Spinal Epidural Hematoma

Another dreaded complication of epidural and spinal anesthesia is the spinal epidural hematoma. Fortunately, spinal epidural hematomas occur in less than 1 in 10,000 procedures.[50] The incidence of spinal epidural hematoma varies from 1 in 150,000 to 1 in 220,000.[51] Between 1906 and 1994 a total of 61 cases of spinal epidural or subdural hematoma in association with neuraxial blockade were published.[51]

Spinal epidural hematomas result from a multitude of factors, including trauma from needle insertion or catheter placement into the epidural or subarachnoid spaces, preexisting vascular anomalies (e.g., arteriovenous malformations), or neoplastic diseases, or they may develop spontaneously. Spontaneous spinal epidural hematomas are more frequent, especially in conjunction with the administration of anticoagulants, than hematomas secondary to neuraxial anesthesia.[51, 52]

Risk factors for epidural hematomas are impaired coagulation; heparin therapy (intravenous and subcutaneous); thrombocytopenia (platelet count of less than 100,000 μl); chronic alcohol abuse; chronic renal insufficiency; hepatic insufficiency; and administration of aspirin, indomethacin, urokinase, dextran, or ticlopidine. Pregnant women and patients with anatomic abnormalities of the spinal cord are at increased risk. Difficult insertions of a spinal or epidural needle and several attempts increase the likelihood of creating an epidural hematoma because there is a greater probability of damaged blood vessels. The chance of a bloody tap when epidural anesthesia is attempted is 1–10%.[51, 53, 54] However, during pregnancy the incidence may be as high as 18%.[51]

A consistent risk factor for spinal epidural hematoma is impaired blood coagulability prior to the initiation of neuraxial anesthesia. Marked coagulopathies remain absolute contraindications. However, regional anesthesia may be instituted with mild impairment in coagulation if the benefits greatly outweigh the risks.[51, 55] Some authors conclude that low-dose heparin prophylaxis is not a contraindication to spinal or epidural anesthesia.[51, 56, 57] Yet, there are a few reports of spinal epidural hematoma in patients who were administered low-dose unfractionated heparin and low-molecular-weight heparins.[51, 56, 58–60] In patients receiving low-molecular-weight heparins, neuraxial blockade should be delayed 10–12 hours after the last dose of enoxaparin. The catheter should not be removed until 10–12 hours have elapsed after the last dose.[60] A more controversial topic is removal of an indwelling epidural catheter or spinal catheter in the presence of impaired coagulation parameters. The most prudent practice would be to follow the same recommendations as for its placement.[61] Multiple studies have demonstrated the safety of intravenous heparin or subcutaneous heparin when an epidural or spinal catheter is in place without increased incidence of epidural spinal hematoma.[52, 56, 62, 63] The occurrence of spinal epidural hematomas with subsequent use of low-dose heparin (unfractionated or low-molecular-weight heparins) after regional anesthesia is infrequent.[58, 61, 64–66] Patients receiving a fibrinolytic agent should be considered at high risk for a spinal hematoma, and epidural or subarachnoid anesthesia should be avoided in these patients.[57, 67, 68] No increased risk has been identified in patients receiving aspirin or nonsteroidal anti-inflammatory agents who undergo an epidural or spinal anesthetic.[69]

To limit the risk of spinal hematoma, one should use the smallest-bore spinal needle available, an atraumatic technique, and the lowest level of anticoagulation feasible.[53] To minimize the possibility of spinal epidural hematoma after a neuraxial anesthetic technique, we recommend avoidance of neuraxial regional technique if patients have received an anticoagulant or have a known coagulopathy.[53] If preoperative anticoagulation is to be initiated, we favor postponing the surgery for 24 hours if a bloody tap does inadvertently occur. We recommend allowing a minimal period of 60–120 minutes post epidural or spinal anesthesia before institution of anticoagulation. We also recommend removal of an epidural or spinal catheter before the next scheduled anticoagulant dose or allowing reversal of anticoagulation before its removal. But most important, close monitoring of the neurologic status is needed in patients receiving a neuraxial anesthetic, especially for those with a greater susceptibility to developing spinal epidural hematomas.

Spinal Epidural Abscess

Another rare and potentially devastating complication of spinal epidural anesthesia is a spinal epidural abscess. The incidence of spinal epidural abscess is estimated at 0.7% following epidural anesthesia.[70] Most spinal epidural abscesses develop in the posterior lateral lumbar and thoracic epidural regions, as the epidural spaces are widest in these areas. The abscess is rarely located in the anterior epidural space. The epidural space extends from the foramen magnum to the sacral hiatus and the potential for spread may be quite high. It may involve multiple segments.[71, 72] The spinal epidural abscess may be secondary to an epidural needle or catheter and contaminated injectate, but is more likely to occur from hematogenous spread.[72, 73] Some studies have evaluated whether culture-positive epidural catheters are related to epidural abscesses.[70, 74, 75] Despite a 5% catheter infection rate, no patient was found with a spinal epidural abscess.[75] No patient required emergent surgical laminectomy and each patient had MRI resolution of the epidural infection.[74] The presence of inflammation and erythema at the catheter site appears to be the strongest predictors of epidural catheter infection, while infections at other sites, antibiotic therapy, duration of epidural analgesia, and insertion site were risk factors.[75] In cases of epidural space infection associated with deep catheter infection, catheter removal and intravenous antibiotics are recommended. Cancer and immunosuppressed patients, intravenous drug abusers, diabetics, and individuals with prolonged epidural catheterization are at a greater risk for developing epidural contaminations and spinal epidural abscesses.[76] Chronic epidural catheter placement can lead to epidural abscesses and may present in an insidious fashion, unlike an acute epidural abscess. Patients with reflex sympathetic dystrophy and diabetes may have a greater predisposition for spinal epidural abscesses.[77] Regional anesthesia is absolutely contraindicated when abscesses or infected wounds exist at the proposed insertion site, but distant infections with or without bacteremia is more controversial. Antibiotic prophylaxis before insertion of the epidural may decrease the risk of spinal epidural abscess.[73] In obstetric patients with bacteremia from chorioamnionitis who subsequently undergo epidural analgesia, epidural abscesses rarely occur.[78] Seeding of the epidural space from a diagnostic or anesthetic lumbar puncture is exceedingly rare.[79] Other etiologies for a spinal epidural abscess include direct extension from a local process, from a lymphatic spread, and postoperatively from a surgery such as laminectomy. Seeding of the epidural space from hematogenous spread can occur as a result of bacteremia from infection of the skin, urinary tract, pharynx, and lung.[71, 72, 80] Concurrent infection and trauma to the vertebral column are factors that increase the risk of spinal epidural abscess formation.[71, 72]

Infectious organisms most commonly cultured from the epidural abscesses are *Staphylococcus aureus* (50–60%), coagulase-negative staphylococci, and gram-negative bacilli.[76] Other pathogens include *Streptococcus pneumoniae*, *Staphylococcus epidermidis*, *Listeria monocytogenes*, *Mycobacterium tuberculosis*, and rarely fungi in compromised hosts.

When a triad of fever, localized back pain, and tenderness exists, a diagnosis of spinal epidural abscess must be considered. Leukocytosis and elevated erythrocyte sedimentation rate is found in 85% of patients.[72] If a catheter is present, a culture from the exit site and luminal aspiration may be warranted. If the catheter appears to be the most likely site of infection, the catheter should be removed and the tip cultured. Blood cultures should be obtained to exclude bacteremia. Radiographic results may be normal or demonstrate osteomyelitis, compression fractures, and paravertebral masses. Enhanced MRI of the spine is the gold standard for the diagnosis of a spinal epidural abscess.

Treatment requires prompt diagnosis to minimize neurologic injury. Emergent surgical drainage plus parenteral antibiotics is favored in cervical and thoracic spinal epidural abscesses.[81] Medical treatment alone may be all that is required for certain patients in the absence of neurologic deficits.[77, 82]

Anterior Spinal Artery Syndrome

Spinal cord infarction is a rare postoperative complication after either regional or general anesthesia. Postoperative spinal cord stroke in association with an epidural anesthetic is estimated to occur in 1 in 11,000 procedures,[83, 84] and in patients undergoing aortic vascular surgery the incidence ranges from 0.5% to 40%.[85–87] Procedures that increase the risk include aortic, lumbar disk, and scoliosis surgery.[88]

Paraplegia after epidural anesthesia has been attributed to neurotoxic effects of local anesthetics injected into the intrathecal space, inadvertent arterial damage by the epidural or spinal needle, and vasoconstrictive effect of additives.[83] Likewise, arachnoiditis and patient position have been identified as factors for postoperative paraplegia.[83, 89–91]

Ischemia to the spinal cord can occur by prolonged hypotension,[42] direct trauma to the supplying radicular spinal arteries,[92] or an increase in intraspinal pressure. Cross clamping of the aorta decreases mean arterial pressure, further limiting spinal cord perfusion and exacerbating spinal cord ischemia. With an epidural injection it is possible to elevate the epidural pressure and transmit an elevated compression pressure to the subarachnoid space, thereby worsening spinal cord perfusion. In pregnant women, inferior vena cava compression secondary to hyperlordosis, surgical packing, or a gravid uterus[83, 91] may decrease spinal cord perfusion, and small fluid injections into the epidural space can elevate the epidural pressure and subsequently the cerebrospinal fluid (CSF) pressure by 14 cm H_2O.[93] Vasoconstrictors as additives to local anesthetics may reduce spinal cord blood flow.[94, 95] However, Kazody et al. were unable to determine any effect on spinal cord blood flow with injection of 0.2 mg of epinephrine or 5 mg of phenylephrine in the dog intrathecal space.[96] Lidocaine also was not found to influence spinal cord blood flow directly.[95, 97] After intra-aortic balloon pump placement, a risk of paraplegia exists if a thoracic dissection occurs.[6] A hyperlordotic position during surgery may predispose patients to this syndrome.[91] Spinal venous infarction is believed to occur as the hyperextension obstructs inferior vena cava flow, thereby increasing distal venous pressure to the intraspinal veins and causing spinal cord ischemia.[90]

The spinal artery syndrome has been identified as a complication of celiac plexus blocks[92, 98–101] and lumbar sympathetic blocks.[102] It is not clear if the etiology is from arterial spasm due to alcohol or direct trauma by the needle; fluoroscopy does not seem to reduce this unfortunate complication.[98] Other potential causes include hematoma formation due to aortic puncture, direct arterial alcohol injection, intramural injection of alcohol, diffusion of alcohol into the spinal cord, spread of alcohol into the epidural space, sclerosis of the artery of Adamkiewicz, and a local inflammatory reaction causing thrombosis of the feeding arteries of Adamkiewicz.[92]

Techniques to minimize the risk of spinal cord infarction include bypass shunts to provide blood to the lower extremities, CSF drainage techniques, extracorporeal bypass, and preservation of the native aorta with its intercostal arteries. CSF drainage theoretically improves spinal cord perfusion if the CSF pressure is less than mean arterial pressure.[86] However, this has not consistently altered the outcome.[85, 103] Somatosensory evoked potentials (SSEPs) may assist in the evaluation of these patients.[104] SSEP monitoring has drawbacks because it is possible to have spinal cord ischemia without any alteration in the SSEPs. Furthermore, SSEPs are affected by anesthetics, hypothermia, hypoxia, and hypotension, limiting their usefulness. Corticosteroids reduce spinal cord edema, decrease chemical mediators, scavenge free radicals, and may limit the incidence of spinal cord injury.[104] The only truly preventive method is a short cross-clamp period with maintenance of oxygenation and hemodynamic parameters.

Treatment of spinal cord infarction remains symptomatic and the prognosis is poor.[42, 105] Recommendations to possibly prevent anterior spinal artery syndrome during anesthesia include avoiding a hyperlordotic position, administering small epidural doses to minimize epidural pressure elevations, and avoiding epidural anesthesia in patients with spinal stenosis.[91]

Iatrogenic Neurologic Complications of Spinal Anesthesia

Backache

Backache is a frequent complication after neuraxial anesthesia. Backaches are usually self-limited and resolve after several days. Approximately 20% of patients experience backache after an epidural anesthetic, whereas 7% of patients develop backache after spinal anesthesia.[52, 55, 106] Backache is not an exclusive complication of regional anesthesia, as obstetric patients experience backache 40% of the time without an epidural, 12% have backache after general anesthesia, and 30% experience backache after pudendal nerve blocks.[106–108]

The backache may be related to the patient's age and sex, needle trauma, interspinous ligament injection, supraspinous hematoma, surgical position, and length of surgery.[109, 110] With longer surgeries and a lithotomy position, a greater stretching of the tissues occurs and a greater incidence of backache is expected.[109] Intraoperative muscle relaxation with regional anesthesia or neuromuscular blockade with general anesthesia may allow unusual positioning and facilitate injury to the connective tissues of the back.[109] Women are at greater risk for developing backache.[109, 111] Furthermore, the greater number of attempts at either spinal or epidural placement quadruples the incidence of backache,[112] and using blunter needles compared with sharp needles increases the incidence.[55, 107]

Postdural Puncture Headache

Postdural puncture headache (PDPHA) is a frequent complication of regional neuraxial anesthesia. PDPHA is believed to occur from decreased CSF pressure due to a persistent CSF leak from a dural hole. The incidence depends on the patient's age and sex, needle size, orientation of the needle, and presence of pregnancy. Obesity may decrease the risk of PDPHA.[113, 114]

A positional frontal or occipital headache exacerbated by assuming an erect posture and relieved in the supine position characterizes PDPHA. Headaches usually occur within 1–5 days after dural puncture. Rapidity of onset depends on the amount of CSF lost during and after the dural puncture; 65% of patients report headaches within 24 hours, whereas 92% present with headaches within 48 hours of the dural puncture.[115] Most headaches last only 3–5 days and resolve without intervention in most patients within 2 weeks. PDPHA may be associated with nausea, vomiting, neck and scapular discomfort, photophobia, blurred vision, diplopia, tinnitus, and hypoacusis.[115] PDPHAs rarely result in seizures.[116]

Pregnancy increases the risk of PDPHA. Age is inversely related,[115] and needle diameter is directly related to the chance of developing PDPHA.[117, 118] Nonobese patients are at higher risk of PDPHA (45% versus 25%).[113] The decreased incidence of PDPHA in obesity is due to a large panniculus acting like an abdominal binder, increasing the intra-abdominal and venous pressure and limiting the amount of CSF leakage.[113] When using a small-bore spinal needle, the incidence of PDPHA is 2–10% (25- or 26-gauge Quincke).[108] The pencil-point spinal needles (Gertie Marx [International Medical Development, Park City, Utah], Sprotte [Pajunk, Gelslinger, Germany], Whitacre [Becton-Dickinson, Rutherford, NJ]) decrease the incidence of PDPHA because these needles spread dural fibers in contrast to the sharp cutting spinal needles (Spinocan [B. Braun Medical, Bethlehem, PA], Quincke [Becton-Dickinson], Atraucan [B. Braun Medical]) that incise the dural fibers, creating larger tears.[117, 119–123] Needle orientation also influences the incidence of PDPHA.[115, 124] When the needle bevel is inserted parallel to the dural fibers, the fibers are spread, and a reduction in PDPHA is expected in contrast to perpendicularly incising the dural fibers.[124, 125] A paramedian approach to the subarachnoid space reduces the incidence of PDPHA by creating a dural flap that reseals the hole and limits CSF leakage. Increasing the number of punctures increases the number of dural holes and the incidence of PDPHA.[126, 127] Continuous spinal anesthesia may decrease the incidence of PDPHA by causing an inflammatory reaction at the site of the dural tear and facilitating early repair. In nonpregnant patients, continuous spinal anesthesia may decrease the incidence of PDPHA to less than 1%.[128] However, in the obstetric patient placement of a spinal catheter for less than 24 hours does not decrease the incidence of PDPHA.[129–131]

Conservative management of PDPHA involves bed rest, abundant caffeinated products (coffee, tea, soft drinks), intravenous caffeine sodium benzoate, and adequate hydration. Intravenous and oral caffeine were effective in controlling 80% of PDPHAs.[108] Opioids given by the epidural, spinal, intramuscular, or intravenous route may abolish or reduce the severity of the PDPHA and may lessen the need for an epidural blood patch (EBP).[132]

The most efficacious therapy is an EBP, which tamponades further CSF leakage. An EBP induces clot formation in the epidural space, directly patching the dural hole.[133] An EBP is accomplished by identifying the epidural space and then administering 15–25 ml of autologous blood as close to the prior dural puncture as possible. The injection is halted when the patient experiences paresthesias or interscapular pain. Fifteen milliliters of blood covers 8–10 spinal segments, with more spread in a cephalad direction.[134] The efficacy of EBP diminishes when administered within the first 24 hours of PDPHA (71% failure rate versus 4% failure).[108, 133] The success of an EBP ranges from 60% to 89% with the first patch, and 97% after a second patch.[115, 133, 135]

The immediate resolution of symptoms is due to the increased volume and pressure within the epidural space reducing further CSF loss and caudal traction on the brain structures.[133] Prophylactic EBP through an indwelling epidural catheter has been tried in some centers and may reduce the development of PDPHA by half.[136] Saline infusions or saline boluses through an epidural catheter may also tamponade the CSF leak.[108, 137]

Complications from EBPs are rare and include backache, neckache, dizziness, auditory disturbances, signs of meningeal irritation, epidural infection, and nerve root compression. Backache and mild temperature elevations are the most common side effects of EBPs.[135] If autologous blood is injected into the subarachnoid space, there is a risk of adhesive arachnoiditis.

If a headache persists after two EBPs, the diagnosis of a PDPHA should be reconsidered and a further evaluation conducted. Protracted migraines, cluster or tension headaches, meningitis, cortical vein thrombosis, pseudotumor cerebri, intracranial tumor, subarachnoid or intracerebral hemorrhage,[138] and preeclampsia or eclampsia[108] should be considered in the differential diagnosis.

Vestibuloauditory and Ocular Complications of Anesthesia

Closely related to PDPHA are vestibuloauditory and ocular complications as a result of dural puncture. Transient hearing loss can occur after spinal anesthesia, lumbar puncture, or myelography. The incidence of hearing loss and tinnitus varies from 0.4% to 8%.[139, 140] Audiometric disturbances are found in 40% of patients after a dural puncture. Unilateral or bilateral hearing loss presents within the first 2 days after a spinal anesthetic. Hearing loss is usually transient and resolves within a few days.[141, 142] A higher incidence of hearing deficit occurs in patients undergoing dural puncture with larger-bore spinal needles.[142] The proposed mechanism for the altered auditory acuity is the persistent CSF leak creating a decrease in the CSF pressure. Due to the direct connection between the CSF and perilymph, a decrease in CSF pressure alters the pressure within the cochlea,[139, 143] modifying the relationship of the hair cells and dampening auditory inputs. Another explanation is that a labyrinthine hydrops creates a hypoacusis similar to Ménière's disease. Altered hearing has been observed after epidural injections.[144] Again the effect is self-limited, lasting at times less than 10 minutes. However, in this instance, a greater epidural pressure, rather than a negative pressure, is transmitted to the perilymph, which distorts the hair cell relationship. Because the etiology is similar to PDPHA, an EBP is appropriate.[140, 145, 146] Others have used dextran and histamine analogues believing that the hearing impairment may be due to ischemia and altered blood viscosity.[143]

Double vision may be identified after spinal, epidural, and general anesthesia. Diplopia can occur with inadequate reversal of muscle paralysis. Blurred vision may occur after atropine administration. Approximately 4 minutes of ischemia or hypoxemia is all that is required to result in retinal ischemia and blindness.[38] Retinal ischemia may result from improper positioning of the head in the prone position or externally applied ocular pressure during face mask ventilation. The increased intraocular pressure can exceed the central retinal artery pressure and cause blindness. Transient blindness has also been reported with the use of ketamine[147] and with glycine after prostatic resection.[148] Central retinal artery occlusion and corneal edema have also been associated with loss of visual acuity postoperatively.[149] However, the most common ocular complication is corneal abrasions during airway management.[149]

Visual alterations after spinal anesthesia are usually seen in conjunction with PDPHA. Traction on cranial nerves III, IV, and VI causes visual disturbances. The abducens nerve (cranial nerve VI) is the most frequently affected. Two cases of blindness have been reported after patients received epidural injections.[150, 151] The increased epidural pressure may be transmitted to the intracranial vault, causing increased retinal venous pressure resulting in retinal hemorrhage and blindness.[150, 151] Funduscopy demonstrates retinal and preretinal hemorrhages.[151] Prognosis of the blindness is generally good with spontaneous resolution within 6 weeks.[151]

Other neuro-ophthalmologic and cranial nerve complications associated with central neurologic blocks include Horner's syndrome and trigeminal and facial nerve palsies. Horner's syndrome may occur in up to 4% of obstetric epidurals[152] or in association with interscalene, supraclavicular, and stellate ganglion nerve blocks and intraoral local anesthetic injections. Sporadic cases of Horner's syndrome have been reported without high epidural blockade.[152, 153] Trigeminal and facial neuropathy can occur after epidurals and usually are associated with a Horner's syndrome and high anesthetic sensory levels.[154] Facial palsy may result from increased CSF pressure associated with the epidural injection and a compromise of the vascular supply to the facial nerve.

Meningitis

Meningitis is a rare complication of regional anesthesia. The etiology includes introduction of skin pathogens from within the hollow needle, contaminated injectate, contaminated equipment (needles, syringes, catheters), and hematogenous sources. Aseptic meningitis can occur from viruses, disinfectants, detergents, and foreign material from the needle. Spontaneous meningitis with preexisting bacteremia (14%) is more frequent than a lumbar puncture–induced meningitis (2%).[155] Sepsis is a relative contraindication for regional anesthesia due to the risk of contaminating the epidural or intrathecal space. However, data suggesting that regional anesthesia before or during bacteremia is a risk factor for meningitis are scarce.[156]

Chorioamnionitis may increase the likelihood of meningitis in parturients who subsequently receive a regional anesthetic. These patients are frequently bacteremic and the risk of seeding into the subarachnoid space is a concern. However, the performance of a neuraxial technique in septic patients does not appear to increase the risk of meningitis.[78, 157] Nonetheless, in a febrile patient, many authors recommend prophylactic antibiotics before regional anesthesia.[156]

Meningitis has also been identified as a complication of combined spinal-epidural anesthesia[158, 159] or as a consequence of spinal anesthesia alone.[159, 160] Thus, patients receiving a combined spinal-epidural anesthetic should be closely evaluated in the postoperative period for meningitis.

Meningitis is rare after epidural anesthesia.[161, 162] Scott and Hibbard had no cases of meningitis after 505,000 epidurals.[163] Whether meningitis occurs from hematogenous spread or as a direct result of the epidural is difficult to assess. There are scattered reports of subarachnoid infection associated with prolonged epidural catheterization in chronic pain patients.[161]

A viral meningitis may be a concern when regional anesthesia is used in patients with herpes simplex virus type II, human immunodeficiency virus, and other viral diseases. Herpes simplex virus type II affects 0.5–1.0% of pregnant women, and patients with active genital herpes simplex virus may require a cesarean section to minimize neonatal risk during delivery. Currently, no increased risk of viral meningitis has been identified,[164–167] allowing the mother and fetus to avoid the risks of a general anesthetic.

Chemical meningitis can occur from intrathecal agents. Manufacturers critically evaluate their products before approval for subarachnoid administration to ensure safety. However, agents once thought to be safe may be neurotoxic. Before the 1940s, aseptic meningitis had a frequency of 1 in 400 spinal anesthetics.[158] The majority of aseptic meningitides reported before the 1980s were frequently associated with reusable regional anesthetic trays. These reusable trays required chemical decontamination and when poorly rinsed, trace particles of detergents on the spinal needles or syringes led to a chemical irritation of the meninges.[168] With the advent of combined spinal-epidural anesthesia, the introduction of metallic particles into the intrathecal space may occur. During combined spinal-epidural anesthesia, the spinal needle is introduced through an epidural needle, a procedure that is associated with friction and the ability to create metallic fragments that when injected intrathecally may pose a risk for meningeal inflammation.[169, 170] Nickel, a component of these needles, has been found to produce necrotic abscesses in rats.[169] Metal particles present as a result of the normal manufacturing process are not liberated when injecting solutions or when using a needle-through-needle technique.[162, 171] Some investigators have been unable to confirm damage to the epidural or spinal needle when using combined spinal-epidural anesthesia.[162, 172] Aseptic meningitis appears to have an acute onset within 24 hours of the dural puncture and a self-limiting course, yet appropriate antibiotic therapy should still be initiated.

Precautions should be taken whenever regional anesthetics are employed to ensure strict aseptic conditions because the CSF is an excellent culture medium with limited defenses. Thus, a sterile procedure should be followed, including caps, masks, and sterile gloves.[173] Common practice includes preparation of the site with an aseptic solution and, before needle insertion, removal of excess solution to minimize meningeal contamination from the preparation solution. Disposable trays are now standard, minimizing the risk of chemical meningitis. Some authors recommend an introducer needle as a conduit for the spinal needle to limit contact of the spinal needle with the skin.[173] Bacterial filters through which injectates are administered before entry into the epidural catheter may lessen contamination, but no studies have evaluated the efficacy of this practice.[161, 174]

Cauda Equina Syndrome

Cauda equina syndrome has resurfaced as a complication since the reintroduction of continuous spinal anesthesia in the early 1990s.[175–178] The Food and Drug Administration issued a caution and ordered an elimination of small-bore spinal microcatheters. The cauda equina syndrome associated with continuous spinal anesthesia results from neurotoxicity of the local anesthetic[42] and not from the catheters. Other etiologies to consider include trauma, arachnoiditis, epidural hematoma, spinal cord ischemia, tumors and other compressive lesions, and prolonged hypotension.[179]

Prolonged neurologic deficits after epidural or unintentional subarachnoid injections of chloroprocaine resembling cauda equina syndrome have been reported.[180–184] The dose of epidurally injected chloroprocaine ranged from 360 to 840 mg with or without epinephrine. Neurologic deficits were likely related to the inadvertent subarachnoid injection of high doses of chloroprocaine intended for epidural anesthesia. Symptoms progressively improved over the initial 48 hours; few patients had complete resolution of neurologic symptoms within 5 years.[180–182] Chloroprocaine was evaluated more closely to determine whether the local anesthetic itself or its additives were toxic. In 1967 and 1968, chloroprocaine contained sodium bisulfite (antioxidant) and methylparaben (preservative). In 1971, methylparaben was removed from the 2% and 3% solutions and marketed as Nesacaine CE for epidural and caudal use. Initially, some thought the toxicity to be related to the pH (2.7–4.0) of this local anesthetic or its hyperbaricity causing osmotic damage.[184] In animal studies, chloroprocaine caused permanent neurologic dysfunction with evidence of impaired nerve conduction, axonal degeneration, and perineural adhesions.[184, 185] Histopathologic changes involved the subpial spinal cord areas in close proximity to the injection site and suggested more of a neurotoxic effect as opposed to a vascular etiology. No changes were seen in dogs administered bupivacaine, saline, or saline titrated to a pH of 3.0.

More recent studies have reevaluated whether local anesthetics are toxic to nerves,[46, 180, 185–188] and investigators have developed models of subarachnoid local anesthetic distribution to further understand the pathophysiology of spinally administered agents.[189] Bupivacaine and mepivacaine are the least toxic, lidocaine is moderately toxic, and procaine and tetracaine are the most damaging to nerves.[46] Local anesthetics precipitate nerve edema, increase endoneural fluid pressure, reduce nerve blood flow, and facilitate nerve ischemia. Application of 3% chloroprocaine and 1% tetracaine to rat vagus nerves resulted in subperineurial and endoneural edema, Schwann's cell necrosis, axonal dystrophy, and wallerian degeneration.[190] Ester local anesthetics (rather than amides, additives and acidotic solutions) exhibit a greater propensity to induce these changes, indicating that the local anesthetics themselves are neurotoxic. However, persistent neurologic deficits were not seen in rabbits with concentrations of tetracaine, lidocaine, bupivacaine, chloroprocaine, chloroprocaine plus 0.2% bisulfite used in clinical practice, but neurologic deficits developed with higher concentrations of tetracaine (8%), lidocaine (32%), and bisulfite.[188]

Factors affecting the concentration of a local anesthetic include baricity, rate of injection, catheter tip direction (cephalad versus sacral), multiorificed versus end-hole catheter, and concentration of the injected local anesthetic. In supine patients, injecting agents of greater baricity results in a greater concentration of local anesthetic pooling in the dependent regions, facilitating cauda equina injury. Faster injections through a catheter increase the distribution of the local anesthetic and decrease its concentration in dependent regions. The type of spinal catheter also influences the distribution, as multiorificed side-port catheters exhibit greater cephalad spread and lesser sacral pooling of local anesthetic when compared with end-hole spinal catheters. The type and concentration of the local anesthetic influences neural toxicity. When 5% lidocaine is injected into a sacrally directed catheter, the concentration increased from 2.0% to 3.4% after three injections. Nerves exposed to a 5% concentration demonstrated no recovery of action potential, whereas nerves exposed to 1.5% lidocaine showed no irreversible effects,[189] demonstrating a dose-dependent neurotoxicity.[189, 191, 192] Permanent neurologic effects are seen with subarachnoid administrations of 4–32% lidocaine. The presence of 7.5% glucose does not appear to influence osmotic neurologic injury.[193] Using bupivacaine for spinal anesthesia and using the lowest concentration of local anesthetic possible may reduce the incidence of cauda equina syndrome.[191]

Transient Radicular Irritation

TRI is another complication of spinal anesthesia.[194–201] Patients report a sharp, cramping, radiating, aching, or dull pain 2–20 hours after spinal anesthesia. The pain, usually bilateral, involves the back, buttocks, and thighs and may radiate to the knees. For many patients, this pain is worse than the incisional pain. The pain lasts less than a week in most cases,[197, 199, 201] is not associated with bowel or bladder dysfunction, and sensorimotor examination results are normal. The incidence of TRI may be as high as 37%[199, 202] but is probably less than 10%[197, 201] when hyperbaric lidocaine is administered. TRI occurs mostly in patients who have received a hyperbaric lidocaine spinal anesthetic. Decreasing the concentration of spinal lidocaine (2% versus 5%) and excluding dextrose do not lessen the incidence of TRI.[202] TRI has occurred with intrathecal doses of 0.5% tetracaine in 7.5% dextrose, with hypobaric lidocaine, with procaine, and rarely with hyperbaric bupivacaine.[199] The addition of epinephrine does not appear to influence the presentation of TRI.

Maldistribution of the local anesthetic and an increased concentration experienced by the cauda equina nerve roots are other factors potentiating TRI. TRI may occur from a restriction in flow secondary to the newer small-bore pencil-point needles. Slow injections (2 ml per minute) via a Whitacre pencil-point spinal needle (25- or 27-gauge) showed greater sacral concentration than a fast injection rate (2 ml per 10 seconds).[195] The Quincke spinal needle (25-gauge) did not show a maldistribution with a slow injection rate. Repeated spinal injections after a failed attempt exaggerate the nerve exposure to the local anesthetic in the dependent portion and increase the likelihood of neurotoxicity.[194] The pooling of the anesthetic in the sacral dermatomes increases the concentration around the L5–S1 roots, facilitating nerve injury. Additional stretching of the cauda equina by the lithotomy position and decreasing the vascular supply further precipitates injury. TRI after epidural anesthesia with lidocaine has been reported.[203]

Nonsteroidal anti-inflammatory drugs may be used as analgesics for the treatment of TRI, but it appears that the discomfort is self-limited and resolves with minimal intervention. Prevention of TRI requires identification of the procedures that increase its probability. When performing single-shot spinal anesthesia, avoidance of lidocaine may be warranted, especially if small-bore pencil-point spinal needles are used. If lidocaine is chosen, a concentration of less than 2% is recommended. Also, if the surgery is performed in a lithotomy position, using a safe local anesthetic, it is hoped, will decrease the incidence of TRI. Finally, predilution of the intrathecal local anesthetic or using larger spinal needles may further decrease the chance of TRI.[204, 205] As with any postoperative neurologic injury, the diagnosis of direct neural injury, bleeding, abscess, ischemia, and meningitis must be excluded.

Miscellaneous Neurologic Complications Associated with Anesthesia

Malignant Hyperthermia

Malignant hyperthermia (MH) is a hypermetabolic disorder of skeletal muscle characterized by abnormal intracellular calcium transportation at the sarcoplasmic reticulum resulting in intracellular hypercalcemia, acidosis, membrane destruction, and cell death.[206] Intraoperative MH presents after a triggering agent, usually an inhalational agent with or without succinylcholine, is administered. Incidentally, enflurane and isoflurane are less likely to trigger MH than halothane.[207] The incidence of MH is estimated to be between 1 in 14,000 and 1 in 200,000 anesthetics.[207–209] Ording found an overall incidence of 1 in 250,000 procedures, but 1 in 62,000 anesthetics when inhalational agents and succinylcholine were administered.[207] The commonly cited incidence is 1 in 50,000 in adults and 1 in 15,000 in children.[210] Patients may have received a prior anesthetic without developing MH.

Initial signs of MH include tachycardia, tachypnea, and hypercarbia. Muscle rigidity develops, and body temperature increases by 1–2°C every 5 minutes. Patients may appear mottled, diaphoretic, and cyanotic. Sympathetic discharge, acidosis, and hyperkalemia result in hypertension and cardiac arrhythmias. Hackl et al. found that generalized rigidity, ventricular arrhythmias, cyanosis, and myoglobinuria were significantly more predictive for developing MH than other clinical signs such as masseter muscle rigidity and tachycardia.[211] Increase in body temperature is a late sign of MH. Blood gases show a mixed metabolic and respiratory acidosis without significant oxygen desaturation. Hyperkalemia, hypercalcemia, lactic acidemia, and myoglobinuria are typical in MH, with creatine kinase levels reaching 20,000 U in the first 12–24 hours.

CNS involvement in fulminant MH is secondary to the elevated temperature, acidosis, and hypoxia. Acute cerebral edema leading to unresponsiveness, fixed and dilated pupils, generalized convulsions, areflexia, and coma may occur.[208, 212] These neurologic findings are late in the sequence of MH and indicate poor survival.

With greater education and awareness, the current mortality of MH is less than 10%.[209] Routine intraoperative monitoring of the end-tidal carbon dioxide levels has allowed earlier diagnosis and treatment of MH, with a reduction in mortality. Ellis evaluated MH over three time intervals (1971–1976, 1977–1981, and 1982–1987) and found the mortality from fulminant MH to be 100%, 53%, and 54%, respectively.[209]

Definitive diagnosis of MH involves a caffeine halothane contracture test from a muscle biopsy, which may be performed under regional anesthesia or using a nontriggering general anesthetic. A family history of anesthetic-related death should heighten the possibility of MH, especially if a history of being "packed in ice" is given. Another indicator may be the development of masseter muscle rigidity after exposure to succinylcholine. Two-thirds of such children were found to have MH on muscle biopsy.[211, 213–215] One percent of children developed masseter muscle rigidity after a halothane-succinylcholine induction, possibly making masseter muscle rigidity the most common manifestation of MH in children.[213, 216] The rigidity may last for a few minutes, and difficulty in opening the jaw occurs despite the nerve stimulator showing a peripheral flaccid paralysis.[210, 216] Repeat doses of succinylcholine do not relieve the rigidity. If masseter muscle rigidity occurs, some authors recommend cancellation of elective nonemergent surgery and further MH testing.[213, 216] However, with improvement in diagnosis and management of MH, others recommend continuation of surgery with nontriggering anesthetic agents, close monitoring of end-tidal carbon dioxide levels and the patient's temperature, with immediate capability to initiate intravenous dantrolene sodium therapy intraoperatively and postoperatively.[210] If dantrolene sodium is not administered, aggressive hydration and diuresis should be ensured postoperatively to prevent myoglobinuric renal insufficiency. Patients who develop masseter muscle rigidity should be advised to undergo muscle biopsy and eliminate succinylcholine in subsequent anesthetics.[213] Not all rigidity is masseter muscle rigidity; other considerations include inadequate dosage of succinylcholine, inadequate time to allow succinylcholine to work, temporomandibular joint dysfunction, and myotonic dystrophy.[210]

Table 5.1. Selected Malignant Hyperthermia–Susceptible Diseases

Central core myopathy
Myotonia congenita
King's syndrome
Schwartz-Jampel syndrome
Duchenne's muscular dystrophy
Hyperkalemic periodic paralysis
Osteogenesis imperfecta
Arthrogryposis multiplex
Becker's muscular dystrophy

Certain physical features and clinical syndromes may carry a greater risk of developing MH (Tables 5.1 and 5.2). MH may be autosomal dominant with reduced penetrance and variable expressivity.[208]

Dantrolene sodium is the only effective therapy; the initial intravenous dose is 2.5 mg per kg to a maximum cumulative dose of 10 mg per kg. Dantrolene sodium attenuates calcium release without altering calcium uptake and is believed to act at the terminal cisterna or transverse tubules of the sar-

Table 5.2. Malignant Hyperthermia and Coexisting Physical Features

Ptosis
Congenital hernias
Strabismus
Recurrent joint dislocations
Kyphoscoliosis
Pectus excavatum/carinatum
Cryptorchidism
Short stature

Note: For additional information, refer to references 212, 217–222.

coplasmic reticulum. Additional management includes discontinuation of the volatile inhalational agents; hyperventilation with 100% oxygen; correction of acidosis with sodium bicarbonate, decreasing body temperature by iced gastric, urinary, and peritoneal lavage; and forced diuresis to avoid myoglobinuric renal failure. Patients are at risk for developing disseminated intravascular coagulation. MH can reoccur within the first 24–36 hours postoperatively, necessitating further dantrolene administration.

It is important to remember that not all elevations in temperature or heart rate during anesthesia are due to MH; other entities may be responsible. Sepsis, thyrotoxicosis, and pheochromocytoma are other diseases that may cause intraoperative symptoms that mimic MH. Also, hypoxic brain damage can lead to postoperative temperature instability, elevated creatine kinase concentration, and convulsions.

Neuroleptic Malignant Syndrome

Neuroleptic malignant syndrome (NMS) is clinically similar to MH. NMS presents with hyperthermia, muscle rigidity, diaphoresis, delirium, acidosis, leukocytosis, elevated creatine kinase level, and autonomic instability. NMS is triggered by phenothiazines and butyrophenones and may follow withdrawal of drugs for treatment of Parkinson's disease.[210] NMS has not been identified as a risk factor for MH, and droperidol has not been identified as a triggering agent for MH. Patients with NMS who require electroconvulsive therapy should undergo electroconvulsive therapy without the administration of succinylcholine or other triggering agents.[210] A full discussion of NMS is included in Chapter 12.

Pseudocholinesterase Deficiency

Besides MH, another inheritable disorder is pseudocholinesterase deficiency. This enzyme deficiency is an etiology of postoperative neuromuscular weakness. Pseudocholinesterase hydrolyses acetylcholine as well as succinylcholine, mivacurium, and ester-linked local anesthetics. Therefore, a deficiency of this enzyme results in abnormally prolonged muscle relaxation when succinylcholine and mivacurium are administered.[223] Mivacurium is a short-acting nondepolarizing muscle relaxant that, like succinylcholine, requires pseudocholinesterase for degradation.

There are multiple genetic variants resulting in a spectrum of enzymatic activity. Homozygous deficiency results in the most prolonged muscle blockade (EaEa, EfEf), whereas heterozygous abnormality (silent, fluoride, atypical genes) moderately extends neuromuscular blockade. The activity of pseudocholinesterase is determined by a dibucaine test. Dibucaine normally inhibits the enzyme with a normal dibucaine number of 80. With a homozygous deficiency, the degree of inhibition decreases to less than 20% and thus a dibucaine number of 20. The other gene variants have dibucaine numbers between 40 and 70. The dibucaine number is not an indicator of the quantity of pseudocholinesterase enzyme but of the quality of enzyme action. There are acquired conditions that decrease pseudocholinesterase activity, but usually this is not clinically significant until there is a reduction to 75% of the enzyme activity levels. Associated disorders that may result in sensitivity to succinylcholine include pregnancy, liver disease, uremia, collagen vascular disease, debilitating disease, alcoholism, obesity, and thyrotoxicosis. Certain drugs may also limit the efficacy of this enzyme and include echothiophate, anticholinesterases, monoamine oxidase inhibitors, organophosphate insecticides, and chlorpromazine. Plasmapheresis, extracorporeal circulation, burns, and radiation therapy also can decrease the activity of pseudocholinesterase and prolong neuromuscular weakness.[224]

After administration of a normal dose of succinylcholine (1–2 mg per kg), the associated neuromuscular block usually resolves within 5 minutes. If an abnormal enzyme is present, the muscle weakness may be prolonged for up to 5 hours with succinylcholine and up to 6 hours with mivacurium. Management includes continuation of mechanical ventilation until residual muscle weakness has resolved and the patient can regain control of ventilation. Transfused blood may contain pseudocholinesterase in sufficient quantities to metabolize the succinylcholine and improve the weakness. Administration of reversal agents (anticholinesterases) tends to worsen the weakness, with initial improvement followed by intensification of the neuromuscular block. The most appropriate management is a tincture of time to allow spontaneous recovery of neuromuscular strength. This involves continuation of mechanical ventilation and appropriate sedation.

Occasionally, in the postanesthesia care unit, the issue of prolonged neuromuscular blockade does arise and results in continued mechanical ventilation or a replacement of an endotracheal tube on an urgent basis. Inadequate reversal of neuromuscular blockers is the most common cause for residual muscle weakness in the postanesthesia care unit and can result in hypoxia, hypercarbia, cardiac arrhythmias, and altered mental status. Typically, patients have a discoordinated respiratory pattern, shallow respirations, and weak limbs and are extremely anxious. With the use of intermediate to short-acting agents (atracurium, cis-atracurium, rocuronium, vecuronium, mivacurium), fewer incidents of recurarization and muscle weakness occur. Prolonged muscle blockade may occur from drug interactions and metabolic disturbances. Certain antibiotics (neomycin, streptomycin, clindamycin and other aminoglycosides, and polymyxins) and antiarrhythmics (lidocaine, procainamide, quinidine) may prolong the muscle blockade.[224] Hypothermia, hypokalemia, hypocalcemia, acidosis, and hepatic and renal insufficiency are other causes of prolonged muscle weakness in the postoperative period.

Patients with myasthenia gravis pose a unique challenge to the anesthesiologist because a narrow spectrum between central cholinergic crisis and myasthenic crisis exists. Traditionally, neuromuscular blocking agents are avoided in patients with myasthenia gravis, as the extreme sensitivity to nondepolarizing muscle relaxants can require postoperative mechanical ventilatory support. These patients are exquisitely sensitive to muscle relaxants; the dose required to produce neuromuscular blockade is reduced by approximately 75% compared with normal individuals. Criteria that may make postoperative controlled ventilation more likely include a disease duration over 6 years, presence of chronic obstructive pulmonary disease, a pyridostigmine dose of more than 750 mg per day, and a vital capacity of less than 2.9 liters.[225] Continuation of the patient's current anticholinesterase regimen on the day of surgery optimizes muscular strength. These patients may be intubated without muscle relaxants or with carefully titrated doses of neuromuscular blockers to limit muscle weakness at the conclusion of surgery. If muscle relaxants are required, the dose should be reduced by one-half to two-thirds, with close monitoring using a peripheral nerve stimulator for maintenance and reversal of muscle paralysis.[225] It is imperative to ascertain that adequate muscle strength has returned prior to extubation, and if necessary, mechanical ventilation should be continued until such time. Excessive anticholinesterase drugs may result in potentiation of skeletal muscle weakness and central cholinergic crisis. Presence of salivation, miosis, bradycardia, and accentuated muscle weakness may indicate this etiology. Therapy involves administration of atropine.

Atlantoaxial Instability

Cervical spine instability places patients with rheumatoid arthritis and Down syndrome at high risk for cervical spinal cord injury during direct laryngoscopy and surgical positioning. It is common practice to place individuals in a "sniffing" position prior to intubation. This mandates lower cervical spine flexion and occipitoatlantoaxial extension to align the oral-pharyngeal-laryngeal axis. In patients with cervical spine instability (cervical osteoarthritis, cervical osteomyelitis, trisomy 21, rheumatoid arthritis, ankylosing spondylitis), this maneuver may induce atlantoaxial subluxation and cervical spinal cord impingement, resulting in tetraplegia. Patients with conditions such as Morquio's syndrome, Klippel-Feil syndrome, Down syndrome, osteogenesis imperfecta, neurofibromatosis, and disproportionate dwarfism may have odontoid hypoplasia and are at risk for subluxation.[226] Atlantoaxial instability occurs in 10–20% of patients with Down syndrome.[227] Some centers recommend cervical spine radiographs before elective surgery in all children with Down syndrome.[226, 228, 229]

In rheumatoid arthritis, the cervical spine is frequently involved, with up to 40–70% of patients having symptoms related to neck instability.[226] Abnormal radiographs are present in up to 86% of patients with rheumatoid arthritis; males with rheumatoid arthritis, subcutaneous nodules, and a long duration of disease are more likely to experience atlantoaxial subluxation.[226] Preoperative radiographic studies should be considered in these patients prior to elective anesthesia. Ankylosing spondylitis also places patients at greater risk of neurologic sequelae if careful laryngoscopy and positioning are not followed. Patients with ankylosing spondylitis are typically fused in a flexed position and may undergo extension injury easily. Movement of the fused spine can result in epidural hemorrhage,[226] and these patients benefit from being positioned in a flexed manner. Atlantoaxial subluxation and cervical osteomyelitis may occur as a complication of tonsillectomy and adenoidectomy, and these patients may present postoperatively with neck pain.[230]

Intubation of a patient with unstable cervical spine is a dilemma because significant cervical spine movement occurs with normal direct laryngoscopy. These cervical spine movements are not reduced with soft or hard collars, so intubation should be performed in a neutral head position with manual in-line traction. The in-line traction does result in radiographic distraction and lengthening of the spinal cord, but clinically no adverse neurologic incidents occur. It is important to remember that common anesthetic techniques to maintain airway patency result in stress on the cervical spine. Maneuvers such as a chin lift, jaw thrust, and placement of oral and nasopharyngeal airways may induce strain on the atlantoaxial joint. Also, cricoid pressure may result in posterior displacement of the spine and must be carefully applied in rapid sequence intubations in high-risk populations for cervical instability. Awake intubation techniques may be superior as postintubation neurologic assessments can be performed.

Conclusion

Neurologic complications secondary to general or regional anesthesia are infrequent and may involve the central or peripheral nervous system. These complications can result in potentially devastating injuries, and it is imperative to quickly diagnose and manage the complications as they arise.

References

1. Dyer CB. Ashton CM, Teasdale TA. Postoperative delirium: a review of 80 primary data-collection studies. Arch Intern Med 1995;155:461.
2. Rosenberg H, Goldberg M. Postoperative Emotional Responses. In N Gravenstein, RR Kirby (eds), Complications of Anesthesiology (2nd ed). Philadelphia: Lippincott–Raven, 1996;431.
3. Marcantonio ER, Goldman L, Mangione CM, et al. A clinical prediction rule for delirium after noncardiac surgery. JAMA 1994;271:134.
4. Siebert CP. Recognition, management, and prevention of neuropsychological dysfunction after operation. Int Anesthesiol Clin 1986;24:39.
5. Chonchubhair AN, Valacio R, Kelly J, O'Keeffe S. Use of the abbreviated mental status to detect postoperative delirium in the elderly people. Br J Anaesth 1995; 75:481.
6. Shaw PJ. Neurologic complications of cardiovascular surgery: II. Procedures involving the heart and thoracic aorta. Int Anesthesiol Clin 1986;24:159.
7. Parikh SS, Chung F. Postoperative delirium in the elderly. Anesth Analg 1995;80:1223.
8. Crosby G. Impaired Central Nervous System Function. In JL Benumof, LJ Saidman (eds), Anesthesia and Perioperative Complications. St. Louis: Mosby–Year Book, 1992;356.
9. Tune LE, Holland A, Folstein MF, et al. Association of postoperative delirium with raised serum levels of anticholinergic drugs. Lancet 1981;2:651.
10. Naber D, Sand P, Heigl B. Psychopathological and neuropsychological effects of 8 days' corticosteroid treatment. Psychoneuroendocrinology 1996;21:25.
11. Travlos A, Hirsch G. Steroid psychosis: a cause of confusion on the acute spinal cord injury unit. Arch Phys Med Rehabil 1993;74:312.
12. Van Der Mast RC, Fekkes D, Moleman P, Pepplinkhuizen L. Is postoperative delirium related to reduced plasma tryptophan? Lancet 1991;338:851.
13. Hindman BJ. Perioperative stroke: the non-cardiac surgery patient. Int Anesthesiol Clin 1986;24:101.
14. Hart R, Hindman B. Mechanisms of perioperative cerebral infarction. Stroke 1982;13:766.
15. Furlan AJ, Breuer AC. Central nervous system complications of open heart surgery. Stroke 1984;15:912.

16. Carney WI, Stewart WB, DePinto DJ, et al. Carotid bruit as a risk factor in aortoiliac reconstruction. Surgery 1977;81:567.
17. Treiman RL, Foran RF, Cohen JL, et al. Carotid bruit: a follow-up report on its significance in patients undergoing an abdominal aortic operation. Arch Surg 1979; 114:1138.
18. Sieber FE, Toung TJ, Diringer MN, Wang H. Factors influencing stroke outcome following carotid endarterectomy. Anesth Analg 1990;70:S370.
19. Porter J, Hart S, Keohane C. Unexpected neurological deficits following recovery from anaesthesia. Can J Anaesth 1994;41:317.
20. Skillman JJ. Neurologic complications of cardiovascular surgery: I. Procedures involving the carotid arteries and abdominal aorta. Int Anesthesiol Clin 1986;24:135.
21. Garg BP, Bruno A, Biller J. Moyamoya Disease and Cerebral Ischemia. In H Hunt Batjer (ed), Cerebrovascular Disease. Philadelphia: Lippincott–Raven, 1997; 489.
22. Nielson TG, Sillesen H, Schroeder TV. Seizures following carotid endarterectomy in patients with severely compromised cerebral circulation. Eur J Vasc Endovasc Surg 1995;9:53.
23. Brown DL, Ransom DM, Hall JA, et al. Regional anesthesia and local anesthetic-induced systemic toxicity: seizure frequency and accompanying cardiovascular changes. Anesth Analg 1995;81:321.
24. Wijdicks EFM. Neurologic complications in critically ill patients. Anesth Analg 1996;83:411.
25. Miller G, Eggli KD, Contant C, et al. Postoperative neurologic complications after open heart surgery on young infants. Arch Pediatr Adolesc Med 1995;149:764.
26. Kroll DA, Caplan RA, Posner K, et al. Nerve injury associated with anesthesia. Anesthesiology 1990;73:202.
27. Parks BJ. Postoperative peripheral nerve neuropathies. Surgery 1973;74:348.
28. Thompson GE, Lui ACP. Perioperative Nerve Injury. In JL Benumof, LJ Saidman (eds), Anesthesia and Perioperative Complications (2nd ed). St. Louis: Mosby–Year Book, 1992;160.
29. Abram SE, Hogan QH. Complications of Nerve Blocks. In JL Benumof, LJ Saidman (eds), Anesthesia and Perioperative Complications (2nd ed). St. Louis: Mosby–Year Book, 1992;52.
30. Nakata DA, Stoelting RK. Positioning. In JD Martin, MA Warner (eds), Positioning in Anesthesia and Surgery (3rd ed). Philadelphia: Saunders, 1997;293.
31. Selander D, Dhuner KG, Lundborg G. Peripheral nerve injury due to injection needles used for regional anesthesia. Acta Anaesthesiol Scand 1977;21:182.
32. Britt BA, Joy N, Mackay MB. Anesthesia-Related Trauma Caused by Patient Malpositioning. In N Gravenstein, RR Kirby (eds), Complications in Anesthesiology (2nd ed). Philadelphia: Lippincott–Raven, 1996;365.
33. Sy WP. Ulnar nerve palsy possibly related to use of automatically cycled blood pressure cuff. Anesth Analg 1981;60:687.
34. Zylicz Z, Nuyten FJJ, Notermans SLH, Koene RAP. Postoperative ulnar neuropathy after kidney transplantation. Anaesthesia 1984;39:1117.
35. Alvine FG, Shurrer ME. Postoperative ulnar-nerve palsy. J Bone Joint Surg Am 1987;69:255.
36. Stoelting RK. Postoperative ulnar nerve palsy—is it a preventable complication? Anesth Analg 1993;76:7.
37. Dawson DM, Krarup C. Perioperative nerve lesions. Arch Neurol 1989;46:1355.
38. Dornette WHL. Compression neuropathies: medical aspects and legal implications. Int Anesthesiol Clin 1986;24:200.
39. Lederman RJ, Breuer AC, Hanson MR, et al. Peripheral nervous system complications of coronary artery bypass graft surgery. Ann Neurol 1982;12:297.
40. Kirsh MM, Magee KR, Gago O, et al. Brachial plexus injury following median sternotomy incision. Ann Thorac Surg 1971;11:315.
41. Bickler PE, Schapera A, Bainton CR. Acute radial nerve injury from use of an automatic blood pressure monitor. Anesthesiology 1990;73:186.
42. Kane RE. Neurologic deficits following epidural or spinal anesthesia. Anesth Analg 1981;60:150.
43. Warner MA, Martin JT, Schroeder DR, et al. Lower-extremity motor neuropathy associated with surgery performed on patients in a lithotomy position. Anesthesiology 1994;81:6.
44. Yuen EC, Layzer RB, Weitz SR, Olney RK. Neurologic complications of lumbar epidural anesthesia and analgesia. Neurology 1995;45:1795.
45. McQuarrie HG, Harris JW, Ellsworth HS, et al. Sciatic neuropathy complicating vaginal hysterectomy. J Obstet Gynecol 1972;113:223.
46. Gentili F, Hudson AR, Hunter D. Clinical and experimental aspects of injection injuries of peripheral nerves. Can J Neurol Sci 1980;7:143.
47. Steward DJ. Eutectic mixture of local anesthetics (EMLA): what is it? What does it do? J Pediatr 1993; 122:S21.
48. Tse S, Barrington K, Byrne P. Methemoglobinemia associated with prilocaine use in neonatal circumcision. Am J Perinatol 1995;12:331.
49. Vandam LD. Complications of Spinal and Epidural Anesthesia. In FK Orkin, LH Cooperman (eds), Complications of Anesthesiology. Philadelphia: Lippincott, 1983;75.
50. Horlocker TT, Wedel DJ, Schlicting JL. Postoperative epidural analgesia and oral anticoagulant therapy. Anesth Analg 1994:79;89.
51. Vandermeulen EP, Van Aken H, Vermylen J. Anticoagulants and spinal-epidural anesthesia. Anesth Analg 1994;79:1165.
52. Rao TL, El-Etr AA. Anticoagulation following placement of epidural and subarachnoid catheters: an evaluation of neurologic sequela. Anesthesiology 1981;55:618.

53. Owens EL, Kasten GW, Hessel EA. Spinal subarachnoid hematoma after lumbar puncture and heparinization. Anesth Analg 1986;65:1201.
54. Ganjoo P, Singh AK, Mishra VK, et al. Postblock epidural hematoma causing paraplegia. Reg Anesth 1994;19:62.
55. Odoom JA, Sih IL. Epidural analgesia and anticoagulant therapy. Experience with one thousand cases of continuous epidurals. Anaesthesia 1983;38:254.
56. Bergqvist D, Lindblab B, Matzsch T. Low molecular weight heparin for thromboprophylaxis and epidural/spinal anaesthesia—is there a risk? Acta Anaesth Scand 1992;36:605.
57. Dickman CA, Shedd SA, Spetzler RF, et al. Spinal epidural hematoma associated with epidural anesthesia: complications of systemic heparinization in patients receiving peripheral vascular thrombolytic therapy. Anesthesiology 1990;72:947.
58. Metzger G, Singbartl G. Spinal epidural hematoma following epidural anesthesia versus spontaneous spinal subdural hematoma. Two case reports. Acta Anaesth Scand 1991;35:105.
59. Sternlo JE, Hybbinette CH. Spinal subdural bleeding after attempted epidural and subsequent spinal anesthesia in a patient on thromboprophylaxis with low molecular weight heparin. Acta Anaesth Scand 1995;39:557.
60. Hynson JM, Katz JA, Bueff HU. Epidural hematoma associated with enoxaparin. Anesth Analg 1996:82;1072.
61. Horlocker TT. When to remove a spinal or epidural catheter in an anticoagulated patient. Reg Anesth 1993;18:264.
62. Ellison N, Jobes DR, Scwartz J. Implications of anticoagulant therapy. Int Anesthesiol Clin 1982;20:121.
63. Baron HC, LaRaja RD, Rossi G, Atkinson D. Continuous epidural analgesia in the heparinized vascular surgical patient: a retrospective review of 912 patients. J Vasc Surg 1987;6:144.
64. DeAngelis J. Hazards of subdural and epidural anesthesia during anticoagulant therapy: a case report and review. Anest Analg 1972;51:676.
65. Janis KM. Epidural hematoma following postoperative epidural analgesia: a case report. Anesth Analg 1972; 51:689.
66. Ruff RL, Dougherty JH. Complications of lumbar puncture followed by anticoagulation. Stroke 1981; 12:879.
67. Onishchuk JL, Carlsson C. Epidural hematoma associated with epidural anesthesia: complications of anticoagulant therapy. Anesthesiology 1992;77:1221.
68. Martinez-Palli G, Sala-Blanch X, Salvado E, et al. Epidural hematoma after epidural anesthesia in a patient with peripheral vascular disease. Reg Anesth 1996;21:342.
69. Horlocker TT, Wedel DJ, Offord KP. Does preoperative antiplatelet therapy increase the risk of hemorrhagic complications associated with regional anesthesia? Anesth Analg 1990;70:631.
70. Holt HM, Anderson SS, Gahrn-Hansen B, Siboni K. Infections following epidural catherization. J Hosp Infect 1995;30:253.
71. Baker AS, Ojemann RG, Swartz MN, Richardson EP. Spinal epidural abscess. N Engl J Med 1975;293:463.
72. Verner EF, Musher DM. Spinal epidural abscess. Med Clin North Am 1985;69:375.
73. Jakobsen KB, Christensen MK, Carlsson PS. Extradural anaesthesia for repeated surgical treatment in the presence of infection. Br J Anaesth 1995;75:536.
74. DuPen SL, Peterson DG, Williams A, Bogosian AJ. Infection during chronic epidural catherization: diagnosis and treatment. Anesthesiology 1990;73:905.
75. Darchy B, Forceville X, Bavoux E, et al. Clinical and bacteriologic survey of epidural analgesia in patients in the intensive care unit. Anesthesiology 1996;85:988.
76. Miller JR, Jubelt B. Bacterial Infections of the Central Nervous System. In LP Rowland (ed), Merritt's Textbook of Neurology (9th ed). Baltimore: Williams & Wilkins, 1995;102.
77. Wang JS, Fellows DG, Vakharia S, et al. Epidural abscess—early magnetic resonance imaging detection and conservative therapy. Anesth Analg 1996;82:1069.
78. Goodman EJ, DeHorta E, Taguiam JM. Safety of spinal and epidural anesthesia in parturients with chorioamnionitis. Reg Anesth 1996;21:436.
79. Loarie DJ, Fairley HB. Epidural abscess following spinal anesthesia. Anesth Analg 1978;57:351.
80. Heusner AP. Nontuberculous spinal epidural infections. N Engl J Med 1948;239:845.
81. Mampalam TJ, Rosegay H, Andrews BT, et al. Nonoperative treatment of spinal epidural infections. J Neurosurg 1989;71:208.
82. Darouiche RO, Hamill RJ, Greenberg SB. Bacterial spinal epidural abscess: review of 43 cases and literature survey. Medicine 1992;71:369.
83. Amoiridis G, Wohrle JC, Langkafel M, et al. Spinal cord infarction in a patient in the hyperlordotic position. Anesthesiology 1996;84:228.
84. Usubiaga JE. Neurological complications following epidural anesthesia. Int Anesthesiol Clin 1975;13:50.
85. Mutch WAC, Thiessen DB, Girling LG, Graham MR. Neuroanesthesia adjunct therapy (mannitol and hyperventilation) is as effective as cerebrospinal fluid drainage for prevention of paraplegia after descending thoracic aortic cross-clamping in the dog. Anesth Analg 1995;81:800.
86. McCullough JL, Hollier LH, Nugent M. Paraplegia after thoracic aortic occlusion: influence of cerebrospinal fluid drainage. J Vasc Surg 1988;7:153.
87. Fitzgibbon DR, Glosten B, Wright I, et al. Paraplegia, epidural analgesia, and thoracic aneurysmectomy. Anesthesiology 1995;83:1355.
88. Dommisse GF. The arteries, arterioles, and capillaries of the spinal cord. Surgical guidelines in the prevention of postoperative paraplegia. Ann R Coll Surg Engl 1980;62:369.

89. Adriani J, Naragi M. Paraplegia associated with epidural anesthesia. South Med J 1986;79:1350.
90. Bromage PR. Spinal cord infarction after surgery in a patient in the hyperlordotic position. Anesthesiology 1996;85:429.
91. Skouen JS. Paraplegia following epidural anesthesia. Acta Anaesth Scand 1985;72:437.
92. Cherry DA, Lamberty J. Paraplegia following coeliac plexus block. Anaesth Intensive Care 1984;12:59.
93. Shah JL. Influence of cerebrospinal fluid on epidural pressure. Anaesthesia 1981;36:627.
94. Davies A, Solomon B, Levene A. Paraplegia following epidural anaesthesia. BMJ 1958;2:654.
95. Dohi S, Matsumiya N, Takeshima R, Naito H. The effects of subarachnoid lidocaine and phenylephrine on spinal cord and cerebral blood flow in dogs. Anesthesiology 1984;61:238.
96. Kazody R, Palahniuk RJ, Wade JG, Cumming MO. The effect of subarachnoid epinephrine and phenylephrine on spinal cord blood flow. Can Anaesth Soc J 1984;31:503.
97. Kazody R, Swartz J, Palahniuk RJ, et al. Spinal cord blood flow following subarachnoid lidocaine. Can Anaesth Soc J 1985;32:472.
98. Woodham MJ, Hanna MH. Paraplegia after coeliac plexus block. Anaesthesia 1989;44:487.
99. Galizia EJ, Lahiri SK. Paraplegia following coeliac plexus block with phenol. Br J Anaesth 1974;46:539.
100. Thompson GE, Bridenbaugh LD, Artin RY. Abdominal pain and alcohol celiac plexus nerve block. Anesth Analg 1977;56:1.
101. Lo JN, Buckley JJ. Spinal cord ischemia: a complication of celiac plexus block. Reg Anesth 1982;7:66.
102. Parris WCV, Kirshner HS. Motor paralysis of the lower extremities following lumbar sympathetic block. Anesthesiology 1993;78:981.
103. Crawford ES, Svensson LG, Hess KR, et al. A prospective randomized study of cerebrospinal fluid drainage to prevent paraplegia after high-risk surgery on the thoracoabdominal aorta. J Vasc Surg 1991;13:36.
104. Shenaq SA, Svensson LG. Paraplegia following aortic surgery. J Cardiothorac Vasc Surg 1993;7:81.
105. Harrison PD. Paraplegia following epidural analgesia. Anaesthesia 1975;30:778.
106. Moir DD, Davidson S. Postpartum complications of forceps delivery performed under epidural and pudendal nerve block. Br J Anaesth 1972;44:1197.
107. Grove LH. Backache, headache, and bladder dysfunction after delivery. Br J Anaesth 1973;45:1147.
108. Chadwick HS, Bonica JJ. Complications of Regional Anesthesia. In JJ Bonica, JS McDonald (eds), Principles and Practice of Obstetrical Anesthesia and Analgesia. Baltimore: Williams & Wilkins, 1995;538.
109. Cotev S, Robin GC, Davidson JT. Back pain after epidural analgesia. Anesth Analg 1967;46:259.
110. Crawford JS. Some maternal complications of epidural analgesia for labour. Anaesthesia 1985;40:1219.
111. MacArthur C, Lewis M, Knox EG, Crawford JS. Epidural anesthesia and long term backache after childbirth. BMJ 1990;301:9.
112. Shutt LE. Backache after spinal anesthesia. Reg Anesth 1995;20:253.
113. Faure E, Moreno R, Thisted R. Incidence of postdural puncture headache in morbidly obese parturients. Reg Anesth 1994;19:361.
114. Heyman HJ, Salem MR, Joseph NJ. Maternal obesity and headache following unexpected dural puncture. Anesthesiology 1990;73:A971.
115. Lybecker H, Djernes M, Schmidt JF. Postdural puncture headache (PDPH): onset, duration, severity, and associated symptoms. Acta Anaesthesiol Scand 1995;39:605.
116. Shearer VE, Jhaveri H, Cunningham FG. Puerperal seizures after post-dural puncture headache. Obstet Gynecol 1995;85:255.
117. Halpern S, Preston R. Postdural puncture headache and spinal needle design. Anesthesiology 1994;81:1376.
118. Dittmann M, Schaefer HG, Renkl F, Greve I. Spinal anaesthesia with 29 gauge Quincke point needles and post dural puncture headache in 2,378 patients. Acta Anaesth Scand 1994;38:691.
119. Lynch J, Arhelger S, Krings-Ernst I. Post-dural puncture headache in young orthopaedic in-patients: comparison of a .33mm (29-gauge) Quincke-type with a .7mm (22-gauge) Whitacre spinal needle in 200 patients. Acta Anesth Scand 1992;36:58.
120. Ross AW, Greenhalgh C, McGlade DP, et al. The Sprotte needle and postdural puncture headache following caesarean section. Anaesth Intensive Care 1993;21:280.
121. Muller B, Adelt K, Reichmann H, Toyka K. Atraumatic needle reduces the incidence of post-lumbar puncture syndrome. J Neurol 1994;241:376.
122. Peterman S. Postmyelography headache rates with Whitacre versus Quincke 22-gauge spinal needles. Radiology 1996;200:771.
123. Buettner J, Wresch KP, Klose R. Postdural puncture headache: comparison of 25-gauge Whitacre and Quincke needles. Reg Anesth 1993;18:166.
124. Norris MC, Leighton BL, DeSimone CA. Needle bevel direction and headache after inadvertent dural puncture. Anesthesiology 1989;70:729.
125. Mihic DN. Postspinal headache and relationship of needle bevel to longitudinal dural fibers. Reg Anesth 1985;10:76.
126. Seeberger MD, Kaufmann M, Staender S, et al. Repeated dural punctures increase the incidence of postdural puncture headache. Anesth Analg 1996;82:302.
127. Carson DF, Serpell MG. Clinical characteristics of commonly used spinal needles. Anaesthesia 1995;50:523.
128. Denny N, Masters R, Pearson D, et al. Postdural puncture headache after continuous spinal anesthesia. Anesth Analg 1987;66:791.
129. Blaise GA, Cournoyer S, Perrault C, et al. Spinal catheter does not reduce the post-dural puncture

headache after caesarean section. Can J Anaesth 1992;39:633.
130. Liu N, Montefiore A, Kermarec N, et al. Prolonged placement of spinal catheters does not prevent postdural puncture headache. Reg Anesth 1993;18:110.
131. Norris MC, Leighton BL. Continuous spinal anesthesia after unintentional dural puncture in parturients. Reg Anesth 1990;15:285.
132. Eldor J. The timing of opioid administration in postdural puncture headache. Reg Anesth 1994;19:222.
133. Taivainen T, Pitkanen M, Tuominen M, Rosenberg PH. Efficacy of epidural blood patch for postdural puncture headache. Acta Anaesth Scand 1993;37:702.
134. Szeinfeld M, Ihmeidan IH, Moser MM, et al. Epidural blood patch: evaluation of the volume and spread of blood injected into the epidural space. Anesthesiology 1986;64:820.
135. Abouleish E, Vega S, Blendinger I, Tio T. Long-term follow-up of epidural blood patch. Anesth Analg 1975; 54:459.
136. Colonna-Romano P, Shapiro BE. Unintentional dural puncture and prophylactic epidural blood patch in obstetrics. Anesth Analg 1989;69:522.
137. Craft JB, Epstein BS, Coakley CS. Prophylaxis of dural-puncture headache with epidural saline. Anesth Analg 1973;52:228.
138. Umstad MP, Ross AW, Adey FD. Headache following epidural analgesia. Aust N Z J Obstet Gynaecol 1992; 32:79.
139. Day CJ, Shutt LE. Auditory, ocular, and facial complications of central neural block. Reg Anesth 1996;21:197.
140. Narchi P, Veyrac P, Viale M. Long-term postdural puncture auditory symptoms: effective relief after epidural blood patch. Anesth Analg 1996;82:1303.
141. Wang LP, Fog J, Bove M. Transient hearing loss following spinal anaesthesia. Anaesthesia 1987;42:1258.
142. Fog J, Wang LP, Sundberg A, Mucchiano C. Hearing loss after spinal anesthesia is related to needle size. Anesth Analg 1990;70:517.
143. Wemama JP, Delecroix M, Nyarwaya JB, Krivosic-Horber R. Permanent unilateral vestibulocochlear dysfunction after spinal anesthesia. Anesth Analg 1996; 82:406.
144. Hardy PAJ. Hypoacousis following epidural injection. Br J Anaesth 1986;58:572.
145. Lee CM, Peachman FA. Unilateral hearing loss after spinal anesthesia treated with epidural blood patch. Anesth Analg 1986;65:312.
146. Lybecker H, Anderson T. Repetitive hearing loss following dural puncture treated with autologous epidural blood patch. Acta Anaesth Scand 1995;39:987.
147. Fine J, Weissman J, Finestone SC. Side effects after ketamine anesthesia: transient blindness. Anesth Analg 1974;53:72.
148. Defalque RJ, Miller DW. Visual disturbances during transurethral resection of the prostate. Can Anaesth Soc J 1975;22:620.
149. Snow JC, Kripke BJ, Norton ML, et al. Corneal injuries during general anesthesia. Anesth Analg 1975;54:465.
150. Victory RA, Hassett P, Morrison G. Transient blindness following epidural analgesia. Anaesthesia 1991;46:940.
151. Ling C, Atkinson PL, Munton CGF. Bilateral retinal haemorrhages following epidural injection. Br J Ophthalmol 1993;77:316.
152. Clayton KC. The incidence of Horner's syndrome during lumbar extradural for elective caesarean section and provision of analgesia during labour. Anaesthesia 1983;38:583.
153. Sprung J, Haddox D, Maitra-D'Cruze AM. Horner's syndrome and trigeminal nerve palsy following epidural anaesthesia for obstetrics. Can J Anaesth 1991;38:767.
154. Shigematsu T. Trigeminal nerve palsy after lumbar epidural anesthesia. Anesth Analg 1985;64:646.
155. Eng RH, Seligman SJ. Lumbar puncture-induced meningitis. JAMA 1981;245:1456.
156. Chestnut DH. Spinal anesthesia in the febrile patient. Anesthesiology 1992;76:667.
157. Bader AM, Gilbertson L, Kirz L, Datta S. Regional anesthesia in women with chorioamnionitis. Reg Anesth 1992;17:84.
158. Harding SA, Collis RE, Morgan BM. Meningitis after combined spinal-extradural anaesthesia in obstetrics. Br J Anaesth 1994;73:545.
159. Cascio M, Heath G. Meningitis following a combined spinal-epidural technique in a labouring term parturient. Can J Anaesth 1996;43:399.
160. Stallard N, Barry P. Another complication of the combined extradural-subarachnoid technique. Br J Anaesth 1995;75:370.
161. Ready LB, Helfer D. Bacterial meningitis in parturients after epidural anesthesia. Anesthesiology 1989;71:988.
162. Hargreaves J. Metal particle generation caused by the combined spinal-extradural technique. Br J Anaesth 1993;70:706.
163. Scott DB, Hibbard BM. Serious non-fatal complications associated with extradural block in obstetric practice. Br J Anaesth 1990;64:537.
164. Lee JJ, Parry H. Bacterial meningitis following spinal anaesthesia for caesarean section. Br J Anaesth 1991; 66:383.
165. Crosby ET, Halpern SH, Rolbin SH. Epidural anaesthesia for caesarean section in patients with active recurrent genital herpes simplex infections: a retrospective review. Can J Anaesth 1989;36:701.
166. Ravindran RS, Gupta CD, Stoops CA. Epidural analgesia in the presence of herpes simplex virus (type 2) infection. Anesth Analg 1982;61:714.
167. Ramanthan S, Sheth R, Turndorf H. Anesthesia for cesarean section in patients with genital herpes infections: a retrospective study. Anesthesiology 1986;64: 807.
168. Bert AA, Laasberg LH. Aseptic meningitis following spinal anesthesia complication of the past? Anesthesiology 1985;62:674.

169. Eldor J. Metallic particles in the spinal-needle technique [letter]. Reg Anesth 1994;19:219.
170. Eldor J, Brodsky V. Danger of metallic particles in the spinal-epidural spaces using the needle-through-needle approach. Acta Anesth Scand 1991;35:461.
171. Molin JD, Knape KG, Herman NL, Husain FJ. No metal particle contamination of epidural or subarachnoid spaces using needle-through-needle techniques. Anesthesiology 1992;77:A1031.
172. Carrie LES. Metallic fragments and the combined spinal-extradural technique. Br J Anaesth 1991;67:662.
173. Roberts SP, Petts HV. Meningitis after obstetric spinal anesthesia. Anaesthesia 1990;45:376.
174. Abouleish E, Amortegui A, Taylor F. Are bacterial filters needed in continuous epidural analgesia for obstetrics? Anesthesiology 1977;46:351.
175. Schell RM, Brauer FS, Cole DJ, Applegate RL. Persistent sacral nerve root deficits after continuous spinal anaesthesia. Can J Anaesth 1991;38:908.
176. Denny NM. Continuous spinal anaesthesia and cauda equina syndrome [letter]. Anaesthesia 1995;50:474.
177. Peyton P. Cauda equina syndrome and continuous spinal anesthesia [letter]. Anesthesiology 1993;78:214.
178. Rigler ML, Drasner K, Krejcie TC, et al. Cauda equina syndrome after continuous spinal anesthesia. Anesth Analg 1991;72:275.
179. Jaradeh S. Cauda equina syndrome: a neurologist's perspective. Reg Anesth 1993;18:473.
180. Ravindran RS, Turner MS, Muller J. Neurologic effects of subarachnoid administration of 2-chloroprocaine-ce, bupivacaine, and low pH normal saline in dogs. Anesth Analg 1982;61:279.
181. Reisner LS, Hochman BN, Plumer MH. Persistent neurologic deficit and adhesive arachnoiditis following intrathecal 2-chloroprocaine injection. Anesth Analg 1980;59:452.
182. Moore DC, Spierdijk J, vanKleef JD, et al. Chloroprocaine neurotoxicity: four additional cases. Anesth Analg 1982;61:155.
183. Allen PR, Johnson RW. Subarachnoid injection during extradural analgesia for labour using 2-chloroprocaine. Anaesthesia 1979;34:874.
184. Ravindran RS, Bond VK, Tasch MD, et al. Prolonged neural blockade following regional anesthesia with 2-chloroprocaine. Anesth Analg 1980;59:447.
185. Barsa J, Batra M, Fink BR, Sumi SM. A comparative in vivo study of local neurotoxicity of lidocaine, bupivacaine, 2-chloroprocaine, and a mixture of 2-chloroprocaine and bupivacaine. Anesth Analg 1982;61:961.
186. Steen PA, Michenfelder JD. Neurotoxicity of anesthetics. Anesthesiology 1979;50:437.
187. Lambert LA, Lambert DH, Strichartz GR. Potential neurotoxicity of lidocaine and dextrose solutions used for spinal anesthesia. Reg Anesth 1992;35S:164.
188. Ready BL, Plumer MH, Haschke RH, et al. Neurotoxicity of intrathecal local anesthetics in rabbits. Anesthesiology 1985;63:364.
189. Drasner K. Models for local anesthetic toxicity from continuous spinal anesthesia. Reg Anesth 1993;18:434.
190. Myers RR, Kalichman MW, Reisner LS, Powell HC. Neurotoxicity of local anesthetics: altered perineural permeability, edema, and nerve fiber injury. Anesthesiology 1986:64:29.
191. Lambert LA, Lambert DH, Strichartz GR. Irreversible conduction block in isolated nerve by high concentration of local anesthetic. Anesthesiology 1994;80:1082.
192. Bainton CR, Strichartz GR. Concentration dependence of lidocaine-induced irreversible conduction loss in frog nerve. Anesthesiology 1994;81:657.
193. Sakura S, Chan VW, Ciriales R, Drasner K. The addition of 7.5% glucose does not alter the neurotoxicity of 5% lidocaine administered intrathecally in the rat. Anesthesiology 1995;82:236.
194. Schneider M, Ettlin T, Kaufmann M, et al. Transient neurologic toxicity after hyperbaric subarachnoid anesthesia with 5% lidocaine. Anesth Analg 1993;76:1154.
195. Beardsley D, Holman S, Gantt R, et al. Transient neurologic deficit after spinal anesthesia: local anesthetic maldistribution with pencil point needles? Anesth Analg 1995;81:314.
196. Pollock JE, Neal JM, Stephenson CA, Wiley CE. Prospective study of the incidence of transient radicular irritation in patients undergoing spinal anesthesia. Anesthesiology 1996;84:1361.
197. Sjostrom S, Blass J. Severe pain in both legs after spinal anaesthesia with hyperbaric 5% lignocaine solution. Anaesthesia 1994;49:700.
198. Sumi M, Sakura S, Kosaka Y. Intrathecal hyperbaric .5% tetracaine as a possible cause of transient neurologic toxicity. Anesth Analg 1996;82:1076.
199. Hampl KF, Schneider MC, Ummenhofer W, Drewe J. Transient neurologic symptoms after spinal anesthesia. Anesth Analg 1995;81:1148.
200. Pinczower GR, Chadwick HS, Woodland R, Lowmiller M. Bilateral leg pain following lidocaine spinal anaesthesia. Can J Anaesth 1995;42:217.
201. Tarkkila P, Huhtala J, Tuominen M. Transient radicular irritation after spinal anaesthesia with hyperbaric lignocaine. Br J Anaesth 1995;74:328.
202. Pollock JE, Mulroy MF, Stephenson C. Spinal anesthesia and the incidence of transient radicular irritation. Anesthesiology 1994;81:A1029.
203. Wong CA, Benzon H, Kim C. Bilateral radicular pain after epidural lidocaine [letter]. Reg Anesth 1996; 21:600.
204. Lambert LA, Lambert DH. 5% Lidocaine safety debate continues [letter]. Anesthesia Patient Safety Foundation Newsletter 1996;11:22.
205. Carpenter RL. Hyperbaric lidocaine spinal anesthesia: do we need an alternative? Anesth Analg 1995;81:1125.
206. Gronert GA, Mott J, Lee J. Aetiology of malignant hyperthermia. Br J Anaesth 1988;60:253.
207. Ording H. Incidence of malignant hyperthermia in Denmark. Anesth Analg 1985;64:700.

208. Britt BA, Kalow W. Malignant hyperthermia: a statistical review. Can Anaesth Soc J 1970;17:293.
209. Ellis FR, Halsall PJ, Christian AS. Clinical presentation of suspected malignant hyperthermia during anaesthesia in 402 probands. Anaesthesia 1990;45:838.
210. Rosenberg H, Fletcher J, Seitman D. Pharmacogenetics. In PG Barash, BF Cullen, RK Stoelting (eds), Clinical Anesthesia (2nd ed). Philadelphia: Lippincott, 1992;589.
211. Hackl W, Mauritz W, Schemper M, et al. Prediction of malignant hyperthermia susceptibility: statistical evaluation of clinical signs. Br J Anaesth 1990;64:425.
212. Gronert GA. Malignant hyperthermia. Anesthesiology 1980;53:395.
213. Rosenberg H, Fletcher JE. Masseter muscle rigidity and malignant hyperthermia susceptibility. Anesth Analg 1986;65:161.
214. Allen GC, Rosenberg H. Malignant hyperthermia susceptibility in adult patients with masseter muscle rigidity. Can J Anaesth 1990;37:31.
215. Flewellen EH, Nelson TE. Halothane-succinylcholine induced masseter spasm: indicative of malignant hyperthermia susceptibility? Anesth Analg 1984;63:693.
216. Schwartz L, Rockoff MA, Koka BV. Masseter spasm with anesthesia: incidence and implications. Anesthesiology 1984;61:772.
217. Eng GD, Epstein BS, Engel WK, et al. Malignant hyperthermia and central core disease in a child with congenital dislocating hips. Arch Neurol 1978;35:189.
218. Frank JP, Harati Y, Butler IJ, et al. Central core disease and malignant hyperthermia syndrome. Ann Neurol 1980;7:11.
219. Rosenberg H, Heiman-Patterson T. Duchenne's muscular dystrophy and malignant hyperthermia: another warning. Anesthesiology 1983;59:362.
220. Kelfer HM, Singer WD, Reynolds RN. Malignant hyperthermia in a child with Duchenne muscular hypertrophy. Pediatrics 1983;71:118.
221. Rampton AJ, Kelly DA, Shanahan EC, Ingram GS. Occurrence of malignant hyperpyrexia in a patient with osteogenesis imperfecta. Br J Anaesth 1984;56:1443.
222. McPherson EW, Taylor CA. The King syndrome: malignant hyperthermia, myopathy, and multiple anomalies. Am J Med Genet 1981;8:159.
223. Petersen RS, Bailey PL, Kalameghan R, Ashwood ER. Prolonged neuromuscular block after mivacurium. Anesth Analg 1993;76:194.
224. Bevan DR, Donati F. Muscle Relaxants. In PG Barash, BF Cullen, RK Stoelting (eds), Clinical Anesthesia (2nd ed). Philadelphia: Lippincott, 1992;481.
225. Stoelting RK, Dierdorf SF. Skin and Musculoskeletal Disease. In RK Stoelting, SF Dierdorf (eds), Anesthesia and Co-Existing Disease (3rd ed). New York: Churchill Livingstone, 1993;427.
226. Crosby ET, Lui A. The adult cervical spine: implications for airway management. Can J Anaesth 1990; 37:77.
227. Harley EH, Collins MD. Neurologic sequela secondary to atlantoaxial instability in Down syndrome. Implications in otolaryngologic surgery. Arch Otolaryngol 1994;120:159.
228. Litman RS, Zerngast BA, Perkins FM. Preoperative evaluation of the cervical spine in children with trisomy-21: results of a questionnaire study. Paediatr Anaesth 1995;6:355.
229. Williams JP, Somerville GM, Miner ME, Reilly D. Atlanto-axial subluxation and trisomy-21: another perioperative complication. Anesthesiology 1987;67:253.
230. Baker LL, Bower CM, Glasier CM. Atlanto-axial subluxation and cervical osteomyelitis: two unusual complications of adenoidectomy. Ann Otol Rhinol Laryngol 1996;105:295.

Chapter 6

Complications of Organ Transplantation

John C. Andrefsky and Jeffrey I. Frank

Objectives

- To recognize the neurologic side effects of immunosuppressive agents
- To appreciate that most neurologic side effects of immunosuppressive agents are reversible with discontinuance or lowering of the dosage
- To recognize that each type of organ failure and transplantation procedure predisposes patients to specific neurologic complications
- To appreciate the postoperative neurologic sequelae of each type of transplantation
- To understand that central nervous system (CNS) infections appear at predictable time intervals after transplantation and immunosuppression
- To learn that many CNS infections lack specific neurologic findings, and further diagnostic procedures should be pursued if the physician has a high index of suspicion

Neurologic complications are commonly encountered in patients with end-organ failure awaiting an organ transplant or in those who have been fortunate enough to receive one. Many of the complications are iatrogenic, due directly or indirectly to a medication necessary to allow tolerance of the transplanted organ or a consequence of the surgical transplant procedure itself. However, particularly with transplant patients, *iatrogenic* does not define these complications as avoidable. On the contrary, most are part and parcel of caring for these patients.

This chapter focuses on the neurologic complications of organ transplantation, emphasizing those definable as iatrogenic. Some noniatrogenic complications are discussed to provide a more thorough analysis of the differential diagnosis that should be considered with certain presenting neurologic syndromes in this patient group.

Complications of immunosuppression are presented first because those are the most important iatrogenic complications in organ transplant recipients. The second section is devoted to complications organized by organ systems failing or transplanted. The space limitations of this chapter preclude an exhaustive overview of the subject. Rather, this narrative highlights the most critical issues and diagnostic and therapeutic considerations. The references are similarly restricted to those most pertinent. However, it is our hope that this chapter will enable clinicians to become more familiar with the neurologic complications that define the risk side of the complex decisions and care devoted to patients before, during, and after organ transplantation.

Complications Secondary to Immunosuppressive Agents

Immunosuppressive agents are employed in organ transplant recipients to prevent and control organ rejection. Historically, corticosteroids were the cornerstone of immunosuppressive therapy, predisposing patients to infections from normal and opportunistic pathogens due to suppression of both cellular and humoral immunity. Fortunately, newer agents allow more selective effects on the immune system, enabling better prevention and treatment of rejection with fewer complications.

Knowledge of the neurologic side effects of immunosuppressive agents assists clinicians in the timely diagnosis and treatment of neurologic symptoms. Anticipation and recognition of these syndromes allow physicians to accurately assess the need for further diagnostic tests. In most cases, the symptoms resolve with discontinuance or reduction of the dosage. Occasionally, failure to promptly recognize these side effects may lead to permanent neurologic dysfunction.

Cyclosporin

Cyclosporin (CsA) is the most commonly used posttransplant immunosuppressive agent. It reduces the production and release of lymphocytes and blocks antigen-induced T-cell activation. The most important and frequent neurologic toxicity of CsA involves the CNS.

The initial signs of CNS neurotoxicity from CsA are tremulousness and restlessness, with tremor observed in 40–100% of patients.[1] The tremor is a fine finger tremor whose intensity diminishes with time. Acute confusional state occurs in approximately 5% of patients, manifesting as two distinct syndromes.[2] One syndrome is characterized by a decreased level of consciousness, confusion, cortical blindness, and visual hallucinations and has been reported in liver, kidney, and bone marrow transplant (BMT) patients. The second syndrome is characterized by ataxia, cerebellar tremor, and focal weakness and occurs in BMT patients only. The exact pathogenesis is unknown, but certain factors such as hypocholesterolemia, hypomagnesemia, beta-lactam antibiotics, corticosteroids, hypertension, uremia, and prior cranial irradiation are reported risk factors for development of CsA neurotoxicity.[3] The toxicity usually begins within 2 weeks and is seen more frequently after intravenous administration.[1] Toxicity secondary to CsA can occur at normal or low CsA levels but is more frequently seen with high levels. Almost all symptoms and signs secondary to CsA toxicity improve partially or completely with decreased dosage or discontinuance of the medication.[4]

Approximately 6% of patients taking CsA have seizures, focal or generalized, and they are usually associated with high CsA levels. BMT patients are at particularly high risk for seizures because they have often received total body irradiation, intrathecal methotrexate, and other chemotherapeutic agents that lower the seizure threshold. Migraine-like headaches can occur in post–liver transplant patients receiving CsA and seem to respond to a decreased CsA dosage or propranolol. A syndrome of visual hallucinations with or without cortical blindness can occur with increased T2 signal in the parieto-occipital white matter, which resolves over months with tapering of the dose. Other neurologic complications secondary to CsA that have been described include psychosis, speech apraxia, neuropathy, central pontine myelinolysis (CPM), mutism, action myoclonus, paresthesias, and acute cerebellar edema with brain stem compression.

FK506

FK506 (tacrolimus) is a relatively new immunosuppressive agent that inhibits cytokine synthesis and blocks T-cell development. The most common neurotoxicity is a fine hand tremor.[5] Even with FK506 levels in the normal range, dose reduction may reduce or abolish the hand tremor. Some patients, however, have persistent tremors despite the dosage reduction. Paresthesias of the hands and feet can occur in up to 25% of the patients.[5]

Psychosis, confusion, mood swings, bizarre behavior, and inappropriate crying can occur with FK506, and the symptoms resolve with medication discontinuance or dose reduction.[6] Akinetic mutism, speech apraxia, aphasia, and hemiplegia have also been reported. Generalized and partial seizures are less common than with CsA.[6]

Cortical blindness with magnetic resonance imaging (MRI) changes similar to CsA toxicity has been reported, with complete recovery of vision after the FK506 was changed to CsA.

FK506 has been associated with three cases of chronic demyelinating sensorimotor polyneuropathy that resembled chronic inflammatory demyelinating polyneuropathy (CIDP).[7–9] The patients all developed neuropathy 2–10 weeks after FK506 exposure. Their initial complaints were painful dysesthesias or paresthesias with asymmetric weakness on examination that became symmetric with time. The cerebrospinal fluid (CSF) showed 0 or 1 white blood cells/HPF (high-power field), normal glucose concentration, and normal or slightly elevated protein concentration at 100–120 mg per dl. Nerve conduction studies were consistent with a predominately demyelinating polyneuropathy. The patients received plasmapheresis and intravenous immunoglobulin (IVIG) and showed significant improvement in their signs and symptoms. A patient with subacute demyelinating sensorimotor neuropathy not associated with other causes has been reported.[8] The neuropathy permanently resolved with a decreased FK506 dosage without any plasmapheresis or IVIG treatment.

OKT3

OKT3 is a monoclonal antibody that suppresses T-cell activity by blocking the CD3 antigen found on the cell surface. The most commonly reported side effect is a flu-like illness beginning within 1 hour of OKT3 administration, and this occurs in 50–80% of patients.[7–9]

The two most common neurologic side effects are aseptic meningitis and toxic encephalopathy. The aseptic meningitis is characterized by meningismus, fever, headache, CSF pleocytosis (neutrophil predominance), mildly elevated CSF protein levels, normal CSF glucose levels, and negative CSF culture results for bacteria or fungi.[8–10] These symptoms occur between the first dose and 16 days after completion of OKT3 administration and resolve within several days independent of discontinuance of the medication. Toxic encephalopathy occurs in approximately 10% of patients. Decreased level of consciousness and CSF pleocytosis are commonly associated with the encephalopathy, which resolves slowly and may take 2 weeks to clear. Seizures, psychosis, myoclonus, and brain edema are sporadic accompaniments to the syndrome.

Visual loss after OKT3 administration has been reported in at least two patients and is thought to be secondary to toxicity of the outer retina.[11] In one patient, the vision improved to 20/200 in both eyes from light perception in both eyes after a 19-day course of OKT3 caused the vision loss.[11] The other patient died, and no follow-up examinations were documented. Papilledema with increased CSF pressure has also been reported.[12] One patient experienced a transient hemiparesis, papilledema, and increased CSF pressure after two doses of OKT3.[13] The hemiparesis and papilledema resolved within 2 weeks after the second OKT3 dose.

Corticosteroids

Corticosteroids are employed for chronic immunosuppression and exert their effect by reducing the immunologic activities of both the cellular and humoral systems. Corticosteroids cause neurologic side effects by direct toxicity, increasing the susceptibility of patients to opportunistic infections, and electrolyte abnormalities secondary to immediate effects or provocation of adrenal insufficiency from rapid discontinuation.

The most common direct neurologic side effects are myopathy and psychosis.[4] The onset of muscle weakness and wasting is subacute, involving the proximal lower extremities first. As the symptoms worsen over weeks, eventually all limb musculature become involved. Muscle stretch reflexes and creatine kinase levels are normal. The usual treatment is to decrease the corticosteroid dose in half or wean the drug over weeks to months. Improvement in the weakness usually begins within weeks and resolves over months. Some clinicians have advocated switching the corticosteroid to a nonfluorinated type.

Many patients develop mild psychiatric symptoms that include euphoria, insomnia, anxiety, and difficulty with concentration. Fewer patients develop more severe symptoms such as delirium and acute psychosis. These complications usually develop in patients on 40 mg per day of prednisone and occur 2–4 weeks after commencement[9–14]; however, it has occurred within days. The symptoms are treated by decreasing the dose, weaning the medication over weeks, or changing to dexamethasone. Major tranquilizers such as thioridazine or chlorpromazine are effective if severe agitation requires treatment. The length of treatment is empiric if the psychosis resolves. Some have also used lithium carbonate to prevent corticosteroid-induced mood disorders and psychosis with variable success, and this approach may be best tailored to patients with a past history of significant mood disorder.[9–14]

Corticosteroids may cause encephalopathies secondary to metabolic disturbances such as hyperglycemia and hypernatremia from glucocorticoid excess. These disturbances are often seen in diabetic patients, who may experience labile glucose levels while on corticosteroids. Hyponatremia from abrupt discontinuance or rapid weaning of corticosteroids may also occur, causing encephalopathy. Long-term corticosteroid use predisposes patients to *Pneumocystis carinii* pneumonia, which often causes hypoxia with a secondary hypoxic encephalopathy.

Complications Secondary to Transplantation Procedures

Immunosuppressive agents cause a wide range of neurologic and systemic complications that increase the morbidity and mortality of transplant patients. These patients also suffer neurologic complications secondary to underlying disease states and their treatments. Encephalopathies, cerebral infarction, and hypoxic ischemic episodes commonly occur in patients with renal, cardiac, and hepatic failure. Although physicians are improving the procedures used, many patients still suffer debilitating neurologic injuries post-transplant. Postoperative complications related to specific organ transplantation can often be treated without any permanent sequelae if they are anticipated and recognized promptly.

Renal Transplantation

Before transplantation, patients with end-stage renal disease requiring hemodialysis often have underlying diseases that predispose them to neurologic complications. They suffer from hypertension, atherosclerosis, uremia, diabetes, and connective tissue diseases. These patients are at high risk for cerebrovascular complications such as cerebral infarctions and intracerebral hemorrhages. They also experience encephalopathy secondary to renal dysfunction and inability to metabolize medications normally.

Two major complications may arise from the renal transplant procedure: cutaneous neuropathies and spinal cord infarction. Both femoral and lateral femoral cutaneous neuropathies secondary to retraction during the procedure have been reported.[10–15] In some patients, the spinal cord receives its blood supply from the iliac arteries. During revascularization of the donor kidney, patients may suffer spinal cord ischemia secondary to interruption of these feeding arteries to the spinal cord.[11–16]

Cerebral infarction and hemorrhage occur in up to 9.5% of renal transplant patients and are associated with premorbid risk factors such as hypertension and diabetes, immunosuppressive medication, and postoperative physiologic changes. Although post-transplant corticosteroid use has declined, it is efficacious when patients are experiencing acute rejection. Corticosteroids can cause hyperlipidemia, a hypercoagulable state, and poor blood sugar control. Postoperatively, patients may experience hypertension related to activation of the renin-angiotensin-aldosterone system, graft kidney pathology, and CsA administration.[12–17] CsA is thought to cause hypertension by direct nephrotoxicity and increased resistance in the afferent arteriole, which leads to volume-dependent hypertension.[13–18]

Clinicians may decrease the risk of cerebrovascular complications by controlling the cerebrovascular risk factors after surgery. This can be accomplished by lowering the dosage of immunosuppression and the anticipatory treatment of hypertension. The hypertension associated with CsA can be treated with diuresis and calcium channel blockers.[13–18]

Besides premorbid risk factors and postoperative hypertension, renal transplant patients experience coagulopathies more often than any other type of transplant patient. Within the first 3 weeks, rebound hypercoagulability secondary to rapid correction of impaired platelet aggregation and thrombin generation caused by preoperative uremia can occur.[14–19] Decreased fibrinolytic activity during the first 2 months and increased inhibition of plasminogen activation in the first 2 years after transplant contribute to the hypercoagulable state.[15–20] However, physicians have not been able to quantify the stroke risk that the previously mentioned factors have on these patients. In the future, anticoagulant and platelet antiaggregate therapy may be routinely used to decrease the risk of postoperative stroke.

Renal transplant patients are at high risk for encephalopathy because they often have underlying structural CNS lesions in combination with decreased urinary excretion of drugs. Electrolyte abnormalities, acid-base disturbances, uremia, and deranged glucose metabolism often coexist in the encephalopathic patient postoperatively. The cause of the encephalopathy is usually multifactorial and improves as the patient's metabolic status improves. Immediately after surgery, clinicians should consider malignant hypertension, infection, acute rejection, impaired drug metabolism, or any of the metabolic factors noted previously as a cause of encephalopathy. Impaired excretion of phenytoin can lead to high levels of free phenytoin, which has been implicated in encephalopathy. Pain medications and sedatives administered after surgery may contribute significantly to the patient's abnormal mental status.

Cardiac Transplantation

Heart transplant patients are at risk for cerebrovascular complications because many of the cardiac abnormalities are important stroke risk factors, such as valvular heart disease, congenital heart defects, atherosclerotic cardiovascular disease, and cardiomyopathies. These conditions can lead to cerebral infarctions secondary to emboli, chronic global hypoperfusion, and acute hypoxic ischemic encephalopathy from an arrest episode.

As a bridge to transplantation, physicians sometimes use left ventricular assist devices in patients with cardiovascular failure. The most widely used left ventricular assist device is the Novacor left ventricular assist system (Baxter Healthcare Corporation, Novacor Division, Oakland, CA). This system has an external pump that connects the left ventricle and ascending aorta in series. Blood flows from the left ventricle through the pump to the aorta. In 68 patients with the left ventricular assist system, seven had presumed cerebral embolism, with one having a persistent neurologic deficit.[16–21]

In the Thermo Cardiosystems (Woburn, MA) HeartMate 1000 IP left ventricular assist device, the interior surface is textured to promote the growth of densely adherent neointima.[17–22] This intima eliminates the interaction between the device and blood elements, which reduces the risk of emboli formation. In the absence of infection, none of the first 57 patients experienced a cerebral embolus. No clot-related problem occurred in the patients despite the use of multiple anticoagulation regimens.

During the transplant procedure, patients often suffer diffuse cerebral hypoperfusion that may have clinical manifestations as severe as anoxic encephalopathy or as mild as postoperative confusion. The hypoperfusion is usually secondary to the bypass pump but can be related to episodes of postoperative hypotension and hypoxia. In one autopsy series, six of 18 patients showed damage to the Sommer sector only, two of 18 had damage to the dentate nucleus only, and three of 18 had diffuse anoxic injury.[18–23] The bypass pump also predisposes patients to cardiac and air emboli. In three autopsy series, 9–44% of patients autopsied had acute cerebral infarction.[24, 25] Post–cardiac transplant patients are at high risk for cerebral infarction from cardiac emboli from the transplanted organ and atherosclerosis.

Investigators in France have produced a procedure called total orthotopic heart transplantation.[19–26] Although more technically challenging, this technique has several anatomic and physiologic advantages over standard heart transplant procedures, with fewer postoperative emboli as a key advantage. Spontaneous echo contrast and atrial thrombosis are commonly discovered on transesophageal echocardiography post-transplant, and this indicates a high risk of embolic events. Transesophageal echocardiography was used to determine the rate of spontaneous echo contrast and atrial thrombosis in both types of transplant.[26] The presence of spontaneous echo contrast and atrial thrombosis led to a high rate of embolic events.[26] In the 20 patients with the total orthotopic heart transplantation, one showed spontaneous echo contrast and none showed left atrial thrombus. Forty-three of the 75 standard heart transplant patients had spontaneous echo contrast, and 20 of the 43 had an associated left atrial thrombus.[26] Eleven of the 75 standard heart transplant patients experienced an arterial embolus, whereas none of the total orthotopic heart transplantation patients did.[26]

Two types of peripheral nerve injuries can occur secondary to thoracotomies. Patients may experience an injury of the entire or lower brachial plexus secondary to stretching during the procedure. Minimally invasive cardiac surgery involves smaller incisions with the removal of two to three ribs directly over the heart. This procedure involves significantly less stretching of the brachial plexus, which should lead to fewer injuries. Patients have also suffered phrenic nerve injuries post-thoracotomy.

Intracerebral hemorrhages have also been noted after cardiac transplantation. The probable mechanism is postoperative cerebral hyperperfusion in patients whose cerebral autoregulatory response has been disabled by chronic vasodilatation secondary to preoperative chronic hypotension.[20–27] Other proposed mechanisms include uncontrolled hypertension, disseminated intravascular coagulopathy with sepsis, or disturbed homeostasis from consumptive coagulopathy during cardiopulmonary bypass. Lobar hemorrhage has occurred in up to 5% of heart transplant recipients in one series.[28]

Approximately 10–15% of the patients experience seizures after cardiac transplantation. In the immediate postoperative period, seizures are most often due to acute cerebral infarction, anoxic injury, or relative hyperperfusion.[27] Postoperative patients also have a lowered seizure threshold secondary to metabolic abnormalities, infection, and CsA administration. After the postoperative period, seizures may signal opportunistic CNS infection. A thorough workup should be performed to rule out hemorrhage, infarction, or CNS infection in patients with seizures, especially those with partial seizures or lateralizing findings on examination. In postoperative patients who are comatose or have prolonged postictal states, an electroencephalogram should be performed to eliminate the possibility of status epilepticus or suppressed brain activity.

Cardiac transplant patients are often subjected to high levels of immunosuppression, which leads to increased susceptibility to infections and post-transplant lymphoproliferative disorder. CNS opportunistic infections occur up to 3–6 months post-transplant. Meningitis, meningoencephalitis, abscess, and viral encephalitis are the most common diagnosed CNS infections. They are often associated with both lung and systemic foci of infection. In patients with pulmonary aspergillosis and neurologic dysfunction, CNS aspergillosis, a meningoencephalitis, should always be considered. *Cryptococcus* and *Listeria* are the most common causes of meningitis. Toxoplasmosis accounts for approximately 12% of the CNS infections observed after cardiac transplant.

Heart transplant patients are at high risk for viral infection with cytomegalovirus (CMV), herpes simplex virus (HSV), and Epstein-Barr virus. CMV and HSV can cause a viral encephalitis that presents with confusion and progresses to obtundation. Additionally, HSV can cause focal neurologic findings frequently accompanied by seizures and periodic lateralizing epileptiform discharges. Epstein-Barr virus and high levels of immunosuppression may account for the increased frequency of post-transplant lymphoproliferative disorder, which occurs in 4.9% of cardiac transplant patients.

Liver Transplantation

Patients with liver disease can become encephalopathic from the liver failure itself or related metabolic and infectious complications. In fulminant hepatic failure (FHF), the severity of the encephalopathy parallels that of the liver failure. The encephalopathy is graded from 1 (mild confusion but alert) to 4 (comatose). Patients with grade 4 encephalopathy are at the highest risk for developing cerebral edema and increased intracranial pressure (ICP). Fifty percent to 80% of patients with FHF develop cerebral edema, and 30–50% of patients die from related complications.[29–31] Failure to anticipate and recognize increased ICP may lead to delays in treatment with increased morbidity and mortality.

ICP monitoring can warn clinicians of increased ICP and subsequently compromised cerebral perfusion pressure when the neurologic status is poor or cannot be evaluated due to heavy sedation or neuromuscular paralysis. Complications such as intracranial hemorrhage and infection related to the insertion of an ICP monitor are rare. Physicians should administer fresh frozen plasma before, during, and after the insertion of the monitor to decrease the risk of hemorrhage, and of course, it should be performed with sterile technique.

If cerebral edema exists and intracranial hypertension develops in a FHF patient, clinicians should avoid exacerbating the ICP and compromising cerebral perfusion pressure. Common medical complications that increase the ICP include hypercarbia, hypoxia, decreased blood pressure, coughing, and overhydration, especially with hypotonic fluids. Hypoglycemic FHF patients treated with hypotonic fluids should have their serum sodium and osmolarity and fluid status monitored closely because administration of D10W can hypothetically exacerbate cerebral edema.

If the ICP becomes difficult to control, clinicians can use hyperventilation as a temporary treatment. With an arterial partial pressure of carbon dioxide ($PaCO_2$) of less than 25 mm Hg, patients may suffer from excessive cerebral vasoconstriction and consequential cerebral ischemia. Clinicians can use intermittent boluses of mannitol for episodes of sustained ICP, which compromises cerebral perfusion pressure if hyperventilation does not work or as its effect predictably diminishes with time. Prolonged mannitol use may lead to dehydration, hypotension, and hyperosmolarity if the patient's fluid status is not monitored closely and optimized. If the ICP becomes resistant to all medical therapies, thiopental or pentobarbital coma can be used as a means to control ICP or improve tolerance of compromised cerebral perfusion. This extreme measure is very risky, however, and demands experienced anticipatory care.

In chronic liver disease, patients manifest portosystemic encephalopathy, which includes changes in mental status, impaired cognitive function, asterixis, and hyperventilation. These patients are exquisitely sensitive to increased nitrogenous loads from gastrointestinal hemorrhages, renal failure, sepsis, and decreased intravascular volume. Patients receiving medications that are metabolized by the liver can have worsened encephalopathy secondary to decreased clearance.

The management of portosystemic encephalopathy includes removal or treatment of precipitating factors, avoidance of dietary proteins, and lactulose to decrease bowel absorption of nitrogenous products. Physicians should not administer benzodiazepines, narcotics, or chlorpromazine to patients with chronic liver failure. If sedation is needed, an antihistamine should be used.

The benzodiazepine antagonist flumazenil can reverse portosystemic encephalopathy in some patients, but the clinical response is variable. When improvement occurs it usually lasts approximately 1 hour, with the return of the encephalopathy afterward. No improvement of long-term outcome of these patients has been noted.

During the transplant procedure, physicians should anticipate that patients may have increased ICP with a severely compromised cerebral perfusion pressure. Hypovolemia and hypercarbia should in general be avoided and especially during the anhepatic phase in liver transplant patients, in whom cerebral blood flow may be further reduced. Hypotension may develop, leading to a hypoxic-ischemic event. Patients are also at a high risk for cerebral infarction secondary to cardiac, atherosclerotic, or air emboli. The brachial plexus may be injured during the axillary dissection for placement of the femoral axillary venous bypass. Neuropathies may also develop secondary to surgical retraction.

Postoperative patients are at high risk for CPM, noted in 7–19% of the patients in several neuropathologic series.[32, 33] The signs and symptoms of CPM include minimal to flaccid quadriplegia, anarthria, inability to swallow, pseudobulbar palsy, and behavioral changes. MRI scans show hypointense T1 and hyperintense T2 ventral pontine lesions. This condition is thought to be secondary to rapid increases in plasma sodium concentration when correcting hyponatremia or extreme shifts in serum osmolarity. In order to avoid CPM, physicians should correct hyponatremia no faster than 12 mmol per liter per day. Patients may suffer severe morbidity and mortality from CPM, but spontaneous recovery has been reported. No effective therapy exists for this condition.

Multiple metabolic factors in combination with immunosuppression, infection, and fevers lower the seizure threshold. When seizures are present, clinicians should first rule out a CNS infection or hemorrhage as a cause for the seizure. If the patient has one or several self-limited seizures and the underlying cause has been treated, then no further seizure therapy is necessary. If seizures continue from either multiple metabolic causes or a known CNS pathologic process, then anticonvulsant drugs should be instituted and continued.

Treatment of seizures in the liver transplant patient are often problematic, as antiepileptic drugs affect the CsA level, thereby challenging graft survival. When phenytoin, phenobarbital, or carbamazepine are used for seizure control, the CsA level decreases along with the level of immunosuppression. The advantages of phenytoin and phenobarbital are that they can be administered intravenously to rapidly achieve a therapeutic level and then continued orally for long-term seizure treatment. Newer antiepileptic drugs such as felbamate, lamotrigine, and gabapentin may be useful because they have fewer neurologic and systemic side effects. Gabapentin has no enzyme-inducing properties and little interaction with other drugs used in the transplant patient. Most seizures involved in the transplant patient tend to occur in the acute phase of transplantation and resolve as the patient becomes more medically stable. Frequent reassessment of the need for chronic antiepileptic drugs should be done in the spirit of minimizing medication use in these patients. However, long-term antiepileptic drug therapy is warranted in patients with continued seizures.

Bone Marrow Transplantation

BMT is used in the treatment of aplastic anemia and hematologic, lymphoreticular, and solid malignancies. Complications related to underlying disease states and their treatments are beyond the scope of this chapter. Commonly used chemotherapeutic agents predispose patients to encephalopathies, myelopathies, neuropathies, and cerebral vasculopathies. Radiation-induced damage to the CNS can include dementia, ataxia, transverse myelopathy, neuropathies including cranial and brachial plexus, and focal syndromes that simulate recurrent tumors (e.g., radiation necrosis).[34]

BMT involves the destruction of the recipient marrow with cyclophosphamide or total body irradiation, which rarely causes neurologic dysfunction. Cranial irradiation may cause cognitive dysfunction in long-term survivors and predispose patients to seizures. The most common neurologic complication in BMT is metabolic encephalopathy, seen in approximately 37% of patients. Multiple etiologies such as hypoxia, ischemia, hepatic and renal dysfunction, electrolyte imbalance, and infections are responsible for encephalopathy, alone or in combination.

The second most common cause of neurologic complications in BMT patients is CNS infection. Unlike other transplant patients, immunosuppression is maximal around the time of transplant because marrow dysfunction occurs secondary to neoplastic diseases, chemotherapy, or irradiation. Production of the new marrow does not occur for approximately 1 month. During this first period of immunosuppression, patients are particularly vulnerable to bacterial (especially gram-negative), viral (especially HSV), and fungal infections. The patients have derangement of both cell-mediated and humoral immunity for approximately 1 year and are susceptible to mostly viral and parasitic CNS infections.

BMT patients also suffer from cerebral infarctions that are secondary to infective or noninfective bacterial thrombotic endocarditis. Despite low platelet counts in these patients, the rate of intracerebral hemorrhage is low.

Patients receiving either autologous or syngeneic transplantation do not usually require immunosuppression. Patients receiving an allogenic transplant require chronic immunosuppression and are predisposed to a graft-versus-host disease (GVHD). Patients may develop a myositis with clinical features identical to idiopathic polymyositis.[25–35] Patients note the insidious onset of painless weakness of proximal musculature, usually beginning with the legs. With time, all of the proximal muscles become involved, including the neck and pharyngeal musculature. Most patients with myositis from GVHD manifest skin lesions that usually show depigmentation, lichen planus–like lesions, papular squamous plaques, and sclerodermal changes. The classic heliotrope rash of dermatomyositis is not seen in these patients.

The electromyographic examination of myositis shows many brief low-voltage action potentials with fibrillations. Serum transaminases, creatine kinase, and aldolase levels are typically elevated. Muscle biopsy shows monocytic infiltration with fiber necrosis and active phagocytosis.

Myasthenia gravis associated with chronic GVHD has been reported in only seven cases.[35] The clinical features are similar and include fatigable weakness of the limbs and bulbar musculature. Respiratory failure was noted in three of the seven patients. All seven patients had an increased acetylcholine receptor antibody titer that correlated with the disease course in individual patients. No thymic mass was found on postmortem examination or chest computed tomography scan in any patient. Classic electromyographic findings of decremental response to repetitive stimulation were noted in several patients. Single-fiber electromyography showed jitter and blocking typical of a neuromuscular junction transmission defect.

An inflammatory demyelinating polyneuropathy similar to chronic inflammatory demyelinating polyneuropathy has been reported in several studies. Amato et al. reported on polyneuropathies in

BMT patients with acute or chronic GVHD.[36] These patients had diffuse, generalized, proximal and distal limb weakness with hyporeflexia or areflexia and variable sensory loss. Nerve conduction studies showed evidence for demyelination but did not meet strict criteria for chronic inflammatory demyelinating polyneuropathy. Sural nerve biopsies on two of the patients showed loss of large myelinated fibers. This polyneuropathy was noted to resolve as the GVHD improved with immunosuppressive therapy.

Pancreas Transplantation

All patients undergoing pancreas transplant have diabetes mellitus. These patients are at risk for the neurologic complications of diabetes, including stroke, peripheral neuropathy, and diabetic retinopathy.

Most complications related to pancreatic transplant are cerebrovascular in nature and include cerebral infarction, hypoxic ischemic episodes, and spinal cord infarctions. Metabolic encephalopathies, seizures, and peripheral neuropathies, including herpes zoster neuritis and compressive neuropathies, have been noted. The immunosuppression-related events are similar to those seen after cardiac transplant.

Lung Transplantation

The neurologic complications of lung transplant are similar to those involving cardiac transplant. Patients undergoing lung transplant are placed on the bypass pump during surgery. These patients are also at high risk for having a brachial plexopathy secondary to the thoracotomy. Diaphragmatic paralysis, either unilateral or bilateral, has been reported, and these patients usually require temporary ventilatory assistance postoperatively with ultimate success in weaning from mechanical ventilation.

CNS complications after lung transplant have been reviewed by Goldstein et al. at the Cleveland Clinic Foundation.[37] The indications for transplant in these patients included chronic obstructive pulmonary disease, cystic fibrosis, idiopathic pulmonary fibrosis, congenital heart disease, and primary pulmonary hypertension. Severe headache was the most common complaint, followed by seizures, stroke, and confusion. Patients with cystic fibrosis developed seizures 31% of the time after lung transplant compared with 8.3% in the noncystic fibrosis patients. The authors thought that the CNS events were secondary to either CsA toxicity or infection.

Central Nervous System Infections

CNS infections represent a major cause of morbidity and mortality in the transplant patient on chronic immunosuppression. Approximately 5–10% of all transplant patients develop a CNS infection at some point and approximately 44–77% die.[38] Table 6.1 lists the clinical syndromes, laboratory diagnosis, neuroimaging, and treatment of the organisms that most commonly cause CNS infections in immunocompromised patients. The following comments address more global considerations about CNS infections in these patients.

Risk Factors

Transplant patients are exposed to multiple risk factors that modulate the body's response to infection and bypass normal defense mechanisms. Diabetes, malnutrition, liver failure, bone marrow dysfunction, irradiation, and chemotherapy are some of the systemic factors that accentuate the ultimate state of immunosuppression before transplant. Immunosuppressive drugs, which represent the major risk factor for opportunistic infections, variably blunt both the humoral and cellular response of the body to infection. Surgery, catheter placement, intubation, and foreign body implantation that violate mucocutaneous and skin barriers represent the major etiologies for hospital-acquired infection. Donor organs may carry bacterial or viral infection to the recipient and directly seed the circulation or a specific body cavity.

Diagnostic Clues and Considerations

The rapid diagnosis and treatment of CNS infections afford patients the best opportunity for improved outcome and survival. Physicians must be able to recognize the early signs and symptoms of

Table 6.1. Organisms that Most Commonly Cause Central Nervous System Infections in Immunocompromised Patients

Organism	Clinical Signs	Laboratory Diagnosis	Neuroimaging	Treatment
Bacterial infections				
Listeria monocytogenes	Acute meningitis: headache and fever, meningismus present in 25–60% of patients; brain abscess	Increased peripheral WBC count, bacteremia; lumbar puncture, WBC 100–100,000 cells/ml; neutrophils 85–95%; protein usually >100 mg/dl; glucose <50% serum; positive Gram's stain and cultures; Gram's stain usually does not confirm diagnosis	CT scan: early, normal; later, mild ventricular dilatation and subarachnoid space enlargement MRI scan: early, T1-weighted images with gadolinium show meningeal enhancement	Ampicillin or penicillin G with gentamicin; if allergic to penicillin, then trimethoprim-sulfamethoxazole
Mycobacterium tuberculosis	Subacute or chronic meningitis: headache, fever, and cranial nerve palsies	Decreased serum sodium (SIADH); lumbar puncture, increased WBC 50–500 cells/ml; early, neutrophils and lymphocytes; later, lymphocytes; protein 100–200 mg/dl; glucose <40 mg/dl; positive culture (may take weeks to become positive); increased CSF pressure	CT scan: plaque-like dural thickening or dural calcifications around basilar cisterns	Isoniazid sensitive *M. tuberculosis:* isoniazid, rifampin, and pyrazinamide; if resistance is suspected consider adding an aminoglycoside within the first 2 weeks of treatment; other drugs that may be added include ethambutol, ethionamide, and ofloxacin
Nocardia asteroides	Brain abscess: headache, fever, focal and nonfocal neurologic signs; multiple abscesses; meningitis; systemic signs of infection especially lung, skin, and kidney	Lumbar puncture: cell counts may be normal or have polymorphonuclear or mononuclear pleocytosis; Gram's stain and culture usually negative; brain biopsy is often required for diagnosis	CT scan: early, normal or subcortical low attenuation that later is better defined; positive ring enhancement with contrast MRI scan: early, T2-weighted images with subcortical hypointensity; later, with central area becoming hyperintense; T1-weighted images with gadolinium with intense rim enhancement	Trimethoprim-sulfamethoxazole with follow-up CT scan of brain to assess efficacy of treatment; brain abscesses often require surgery for debridement
Fungal infections				
Aspergillus	Hemorrhagic infarction: mental status changes, seizures, and focal neurologic signs; brain abscesses; critical period within the first 3 mos; systemic signs of infection especially lung, skin, or paranasal sinus involvement; critical period is 1–4 mos after transplant	Positive biopsy from an infected site; lumbar puncture: CSF may be normal or have a moderate polymorphonuclear or lymphocytic pleocytosis; mild protein elevation	CT scan: cortical, subcortical, or deep; high attenuation (hemorrhagic component) surrounded by low attenuation (edema); low attenuation in a specific vascular distribution with or without hemorrhage	Amphotericin B

Candida	Subacute or chronic meningitis: fever, headache, and meningismus; brain abscess; systemic signs of infection especially endocarditis and sepsis	Biopsy of infected tissue or isolation of fungi from fluid in a closed body cavity; lumbar puncture, WBC cells up to 2,000 cells/ml with polymorphonuclear (acute) and mononuclear (chronic) pleocytosis; increased protein 50–200 mg/dl; decreased glucose; positive CSF culture in 40–45% of cases	—	Amphotericin B and fluconazole
Cryptococcus neoformans	Chronic meningitis: fever, headache, and meningismus; focal neurologic signs are uncommon; systemic signs of infection especially skin and pulmonary sites	Decreased serum sodium (SIADH); lumbar puncture, increased WBC but <500 cells/ml, usually lymphocytes; increased protein up to 500 mg/dl; glucose <50% serum level; positive India ink preparation and cryptococcal antigen; increased CSF pressure	CT scan: usually not useful, but can identify hydrocephalus when present MRI scan: T2-weighted images with multifocal basal ganglia and midbrain hyperintensities that represent cryptococcomas	Amphotericin B and fluconazole
Mucoraceae	Rhinocerebral mucormycosis: early, visual loss, ophthalmoplegia, cranial neuropathies, especially V and VII; late, obtundation, focal deficits; systemic signs of infection especially eschar on palate or paranasal sinus	Biopsy of infected tissue; lumbar puncture, pleocytosis >50% polymorphonuclear cells, increased protein, decreased glucose (rare), cultures almost always negative	Abscess formation or cerebral infarction	Aggressive surgical debridement and amphotericin B
Parasitic infection				
Toxoplasmosis gondii	Meningoencephalitis: low-grade fever, confusion, focal neurologic signs, seizures, and meningismus; brain abscess (deep); systemic signs of infection especially skin, pulmonary, myocardial, and hepatic sites; critical period is 1–4 mos post-transplant	Serum Sabin-Feldman dye test or indirect fluorescent antibody test titers ≥1:1,000 or biopsy of infected tissue; lumbar puncture, increased WBC 10–50 cells/ml, mostly mononuclear; slightly increased protein; glucose usually normal but may be low; CSF pressure may be elevated	CT scan: solitary or multiple ring-enhancing masses with peripheral edema MRI scan: T1-weighted images with isointense slightly hypointense lesions that rim enhance with gadolinium; T2-weighted images with hyperintense lesions	Pyrimethamine and sulfadiazine

Table 6.1. *continued.*

Organism	Clinical Signs	Laboratory Diagnosis	Neuroimaging	Treatment
Viral infections				
Cytomegalovirus	Encephalitis: headache, vomiting, encephalopathy, and seizures; systemic signs of infection especially eye, pulmonary, gastrointestinal, and hepatic sites	Positive urine or blood (buffy coat) or bronchoalveolar fluid for cytomegalovirus; fourfold or greater increase in antibody titer; lumbar puncture, increased WBC 10–1,000 cells/ml; early, polymorphonuclear; late, mononuclear pleocytosis; protein 50–200 mg/dl; glucose normal or slightly low; pressure may be increased or decreased; positive culture	CT scan: hypointense confluent periventricular rim	Intravenous ganciclovir or acyclovir
Epstein-Barr virus	Post-transplant lymphoproliferative disorder: mental status changes, headache with or without focal neurologic signs; critical period is 3–6 mos after transplant	Laboratory stereotactic brain biopsy	CT scan: isointense to moderately hyperintense masses with strong, homogeneous enhancement MRI scan: T1 weighted isointense to slightly hypointense relative to gray matter that strongly and homogeneously enhance with gadolinium; T2 weighted isointense to slightly hyperintense	Decrease the immunosuppressive dosage, administer dexamethasone and cranial radiation
Papovavirus (JC virus)	Progressive multifocal leukoencephalopathy: dementia, confusion over days to weeks, hemiparesis, aphasia, cortical blindness, dysarthria	Lumbar puncture, usually normal but may have mildly increased protein	CT scan: hypodense, nonenhancing subcortical lesions MRI scan: T2-weighted images show multifocal oval or round white matter hyperintensities in the parieto-occipital area	No effective treatment
Varicella-zoster virus	Diffuse meningoencephalitis: delirium, headache, and meningismus; focal meningoencephalitis, headache, meningismus, and focal findings; systemic signs of infection especially prior skin rash	Brain biopsy with Cowdry type A intranuclear inclusion bodies on microscopic examination or visualization of herpesvirus nucleocapsids by electron microscopy; lumbar puncture, increased WBC 0–2,795 cells/ml (80% had <100 cells) with a lymphocyte predominance; increased protein 100–175 mg/dl	MRI scan: T2-weighted images multiple ovoid areas of high signal intensity in the deep and subcortical white matter	Intravenous acyclovir

CSF = cerebrospinal fluid; SIADH = syndrome of inappropriate diuretic hormone; CT = computed tomography; MRI = magnetic resonance imaging; WBC = white blood cell count.

systemic infection of both normal and opportunistic pathogens. Most opportunistic infections that invade the CNS spread via the hematogenous or pulmonary routes and leave diagnostic clues in the form of lung or skin involvement. Some infections begin on mucocutaneous membranes and invade the CNS locally or via the hematogenous route. The physician's best tools in the diagnoses of CNS infection are a strong clinical suspicion and the presence of systemic infection.

The most common symptoms and signs of CNS infection in transplant patients are fever, headache, encephalopathy, meningismus, and mild focal findings.[38] These abnormalities may be striking, mild, or absent even in some cases of advanced CNS infection. The encephalopathy may evolve rapidly or slowly, and both temporal problems should prompt an expeditious diagnostic workup for CNS involvement. Meningismus in the immunocompromised patient may be absent in acute, subacute, or chronic meningitis because these patients have a blunted immunologic response that delays or prevents the development of meningeal inflammation.

Another diagnostic clue to the etiology of a CNS infection is the specific syndrome present. The presence of an acute, subacute, or chronic meningitis, encephalitis, or focal infection combined with the time interval from transplant can help the clinician to accurately predict the causative organism.

Immunosuppression Duration and Infection Risk

It is most useful to consider the potential infections or organisms based on the duration of immunosuppression. Three distinct periods help stratify the CNS infection risk: (1) less than 1 month, (2) from 1 to 6 months, and (3) greater than 6 months.[4] Exceptions to the time table for stratifying infection risk are often caused by exposure to an excessive epidemiologic hazard such as endemic infection or exposure during hospitalizations from the environment or health care personnel.

During the first month post-transplant, the greatest risks come from infections that were present in the recipient before the transplant or in a contaminated graft. These infections are usually routine, and there is no associated high risk during this period for CNS infections. The primary etiologies during the first period include *Mycobacterium tuberculosis, Strongyloides stercoralis*, or one of the following geographically restricted systemic mycoses: *Histoplasma capsulatum, Blastomyces dermatitidis*, or *Coccidioides immitis*.

From 1 to 6 months post-transplant, patients are at the peak of their drug-induced immunosuppression and viruses, especially CMV, Epstein-Barr virus, hepatitis viruses, and the human immunodeficiency virus can immunosuppress patients even further. This is the highest risk period for CNS infections, most importantly from viruses and opportunistic organisms.

During the third period, more than 6 months after transplant, the patient is at risk for three types of infections: (1) infections from pathogens that affect the general community, (2) recrudescence of a chronic viral infection with progression secondary to immunosuppression, and (3) opportunistic infections in patients with chronic rejection receiving prolonged high-dose immunosuppression.

General Diagnostic Issues Regarding Pathogens

Listeria monocytogenes is the most likely cause of acute bacterial meningitis in the transplant patient. In neutropenic patients, gram-negative meningitis is common. In asplenic patients, acute meningitis is often caused by pneumococcus, meningococcus, or *Haemophilus influenzae*.

Subacute meningitis, which progresses over 2–10 days, is most often caused by *L. monocytogenes* or *M. tuberculosis*. Chronic meningitis, which progresses over greater than 10 days, is most likely secondary to *Cryptococcus* but other organisms such as *M. tuberculosis, L. monocytogenes, Candida, H. capsulatum*, or *C. immitis* are causative as well.

Meningoencephalitis in an immunocompromised patient can be caused by many different organisms. Physicians should have a high clinical suspicion for *Listeria*, the herpes virus group including CMV, and zoster, and the papovaviruses (JC virus). Parasitic infections such as toxoplasmosis and fungal infections including cryptococcosis, aspergillosis, and candidiasis may also cause meningoencephalitis.

Focal CNS infections are usually caused by a fungal or parasitic infection such as toxoplasmosis, cryptococcosis, and aspergillosis. Both *Nocardia* and *Listeria* brain abscesses have been reported in the literature.

Conclusion

Immunosuppressive therapy is the most common source of iatrogenic complications in organ transplant patients. Therapy causes a predisposition to infection and other more direct toxic effects on the nervous system. Surgical complications are less frequent and usually less consequential. A working knowledge of these potential complications allows an anticipatory approach to recognizing and minimizing the severity and duration of the iatrogenic problem.

References

1. Wijdicks EF, Wiesner RH, Krom RA. Neurotoxicity in liver transplant recipients with cyclosporin immunosuppression. Neurology 1995;45:1962.
2. Walker RW, Brochstein JA. Neurologic complications of immunosuppressive agents. Neurol Clin 1988;6:261.
3. Kahan BD. Cyclosporine. N Engl J Med 1989;321:1725.
4. Patchell RA. Neurological complications of organ transplantation. Ann Neurol 1994;36:688.
5. Neuhaus P (Berlin), Pichlmayr R (Hannover), Williams R (London). Randomised trial comparing tacrolimus (FK506) and cyclosporin in prevention of liver allograft rejection. Lancet 1994;344:423.
6. Wijdicks EFM, Wiesner RH, Dahlke LJ, Krom AF. FK506-induced neurotoxicity in liver transplantation. Ann Neurol 1994;35:498.
7. Wilson John R, Conwit RA, Eidelman BH, et al. Sensorimotor neuropathy resembling CIDP in patients receiving FK506. Muscle Nerve 1994;17:528.
8. Bronster DJ, Yonover P, Stein J, et al. Demyelinating sensorimotor polyneuropathy after administration of FK506. Transplantation 1996;59:1066.
9. DeGroen PC, Aksamit AJ, Rakela J, et al. Central nervous system toxicity after liver transplantation. N Engl J Med 1987;317:861.
10. Emmons C, Smith J, Flanigan M. Cerebrospinal fluid inflammation during OKT3 therapy [letter]. Lancet 1986;2:510.
11. Dukar O, Barr CC. Visual loss complicating OKT3 monoclonal antibody therapy. Am J Ophthalmol 1993; 115:781.
12. Strominger MB, Liu GT, Schatz NJ. Optic disk swelling and abducens palsies associated with OKT3. Am J Ophthmal 1995;119:664.
13. Osterman JD, Trauner DA, Resnik VM, Lemire J. Transient hemiparesis associated with monoclonal CD3 antibody (OKT3) therapy. Pediatr Neurol 1993;9:482.
14. Kaufmann MW, Casadonet PE, Peselow ED. Steroid psychosis. N Y State J Med 1981;81:1795.
15. Junaid I, Kwan JTC, Lord RHH. Femoral neuropathy in renal transplantation. Transplantation 1993;56:240.
16. Jablecki CK, Aguilo JJ, Piepgras DG, et al. Paraparesis after renal transplantation. Ann Neurol 1977;2:154.
17. Raman GV. Post transplant hypertension. J Hum Hypertens 1991;5:1.
18. Curtis JJ. Cyclosporine and posttransplant hypertension. J Am Soc Nephrol 1992;2:S243.
19. von Kaulla KN, von Kaulla E, Wasantapruck S, et al. Blood coagulation in uremic patients before and after hemodialysis and transplantation of the kidney. Arch Surg 1966;92:184.
20. Wardle EN, Menon IS, Uldall PR, et al. Proteins and fibrinolysis in recipients of renal allografts. J Clin Pathol 1971;24:124.
21. McCarthy PM, Portner, PM, Tobler HG, et al. Clinical experience with the Novacor ventricular assist system. J Thorac Cardiovasc Surg 1991;102:578.
22. Rose EA, Levin HR, Oz MC, et al. Artificial circulatory support with textured interior surfaces. Circulation 1994;90(part 2):II-87.
23. Prayson RA, Estes ML. The neuropathology of cardiac allograft transplantation. Arch Pathol Lab Med 1995; 119:59.
24. Martinez AJ, Puglia J. The neuropathy of liver, heart, and heart-lung transplantation. Transplant Proc 1988; 20:806.
25. Ang LC, Gillett JM, Kaufmann JCE. Neuropathology of heart transplantation. Can J Neurol Sci 1989;16:291.
26. Derumeaux G, Habib G, Schleifer DM, et al. Standard orthotopic heart transplantation versus total orthotopic heart transplantation. Circulation 1995;92(suppl II):II-196.
27. Sila CA. Neurologic Complications Following Heart and Heart-Lung Transplantation. In AS Kapoor, H Laks, JS Schroeder, MH Yacoub (eds), Cardiomyopathies and Heart-Lung Transplantation. New York: McGraw-Hill, 1991;265.
28. Sila CA, Furlan AJ, Stewart RW. Intracerebral hemorrhage complicating cardiac transplantation: hyperperfusion breakthrough [abstract]. Neurology 1989;39 (suppl):161.
29. Gazzard BG, Portmann BC, Murray-Lyon IM, Williams R. Causes of death in fulminant hepatic failure and relationship to quantitative histological assessment of parenchymal damage. Q J Med 1975;176:615.
30. Ware AJ, D'Agostino A, Combes B. Cerebral oedema: a major complication of massive hepatic necrosis. Gastroenterology 1971;61:877.
31. Ede RJ, Williams R. Occurrence and Management of Cerebral Oedema in Liver Failure. In R Williams (ed),

Liver Failure. Edinburgh: Churchill Livingstone, 1986;26.

32. Martinez AJ, Ahdab-Barmada M. The neuropathology of liver transplanation: comparison of main complications in children and adults. Mod Pathol 1993;6:25.
33. Power C. Poland SD, Kassim KH, et al. Encephalopathy in liver transplantation: neuropathology and CMV infection. Can J Neurol Sci 1990;17:378.
34. Delattre JY, Posner JB. The Neurological Aspects of Medical Disorders. In MJ Aminoff (ed), Neurology and General Medicine (2nd ed). New York: Churchill Livingstone, 1995;421.
35. Nelson KR, McQuillen MP. Neurologic complications of graft versus-host-disease. Neurol Clin 1988;6:391.
36. Goldstein LS, Haug M, Perl J II, et al. Central nervous system (CNS) complications following lung transplantation. J Heart Lung Transplant (in press).
37. Amato AA, Barohn RJ, Sahenk Z, et al. Polyneuropathy complicating bone marrow and solid organ transplantation. Neurology 1993;43:1513.
38. Conti DJ, Rubin RH. Infection of the central nervous system in organ transplant recipients. Neurol Clin 1988;6:241.

Chapter 7

Neurologic Complications of Spinal Surgery

Kylene K.H. Huler and Robert Jay Huler

Objectives

- To appreciate that some complications of spine surgery are unavoidable despite the best of preoperative planning, technical execution, and postoperative care
- To prepare for an accurate preoperative discussion of surgical risk and informed consent
- To emphasize the early recognition and treatment of those problems that inevitably occur, thereby minimizing the impact and morbidity
- To understand the anatomic basis for most neurologic complications of spine surgery and thereby anticipate and prevent problems before they occur
- To emphasize the recognition of problems that may occur months to years after otherwise successful surgery
- To develop a broad range of differential diagnoses so that postoperative difficulties are appropriately recognized and managed
- To develop the skills that allow interpretation of complex spinal problems using plain radiography, computed tomography (CT), myelography, and magnetic resonance imaging (MRI) and to identify the indications for each imaging study
- To recognize the utility, diagnostic capacity, and technical limitations of available intraoperative spinal cord and nerve root monitoring techniques including somatosensory evoked potentials (SSEPs) and electromyography

Traditionally, the neurosurgeon would resect disease about the neuraxis; the neurologist would provide clinical and electrophysiologic diagnosis; and the orthopedic surgeon would manage the bone deformities such as scoliosis, kyphosis, spondylolisthesis, fractures, and infection. The traditional divisions between the medical specialties have blurred. Spinal surgery is a new, dynamic, and emerging specialty consisting of orthopedic surgeons and neurosurgeons with similar interests. Both disciplines now perform complex resections about the neuraxis, as well as bone fusion and spine implant surgery. The neurologist has the capability to provide real-time intraoperative electrophysiologic monitoring and interpretation, allowing complex surgery to be performed with relative safety. The neurointensive critical care specialist is often the first to recognize, evaluate, and treat the precarious and fluctuating neurologic status in the spine patient immediately postoperatively.

Complications of spinal surgery are among the most highly litigated in medicine and have great potential for producing catastrophic and permanent sequelae. The emphasis of this chapter is on prevention of complications and the early recognition and treatment of problems that inevitably occur. Preoperative patient consultation and informed consent requires a discussion of surgical risk, and this chapter gives guidelines for use both by surgeon and patient. This work details the surgical approaches and the preoperative, perioperative, and postoperative complications of spinal surgery.

This chapter is organized anatomically, because specific complications occur in either the cervical, thoracic, or lumbar spine with a predilection for either the anterior or posterior surgical approach. Complications are recognized to occur in the immediate intraoperative period and in the early or late postoperative period. An example of an intraoperative complication is the failure to perform an adequate neural decompression. An epidural hematoma with rapid onset of quadriparesis is an example of an early postoperative complication. An example of a late complication is cervical cord compression caused by an iatrogenic pseudomeningocele. With these concepts, there is a decreased focus on the technical aspects of surgery, while emphasizing prevention, recognition, and expeditious management of preventable or treatable neurologic complications of spinal surgery.

All clinical examples and figures cited in this chapter have come from the clinical practice of Robert Jay Huler, M.D.

Overview of Surgical Exposure of the Spine

Cord-level neural elements will not safely tolerate retraction during laminectomy. Therefore, pathology anterior to the conus medullaris or to the thoracic or cervical cord is most safely treated via direct anterior surgical exposure, eliminating the need for neural retraction.

The anterior cervical cord is relatively easily exposed from the clivus to the proximal aspect of the second thoracic vertebral body. Transoral and retropharyngeal exposures are selectively used in the treatment of rheumatoid disease or tumor causing upper cervical cord compression. The most commonly employed surgical approach to the midcervical spine is through an anteromedial exposure between the carotid sheath and sternocleidomastoid muscle laterally, and the trachea, esophagus, and strap muscles medially. Posterior pathology, extensive multiple level cervical spondylotic myeloradiculopathy spanning distances greater than three vertebral bodies or four disk spaces, and intradural tumors are best treated with the cervical laminectomy.

Anterolateral thoracotomy or posterolateral costotransversectomy allow access anterior to the thoracic cord without retraction of neural elements. The exposure obtained with the costotransversectomy is limited when compared with that of an open thoracotomy, and thus may not be suitable for patients with extensive disease or those needing vertebral body reconstruction. The costotransversectomy, however, is a selected alternative to the increased pulmonary morbidity but neurologic safety of the thoracotomy. The thoracic laminectomy has been abandoned as a technique for excision of anterior disk or tumor because of the high incidence of paraplegia.

The cauda equina and lumbar roots tolerate surgical retraction with relative safety. Therefore, disk, tumor, or infection compressing the lumbar spine may be safely managed by either the familiar lumbar laminectomy or an anterior retroperitoneal approach.

Neurologic Complications of Bone Graft Harvest

Bone grafting is necessary in order to obtain a spinal fusion. Unfortunately, persistent donor site pain occurs in 15% of these patients,[1, 2] marring an otherwise excellent outcome. Sensory nerves at risk for injury during iliac crest bone harvest include the lateral femoral cutaneous nerve and the three posterior cluneal nerves.[1, 2]

The lateral femoral cutaneous nerve is superficial and thus commonly injured during routine exposure of the anterior iliac crest. It arises from branches of L1, L2, and L3, and appears 1 cm inferior to the anterior superior iliac spine. The nerve then passes over the lateral surface of the sartorius muscle. The normal course of the nerve is medial and inferior to the anterior superior iliac spine and deep to the inguinal ligament. However, in 10% of patients, the nerve takes an anomalous course over the anterior crest while coursing up to 2 cm lateral to the anterior superior iliac spine.[2] This anomalous position places the nerve at risk for injury during bone graft harvesting from the anterior ileum. Meralgia paresthetica—that is, painful numbness and paresthesias—occurs on the anterolateral thigh in 10% of patients after anterior iliac crest bone harvest.[2] Expectant treatment includes nerve blocks, transcutaneous electrical nerve stimulators, and analgesics. Recalcitrant cases may require neuroma excision.

The three superior cluneal nerves originate above the posterior iliac crest and supply sensation

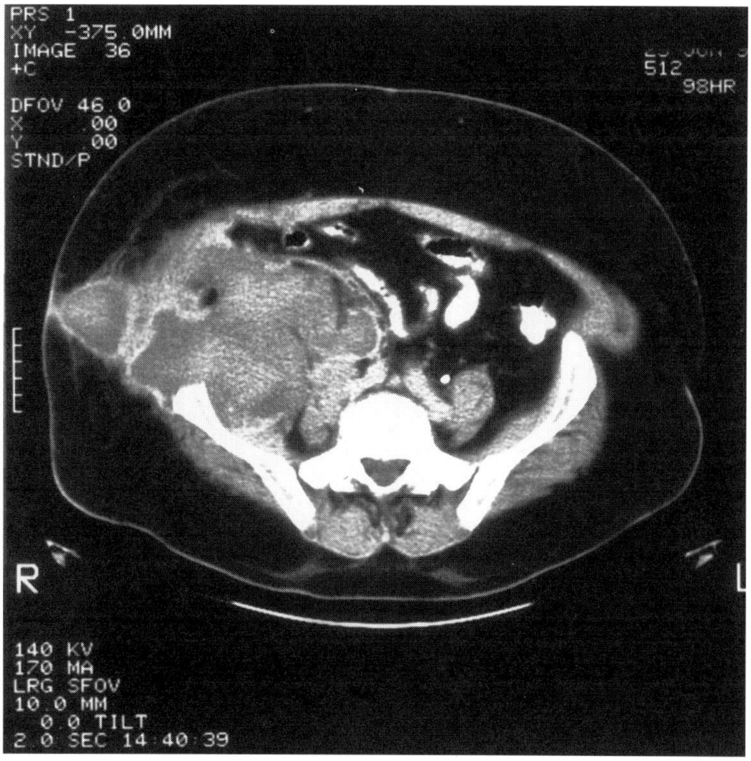

Figure 7.1. This postoperative pelvic computed tomography scan demonstrates a massive right-sided retroperitoneal hematoma in a patient with known type I von Willebrand's disease. The patient underwent harvest of bone graft from the right anterior iliac crest and had received appropriate presurgical management with factor VIII, desmopressin, and platelets. The anterior cervical diskectomy and fusion was uneventful. On the second postoperative day ileus, abdominal rigidity, and a complete right-sided femoral neuropathy was noted. The computed tomography scan documented the iliacus hematoma. Muscle strength returned within 1 year, but the patient remained anesthetic on the anterior thigh.

to the buttock in its middle third.[1, 2] They pierce the lumbodorsal fascia and posterior iliac crest beginning 8 cm lateral to the posterior superior iliac spine. Therefore, an incision placed for posterior ileum bone harvest should not stray greater than 8 cm lateral from the midline.[2] Expectant and symptomatic treatment has been described.

Femoral nerve palsy is a well-reported complication of retroperitoneal, psoas, or iliacus hematoma that may cause direct compression of the femoral plexus. This is documented in people with bleeding disorders and in anticoagulated patients.[3–5] Femoral nerve palsy as a complication of anterior lumbar interbody fusion is further discussed later in this chapter (see "Neurologic Complications Associated with Surgery of the Lumbar Spine"). One of our patients suffered a femoral neuropathy related to bone graft harvest from the anterior ileum. The postoperative pelvic CT scan shown in Figure 7.1 demonstrates a massive right-sided retroperitoneal hematoma in a patient with known type I von Willebrand's disease. The patient underwent harvest of bone graft from the right anterior iliac crest and had received appropriate presurgical management with factor VIII, desmopressin, and platelets. The anterior cervical diskectomy and fusion was uneventful. On the second postoperative day ileus, abdominal rigidity, and a complete right-sided femoral neuropathy was noted. CT scan documented the iliacus hematoma. Muscle strength returned within 1 year, but the patient remained anesthetized on the anterior thigh.

We have had regrettable experiences with four additional patients who required anticoagulation. Two patients suffered massive hematoma related to harvest of anterior iliac crest bone graft. Both patients required anticoagulation for aortic valve replacement. Preoperatively, the warfarin had been discontinued and replaced with heparin. The heparin had been discontinued 12 hours before surgery, and normal coagulation studies were documented. At the urging of the cardiology consultants, the warfarin was resumed on the second postoperative day. Both patients developed hematoma on the fourth postoperative day. Allograft bone is now preferred for all anticoagulated patients and those with bleeding disorders who would otherwise have required structural bone graft harvest from the anterior iliac crest. Two additional patients with valve replacement (one mitral, one aortic) suffered postoperative transient cerebral ischemic events within 2 weeks of otherwise successful surgery. At the time of the transient cerebral ischemic events both patients had resumed warfarin and were adequately anticoagulated. No further sequelae resulted. Despite these near neurologic catastrophes, anticoagulated patients and those with bleeding disorders may undergo successful spine surgery, constituting a satisfying yet challenging portion of the author's (R.J.H.) practice. The surgical indications must be strict, and consultation with a hematologist or cardiologist who understands the needs for intraoperative and postoperative hemostasis is required.

Neurologic Complications of Surgical Positioning

Commonly used patient positions for spinal surgery include sitting, prone, supine, and lateral recumbent. Catastrophic neurologic damage may result from the patient's placement on the operating table. General anesthesia abolishes protective muscle tone and patient feedback. Selected neurologic complications related to the operative position include air embolism and stroke, blindness, quadriplegia, and peripheral nerve palsies.

Craniotomy and cervical spine surgery is facilitated with the head and neck elevated above the level of the heart. The advantages of elevation include improved hemostasis and visualization of the operative field secondary to improved venous drainage and decreased arterial perfusion pressure. Symptomatic air embolism is a feared, although rare complication associated with surgical incisions positioned above the level of the heart.[6–13] The large exposed bleeding surfaces of scoliosis wounds also increase the risk of developing of air embolism.[13–15] The position of greatest risk is a seated position for cervical laminectomy.[6–10, 13] Doppler ultrasound has detected evidence of air embolism in 10–58% of patients while seated for cervical laminectomy.[6, 7] In one study, Doppler ultrasound detected evidence of air embolism in 25% of those seated, 14% of those in supine positions, 10% of those in prone positions, and 8.3% of patients in the lateral recumbent position.[6]

Most commonly, surgically introduced air passes inconsequentially through the alveolar membrane and is expired. Small amounts of air may pass through pulmonary vessels to reach the coronary and cerebral circulation. The rare but serious condition of paradoxic air embolism occurs when venous air is shunted systemically through a right-to-left intracardiac defect, most commonly a patent foramen ovale.[8, 10, 13, 16] The seated position predisposes one to paradoxic embolism because the normal interatrial pressure gradient may be reversed.[10] Of note, a patent foramen ovale has been reportedly found in 18% of volunteers undergoing echocardiography.[17]

Paradoxic air embolism causes audible air bubbles that may be detected by the anesthesiologist's Doppler ultrasound, esophageal stethoscope, or transesophageal echocardiography. Anesthetic monitoring documents the clinical decline, showing a decreased arterial partial pressure of oxygen (PaO_2), decreased end-expired arterial partial pressure of carbon dioxide ($PaCO_2$), and increased arterial $PaCO_2$. Finally, hypotension, tachycardia, cardiac arrest, seizures, coma, quadriplegia, decerebrate rigidity, vegetative state, and death may occur.[8–12, 15, 16] Electroencephalographic changes caused by cerebral emboli and ischemia have been documented.[8] Death results from acute cor pulmonale and arterial hypoxemia, as right ventricular ejection into the pulmonary artery is blocked by air. Air in the coronary arteries causes ischemia and fibrillation.

Before seated surgery, an echocardiogram is used to determine if a patent foramen ovale is present.[11, 17] If shunting is demonstrated, the seated position should not be considered. Intraoperative use of gradient compressive stockings may diminish venous pooling and maintain central venous pressure. Transesophageal echocardiography may be the most sensitive method for detection of intraoperative air bubbles and should be considered for high-risk seated surgery or in those with patent foramen ovale.

Central venous right atrial catheterization or Swan-Ganz catheterization allows intraoperative monitoring and air withdrawal from the heart if significant embolism occurs.[12] Swan-Ganz monitoring can differentiate the hemodynamic effects of brain stem or cord manipulation from air embolism.[12, 18] Transesophageal echocardiography is superior to Swan-Ganz monitoring for early detection of air bubbles. However, Swan-Ganz monitoring can measure both right and left atrial pressures, thus identifying those patients with a patent foramen ovale who are at risk for paradoxic embolism.[15, 18]

If embolism is suspected, the wound should be covered with irrigation and hemostasis achieved. Air may be removed from the heart via the central venous right atrial catheter or Swan-Ganz catheter.[12] Nitrous oxide as an anesthetic must be stopped because it increases the size of the embolus.[11] If symptoms persist, the patient should be placed in the lateral decubitus position, right side up, to trap the air in the right side of the heart and prevent air from entering the coronary arteries and systemic circulation.[11]

Both anterior ischemic optic neuropathy[19] and central retinal artery occlusion[20–22] resulting in blindness have been described following spinal surgery. The mechanism of ischemic optic neuropathy is thought to be hypotension, resulting in infarction of the optic nerve from lowered perfusion pressure[19, 22]; funduscopic examination reveals a normal retina, with a swollen and ischemic optic nerve head.[22] Central retinal artery occlusion has been associated with prone head positioning on the horseshoe headrest, creating increased external ocular pressure resulting in direct compression and necrosis of the retinal vascular supply[19–22]; funduscopic examination reveals an edematous retina with dilated arterioles and engorged veins.[22] Both conditions have been related to intraoperative hypotension, massive blood loss, preexisting microvascular disease, and increased external ocular pressure.[19–22]

Patients at risk for direct laryngoscopy and oral tracheal intubation include those with cervical spine pain, preexisting central cord compression, cervical spondylosis, or myeloradiculopathy. Patients with rheumatoid arthritis, dwarfism, Down syndrome, and congenital anomalies of the head and neck are assumed to be at high risk for cervical anomalies that may cause brain stem or cord compression while under general anesthesia. General anesthesia abolishes protective cervical muscle function and patient feedback, thereby increasing the risk of intolerable neck positioning.

The patient's preoperative cervical spine evaluation must include an assessment for the tolerance of extreme neck positions, the position of neck comfort, and the risk associated with neck extension during intubation. Forced neck extension or passage of the laryngoscope blade may displace fractures. Neck extension during intubation or extremes of neck positioning during surgery may cause cord compression by a spondylotic bone ridge or infolding of redundant ligamentum flavum in patients with preexisting cervical spondylosis (Figure 7.2). This may precipitate a central cord syndrome or quadriplegia. Extremes of positioning may obstruct the carotid or vertebral arteries, resulting in stroke.[23, 24] Neck extension may be avoided through the use of awake fiberoptic endotracheal intubation. If a fiberoptic bronchoscope is not available, awake intubation may be accomplished using the laryngoscope after the upper airway is anesthetized and the neck stabilized. Blind or fiberoptic-guided nasal intubation may be used only in the absence of facial trauma or basilar skull fracture because the endotracheal tube could be placed into a false passage. Transtracheal jet ventilation through a cricothyroidotomy or a tracheostomy may be needed in the presence of severe head and neck trauma or for patients with rheumatoid arthritis or ankylosing spondylitis and severe fixed cervical kyphosis.

Anterior cervical disk surgery is facilitated with the neck in an extended position. Posterior cervical laminectomy is facilitated with the neck flexed. Prone positioning for thoracic or lumbar surgery without use of a head and neck positioning device requires that the neck be rotated to either side. Prone positioning in high-risk patients may be accomplished with the patient awake while intubated. After positioning is complete, the patient is asked to flex and dorsiflex his or her ankles and give the OK sign with the thumb and index finger to ensure comfortable neck position before general anesthesia. As an alternative, intraoperative SSEP and motor evoked potential (MEP) monitoring can quickly prompt the surgeon to correct a neurologically dangerous neck position. After high-risk prone positioning, a lateral cervical spine radiograph can ensure and document neutral neck position before the surgical preparation and drape. After surgical positioning, but before patient draping, this author (R.J.H.) makes a final visual and palpable check of the spine and extremities while questioning the patient's comfort for the upcoming 6–10 hours. If the response is unfavorable, the patient is repositioned.

The radiographs shown in Figure 7.2 demonstrate a 62-year-old patient with severe rheumatoid arthritis. The patient was ambulatory but noted increasing symptoms of "numb and clumsy hands and a drunken gait." Electrical shocks passed into his shoulders and arms while his wife inserted his

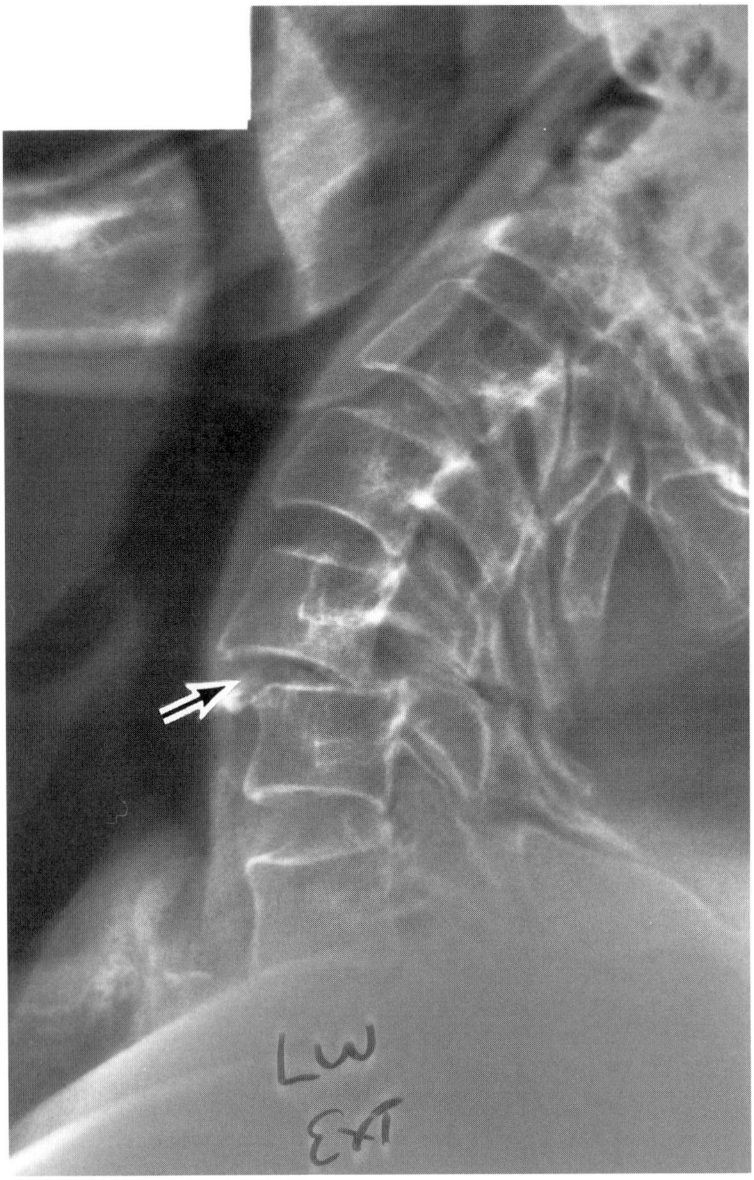

A

Figure 7.2. This 62-year-old patient had severe rheumatoid arthritis. The patient was ambulatory but noted increasing symptoms of "numb and clumsy hands and a drunken gait." Electrical shocks passed into his shoulders and arms while his wife inserted his contact lenses. (A) Subaxial cervical instability with spondylolisthesis (arrow) of C5 on C6. (B and C) Extension and flexion magnetic resonance image scans show severe spondylosis with infolding and buckling of the ligamentum flavum, causing severe cord compression. The cervical cord compression is worsened with the neck held in extension (B) and improved with the neck held in flexion (C). Note the vertical migration of the dens into the foramen magnum seen best with the neck held in extension. Patients with preexisting cervical spondylosis may suffer cord compression attributed to neck extension during endotracheal intubation or surgical positioning. This patient had an awake fiberoptic intubation and the neck was carefully maintained in neutral position during surgery.

contact lenses. Figure 7.2A demonstrates subaxial cervical instability with spondylolisthesis of C5 on C6. Extension and flexion MRI scans (see Figures 7.2B and C) show severe spondylosis with infolding and buckling of the ligamentum flavum causing severe cord compression. The cervical cord compression is worsened with the neck held in extension (see Figure 7.2B) and improved with the neck held in flexion. Note the vertical migration of the dens into the foramen magnum, seen best with the neck held in extension. Patients with preexisting cervical spondylosis may suffer cord compression attributed to neck extension during endotracheal intubation or surgical positioning. This patient had an awake fiberoptic intubation, and the neck was carefully maintained in neutral position during surgery. The postoperative radiograph (see Figure 7.2D) demonstrates multilevel vertebrectomy, strut grafting, and anterior and posterior fusion. An otherwise successful surgery was marred for 3 months

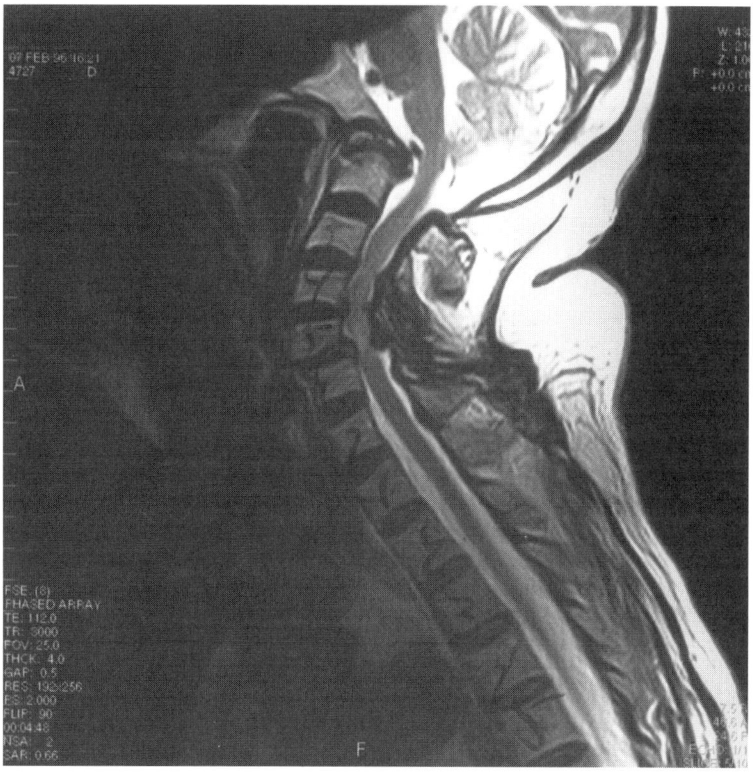
07 FEB 96 16:21
4727 D
A
FSE (8)
PHASED ARRAY
TE: 112.0
TR: 3000
FOV: 25.0
THCK: 4.0
GAP: 0.5
RES: 192/256
ES: 2.000
FLIP: 90
00:04:48
NSA: 2
SAR: 0.66
F

B

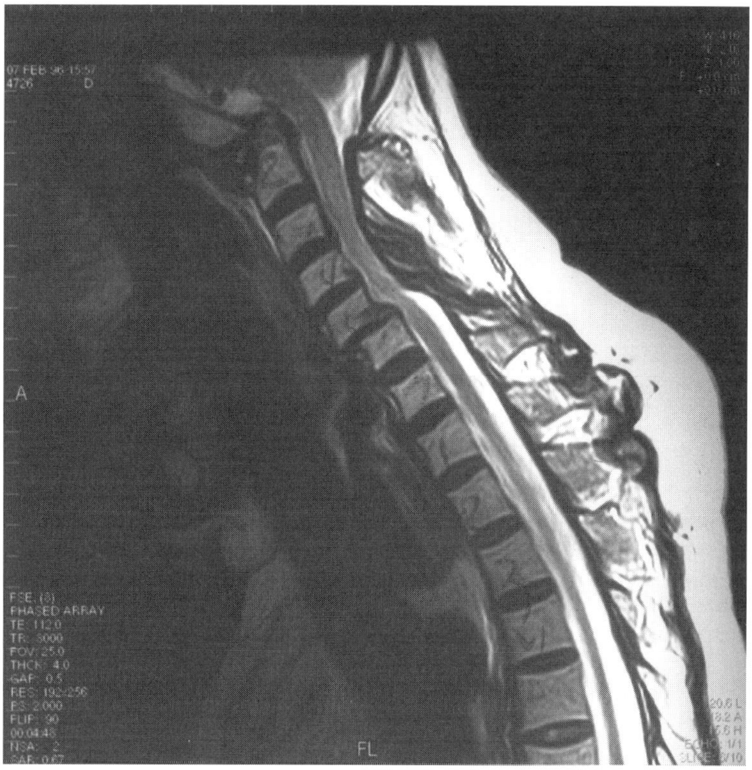
07 FEB 96 15:57
4726 D
A
FSE (8)
PHASED ARRAY
TE: 112.0
TR: 3000
FOV: 25.0
THCK: 4.0
GAP: 0.5
RES: 192/256
ES: 2.000
FLIP: 90
00:04:48
NSA: 2
SAR: 0.67
FL

C

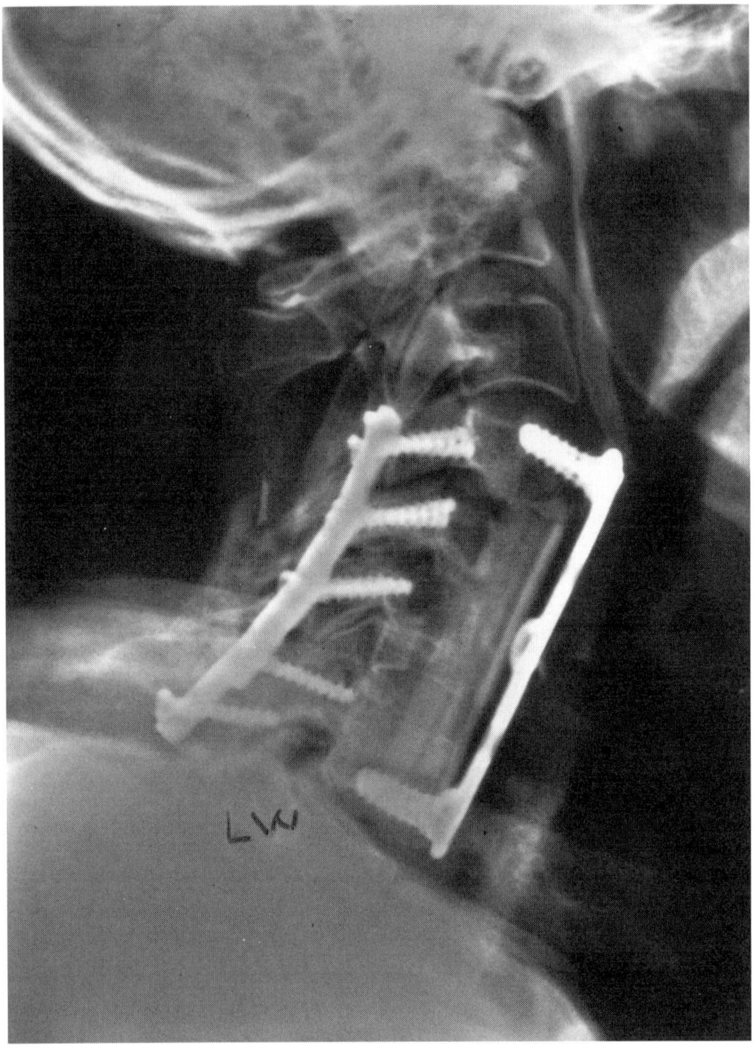

D

Figure 7.2. *continued.* (D) The postoperative radiograph demonstrates multilevel vertebrectomy, strut grafting, and anterior and posterior fusion. An otherwise successful surgery was marred for 3 months by loss of the gag reflex resulting in multiple aspirations, repeated bouts of pneumonia, and eventual tracheostomy. Fortunately, the gag reflex recovered spontaneously.

by loss of the gag reflex, resulting in multiple aspirations, repeated bouts of pneumonia, and eventual tracheostomy. Fortunately, the gag reflex was recovered spontaneously.

Prone, supine, or lateral recumbent positions for spinal surgery may produce compression of peripheral nerves. The following conditions have been reported:

1. In sciatic nerve palsy, the sciatic nerve may be compressed against a buttress while in the kneeling position.[25, 26]
2. In ulnar nerve palsy, a hyperflexed elbow or direct compression may precipitate a cubital tunnel syndrome with ulnar digit paresthesias.[27] The subcutaneous location at the elbow places this nerve at increased risk for injury.
3. In anterior interosseous nerve palsy, this nerve may be compressed at the tendinous origin of the deep head of the pronator teres, resulting in paresis of the flexor pollicis longus and flexor profundus tendons to the index and middle fingers, as well as the pronator quadratus.[28]
4. Axillary nerve palsy has been reported from intraoperative shoulder subluxation, shoulder hyperabduction of more than 90 degrees, or direct compression.[29]

5. Suprascapular nerve palsy results from intraoperative shoulder subluxation, shoulder hyperabduction of more than 90 degrees, or direct compression.[30]
6. In brachial plexus palsy, the lower trunk of the brachial plexus may be injured by prolonged shoulder abduction of more than 90 degrees.[31, 32] Note that in addition, protective muscular tone is lost in the anesthetized patient. The shoulders must therefore be supported to prevent anterior subluxation and stretch injury in the prone patient.[26, 31, 32] When in the lateral recumbent position, the dependent axilla and brachial plexus must be protected from compression with an axillary roll, which is properly placed beneath the upper chest, just distal to the axilla.[33]
7. Finally, in peroneal nerve palsy, the common peroneal nerve is injured and results in footdrop, which may occur in the lateral recumbent position as the patient's dependent leg compresses the nerve against the fibular head. Careful padding and attention to detail are required for prevention.[25, 26, 34]

Neurologic Complications Associated with Surgery of the Cervical Spine

There are a greater variety of neurologic complications associated with anterior, rather than posterior cervical surgery. These complications are related to the more complex anatomy of the anterior neck rather than to the actual neural decompression procedure. Most series comparing anterior and posterior cervical surgery are retrospective, variable, and uncontrolled for preoperative severity of compressive disease and comorbidity. The literature cannot support either surgical approach as superior for the treatment of cervical spondylotic myeloradiculopathy.[35] Preferences for either the anterior or posterior procedure depend on the surgeon's training and patient selection. In general, supine positioning for the anterior exposure of the middle cervical spine is straightforward when compared with the prone or sitting position and skull pin traction needed for cervical laminectomy. By comparison, multilevel cervical laminectomy is a less formidable procedure than multilevel anterior vertebrectomy, which requires extensive anterior soft tissue dissection, structural bone graft, and fusion.[35] For most surgeons and patients, the technical limit for anterior exposure of the midcervical spine is three vertebral bodies and four disk spaces. Therefore, extensive multilevel spondylotic disease may best be treated with posterior laminectomy.[35]

Portions of the midcervical spine may be exposed anteriorly from C2–C3 to T1–T2 with relative ease and in a bloodless fashion. The decompression is usually straightforward because the cord need not be manipulated. The difficulties associated with prone positions are avoided. Complications are many but are usually related to the anatomic soft tissue dissection at the proximal and distal extents of the exposure rather than to decompression of the cervical cord. Sensory branches of the facial nerve may be cut during the skin incision and elevation of the platysma. This creates problematic numbness, especially while shaving. Other complications unique to anterior exposure of the midcervical spine include dislodgment of bone graft into the cord, recurrent laryngeal nerve palsy, superior laryngeal nerve palsy, hypoglossal nerve palsy, Ondine's curse, Horner's syndrome, vertebral artery laceration, stroke, myelopathy, and quadriplegia. Spinal stenosis may occur adjacent to a solid fusion, years after otherwise successful surgery.

Myelopathy and quadriplegia are the most feared complications of anterior cervical surgery. In Flynn's survey of more than 82,000 cases of anterior cervical diskectomy, the incidence of quadriplegia was 0.1%.[36] Estimates from other authors range from 0% to 1.8%.[37–43] Most spinal cord or nerve root injuries are associated with technical misadventures.[36, 44, 45] Risk factors include operative trauma from a plunging instrument or posterior displacement of bone graft into the spinal canal.[46] Krause and Stauffer reported on 10 spinal cord injuries suffered during anterior cervical diskectomy and fusion. Five of these injuries were attributed to plunging instruments, bone graft insertion, or electrocautery on the posterior longitudinal ligament.[46] Also reported is quadriplegia related to a "water hammer" effect created during bone graft impaction.[36, 47] Although the perfectly shaped bone graft would completely fill the operative defect, it would seal the cord from the superficial soft tissues, preventing egress of blood products anterior to the bone graft during impaction. This author (R.J.H.) recommends allowing some space for blood products to vent. This may prevent the water hammer effect and allow drainage of an expanding epidural hematoma.

Recurrent laryngeal nerve palsy may result during the distal extension of the anterior approach below C6, especially from a right-sided incision.[48–50] A right-handed surgeon, however, often prefers the right-sided approach. On the left, the recurrent laryngeal nerve passes under the aortic arch and joins the tracheoesophageal groove in the upper thoracic spine, which is away from the operative field. The left recurrent nerve is therefore relatively protected. On the right, the recurrent laryngeal nerve passes under the subclavian artery. The right recurrent nerve may enter the tracheoesophageal groove as far proximally as C5, crossing through the operative field.[50] In fact, the right recurrent nerve is vulnerable for two reasons. First, as noted, the right recurrent nerve may not be protected in the tracheoesophageal groove as it passes from under the subclavian artery into the neck. Second, and possibly more important, the right-sided nerve may be nonrecurrent, therefore passing directly from the vagus nerve and carotid sheath to the larynx. In this situation, the nerve is vulnerable to direct trauma because it crosses the operative field. A nonrecurrent laryngeal nerve may act as a direct tether to retraction of the carotid sheath. Neuropraxia may result even when the nerve is recognized and protected. If the nerve is not recognized, it may be inadvertently ligated with the inferior thyroid artery in an attempt to improve the surgical exposure. The incidence of a nonrecurrent laryngeal nerve on the right may approach 1%.[51, 52] If the nerve cannot be safely retracted, the right-sided procedure may be aborted and a left-sided approach may be undertaken.[51]

Both the right and left recurrent laryngeal nerves enter the larynx through the cricothyroid membrane along with the inferior thyroid artery and are rarely injured cephalad to the C6 body. Theoretically, to minimize injury to the recurrent laryngeal nerve, planned exposures below the C6 body may be approached from the left. The left recurrent nerve may still be damaged, especially if surgical orientation is lost and dissection strays into the tracheoesophageal groove. We have examined patients with partial vocal cord paralysis from a left-sided surgical exposure. Although difficult to discern from the operative record, one may postulate unintended dissection within the left tracheoesophageal groove.

Temporary hoarseness or sore throat after anterior cervical surgery is common and may be related to surgical or anesthetic manipulation of the trachea. However, recurrent laryngeal nerve palsy may be present in 2.0–3.5% of patients with persistent hoarseness.[51, 53] The incidence of temporary vocal cord palsy may be much higher. Heeneman reported on 85 patients in whom 3% had permanent changes but 11% had at least temporary hoarseness.[53] The possibility of a nonrecurrent laryngeal nerve, as described earlier, should always be foremost in the surgeon's mind. In more than 200 exposures to the midcervical spine, five of our patients (four right-sided exposures, one left-sided exposure) suffered persistent postoperative hoarseness (2.5%). Three patients resolved their deficits within 6 weeks, and two patients suffered permanent recurrent laryngeal nerve palsy (1%). One of these two patients, in fact, resolved his hoarseness. His voice diminishes to a whisper with prolonged conversation, however. His greatest complaint is the inability to be clearly understood over the telephone. Any patient under consideration for additional or repeated anterior cervical surgery should be questioned regarding prolonged hoarseness after the initial surgery. Many surgeons would prefer to do repeat anterior surgery from the contralateral side to the previous operation, thereby avoiding scar tissue during the dissection. If there is a question of prior recurrent laryngeal nerve damage, however, the surgery should be performed ipsilateral to the previous surgery to avoid the catastrophic situation of inducing bilateral nerve damage with resultant asphyxiation. If there is any doubt, the situation may be confirmed preoperatively via direct laryngoscopy. If there is a recurrent nerve palsy, the vocal cord will be paralyzed in a paramedian position.

Superior laryngeal nerve palsy may occur during cephalad retraction and exposure of the C2–C3 disk space while performing an anterior approach to the midcervical spine. The hypoglossal and superior laryngeal nerves both arise from the inferior ganglion of the vagus nerve and are at risk for injury during surgical exposure to the C2–C3 disk space.[48–50, 54] Hoarseness, fatiguing of the voice, or aspiration results from cricothyroid paralysis and laryngeal sensory loss.[51, 53] Direct laryngoscopy shows a more lateral deviation of the vocal cords. The disability from a superior laryngeal nerve palsy may be less profound than that from a recurrent laryngeal nerve palsy.

Hypoglossal nerve palsy may result from the anterior retropharyngeal approach, which is performed to allow an extramucosal exposure of the clivus and upper cervical spine.[48–50, 54] Damage to the hypoglossal and glossopharyngeal nerves may occur in 15% of individuals who undergo this surgical approach.[49, 54, 55] Hypoglossal nerve palsy may also occur from proximal extension of the midcervical approach above the C2–C3 disk space.[49, 50, 54] The hypoglossal nerve exits the condylar foramen 2 cm lateral to the midline. Therefore, transoral procedures must be limited to a total exposure width of 4 cm.[48, 55, 56]

Ondine's curse is a postoperative complication of upper cervical spine surgery characterized by loss of automatic respiration but preserved voluntary breathing. Sleep-induced apnea may result that is reversed with awakening. This rarely reported condition may follow anterior surgery at the C3–C4 disk space.[56–58] Krieger and Rosomoff noted the problem to occur with anterior cervical surgery at the C3–C4 level, the main origin of the phrenic nerves. The respiratory center is in the medulla oblongata, and spontaneous respiration is maintained by both wakefulness and the $PaCO_2$.[57] During sleep, the respiratory drive depends largely on the $PaCO_2$. High cervical surgery may damage the reticulospinal tract, the descending respiratory pathway that is located in the anterolateral quadrant of the spinal cord and extending longitudinally from the first to the fourth cervical vertebrae.[56, 57] Patients may initially be misdiagnosed as having pulmonary emboli, myocardial infarction, or pneumonia.[56]

Horner's syndrome may result from interruption of the sympathetic plexus or superior cervical ganglion, which lies on the anterior surface of the longus coli muscle and lateral aspect of vertebral bodies, as far distally as the third thoracic vertebra.[48, 50] The syndrome consists of ipsilateral mild ptosis with involvement of the smooth muscle of Müller, ipsilateral pupillary constriction, and ipsilateral facial anhydrosis. This condition may result from an extraperiosteal exposure that has been extended too far laterally onto the surface of the longus coli muscle during exposure of the anterior aspect of the cervical disk space. This condition is rare after cervical surgery, occurring in less than 1% of cases.[36]

Intraoperative vertebral artery laceration is a fortunately rare event. Recommendations for emergent treatment include attempts at packing, repair, or ligation.[59–66] The paired vertebral arteries usually originate from their respective subclavian arteries. The vertebral artery enters the foramen transversarium at the sixth cervical vertebra and progresses in a cephalad fashion, lateral to the uncovertebral joints. The artery is located in the anterior one-half of the vertebral body. It exits the foramen transversarium of C1 and turns posteriorly and medially to lie in a groove on the upper border of the posterior ring of C1. The artery exits this groove and enters the spinal canal, penetrating the posterior atlanto-occipital membrane, 12–16 mm from the midline.[50, 55] The paired vessels unite at the lower border of the pons to form the basilar artery. Together, the vertebral and basilar arteries supply the brain stem and cerebellum. The basilar artery terminates by dividing into two posterior cerebral arteries, which complete the circle of Willis.[57]

A hypoplastic vertebral artery is observed in 5–10% of normal angiograms.[67] In 1% of cases the vertebral artery may terminate in a posterior inferior cerebellar artery.[68] However, unilateral extracranial occlusion of a vertebral artery is usually well tolerated. The brain stem may be supplied from the contralateral vertebral artery. In addition, extracranial occlusion of a vertebral artery may be compensated by anastomotic flow to the upper part of the artery via the thyrocervical, deep cervical, and occipital arteries, or retrograde flow from the circle of Willis.[57] However, unilateral intracranial occlusion of a vertebral artery may result in a lateral medullary (Wallenberg's) syndrome.[57] A lateral medullary syndrome by itself is not fatal, and the cerebellum is usually spared.[69] However, delayed cerebellar infarcts resulting from traumatic vertebral artery dissection and subsequent embolization have been reported and should be suspected.[70] Hoshino et al. reported on the safety of planned unilateral vertebral artery ligation during tumor surgery in 15 patients.[60] They noted no postoperative ischemic changes. All patients were evaluated preoperatively by angiography. They concluded that a vertebral artery could be ligated uneventfully when the diameter of the ligated vessel was not larger than the contralateral artery.

There is a 1% incidence of ectatic or medially displaced vertebral arteries that may actually lie within the vertebral body, creating great risk for injury during routine anterior cervical exposure.[61] Oga et al. noted that the vertebral artery may become medially displaced in patients with severe spondylotic changes.[65] CT scan identifies the location of the transverse foramen, but the vertebral artery is not demonstrated. Myelographic enhanced CT scan may demonstrate an extradural mass but cannot differentiate soft tissue from vascular structures. T1-weighted MRI demonstrates a signal void that differentiates solid lesions from vascular anomalies.[61] Epstein and Silvergleid recommend magnetic resonance angiography to demonstrate the blood flow of an aberrant vertebral artery if suspected by unexplained signal voids on preoperative MRI or by foraminal masses noted on myelographic enhanced CT of the cervical spine.[61] Smith et al. analyzed 1,195 anterior cervical operations and reported 10 cases of vertebral artery laceration (0.8%).[62] Golfinos et al. noted four of 1,215 (0.3%) anterior cervical disk surgeries complicated by vertebral artery laceration.[63]

Important surgical landmarks that must be respected during the neural decompression include the anterior longitudinal ligament, the medial border of the uncovertebral joint, and the posterior annulus fibrosis. The amount of disk and bone removal necessary to achieve satisfactory decompression may be measured preoperatively on the axial MRI or CT view. This is compared with the lateral width of the transverse foramen, which provides cephalad passage for the vertebral arteries. The typical width of surgical decompression necessary for the treatment of cervical spondylotic myeloradiculopathy is 20 mm. Bone and disk may be resected with a high-speed pneumatic drill with continuous reference to the anterior longitudinal ligament, which identifies the midline. The width of the decompression may be measured intraoperatively with a 0.75-in. (19-mm) osteotome. An additional 2–3 mm of lateral decompression on either side is performed by undercutting the uncovertebral joint with the Kerrison's punch. The medial border of the uncovertebral joint is well visualized with use of the surgical microscope. The pedicle that identifies the lateral margin of the dissection may be palpated with a probe. Dissection lateral to the uncovertebral joint places the vertebral artery at risk for injury when working in the anterior one-half of the vertebral body. When working in the posterior aspect of the vertebral body, however, it is safe to undercut the uncovertebral joint and thereby increase the lateral exposure. Both the posterior annulus fibrosis and posterior longitudinal ligament are resected to allow visualization of the anterior cervical cord. Bone osteophytes causing cord compression are resected. It is preferable to sacrifice the cortical endplates and bone of the adjacent vertebral bodies rather than attempt blind resection of osteophytes with a Kerrison's punch or curette. The surgical defect created is shaped like the outward flair of a trumpet, and the exposure is widened to 20 mm or more in the posterior aspect of the body.

In patients previously operated on or when performing multiple level vertebrectomy, the anterior longitudinal ligament may have been resected or buried in scar, making identification of the midline especially difficult. Many surgeons find anterior cervical exposure is facilitated by turning the neck away from the operated side. Vigilance is needed during this maneuver to prevent loss of surgical orientation. With the head turned away from the incision, it is possible to inadvertently resect the uncovertebral joint and lateral vertebral body wall on the side opposite the surgical incision, thereby inadvertently exposing the vertebral artery.

Complications related to the superficial soft tissue dissection of the posterior cervical spine include painful sensory neuroma. The greater occipital nerve is the medial branch of the dorsal division of the second cervical nerve. It penetrates the trapezius near the inion. Surgical exposure may damage this nerve, resulting in the formation of a painful neuroma.[48]

The posterior exposure of the craniovertebral junction may endanger the vertebral artery and cause stroke. The artery may be injured when surgical exposure strays greater than 15 mm from the midline.[50, 55, 61] There is a 1% incidence of ectatic, medially displaced vertebral arteries, which may complicate extensive anterior surgery or high posterior surgery.[61] However, arterial injury is more commonly associated with anterior surgery as previously described. Inadvertent vertebral artery laceration from the posterior approach should be more easily repaired.

Neurologic complications unique to the posterior laminectomy include worsened neurologic deficit related to root or cord retraction in an attempt to retrieve anterior disk or osteophyte. Laminectomy in children for intradural tumor is associated with

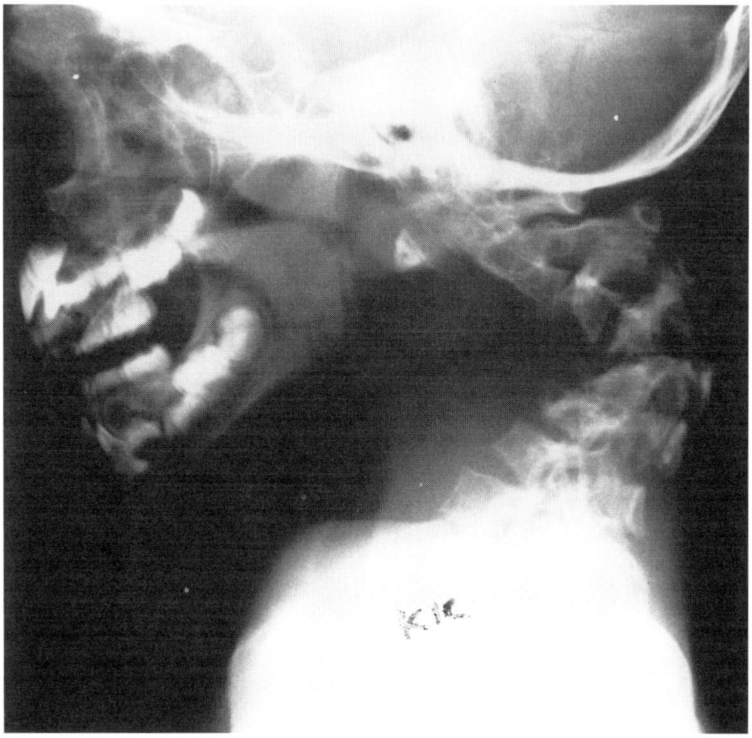

A

Figure 7.3. This 4-year-old child with neurofibromatosis had undergone extensive cervical laminectomy and intradural tumor resection. (A) Severe postlaminectomy kyphosis is shown.

the development of kyphosis and late myelopathy. Posterior surgical reduction of traumatic facet dislocations may be associated with quadriplegia from retropulsed disk into the cord. Persistent cerebrospinal fluid leak may lead to the formation of a pseudomeningocele resulting in late compressive myelopathy.

Postlaminectomy kyphosis can occur after the extensive cervical laminectomy required for the treatment of Arnold-Chiari malformation, congenital stenosis, syrinx, intradural tumor, cervical spondylotic myelopathy, and arteriovenous malformations. Postlaminectomy kyphosis may be minimized in adults by careful preservation of at least 50% of the facet joints.[71, 72] The risk of late kyphosis in children is high, however. Kyphosis may be associated with neurologic deterioration and should be suspected in children who have undergone cervical laminectomy without fusion.[73, 74] Bell et al. studied 89 children who had undergone extensive cervical laminectomy, and 53% developed kyphosis.[73] The 4-year-old child with neurofibromatosis shown in Figure 7.3 had undergone extensive cervical laminectomy and intradural tumor resection. Severe postlaminectomy kyphosis is shown in Figure 7.3A. The subtotal but adequate reduction of the deformity and fusion shown in Figure 7.3B should prevent further progression of the deformity.

Cervical facet dislocation disrupts the posterior elements of the cervical spine but may disrupt the disk as well.[75] Surgical fusion is indicated and is ideally performed through a posterior exposure of the disrupted ligaments and facet joints. However, post-traumatic disk herniation may occur in 80% of patients with bilateral facet dislocation.[75] Eismont et al. have described postoperative quadriplegia that resulted from further displacement of disk material into the spinal cord, associated with posterior reduction of the dislocation under anesthesia.[76] MRI documents the presence of a traumatic disk herniation. If disk disruption is present, anterior diskectomy must precede attempts at posterior reduction or fixation.[75–77]

Persistent cerebrospinal fluid leak may result in wound infection, meningitis, dural cutaneous fistula, or the formation of a pseudomeningocele.

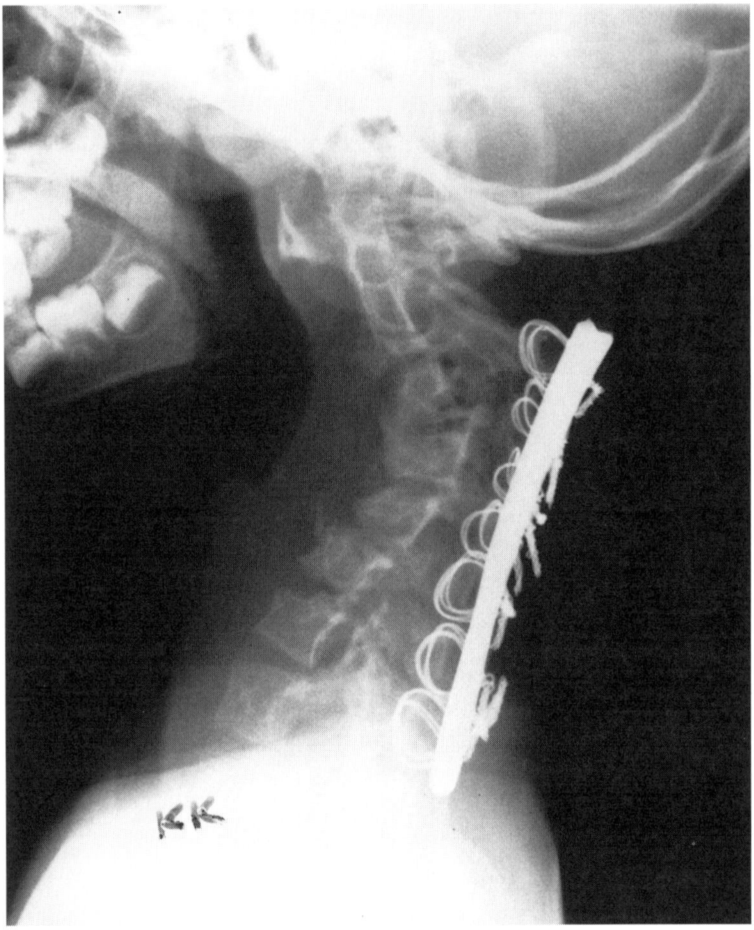

B

Figure 7.3. *continued.* (B) The subtotal but adequate reduction of the deformity and fusion should prevent further progression of the deformity.

The patient shown in Figure 7.4 had a cervical laminectomy for spondylotic myeloradiculopathy. The surgery was initially complicated by a persistent cerebrospinal fluid leak, which required the placement of a lumbar subarachnoid shunt. Despite this, the patient had relief of symptoms until the insidious return of spastic gait and clumsy hands after 10 years. Note the large postoperative cerebrospinal fluid accumulation causing severe cord compression.

Neurologic complications common to both the anterior and posterior exposures are related to the neural decompression rather than to the exposure itself. Quadriparesis or root injury may result from blunt, penetrating, thermal, or electrical injury. Epidural hematoma or retained disk fragment should be suspected in all patients whose condition deteriorates in the postoperative period. A disturbing incidence of sensory motor dissociated fifth cervical radiculopathy may occur.

Yonenobu et al. reported on 384 patents (204 anterior, 180 posterior) treated for cervical spondylotic myeloradiculopathy.[43] Twenty-one (5.5%) suffered neurologic deterioration related to surgery. Thirteen (3.5%) showed signs of C5 root paresis, and eight (2%)of spinal cord dysfunction. Of the eight patients in this study suffering spinal cord injury, three had a compressive epidural hematoma that complicated a posterior laminectomy, bone graft complications resulted in cord injury in three patients, and one patient suffered cord trauma during resection of thickened ossified posterior longitudinal ligament from an anterior approach. One patient suffered hemiparesis after an anterior approach, but the cause was not identified.

In 1981, the Cervical Spine Research Society established a morbidity and mortality committee whose function has been to survey the membership annually and provide statistics for complications. The 5-year experience from 1982 to 1986 included 5,356 surgeries of which 64% of the procedures were approached anteriorly.[78] The incidence of neurologic complications was higher (2.18% versus 0.64%) in the posteriorly treated group.[78] Spinal cord complications were more common in the group of patients undergoing posterior surgery, whereas root complications were more common in patients who were treated with anterior surgery.

Therapeutic measures should be promptly implemented for worsening neurologic deficit in the immediate postoperative patient. For instance, hypotension must be corrected to prevent further cord ischemia. High-dose methylprednisolone at a dosage of 30 mg per kg of body weight followed by 5.4 mg per kg per hour is administered.[79] Lateral cervical spine radiography may determine if bone graft retropulsion into the spinal cord has occurred. MRI, CT, or myelography can identify an epidural hematoma, retained disk fragment, retropulsed bone graft, or aberrant placement of spinal instrumentation. If spinal instrumentation has been used to correct kyphosis, the implants must be removed unless there is no possibility of their presence adding to the neurologic deficit. In the presence of compressive lesions, reoperation is indicated. In the absence of a compressive lesion, corticosteroids are continued while surgery is deferred.

Rare case reports documenting spinal epidural hematoma include spontaneous occurrences or association with vascular anomalies, anticoagulant mediation, trauma, hemophilia, lumbar puncture, and hypertension.[80–82] Reports of postoperative spinal epidural hematoma are extremely rare,[43, 78, 83–85] but may be under-reported. Epidural hematoma should be suspected in any patient who has severe postoperative pain that is out of proportion to that which is expected or in any patient with a progressive neurologic deficit immediately after surgery.

Sagittal MRI or myelography must be performed before the decision is made to proceed with wound exploration for suspected epidural hematoma. This strong recommendation is based on this author's (R.J.H.) experience with three healthy patients who have awakened from uncomplicated surgery with

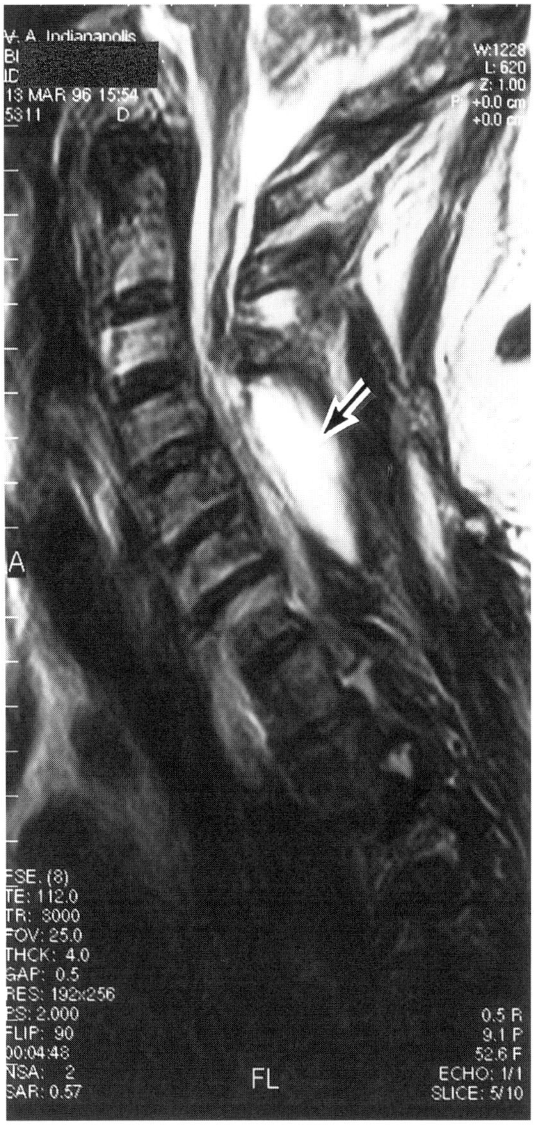

Figure 7.4. This patient had a cervical laminectomy for spondylotic myeloradiculopathy. The surgery was initially complicated by a persistent cerebrospinal fluid leak, which required the placement of a lumbar subarachnoid shunt. Despite this, the patient had relief of symptoms until the insidious return of spastic gait and clumsy hands after 10 years. Note the large postoperative cerebrospinal fluid accumulation (arrow) causing severe cord compression.

either quadriplegia or paraplegia. In all three patients, MRI defined pathology distant from the surgical site, enabling directed, expeditious, and successful management. The patient shown in Figure 7.5 had a routine anterior cervical diskectomy

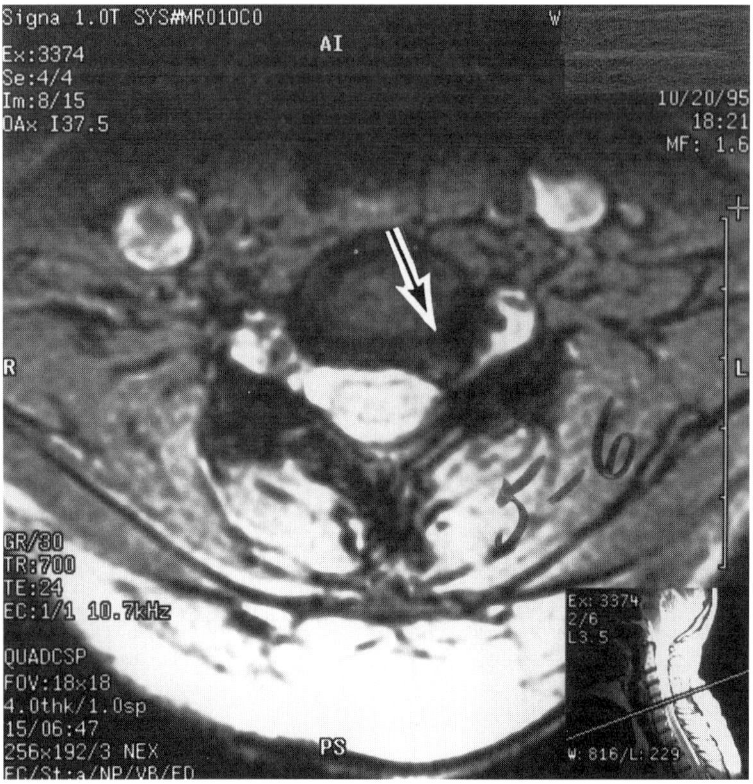

A

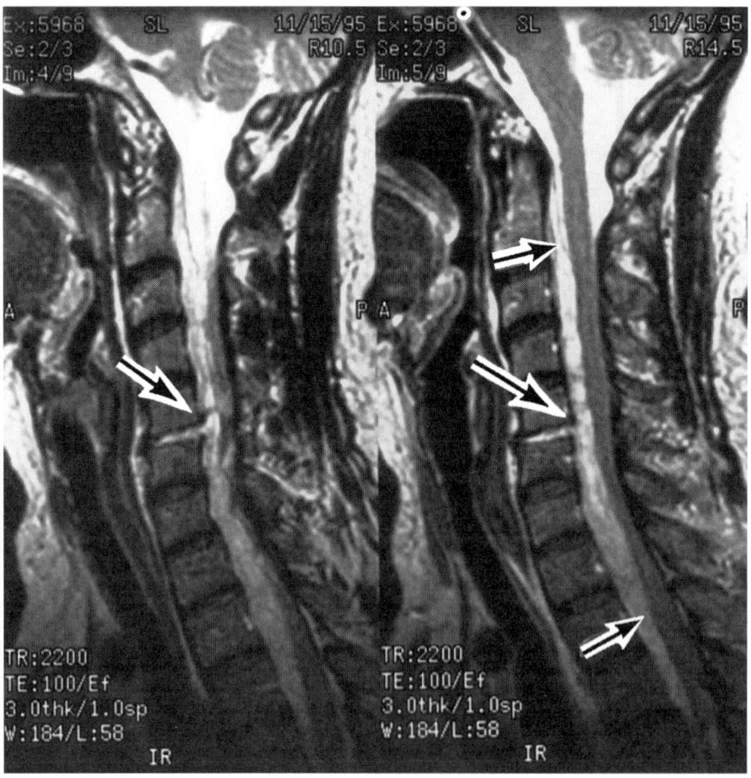

B

Figure 7.5. This patient underwent routine anterior cervical diskectomy without fusion, but became quadriparetic within 30 minutes of arrival in the recovery room. (A) The preoperative magnetic resonance imaging (MRI) scan demonstrates a large left-sided foraminal disk herniation (arrow). (B) The emergent postoperative MRI scan demonstrates an extensive epidural hematoma causing cord compression and extending from the foramen magnum to the fourth thoracic vertebrae. Note the C5–C6 disk excision and blood products emanating from this defect. Because of the extensive nature of the epidural hematoma (arrow), the patient was returned to the operating room for a cervical laminectomy extending from C2–T2. There would have been no chance of decompression of this extensive hematoma through the minimal anterior diskectomy site. The MRI scan, completed within 15 minutes, provided useful information that dictated a different surgical approach that could not have been predicted otherwise. Fortunately, the patient fully recovered.

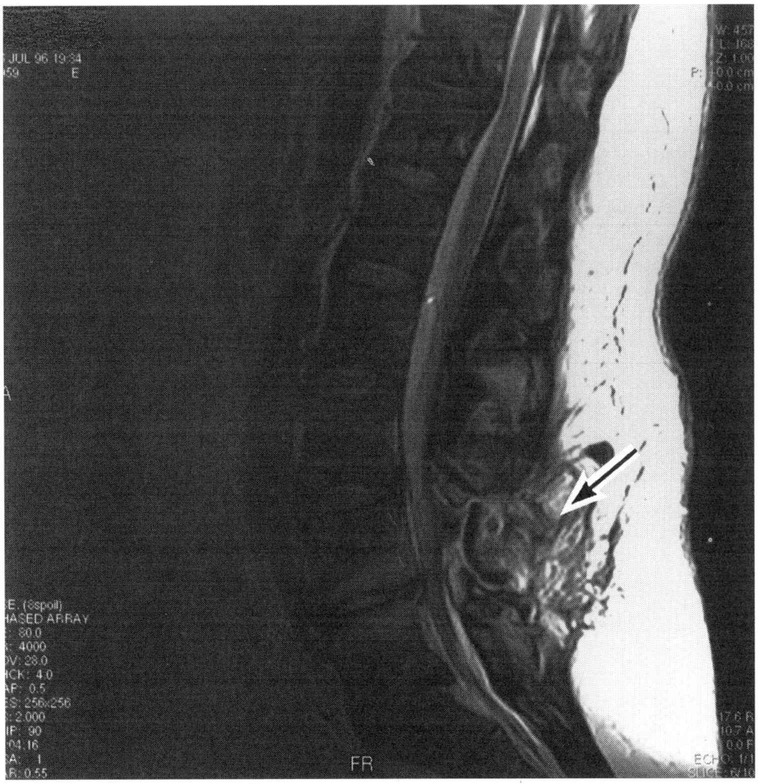

A

Figure 7.6. This patient developed paraparesis, the Brown-Séquard syndrome, and a T11-level sensory deficit within hours after having awakened from an uncomplicated lumbar laminectomy. Three grams of methylprednisolone (30 mg per kg) were administered intravenously. (A) An emergent postoperative magnetic resonance imaging (MRI) scan revealed only the posterior soft tissue defect (arrow) associated with the L4–L5 laminectomy and a T11–T12 disk bulge. However, pathology sufficient to explain the Brown-Séquard syndrome was not identified. The MRI technician was instructed to image further proximal into the thoracic spine, producing the scan seen in B and C. Note the large left-sided T9–T10 disk herniation identified by arrows. The patient was returned to surgery for emergency costotransversectomy and diskectomy. The patient recovered completely within 24 hours. Emergent MRI scan in this patient identified the large thoracic disk herniation, which was retrieved via costotransversectomy. There was no explanation for the untimely occurrence of the thoracic disk herniation.

without fusion, but became quadriparetic within 30 minutes of arrival in the recovery room. The preoperative MRI (see Figure 7.5A) demonstrates a large left-sided foraminal disk herniation. The emergent postoperative MRI (see Figure 7.5B) revealed an extensive anterior epidural hematoma causing cord compression and extending from the foramen magnum to the fourth thoracic vertebrae. Note the C5–C6 disk excision and blood products emanating from this defect. Because of the extensive nature of the epidural hematoma, the patient was returned to the operating room for a cervical laminectomy extending from C2–T2. There would have been no chance of decompression of this extensive hematoma through the minimal anterior diskectomy site. The MRI, completed within 15 minutes, provided useful information that dictated a different surgical approach that could not have been otherwise predicted. Fortunately, the patient has fully recovered.

Two additional patients from this author's (R.J.H.) clinical practice suffered the identical onset of postoperative paraplegia and deserve discussion. The radiographs of only one patient are presented for illustration. The patient shown in Figure 7.6 developed paraparesis, the Brown-Séquard syndrome, and a thoracic 11 level sensory deficit within hours after having awakened from an uncomplicated lumbar laminectomy. Three grams of methylprednisolone (30 mg per kg) were administered intravenously. An emergent postoperative MRI (see Figure 7.6A) revealed only the posterior soft tissue defect associated with the L4–L5 laminectomy and a

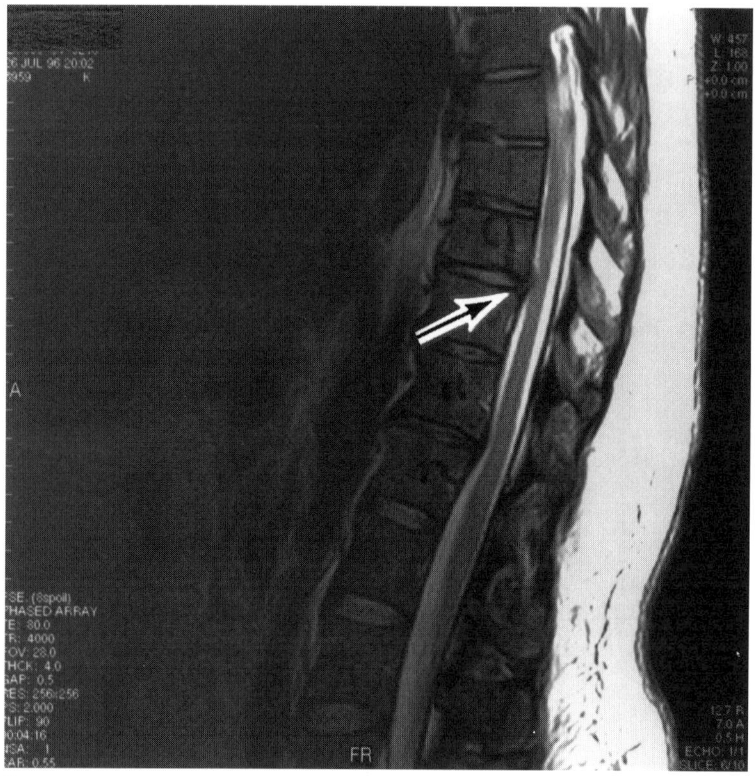

B

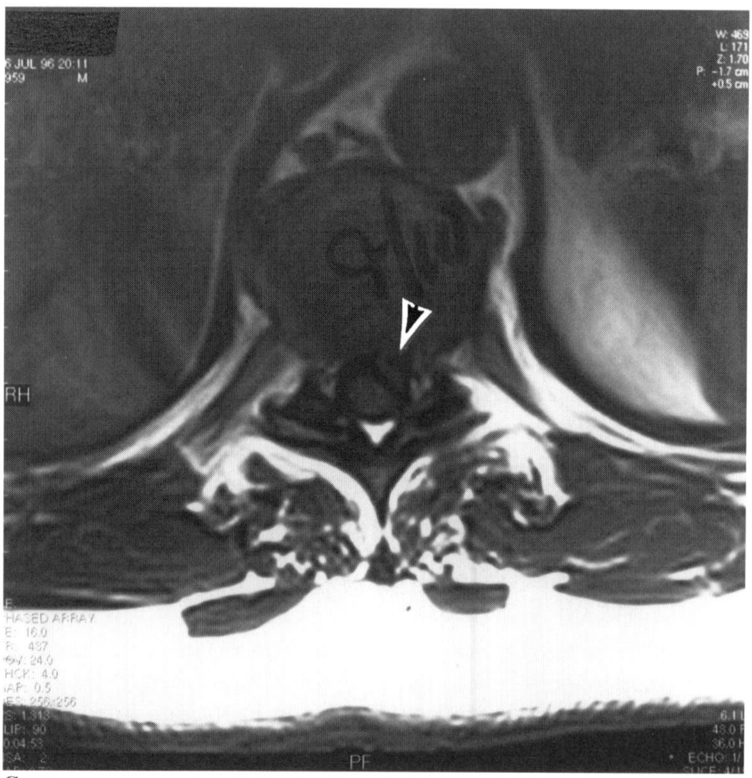

C

Figure 7.6. *continued.*

T11–T12 disk "bulge." However, pathology sufficient to explain the Brown-Séquard syndrome was not identified. The MRI technician was instructed to image further proximal into the thoracic spine, producing the MRI scan seen in Figures 7.6B and C. Note the large left-sided T9–T10 disk herniation. The patient was returned to surgery for emergency costotransversectomy and diskectomy. The patient recovered completely within 24 hours. Emergent MRI in this patient identified the large thoracic disk herniation, which was retrieved via costotransversectomy. There was no explanation for the untimely occurrence of the thoracic disk herniation.

A sensorimotor dissociated C5 or C6 radiculopathy may complicate posterior cervical laminectomy, laminoplasty, or vertebrectomy when used for the treatment of cervical spondylotic myeloradiculopathy. The postoperative course is marred by severe muscle atrophy, weakness, and deltoid or biceps pain in the absence of sensory deficit or myelopathy. The C5 and C6 roots are almost exclusively involved.[43, 86–92] The onset of symptoms may be noted in the recovery room or days thereafter.[88–90] The incidence of this complication is reported to be 4–17%.[89–91] This condition is well described in the Japanese literature,[86–88, 91, 92] but is infrequently discussed in the North American literature.[89, 90] In Yonenobu's study of 384 patients treated for cervical spondylotic myeloradiculopathy, 13 patients suffered a sensorimotor dissociated C5 radiculopathy; eight were associated with anterior surgery and five were associated with laminectomy. The etiology is thought to be related to either incomplete decompression of the nerve roots or to extradural tethering of the C5 or C6 roots that occurs after the stenotic cord decompresses into the surgically created defect.[87, 88, 92] Tsuzuki et al. recommend that posterolateral durotomy accompany cervical laminectomy to prevent extradural tethering of the cervical roots.[87] There is no consensus regarding treatment. The radiculopathy has been reported as self-limiting within 3–12 months.[87, 88] Others recommend repeat imaging studies, and if foraminal stenosis is documented, additional surgery is recommended.[89, 90] This condition is rarely reported after cervical diskectomy, perhaps because the cord does not decompress into the smaller defect, or perhaps because laminectomy or vertebrectomy are preferred by the Japanese for the treatment of severe cervical spondylotic myeloradiculopathy.

Neurologic Complications Associated with Surgery of the Thoracic Spine

The anterior exposure of the thoracic spine was born of the frustration and disastrous neurologic complications that occurred when thoracic laminectomy was used for treatment of pathology anterior to the cord. Thoracotomy is commonly performed for treatment of tumor, thoracic disk herniation, scoliosis, kyphosis, and infection.

The standard anterolateral thoracotomy provides safe exposure for vertebral levels T3–T10. For access to the thoracolumbar junction (T10–L2), a thoracoabdominal exposure of both the chest and retroperitoneal space is required. The diaphragm is the intervening structure between the chest and abdominal cavities. It is divided and then reattached at its periphery. The diaphragm is innervated in centrifugal manner, from the center to the periphery. Therefore, the peripheral detachment of the diaphragm does not cause problematic denervation.[50]

The surgical indications for anterolateral thoracotomy in the management of adolescent spinal deformity include most kyphoses, rigid mature scoliosis curvatures of more than 60 degrees, and curvatures of more than 45 degrees in very skeletally immature children. Ligation of segmental arteries over multiple vertebral segments is often required to mobilize the great vessels and improve visualization of the anterior spine. Surgery is ideally performed using hypotensive anesthesia (mean arterial pressure near 60 mm Hg) for control of hemorrhage.[93, 94] Complete diskectomy, excision of the anterior longitudinal ligament and annulus fibrosis, and bone grafting of the disk spaces are performed so that curve correction may be obtained. Finally, the patient is repositioned prone whereby the posterior thoracic spine is exposed, the deformed spine is corrected, and the metal implants including sublaminar wires and hooks are placed. Intraoperative electrophysiologic monitoring is invaluable and is the standard of care in scoliosis centers. When treating healthy adolescents with idiopathic scoliosis, these combined risks of producing cord ischemia remain acceptable.

The neurologic complications related to the thoracotomy exposure for the anterior thoracic spine are vascular and related to ligation of segmental vessels for exposure. Troublesome post-thoracotomy syndrome pain from intercostal nerve trauma and irritation may occur in 10% of these patients but often responds to intercostal nerve blocks in the pediatric population.

The afferent blood supply to the thoracic cord is derived from the 31 pairs of radicular branches, the intramedullary arteries, and the anastomotic arterial pathways. Lazorthes et al. divide the thoracic cord into three regions based on the origin and quality of vascularity.[95] The richly vascularized cervicothoracic zone includes the cervical cord and first three thoracic segments. The midthoracic zone extends from T4 to T8. Because the blood supply is tenuous, this area is referred to as the watershed zone, and it is uniquely susceptible to ischemic injury.[95] The thoracolumbar zone extends from T9 to L4. The blood supply is abundant to this area. The largest radiculomedullary feeder vessel to this area is the artery of Adamkiewicz. This artery is located on the left side in 60% of patients. It enters between T5 and T8 in 15%, T9 and L2 in 75%, and L1 and L2 in 10% of patients.[95] According to Dommisse, this artery occurs on the left side in 80% of patients between the T7 and L4 levels, with the most common site being T9–T11.[96]

The treatment of spinal deformity carries the potential risk of devastating paraplegia. Fortunately, reports of neurologic complications related to the anterior exposure of the thoracic spine are rare, even after extensive ipsilateral sacrifice of multiple segmental vessels.[97–101] One study documented 1,223 patients who underwent anterior exposure of the thoracic or lumbar spine.[99] Three of 42 patients who underwent high thoracotomy suffered Horner's syndrome (7%). Sixty-one of 665 patients who underwent thoracotomy suffered post-thoracotomy pain syndrome (9%). Two patients having combined anterior and posterior surgery developed paraplegia (0.16%), and three developed stroke (0.25%). Authors of the previous study[99] again reviewed their patients specifically regarding ischemic injury resulting from vessel ligation; 1,197 consecutive patients underwent anterior thoracic procedures, with more than 6,000 segmental vessels ligated. There was no instance of paraplegia related to segmental vessel ligation.[101] Bassett et al. identified radicular arteries using preoperative spinal cord angiography and then studied the relationships of temporary intraoperative occlusion of segmental vessels and the resultant SSEP response.[102] There was no evidence of SSEP changes. Currently, unilateral segmental vessel ligation is widely observed to be a relatively safe procedure in young patients with idiopathic scoliosis.

Unfortunately, paraplegia and cord ischemia are more commonly associated with anterior surgery and segmental vessel ligation surgery for congenital spine deformities such as cord tethering, diastematomyelia, kyphosis, or spinal dysraphism.[103–110] Intraoperative spinal cord monitoring is the current standard of care in such high-risk patients.[102, 111–114] Techniques of sequential temporary and reversible occlusion of the segmental vessels under SSEP monitoring should be employed before permanent vessel ligation in this special subset of high-risk patients.[102, 111]

Bilateral disruption of the segmental blood supply carries high risk. This is documented following aortic cross clamp or dissecting aortic aneurysms with bilateral occlusion of segmental vessels.[111, 115–117] Bilateral thoracic sympathectomy has caused paraplegia.[118] Revision of anterior spinal procedures, when the contralateral segmental vessels have been previously ligated, carries great risk. Extensive spinal resections requiring bilateral sacrifice of segmental vessels also carries risk. The patient shown in Figure 7.7 presented with a previously operated and recurrent malignant pheochromocytoma, epidural metastasis, and paraparesis. A left-sided thoracoabdominal approach was undertaken to avoid scar from the previous operated and irradiated site. Ligation of segmental vessels under SSEP monitoring demonstrated reversible loss of waveform with the removal of temporary ligatures, and the procedure was aborted. The patient was returned to surgery 3 days later for a subtotal tumor resection via a costotransversectomy surgical approach. Despite this, the patient's neurologic condition markedly improved. Preoperative radiography (see Figure 7.7A) revealed extensive placement of vascular clips during the tumor resection surgery 10 years previously. The MRI (see Figure 7.7B) revealed a near complete block at T12. The intraoperative SSEP (see Figure 7.7C) recording demonstrated

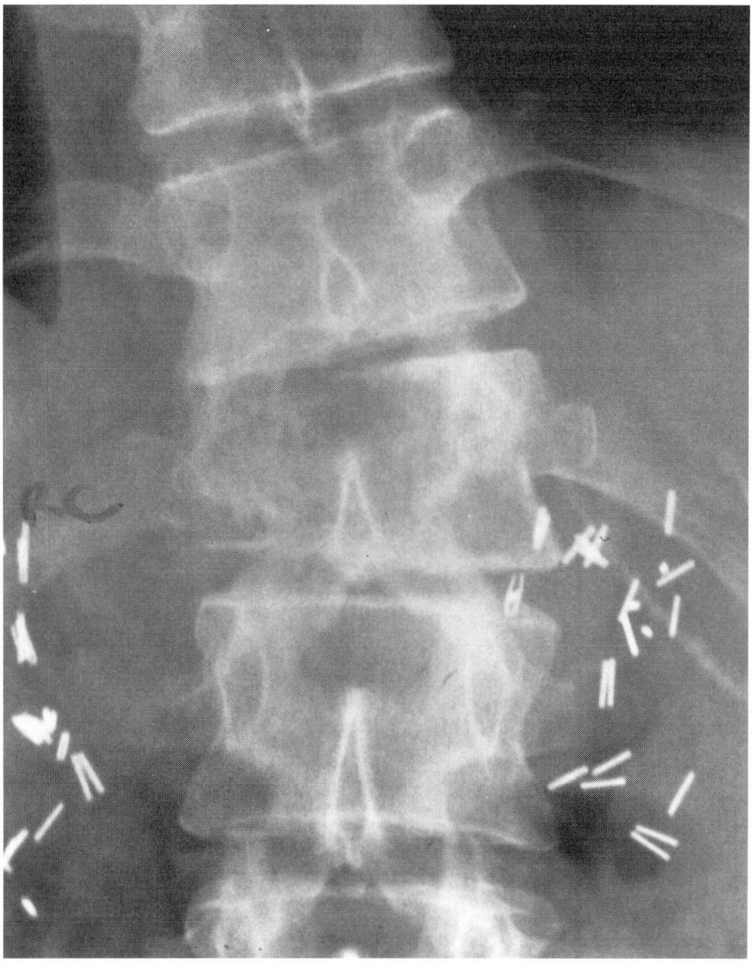

A

Figure 7.7. This patient presented with a previously operated and recurrent malignant pheochromocytoma, epidural metastasis, and paraparesis. A left-sided thoracoabdominal approach was undertaken to avoid scar from the previous operated and irradiated site. Ligation of segmental vessels under somatosensory evoked potential (SSEP) monitoring demonstrated reversible loss of waveform with the removal of temporary ligatures, and the procedure was aborted. The patient was returned to surgery 3 days later for a subtotal tumor resection via a costotransversectomy surgical approach. Despite this, the patient's neurologic condition markedly improved. (A) Preoperative radiography revealed extensive placement of vascular clips during the tumor resection surgery 10 years previously.

the loss of waveform during temporary occlusion of segmental vessels, which was reversible after release of the temporary occlusion. The final laminectomy and reconstruction are shown in Figures 7.7D and E.

Posterior soft tissue dissection of the thoracic spine provides direct and easy access and endangers no vital structures. The incision can be easily extended to include the cervical or lumbar spine, if needed. The wide, extensile exposure is ideal for spinal instrumentation of deformity, fracture, or tumor. Thoracic laminectomy is indicated for intradural tumor resection, vascular malformations, the rare posterior element tumor with cord compression, placement of shunts, and spinal cord stimulators. Preventable neurologic complications of laminectomy are related to ill-advised manipulation of the cord when attempting to gain access to anterior-based pathology. The costotransversectomy technique allows the anterolateral aspect of the spinal canal to be decompressed without manipulation of the cord.[119–123] If the anterior elements are destroyed or kyphosis is present, however, the addition of instrumented posterior fusion is advised. Costotransversectomy entails disarticulation of several inches of rib from under the transverse process. Extrapleural dissection then allows a tangential line of sight into the anterolateral aspect of the spinal canal without manipulation of the cord.

Cord compression due to lesions arising from the anterior elements are rarely improved by laminectomy alone. Thoracic laminectomy for

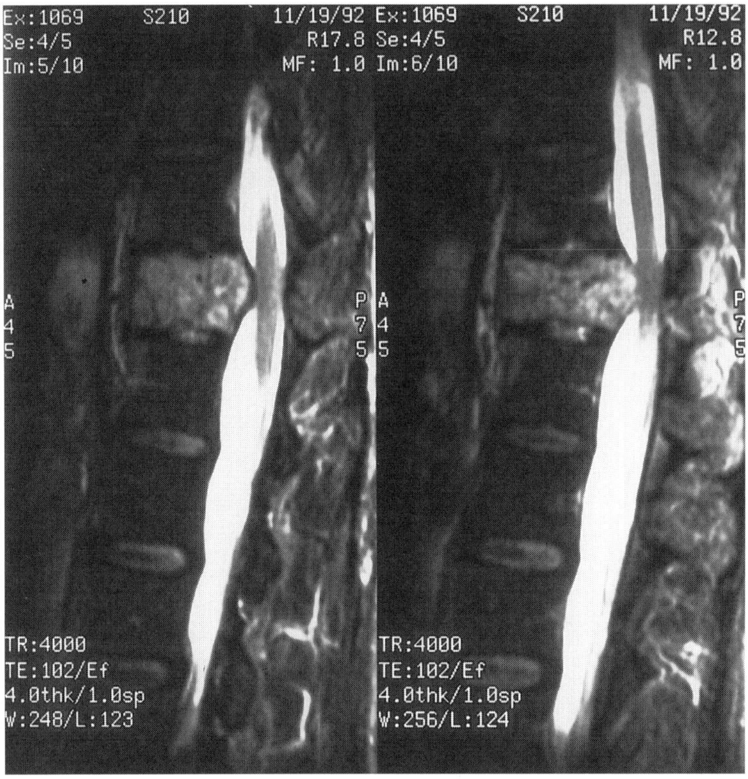

B

Figure 7.7. *continued.* (B) The magnetic resonance imaging scan revealed a near complete block at T12. (C) The intraoperative SSEP recording demonstrated the loss of waveform during temporary occlusion of segmental vessels, which was reversible after release of the temporary occlusion.

disk disease has been abandoned because of the unacceptable incidence of paraplegia associated with the cord manipulation.[119–122, 124] In a review of 135 cases of thoracic laminectomy for disk disease, Arce and Dohrmann found that 58% of patients improved neurologically.[124] Unfortunately, 10% were unchanged, 28% worsened, and 4% died. Animal studies have confirmed neurologic deterioration after laminectomy for anterior epidural masses.[125, 126]

Finally, anterior tumor or retropulsed bone may be associated with anterior column destruction and kyphosis. Removal of the intact posterior column with thoracic laminectomy may cause worsening kyphosis, return of the neurologic deficit, and intractable pain. The 22-year-old patient shown in Figure 7.8 had known osteosarcoma of the femur and presented with 2 days of paraparesis, loss of vibratory sense and proprioception, and spasticity. He underwent thoracic laminectomy for tumor excision and regained the ability to ambulate with a spastic gait. His pain was much improved. Spinal instrumentation was indicated because of preexisting kyphosis, tumor destruction of the anterior vertebral body, and subsequent destabilizing laminectomy. Unfortunately, he died within 6 months from pulmonary metastasis. The posterolateral mass with resultant thoracic cord compression is shown in Figures 7.8A and B. This is an situation where thoracic laminectomy for tumor excision is indicated and may benefit the patient. Manipulation of the neural elements was not required. The laminectomy and reconstruction is shown in Figures 7.8C and D.

Besides death, neurologic injury is the most feared complication associated with the treatment of spinal deformity. Patients at risk for paraplegia may be identified on preoperative physical examination. Scoliosis that is associated with neurologic signs including spasticity, sensory loss, asymmetric reflexes, atypical abdominal reflexes, or high arched cavus foot may be the initial manifestation of occult intraspinal pathology.[127–133] Preoperative total spine myelography or MRI is indicated for patients with

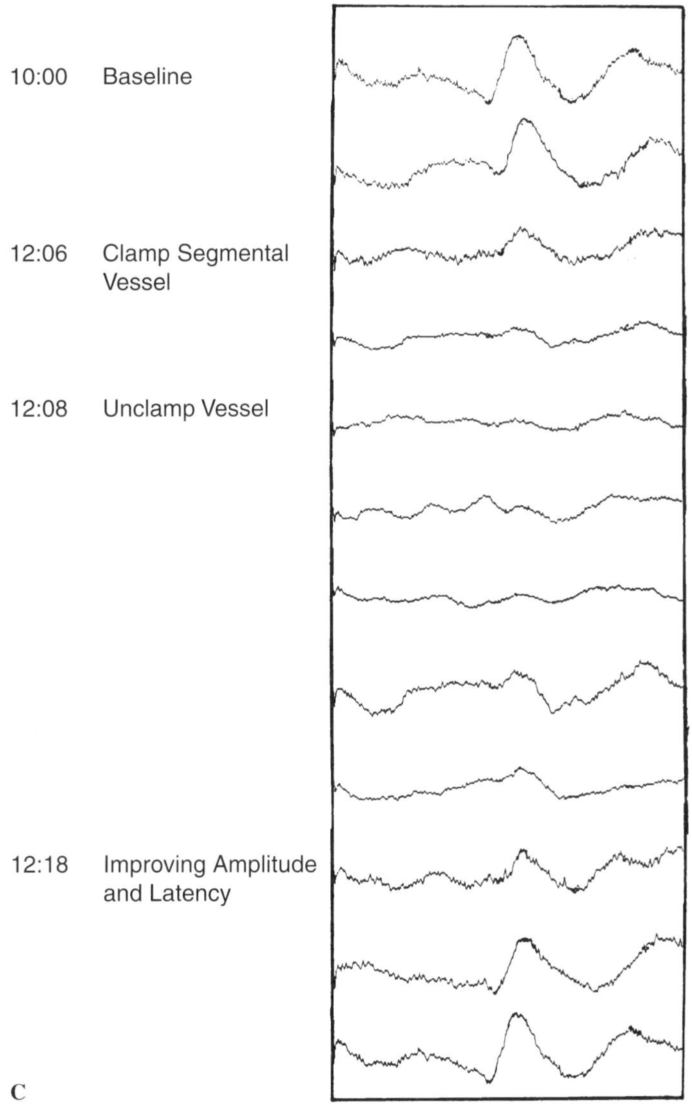

scoliosis and focal neurologic findings,[107, 127–129, 134–136] for patients younger than age 11 with juvenile scoliosis,[137] and for patients with atypical left thoracic curves and evidence of neurologic deficit.[135, 136] Idiopathic scoliosis typically presents with a right thoracic curvature (curve bends away from the cardiac shadow) in more than 95% of cases. Presumed idiopathic left thoracic curvature may be associated with cord tethering, diastematomyelia, or syringomyelia.[131, 135, 136, 138, 139] Treatment of neurogenic scoliosis without treatment of the underlying intraspinal disorder may result in paraplegia.[131, 135, 136, 138, 139]

The child shown in Figure 7.9 presented with a painless left thoracic scoliosis. Ankle spasticity was noted on neurologic examination. On questioning, the mother noted bed-wetting after years of "good behavior." Note the convexity of the left thoracic scoliosis (Figure 7.9A points in the direction of the left ventricle of the heart). The MRI (see Figure 7.9B) demonstrated a conus level diastematomyelia and split cord. The child was referred to the pedi-

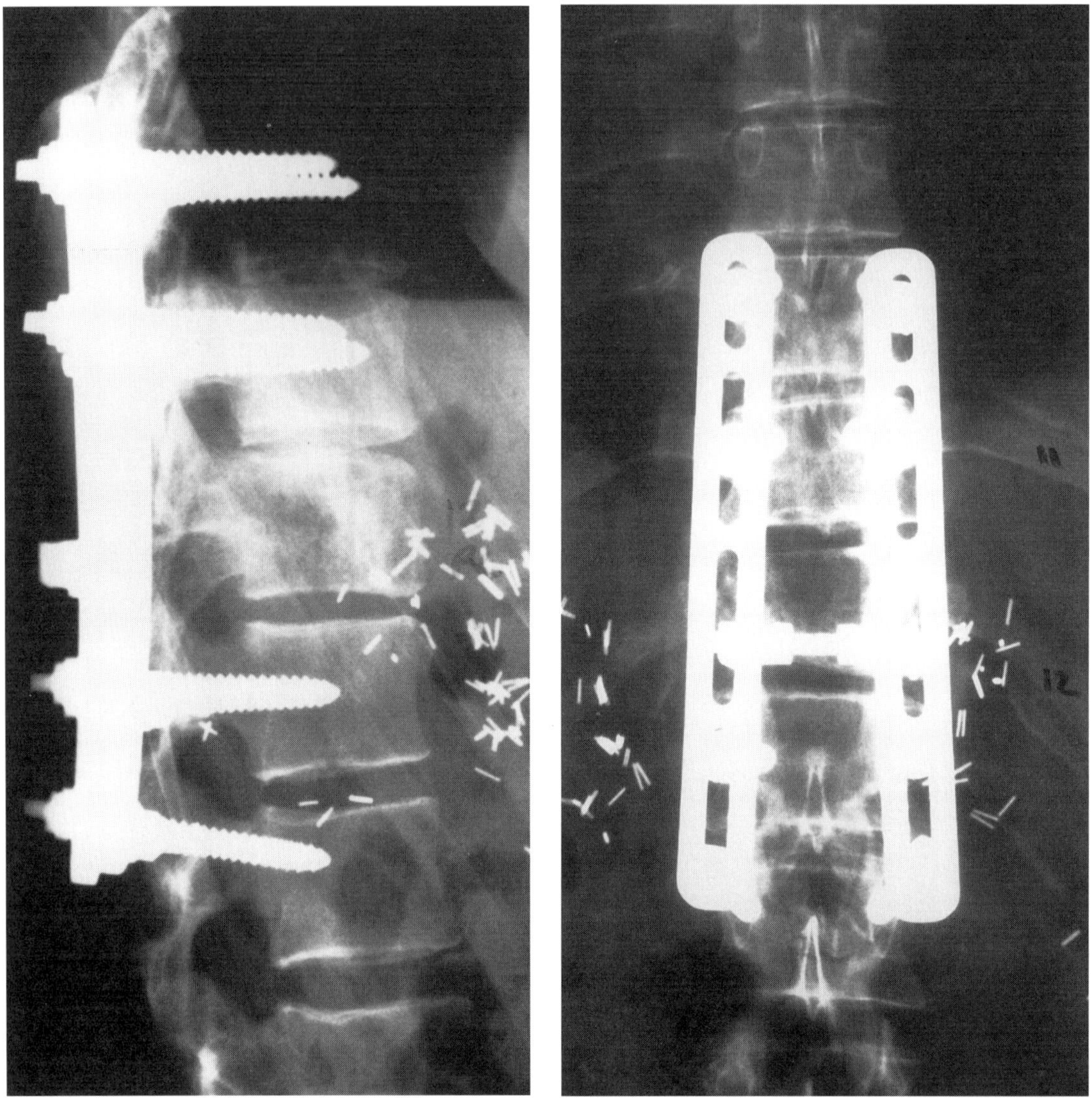

D E

Figure 7.7. *continued.* (D and E) The final laminectomy and reconstruction are shown.

atric neurosurgery service for resection of the diastematomyelia and tethered cord release.

The incidence of spinal cord injury is related to the type of spinal implant, the patient's age, the presence of congenital spinal deformity, and the presence of kyphosis.[140–157] MacEwen et al. reported a 0.72% incidence of cord injury in a mixed population of 7,885 patients treated for scoliosis with Harrington distraction rods.[158] More recent results are reported in the Scoliosis Research Society Morbidity and Mortality reports of 1987 and 1995.[159, 160] In 1987, the incidence of cord injury was 0.26% overall. Spinal cord damage associated with use of the Luque sublaminar wire technique was 0.86%. The Cotrel-Dubousset derotation technique was associated with a 0.60% incidence of cord damage. The Harrington distraction rod technique was associated with cord damage in 0.23% of patients. The 1995 Scoliosis Research Society data revealed 1,633 patients having undergone surgery for idiopathic scoliosis.[160] There were 11 reports of neurologic injury. These included one complete cord injury, four incomplete cord injuries, and five nerve root injuries. The incidence of cord injury, therefore, was 0.3%, which is similar to the 1987 data.[159, 160] An increased risk of neurologic injury was present in patients with severe scoliosis, congenital scoliosis, kyphosis, and preexisting neurologic deficit. In the 1995 data, 211 patients were treated for congenital scoliosis; five of these suffered neurologic injury for an incidence of 2.4%; 332 patients underwent surgery for kyphosis of all etiologies; six of these patients suffered neurologic injury for an incidence of 1.8%.

The radiographs in Figure 7.10 demonstrate commonly used spinal implants. A Harrington rod was used for the treatment of idiopathic scoliosis (see Figure 7.10A). Distraction at the end vertebrae allows deformity reduction of the intervening vertebrae through the pull of intact ligament structures. A Luque rod with sublaminar wires (see Figures 7.10B through D) was used after anterior and posterior resection of breast tumor metastasis. The Luque technique pulls the spine transversely to the rod, and distraction is not possible. However, passage of the sublaminar wire carries risk, especially when an epidural tumor is present. Note the anterior thoracic vertebrectomy with "reinforced concrete" technique using methylmethacrylate bone cement and plate. The Cotrel-Dubousset rod derotation technique (see Figures 7.10E and F) was used for the management of a severe right thoracic scoliosis. The Isola rod technique (see Figures 7.10G through I) was used for the management of a right thoracic scoliosis. This technique incorporates the interchangeable uses of sublaminar wire, hooks, and screws.

If neurologic deficit is evidenced by a decline of 50% in the amplitude of intraoperative SSEP or MEP responses,[102, 111–114] hypotension must be reversed, high-dose corticosteroids administered, and the offending spinal implant loosened or removed. An intraoperative wake-up test may determine if the patient is able to voluntarily move the feet and ankles, because a small percentage of patients demonstrate false-positive results on the intraoperative SSEP.[112] The anesthetic agent is reversed to a level where the patient can follow commands. The patient is then instructed to move the toes, this being a direct test of neurologic integrity. If the SSEP waveform amplitude remains damped to less than 50% and the patient cannot

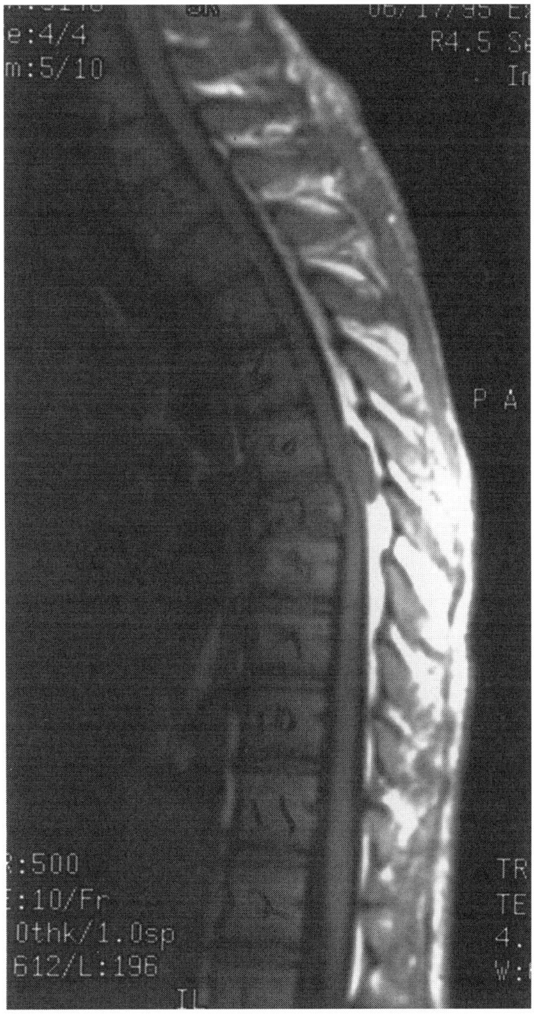

A

Figure 7.8. This 22-year-old patient had known osteosarcoma of the femur and presented with 2 days of paraparesis, loss of vibratory sense and proprioception, and spasticity. He underwent thoracic laminectomy for tumor excision and regained the ability to ambulate with a spastic gait. His pain was much improved. Spinal instrumentation was indicated because of preexisting kyphosis, tumor destruction of the anterior vertebral body, and subsequent destabilizing laminectomy. Unfortunately, he died within 6 months from pulmonary metastasis. (A and B) The posterolateral mass (arrow) with resultant thoracic cord compression. This is an ideal indication where thoracic laminectomy for tumor excision may benefit the patient. Manipulation of the neural elements was not required.

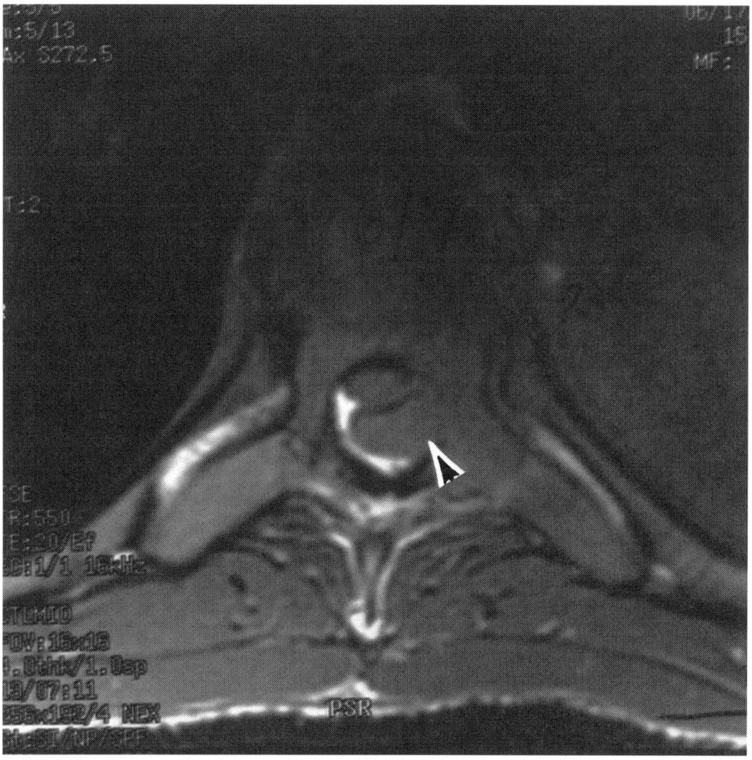

B

Figure 7.8. *continued.*

comply with the intraoperative wake-up test, the risk of postoperative neurologic deficit is likely very high.[102, 111–114] Intraoperative myelography may reveal an epidural hematoma or spinal implant compressing the cord. Unless absolutely certain that the implant or correction of the spinal deformity could not be a cause of the paralysis, it is advisable to remove the implant and observe the patient postoperatively. Once stabilized, the patient can be returned to the operating room for completion of the procedure. Delayed postoperative neurologic deficit may occur up to 7 days later.[161–163] Examples include corticosteroid-dependent cord edema and hypotensive ischemia from which the patient may make a significant recovery.

Syndrome of inappropriate antidiuretic hormone (SIADH) is commonly observed after major spinal fusion and may contribute to postoperative confusion secondary to hyponatremia. SIADH is manifest by water retention and diminished urinary output without evidence of hypovolemia or renal disease.[164–168] SIADH is associated with hyponatremia, serum hypo-osmolality, and an increased urine sodium. Most patients undergoing scoliosis surgery demonstrate a decreased hematocrit on the second to fourth postoperative day associated with dilution, rather than blood loss.[164–167] The clinical picture depends on the degree of water intoxication and hyponatremia. Deaths have occurred from cerebral edema.[168] Osmotic demyelination may occur from too rapid correction of the hyponatremia.[169] Accurate fluid management should replace only blood and insensible losses, preventing fluid overload until diuresis occurs.[167]

Acute hydrocephalus may complicate spine surgery in a child with myelomeningocele.[107] Any spinal procedure may disturb the cerebrospinal fluid balance of formation and absorption. The ventriculoperitoneal shunt could be displaced during an anterior approach to the spine. The child may present with decreased levels of consciousness, seizures, and papilledema. Emergency neurosurgical consultation and shunting is required.

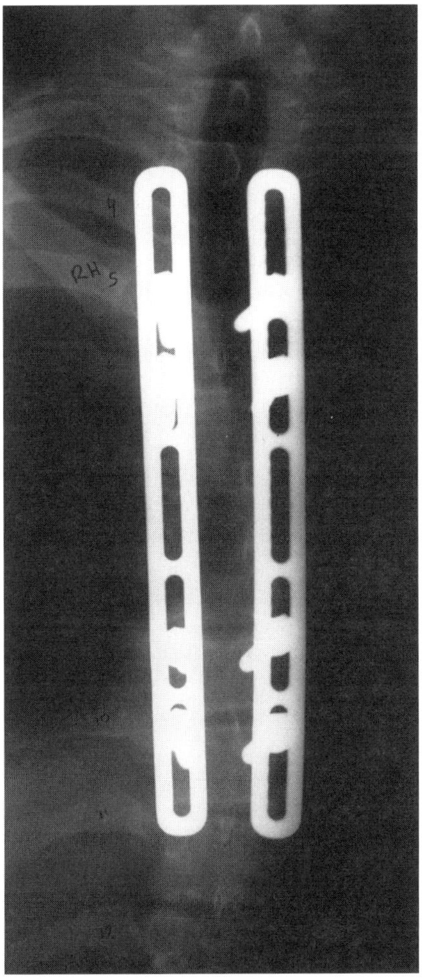

C

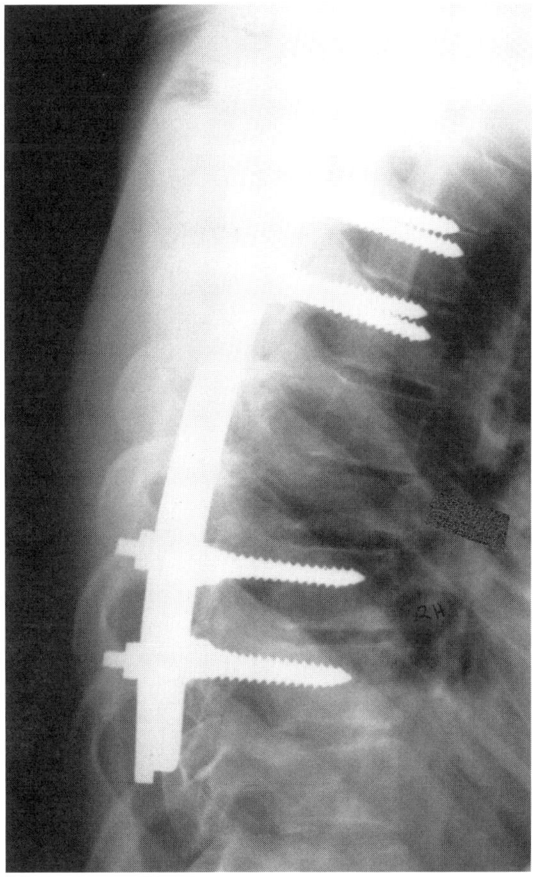

D

Figure 7.8. (C and D) The laminectomy and reconstruction is shown.

Neurologic Complications Associated with Surgery of the Lumbar Spine

Complications of lumbar spine surgery include errors in patient selection, errors in technical execution, intraoperative iatrogenic neural trauma, and postoperative epidural hematoma or abscess. As in the cervical spine, neurologic complications associated with anterior lumbar spine surgery are related to the surgical approach rather than to the neural decompression. Neurologic complications unique to the retroperitoneal approach for the anterior lumbar spine include damage to the superior hypogastric plexus, inadvertent sympathectomy, pelvic splanchnic (parasympathetic) nerve dysfunction, and femoral nerve palsy. Neurologic complications unique to posterior lumbar spine surgery include recurrent disk herniation, iatrogenic instability, and adjacent segment deterioration. Procedures associated with postoperative radiculopathy include malpositioned pedicle screws and treatment of high-grade isthmic spondylolisthesis. The use of intraoperative electromyographic (EMG) monitoring to ensure safe placement of lumbar pedicle screws is discussed. The tenth rib thoracoabdominal approach is the universal approach to the thoracolumbar junction (T10–L2). Optimal exposure for the L1–L2 disk space is via a twelfth rib extrapleural approach. The remainder of the lumbar spine (L2–L5) may be exposed via transperitoneal or retroperitoneal surgery.

The vascular anatomy of the anterior lumbar spine consists of the bifurcation of the common iliac artery and vein, rendering anterior exposure of the L4–L5 disk space technically demanding.[50, 170, 171] Great vessel laceration and thrombotic occlusion of the common iliac system are known and feared complications related to the surgical exposure of the anterior lumbar spine. The lumbar nerve roots exit the intervertebral foramen anteriorly and lie under and within the substance of the psoas muscle before joining to form the femoral plexus. The psoas muscle may be of formidable size, nearly obscuring the anterior surface of the lumbar spine in muscular persons. Femoral nerve palsy after anterior lumbar interbody fusion (ALIF) may result from overly aggressive mobilization of the psoas muscle or postoperative retroperitoneal or psoas hematoma.

The urogenital system is innervated by three nerve plexuses: the sympathetic, parasympathetic, and somatic plexus through the pudendal nerve. ALIF may damage these plexuses. The preaortic sympathetic chain extends from the thoracic spine and lies on the anterior surface of the lumbar spine. The inferior mesenteric ganglion lies at the L3–L4 level. The superior hypogastric plexus lies directly on the anterior surface of the L4–L5 and L5–S1 disk spaces. The superior hypogastric plexus (presacral nerve) contains the sympathetic nerve tissue to the urogenital mechanism.

Penile erection is via parasympathetic control of the seminal muscles and vascular structures.[69, 172] The parasympathetic fibers responsible for erection arrive with the L1–L4 nerve roots, which supply the pelvic splanchnic nerve.[173] Somatic function from S1–S4 is carried via the pudendal nerve.[69, 172, 173] Ejaculation is a combination of sympathetic and parasympathetic activity. Damage to the pelvic splanchnic parasympathetic plexus after ALIF has been reported to cause neurogenic bladder while rectal tone has remained intact.[173] Surgical interruption of the superior hypogastric plexus during ALIF may cause retrograde ejaculation of seminal fluid into the bladder as the sphincter control for closure of the bladder neck with ejaculation is lost.[69, 170–177] This may result in sterility. Sacks noted only two cases of sterility in 200 patients who underwent ALIF.[176] However, Tiusanen et al. noted seven of 40 male patients (17.5%) to develop retrograde ejaculation.[172] Tiusanen et al. observed that

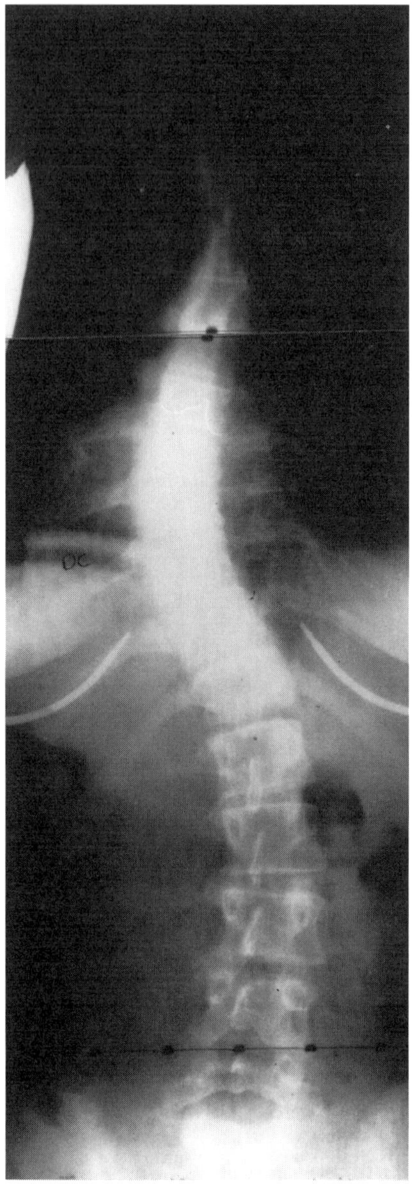

A

Figure 7.9. This child presented with a painless left thoracic scoliosis. Ankle spasticity was noted on neurologic examination. On questioning, the mother noted bed wetting after years of "good behavior." (A) Note the convexity of the left thoracic scoliosis (points in the direction of the left ventricle of the heart). (B) The magnetic resonance imaging scan demonstrated a conus level diastematomyelia and split cord. The child was referred to the pediatric neurosurgery service for resection of the diastematomyelia and tethered cord release.

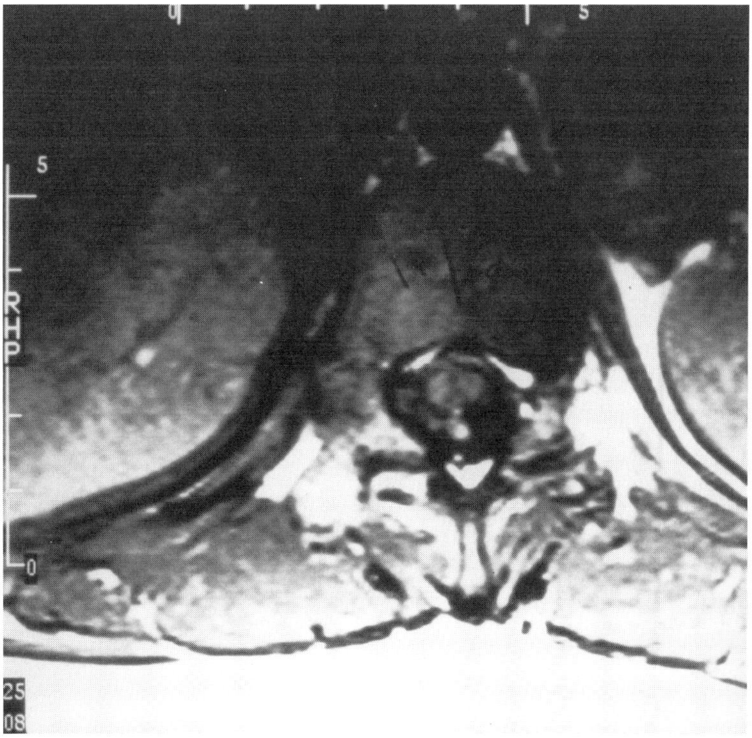

B

the incidence of this complication may be underestimated and no longer recommend ALIF as an option for young male patients. This complication is best treated by avoidance. ALIF for degenerative back pain or repair of pseudoarthrosis is elective. Preoperative patient counseling will determine those young men who would be intolerant of sterility. Alternative fusion options include posterior fusion or posterior lumbar interbody fusion. Women do not have a genital sphincter, and therefore the influence of sympathectomy on genital function is less striking and possibly unrecognized.[173]

Injury to the paraspinous sympathetic chain (T12–L4) may be a common and unavoidable complication of ALIF.[170, 171] The sympathectomy effect causes increased warmth of the ipsilateral leg due to the lack of vasoconstriction. The patient complains, however, of the comparative coolness of the opposite leg. This is not a complication of great significance except that the patient requires preoperative consultation regarding the possibility of the sympathectomy effect.

Femoral nerve palsy is a well-reported complication of retroperitoneal or psoas hematoma that may cause direct compression of the femoral plexus. This is documented in patients with hemophilia, those with bleeding disorders, and those receiving anticoagulation.[3–5] Retroperitoneal hematoma and femoral neuropathy complicating anterior bone graft harvest in a patient with von Willebrand's disease was previously discussed (see Figure 7.1). ALIF as a cause for femoral neuropathy has been reported in only two patients, whereby traction neuropraxia of the femoral nerve was postulated to result from intraoperative stretching of the psoas muscle.[3]

Three additional patients have suffered postoperative femoral neuropathy secondary to traction neuropraxia of the femoral nerve. For each of these three patients, femoral neuropathy was postulated to occur either from vigorous dissection and retraction of the psoas or use of electrocautery in the subperiosteal dissection of the psoas from the anterior vertebral body. One of these three patients was referred for evaluation of a postoperative femoral neuropathy. This 62-year-old patient underwent ALIF of both the L4–L5 and L5–S1 disk spaces. The postoperative course was marred by iliac artery thrombosis and a dysvascular, insensate extremity requiring emergency bypass graft-

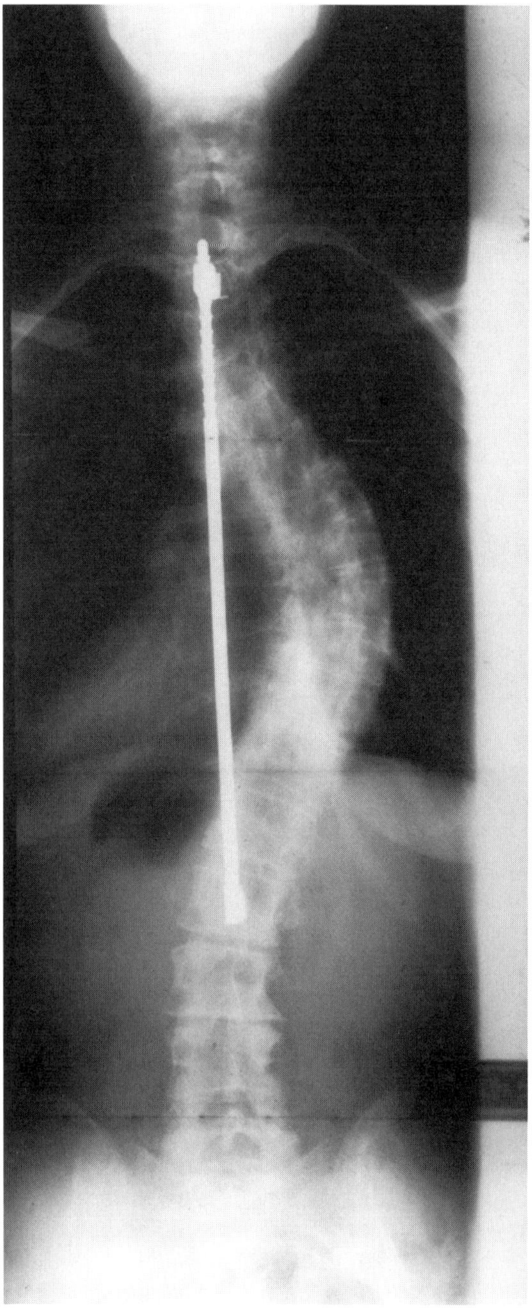

A

Figure 7.10. These radiographs demonstrate commonly used spinal implants. (A) A Harrington rod was used for the treatment of idiopathic scoliosis. Distraction at the end vertebrae allows deformity reduction of the intervening vertebrae through the pull of intact ligament structures. (B through D) A Luque rod with sublaminar wires was used after anterior and posterior resection of breast tumor metastasis. The Luque technique pulls the spine transversely to the rod and distraction is not possible. However, passage of the sublaminar wire carries risk, especially when epidural tumor is present. Note the anterior thoracic vertebrectomy with "reinforced concrete" technique using methylmethacrylate bone cement and plate.

ing. Unfortunately, a complete femoral plexopathy persisted. Vigorous dissection and mobilization of the psoas were thought to be the cause for the palsy. Evaluation of postoperative femoral nerve palsy in the two additional patients revealed a similar clinical history, and the radiographs of one are presented for review.

The 22-year-old man shown in Figure 7.11 suffered a postoperative femoral nerve palsy. He was treated with an extensive retroperitoneal dissection and en bloc spondylectomy for metastatic testicular tumor refractory to chemotherapy regimens. The L4 vertebral body, a large retroperitoneal mass, the abdominal

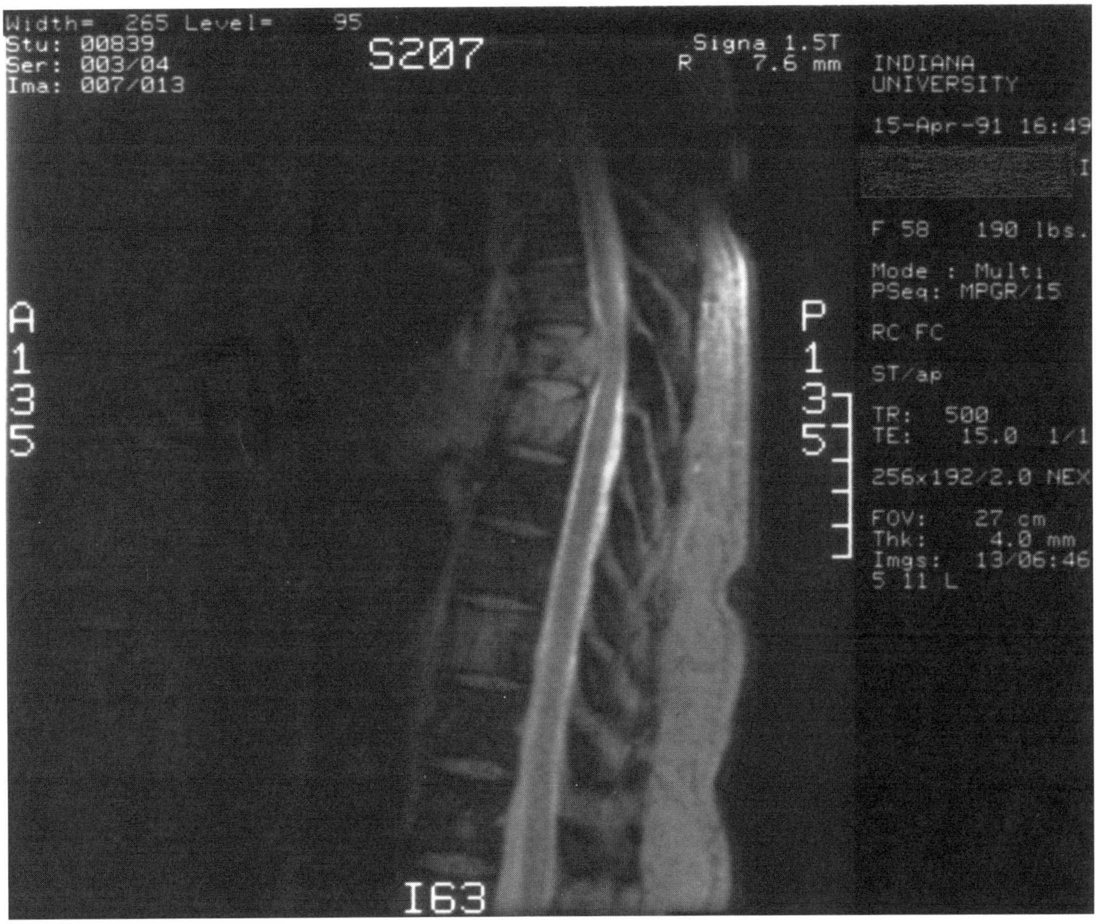

B

aorta, vena cava, and the common iliac vessels were resected. The vascular structures were reconstructed. The patient suffered a complete left-sided femoral neuropathy. Vigorous dissection and retraction of the psoas, or the use of electrocautery for the subperiosteal dissection of the psoas was the likely cause. The patient was treated expectantly with a hinged hip-knee-ankle-foot orthosis and fortunately had remarkable return of function between 9 and 12 months postoperatively. A lytic metastasis to the L4 vertebral body is shown (see Figure 7.11A). Note the extensive retroperitoneal soft tissue mass that fills the left retroperitoneal space. The final resection and reconstruction is shown (see Figures 7.11B and C).

Posterior surgical exposure of the lumbar spine is straightforward, requiring prone positioning and a midline longitudinal incision. There are no vital structures superficial to the lamina. In cases of spina bifida occulta, it is possible to plunge too deeply with a periosteal elevator or electrocautery device, creating an unintended durotomy. Laminectomy, laminotomy, and diskectomy, whether radical, limited, or microsurgical, describe nearly the same operation. These procedures share common bone, soft tissue, and neural anatomy, and therefore have common neurologic complications.

More than 200,000 lumbar laminectomy procedures are performed yearly for disk disease in the United States. A recurrent disk herniation may occur at the same operative site and through the same annular defect.[174] The incidence of a recurrent disk herniation after surgery is common. Reports on the incidence of the recurrent disk herniation vary from 3% to 37%.[178–183] Garfin et al. noted a recurrence rate of 3%.[178] Rish described a recurrence rate of 16–37% for neurosurgeons in his community.[179] Weir and Jacobs reported an 8–11% reoperation rate for recurrence.[180] Williams noted the recurrence rate after

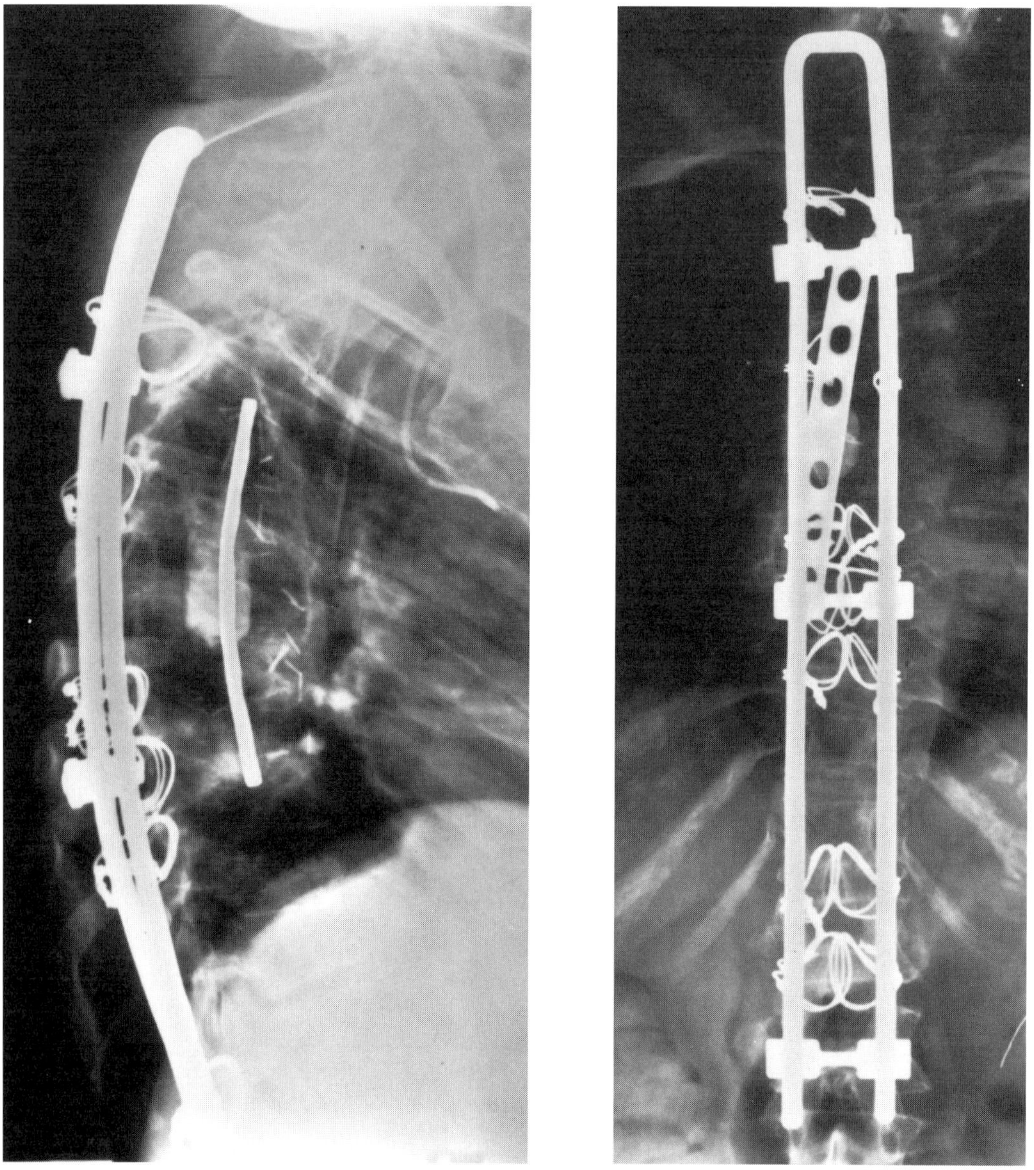

C D

Figure 7.10. *continued.*

microsurgical laminotomy (5–10%) was higher than that after a more complete diskectomy achieved with traditional open laminectomy.[181] McCulloch noted that 5% of patients require repeat surgery within the first year.[183] Not all authors consider the return of sciatica as a complication. The true incidence of recurrent symptoms is probably under-reported for several reasons. First, not all patients require a second operation, and therefore are more difficult to identify from retrospective medical record reviews. Second, symptoms may appear years later, and their association with the original surgery may not be clear.

The possibility of a recurrent herniation should be considered in patients with an initial pain-free interval of days to years who return with sciatica and positive nerve tension signs.[174, 182] The differential diagnosis for the return of severe pain and neurologic deficit may include a massive recurrent disk hernia-

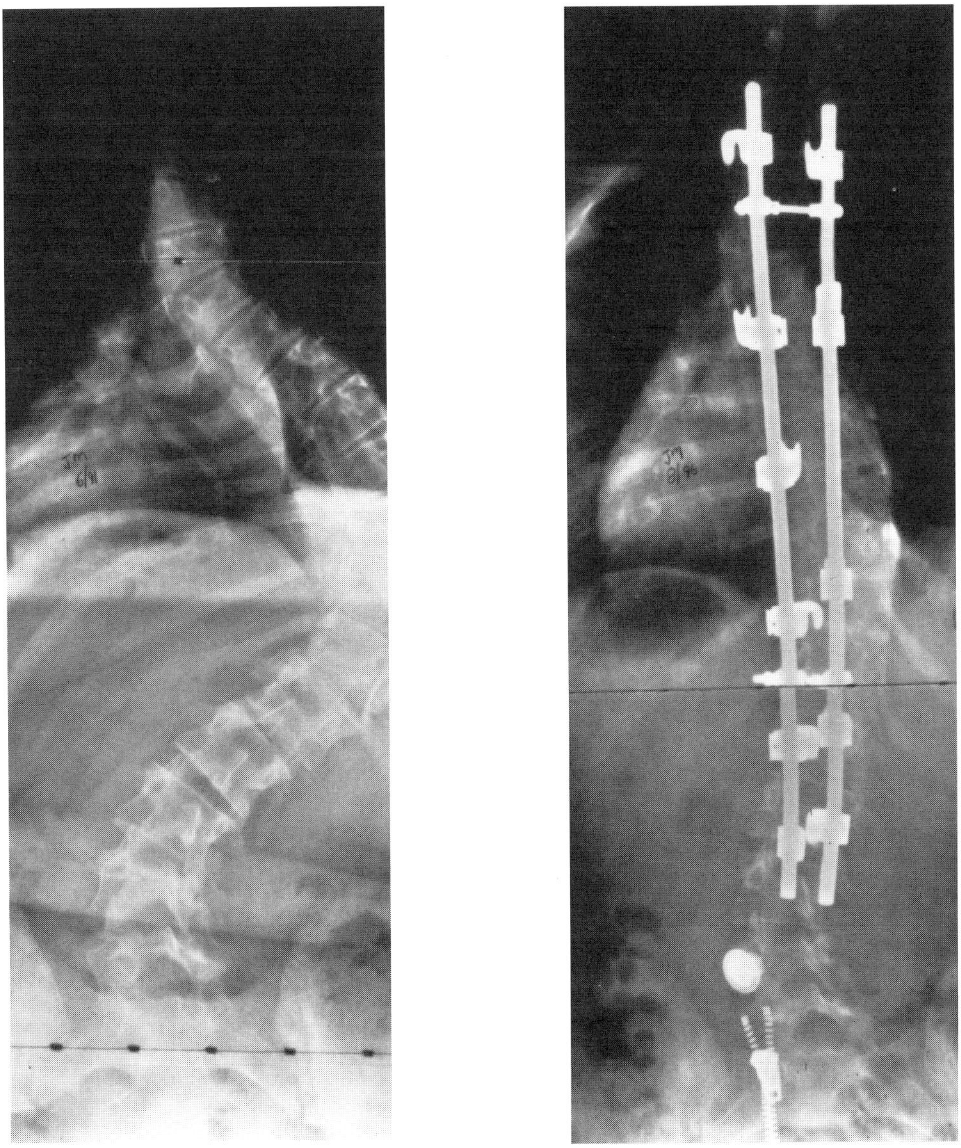

E F

Figure 7.10. (E and F) The Cotrel-Dubousset rod derotation technique was used for the management of a severe right thoracic scoliosis.

tion, epidural hematoma, epidural fibrosis, remote disk disease, postoperative diskitis, or iatrogenic epidural abscess. The MRI should be diagnostic.

Consideration for the diagnosis of recurrent disk herniation is important to prevent a patient from being labeled as having chronic pain when in fact surgically treatable compressive pathology is present. The diagnosis is often made clinically because the postoperative MRI of the lumbar spine is difficult to interpret because of fluid and edema.[184, 185] Many recurrent disk herniations respond poorly to conservative management, including epidural corticosteroid injections and physical therapy. Postoperative epidural scar tethers the normal nerve root excursion, enabling even a small recurrent disk to produce severe symptoms. The reoperation rate may be 50%.[186] If the recurrence occurs within the first few weeks, repeat surgery is technically much less difficult, because epidural scarring has not yet achieved great strength.

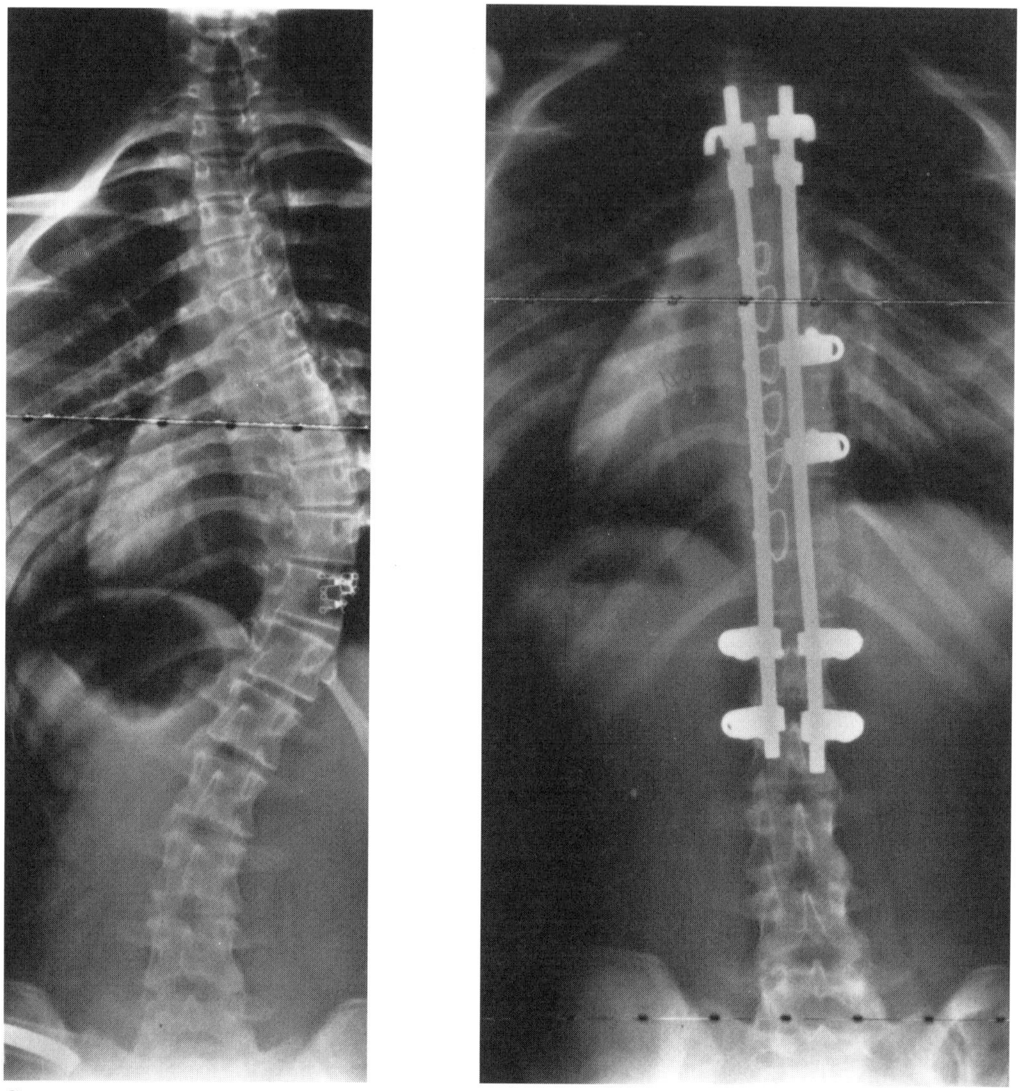

G H

Figure 7.10. *continued.* (G through I) The Isola rod technique was used for the management of a right thoracic scoliosis. This technique incorporates the interchangeable uses of sublaminar wire, hooks, and screws.

The patient shown in Figure 7.12 underwent a successful left-sided lumbosacral laminotomy but suffered return of the identical sciatica and positive nerve tension signs within 6 months of surgery. The postoperative MRI (see Figure 7.12A) could not distinguish epidural scar from a potentially large left-sided lumbosacral disk herniation. The MRI, after administration of intravenous gadolinium contrast (see Figure 7.12B), showed a small but clearly demonstrated recurrent disk herniation with resultant posterior displacement of the left S1 nerve root. Although this could represent normal postoperative changes, the return of nerve tension signs after a pain-free interval are consistent with a recurrent disk herniation.

Adjacent segment deterioration probably accounts for many of the poor long-term results observed after fusion for the degenerative lumbar spine.[187] Fusion of the mobile cervical or lumbar spine causes increased strain on the adjacent unfused segments, predisposing them to early degeneration.[188–199] Fusion of the spine places increased stress on the adjacent and unfused facet joints.[195] Kinematic studies show increased

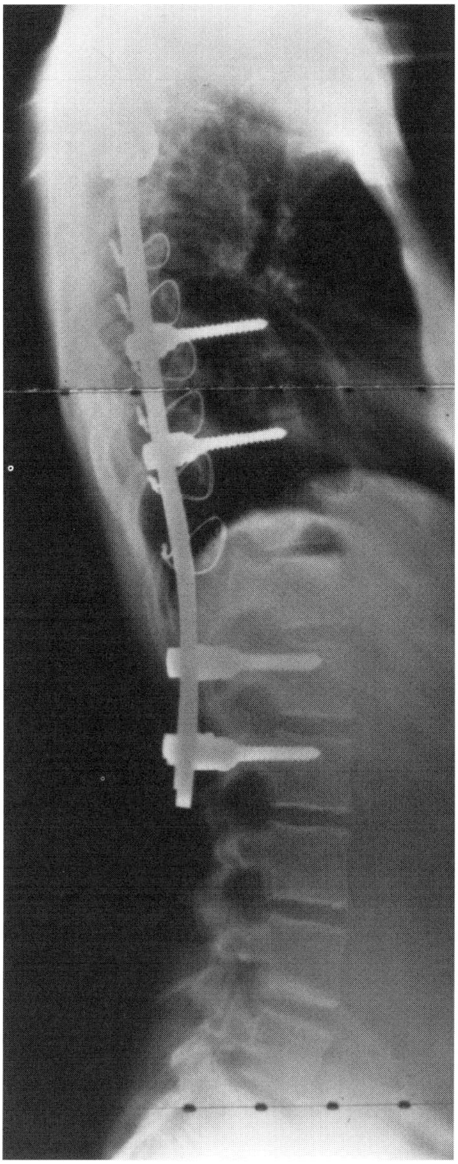

I

motion of the unfused motion segments adjacent to a bone fusion.[195] Lee and Langrana have shown that a bilateral lateral transverse process fusion is biomechanically superior and produces less adjacent segment stress than does a posterior laminar fusion.[195] Rigid spinal instrumentation increases the likelihood of solid arthrodesis and improves the early clinical outcome.[198, 200] However, rigid spinal instrumentation may accelerate adjacent segment deterioration in two ways. The surgical exposure required for accurate pedicle screw placement may cause inadvertent damage to the immediately adjacent unfused facet joint. Second, the ideal spinal implant stiffness has not been determined. A theoretic concern is that the use of rigid implants may increase the rate of deterioration of adjacent segments by increasing the rigidity of the fused segment beyond that expected for normal bone.

Frymoyer et al. presented a 10-year follow-up study of lumbar fusion.[192] In that study, 50% of patients developed claw spurs, 71–83% of patients developed facet subluxation, and 2.5% developed acquired spondylolysis adjacent to a lumbar fusion. Lehmann et al. reported on 94 patients with at least a 20-year follow-up; 42% of patients developed spinal stenosis adjacent to the fusion.[196] Brodsky noted development of severe spinal stenosis adjacent to a solid lumbar fusion.[188] Rahm and Hall noted that 35% of patients developed adjacent segment deterioration after lumbar fusion.[197] The problem also presents after scoliosis fusion.[187, 189–193, 199] Cochran et al. noted an increase in patients who developed low back pain after Harrington instrumentation for scoliosis.[189] In this study, scoliosis fusion below L3 was associated with the highest incidence for the late development of back pain. A 37-year-old patient was treated with a Harrington rod and fusion for scoliosis. Twenty-five years later, the patient presented with severe low back pain and symptoms consistent with neurogenic claudication. The radiograph (Figure 7.13) shows a previous fusion to L4 and the development of adjacent segment deterioration with spondylolisthesis of L4 on L5.

A history of previous fusion and the development of new symptoms of neurogenic claudication are common and nearly diagnostic for adjacent segment deterioration. Radiography confirms the fusion, presence of spinal implants, and adjacent segment degenerative changes. Neural imaging for adjacent segment stenosis in the presence of MRI-incompatible stainless steel implants requires myelography, postmyelogram CT, or CT alone. CT provides insufficient detail in the cervical spine but may be sufficient in the lumbar spine. Even with MRI-compatible titanium implants, postmyelogram CT may be required because of metallic debris created at the time of the initial surgery. MRI poses no danger when stainless steel spinal implants are present, but artifact and signal void obscure neural detail immediately adjacent to the implant. Scatter artifact obscures neural detail immediately under-

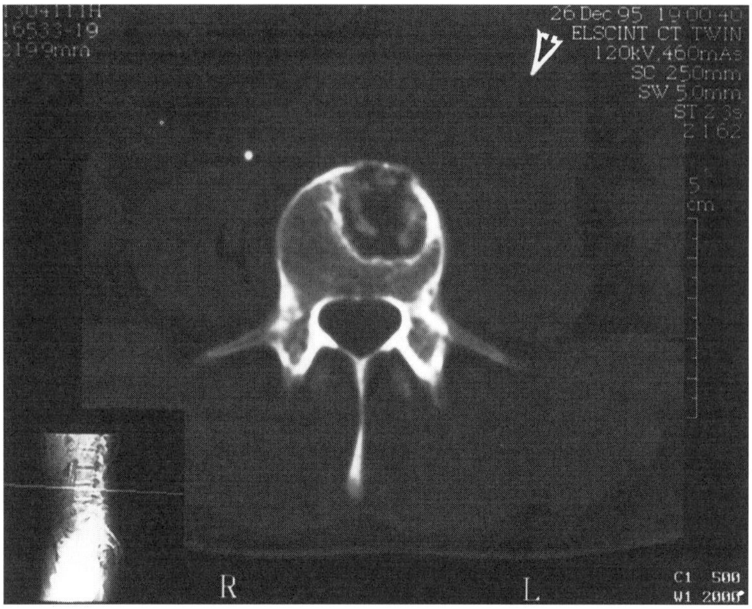

A

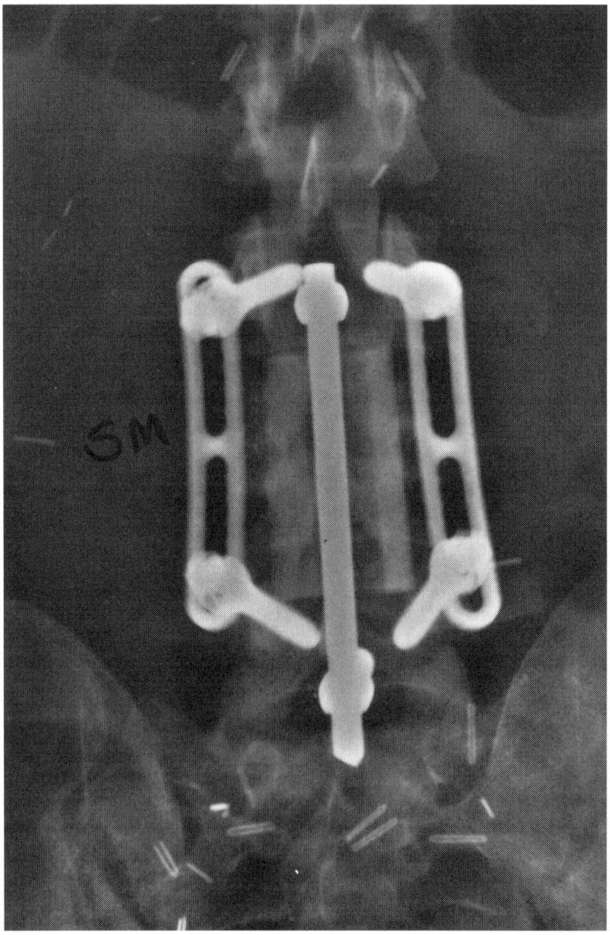

B

Figure 7.11. This 22-year-old man suffered a postoperative femoral nerve palsy. He was treated with an extensive retroperitoneal dissection and en bloc spondylectomy for metastatic testicular tumor refractory to chemotherapy regimens. The L4 vertebral body, a large retroperitoneal mass, abdominal aorta, vena cava, and common iliac vessels were resected. The vascular structures were reconstructed. The patient suffered a complete left-sided femoral neuropathy. Vigorous dissection and retraction of the psoas or the use of electrocautery for the subperiosteal dissection of the psoas was the likely cause. The patient was treated expectantly with a hinged hip-knee-ankle-foot orthosis and fortunately had remarkable return of function between 9 and 12 months postoperatively. (A) A lytic metastasis to the L4 vertebral body is shown. Note the extensive soft-tissue mass (arrow) that fills the left retroperitoneal space. (B and C) The final resection and reconstruction is shown.

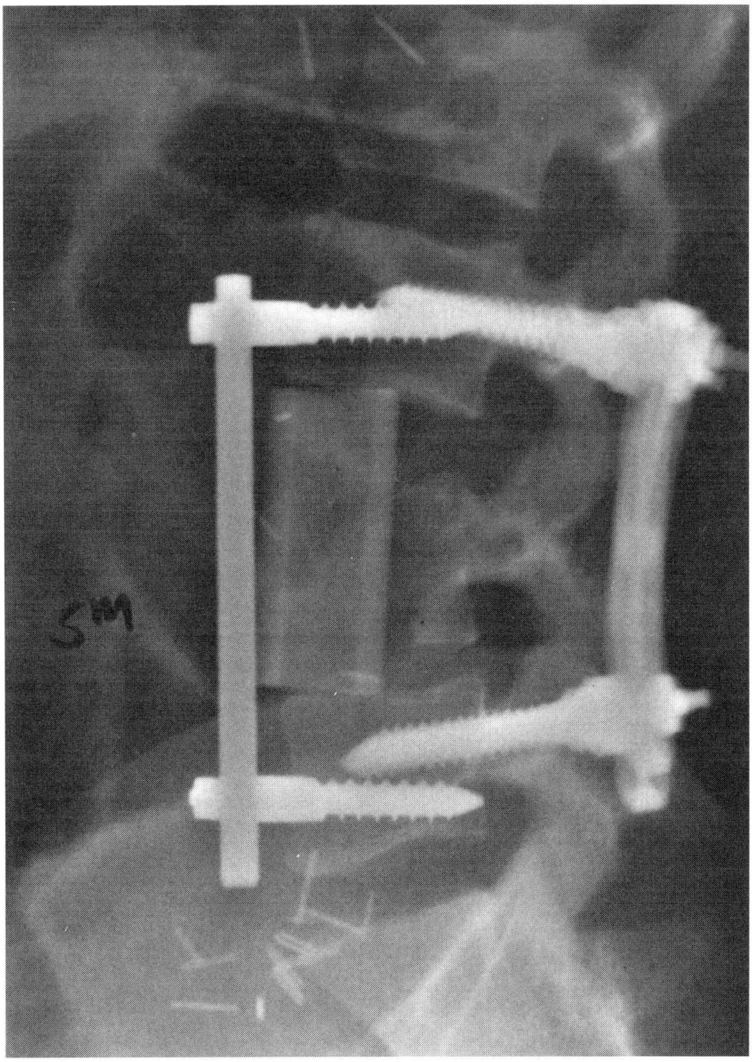

C

neath the fusion mass and plates; however, neural detail of the adjacent segment is well visualized with CT or myelography. Only rarely would stenosis reappear under a solid fusion mass. This possibility would exist only in the presence of pseudoarthrosis, if a bone graft migrated into a laminectomy defect, or if metal implants had migrated within the spinal canal. These causes of late stenosis, however, are rare when compared with the common occurrence of adjacent segment stenosis.

The patient shown in Figure 7.14 was treated with a lumbar fusion in the early 1970s. Severe symptoms consistent with neurogenic claudication returned in 1995. The patient was then treated with lumbar laminectomy, but his symptoms were not improved. Additional radiography and MRI were obtained to determine the cause for the continuing symptoms. Note the spondylolisthesis of L3 on L4 (see Figure 7.14A). Previous fusion of L4 to the sacrum with bone graft spanning the transverse processes is shown (see Figure 7.14B, lower arrow); the first open motion segment is L3–L4. However, the surgeon performed a left-sided laminectomy (see Figure 7.14B, identified by the upper arrow) at L2–L3 rather than L3–L4. The MRI (see Figure 7.14C) shows the persistent stenosis at L3–L4 and the posterior soft tissue defect leading to the errant laminectomy at L2–L3. The patient was returned to surgery,

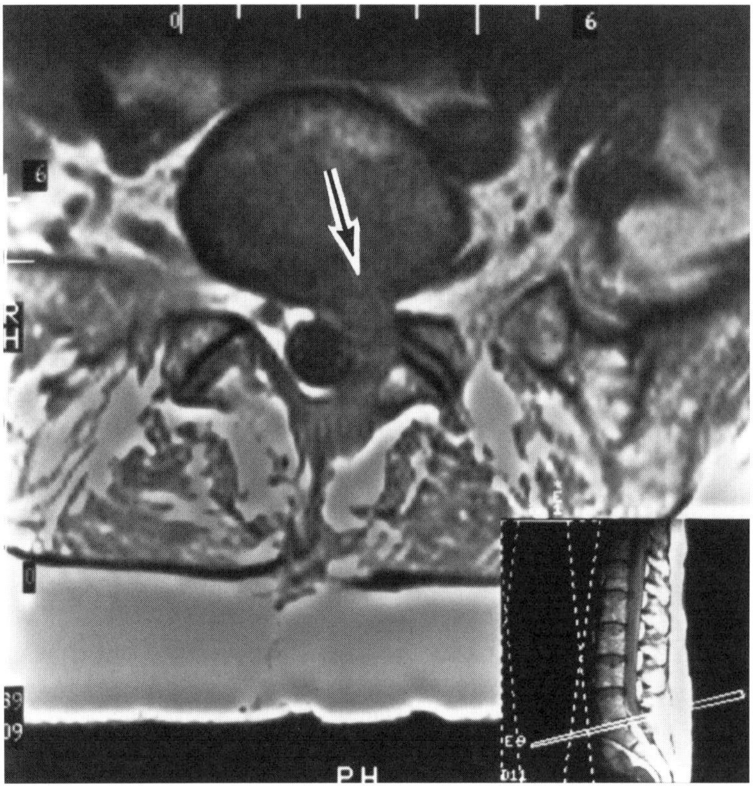

A

Figure 7.12. This patient underwent a successful left-sided lumbosacral laminotomy but suffered return of the identical sciatica and positive nerve tension signs within 6 months of surgery. (A) The postoperative magnetic resonance imaging scan (MRI) cannot distinguish epidural scar from a potentially large left-sided lumbosacral disk herniation (arrow). (B) The MRI scan after administration of intravenous gadolinium contrast shows a small (arrow) but clearly demonstrated recurrent disk herniation with resultant posterior displacement of the left S1 nerve root. Although this could represent normal postoperative changes, the return of nerve tension signs after a pain-free interval are consistent with a recurrent disk herniation.

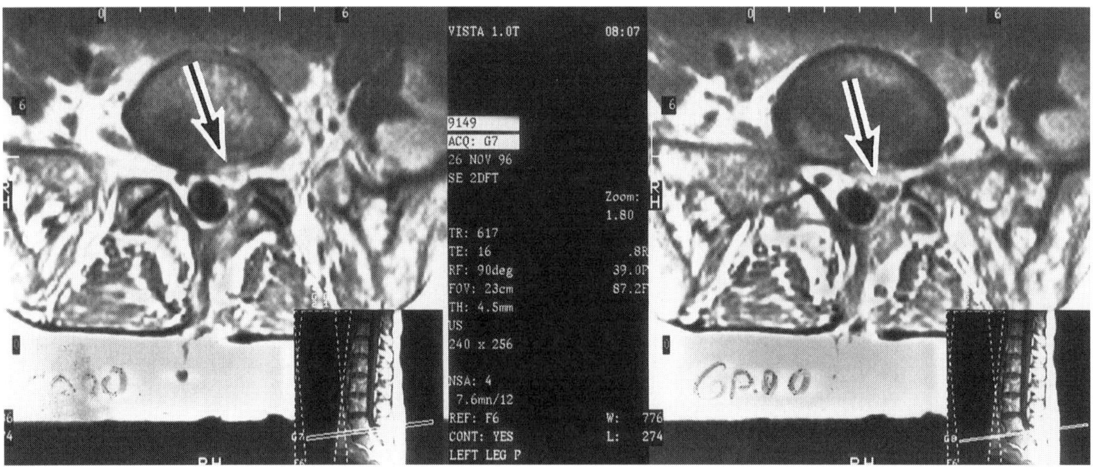

B

and the laminectomy and reconstruction are shown (see Figures 7.14D and E). The patient experienced complete relief of lower extremity neurogenic claudication but awakened from surgery with severe bilateral hand numbness. A follow-up MRI of the patient's cervical spine (see Figure 7.14F) revealed severe spondylotic changes at C4–C5 and C6–C7. The diagnosis of iatrogenic central cord syndrome was made.

Adjacent segment deterioration may be the most significant problem in spinal implant surgery. As discussed, it is a likely cause for the late failures of

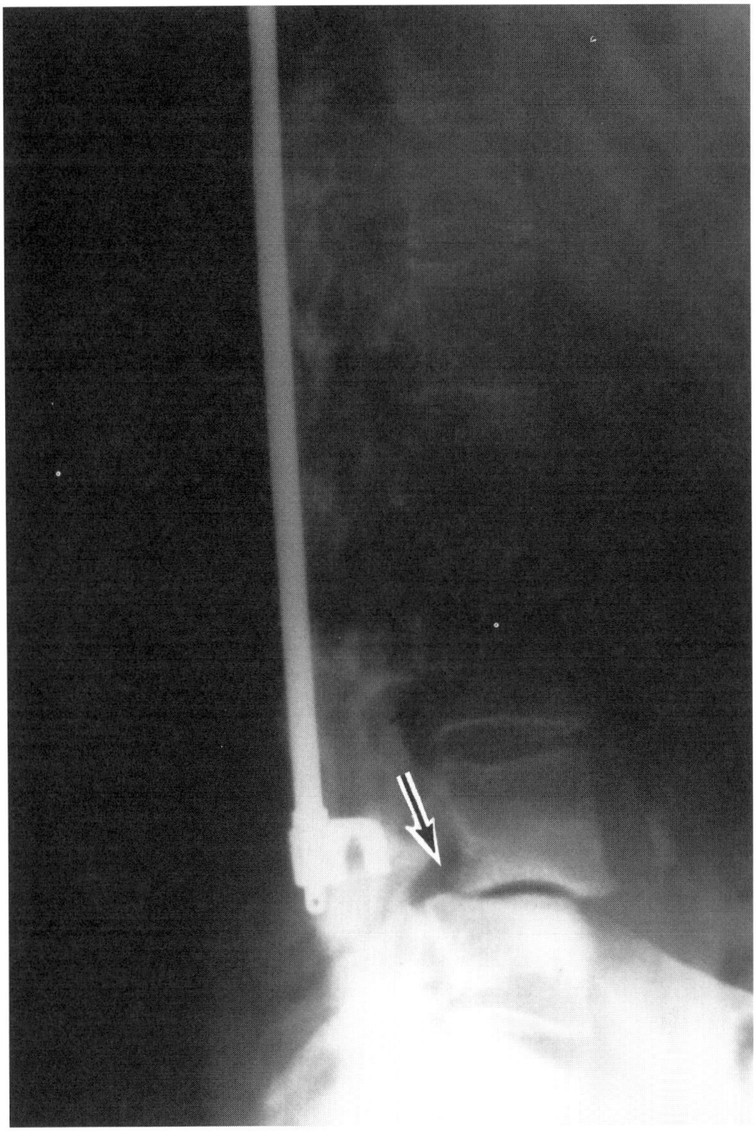

Figure 7.13. This 37-year-old patient was treated with a Harrington rod and fusion for scoliosis. Twenty-five years later, the patient presented with severe low back pain and symptoms consistent with neurogenic claudication. The radiograph shows a previous fusion to L4 and the development of adjacent segment deterioration with spondylolisthesis (arrow) of L4 on L5.

spinal fusion. The magnitude of the problem will surely increase. The use of rigid transpedicular segmental spinal fixation as an aid for lumbar spine fusion was not widespread in North America until the late 1980s. If indeed, the use of rigid spinal implants does accelerate adjacent segment deterioration, a large population of patients having undergone lumbar fusion will shortly come of age, presenting with symptoms of neurogenic claudication. Alternatives to fusion attempt to retain motion in the mobile lumbar spine while treating the painful degeneration or spinal deformity. The artificial lumbar disk, like the artificial hip and knee implants, attempts to preserve normal joint motion but treat painful disk disease. Artificial lumbar disks have been placed in a few select persons, but the procedure is not yet ready for clinical use.[201]

Besides death, cauda equina syndrome (CES) and worsened neurologic deficit are the most feared complications of lumbar spine surgery. CES may be either an urgent indication to proceed with surgery or a devastating complication of routine laminec-

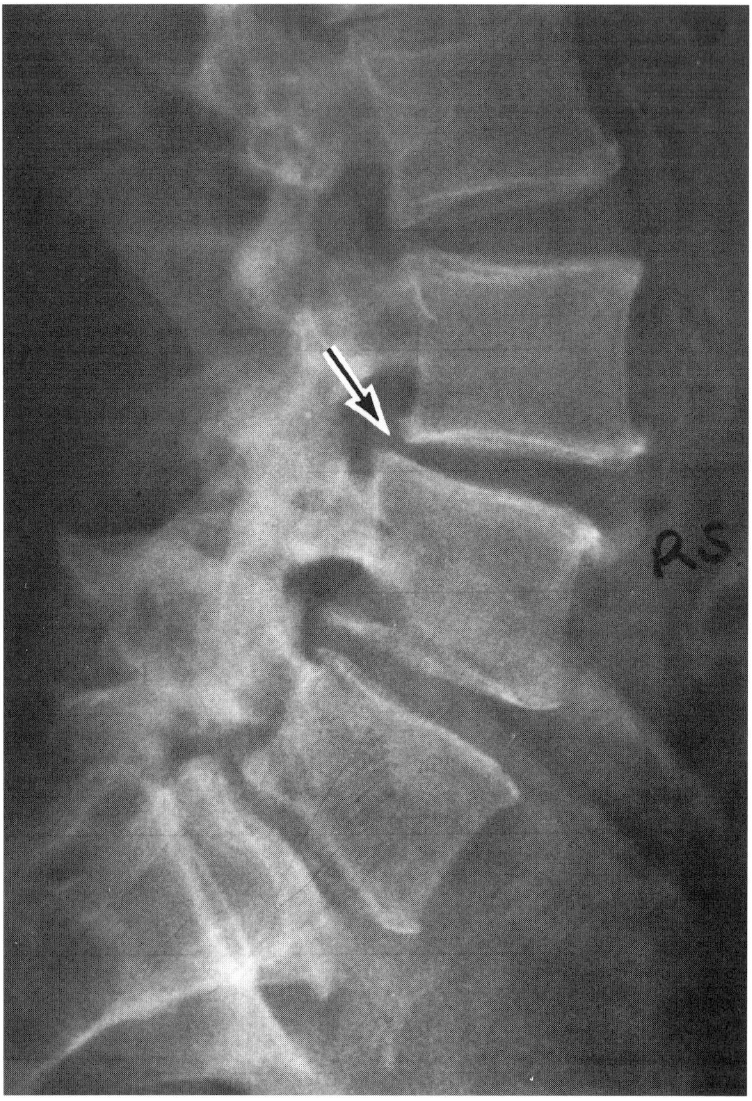

A

Figure 7.14. This patient was treated with a lumbar fusion in the early 1970s. Severe symptoms consistent with neurogenic claudication returned in 1995. The patient was then treated with lumbar laminectomy, but his symptoms were not improved. Additional radiographs and magnetic resonance imaging (MRI) were obtained to determine the cause for the continuing symptoms. (A) Note the spondylolisthesis (arrow) of L3 on L4. (B) Previous fusion L4 to the sacrum with bone graft spanning the transverse processes (lower arrow) is shown; the first open motion segment is L3–L4. However, the surgeon performed a left-sided laminectomy (upper arrow) at L2–L3 rather than L3–L4.

tomy.[179, 186, 202–207] Ramirez and Thisted determined the incidence of acute and major complications in a population of 28,395 patients who underwent diskectomy from 1,690 community hospitals throughout the United States.[186, 205] In this study, the incidence of any neurologic complication was an astounding 29.8%. Eight percent of patients suffered CES, with two-thirds requiring reoperation; 2% suffered a nerve root avulsion; 11% suffered worsening radiculopathy, and of these, 50% required repeat surgery during the same hospitalization.[186, 205] In contrast, McLaren and Bailey reported six cases of postdiskectomy CES in a series of 2,842 lumbar diskectomies (0.21%).[204] Five of these six patients were thought to have inadequate decompression of coexisting spinal stenosis. Spangfort reviewed 2,504 laminectomy procedures and reported five patients who developed postoperative CES, (0.2%).[208] Mayfield reported the incidence of major neurologic complications after lumbar spine surgery to be only 0.2%.[209]

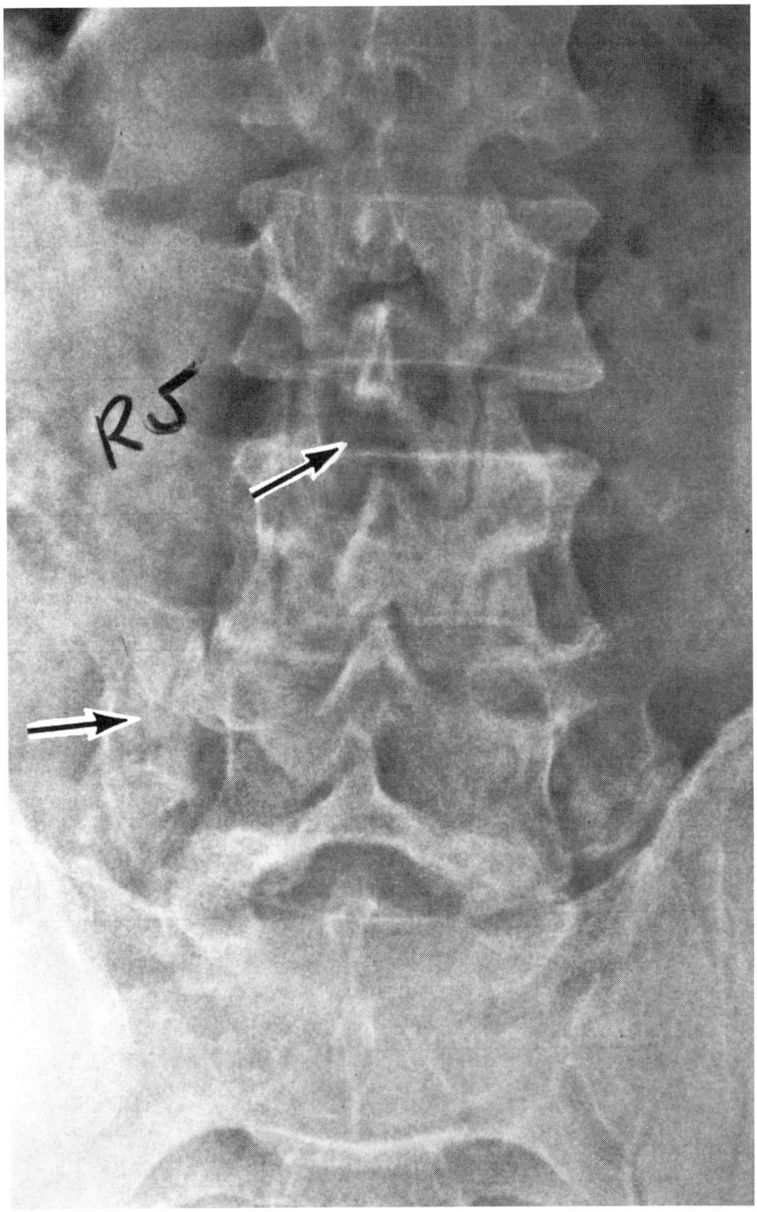

B

Inadequate laminectomy may cause worsened neurologic deficit or CES. Review of the preoperative MRI or CT may show spinal stenosis on the basis of hypertrophy of the ligamentum flavum and facet joints. Unfortunately, in the enthusiasm to achieve even shorter hospital stays and surgical incisions, a microsurgical diskectomy rather than the ncccssary extensive laminectomy may be performed, and the spinal stenosis may remain untreated. Significant spinal stenosis or a huge disk herniation simulating spinal stenosis causes marked compression of the cauda equina. The resulting edema and decreased vascular supply make neural tissue even more susceptible to surgical trauma. Unintended durotomy with cerebrospinal fluid leak, nerve root avulsion, or CES may be precipitated

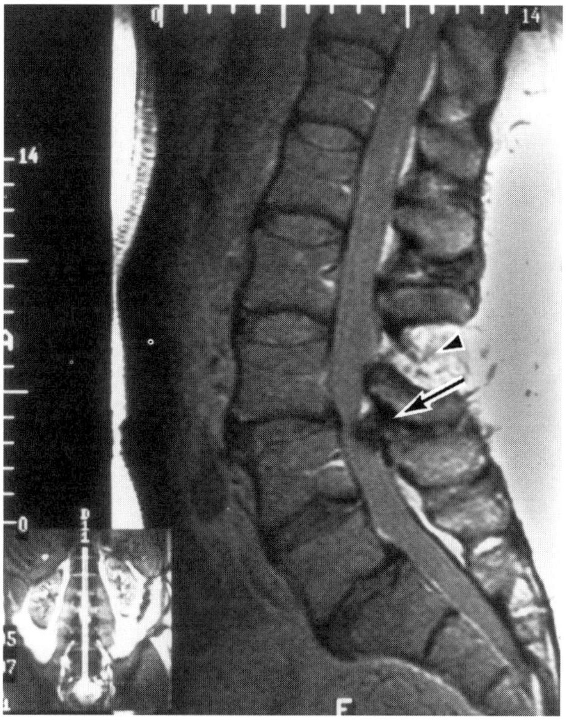

C

Figure 7.14. *continued.* (C) The MRI scan shows the persistent stenosis at L3–L4 (large arrow) and the posterior soft tissue defect (small arrow) leading to the errant laminectomy at L2–L3. (D and E) The patient was returned to surgery, and the laminectomy and reconstruction are shown. The patient experienced complete relief of lower extremity neurogenic claudication but awakened from surgery with severe bilateral hand numbness. (F) A follow-up MRI scan of the patient's cervical spine revealed severe spondylotic changes at C4–C5 and C6–C7. The diagnosis of iatrogenic central cord syndrome was made.

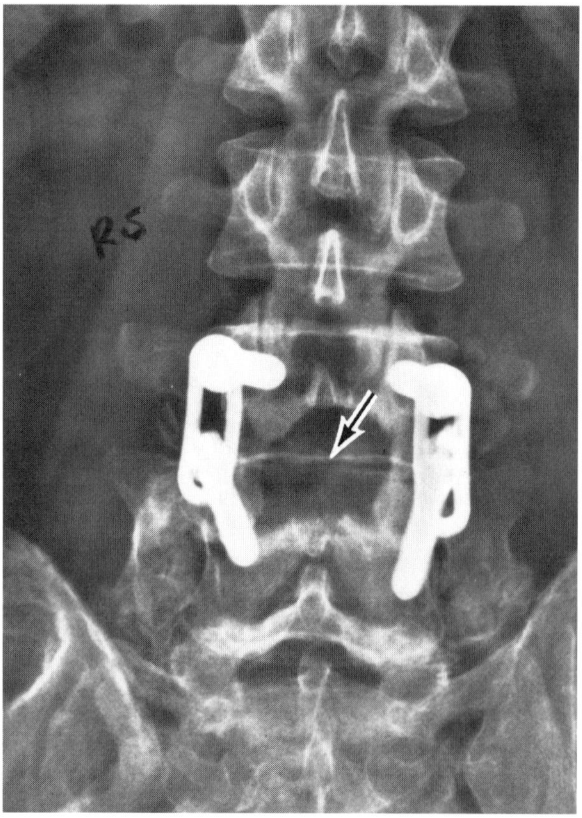

D

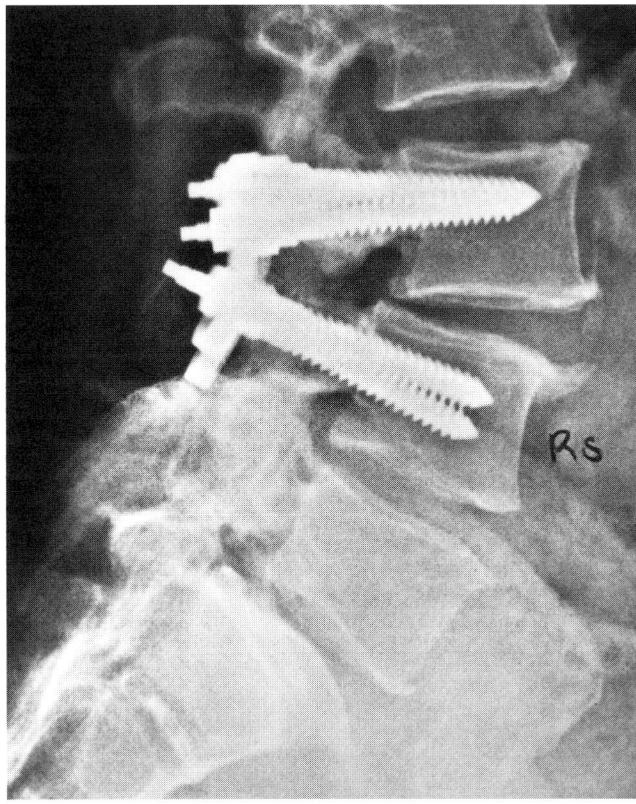

E

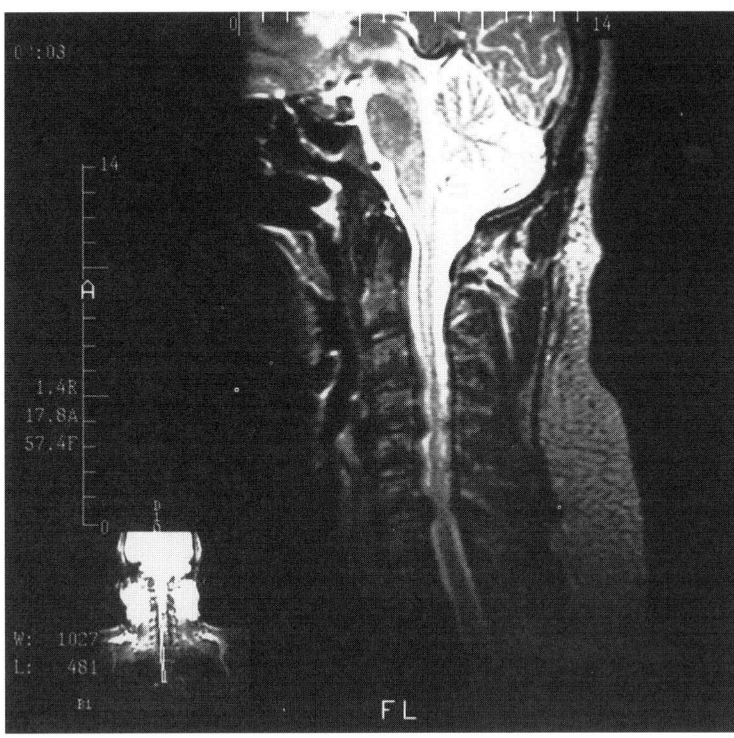

F

when attempting to retract the lateral border of the dura in the unyielding environment of spinal stenosis. In the presence of CES or spinal stenosis, Kostuik et al. recommend complete as opposed to partial laminectomy.[202, 203] After complete laminectomy, it is easier and safer to retract the cauda equina for retrieval of disk material.

Persistent compressive pathology must be suspected in patients with persistent or worsened postoperative symptoms. Potentially treatable causes include persistent stenosis or disk or new compressive pathology from epidural hematoma, migrated fat graft, or swollen hemostatic agent. Free-fat grafts may be applied directly to the exposed posterior dura to act as a barrier to epidural scar formation. These grafts may migrate within the epidural space, causing symptomatic compression mimicking hematoma.[206, 207] Absorbable hemostatic agents are often placed within the epidural space beyond the confines of the exposed laminectomy defect to compress the bleeding epidural venous plexus. These substances may swell in the postoperative period resulting in CES.

Pathology that extends beyond the operative site, such as epidural hematoma or new disk herniation at another intervertebral level, may not be visualized on the emergent postoperative imaging study, which likely focuses on the operated site. Thorough neurologic examination is required to properly direct the viewing field of the postoperative imaging studies (see Figures 7.5 and 7.6).

Treatment of high-grade isthmic spondylolisthesis (more than 50% subluxation of L5 on S1) carries the significant risk of L5 root palsy, and to a lesser extent, CES.[210–222] Central canal stenosis is only rarely associated with an isthmic spondylolisthesis. In the presence of an isthmic (bilateral fracture of the pars interarticularis) spondylolisthesis, the posterior arch, including lamina and spinous process, is fractured at the pars interarticularis and remains posterior as the pedicles and vertebral body slip anteriorly. Essentially, this is a centrally self-decompressing lesion. Radicular symptoms may be severe, however, because the bony hook of the fractured pars interarticularis may create a severe degree of neuroforaminal stenosis; a traction neuropraxia of the exiting nerve root may occur. The absence of central canal stenosis observed in isthmic spondylolisthesis differs markedly from the severe degrees of central canal stenosis observed in patients with degenerative and dysplastic spondylolisthesis. In these cases, the neural arch remains intact and central canal stenosis is severe.[212]

The patient identified in Figure 7.15 suffered back and leg pain consistent with an L4 radiculopathy. Note the isthmic L4 on L5 spondylolisthesis (see Figure 7.15A). The arrow (see Figure 7.15A) identifies a severe degree of neuroforaminal narrowing and also identifies the bony hook of the fractured pars interarticularis. The bony hook caused a traction neuropraxia of the L4 root as it, the vertebral body, and pedicle translated anteriorly. pulling the root as well. The postmyelogram CT (see Figure 7.15B) demonstrates the fractured and loosened lamina. There is no evidence of central canal stenosis as the lamina and posterior arch are pulled away from the dura as the vertebral body and pedicles slip anteriorly.

Figure 7.16 demonstrates how the deformity of an isthmic spondylolisthesis may cause the cauda equina to be tethered anteriorly over the dome of the sacrum while the fifth lumbar roots are tethered, trapped, and displaced by the fractured pars interarticularis and pedicle.[220] Note the absence of central canal stenosis on the midsagittal MRI (see Figure 7.16A). However, the degree of neuroforaminal narrowing with fifth nerve root compression seen in the parasagittal MRI is severe (see Figure 7.16B).

Surgical reduction of the spondylolisthesis deformity with instrumentation and fusion may be indicated in patients with severe deformity. L5 root paresis may occur in 20–30% of patients, however, even when the cauda equina is decompressed and directly visualized during the reduction.[210, 211, 215, 216, 218] In situ fusion without active attempts at reduction of the deformity carries risk as well. Maurice and Morley reported three patients who suffered postoperative CES after in situ fusion.[217] Schoenecker et al. reported a 6% incidence (12 of 189 patients) of CES after in situ fusion performed by experienced surgeons.[221] Schoenecker et al. postulated that the CES was precipitated merely by positioning the patient on the operating table, with unintended reduction of the deformity while under a general anesthetic.

Intraoperative electromyographic monitoring of the L5, S1, and pudendal nerves can monitor for pedicle screw placement, CES, and fifth root radiculopathy and is useful in the management of

Figure 7.15. This patient suffered back and lcg pain consistent with an L4 radiculopathy. (A) Note the isthmic L4 on L5 spondylolisthesis. The arrow identifies a severe degree of neuroforaminal narrowing and also identifies the bony hook of the fractured pars interarticularis. The bony hook caused a traction neuropraxia of the L4 root as it, the vertebral body, and pedicle translated anteriorly, pulling the root as well. (B) The postmyelogram computed tomography scan demonstrates the fractured (arrows) and loosened lamina. There is no evidence of central canal stenosis as the lamina and posterior arch are pulled away from the dura as the vertebral body and pedicles slip anteriorly.

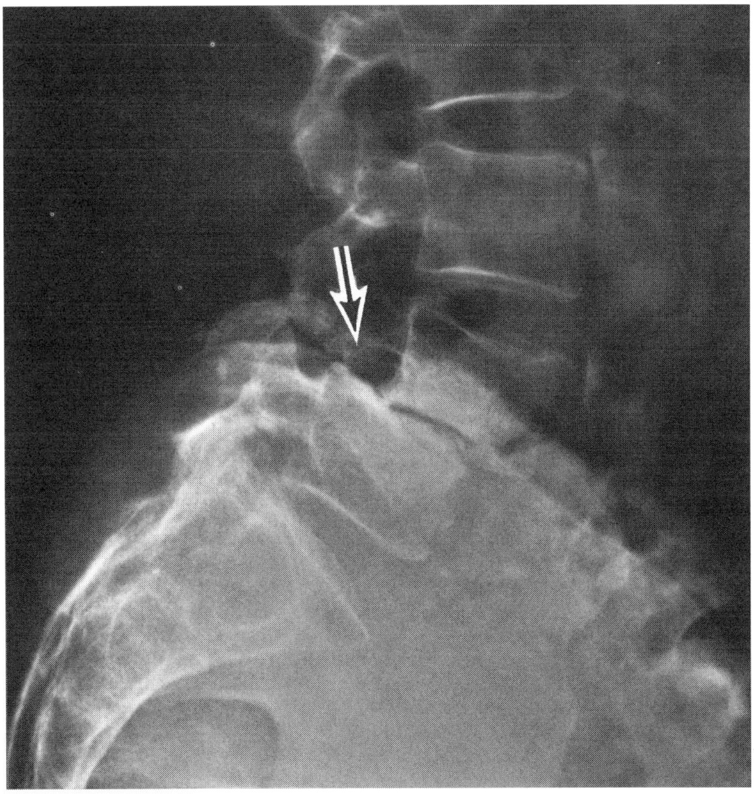

A

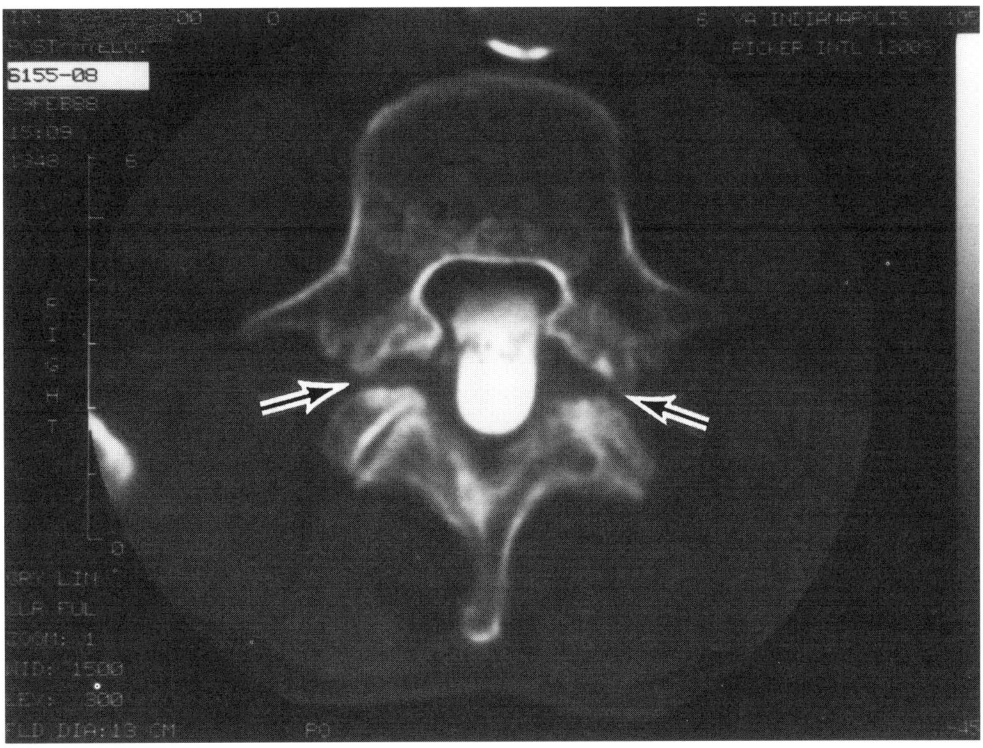

B

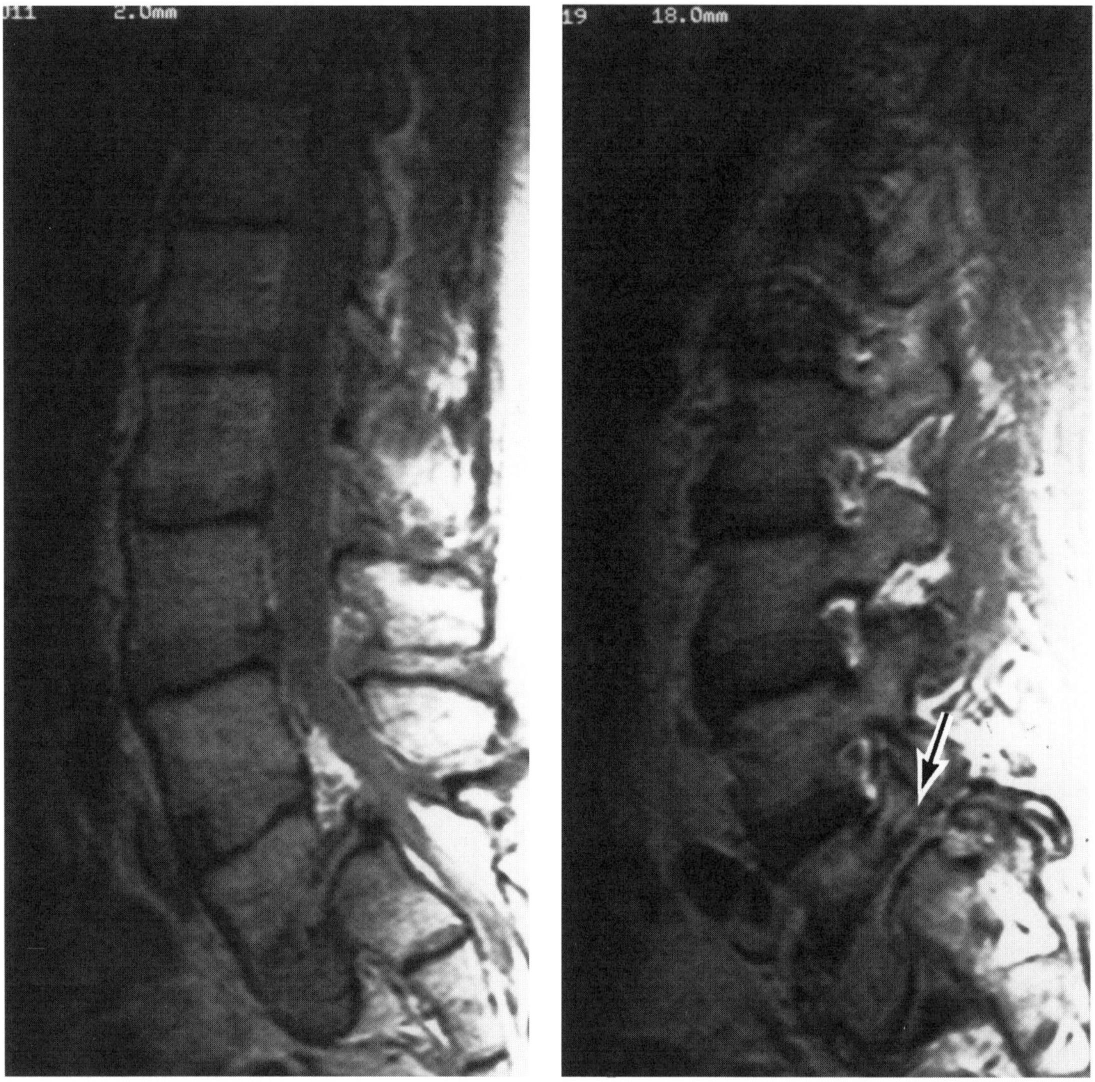

A B

Figure 7.16. The deformity of an isthmic spondylolisthesis may cause the cauda equina to be tethered anteriorly over the dome of the sacrum while the fifth lumbar roots are tethered, trapped, and displaced by the fractured pars interarticularis and pedicle. (A) Note the absence of central canal stenosis on the midsagittal magnetic resonance imaging scan. (B) However, the degree of neuroforaminal narrowing with fifth nerve root compression (arrow) seen in the parasagittal magnetic resonance imaging scan is severe.

such severe deformities.[223] The 11-year-old patient shown in Figure 7.17 was successfully treated with reduction, instrumentation, and fusion of a high-grade isthmic spondylolisthesis (see Figure 7.17A). The procedure was monitored with intraoperative electromyography of the L4, L5, S1, and pudendal nerves. Bursts of motor unit potentials were observed in the external anal sphincter electrodes after the deformity was reduced by 50%, and no further attempts at reduction were performed. The postreduction radiographs are shown (see Figure 7.17B). Active attempts at reduction of high-grade isthmic spondylolisthesis carry high neurologic risk as outlined.

Postoperative pain, increased neurologic deficit, or symptoms unchanged from the preoperative

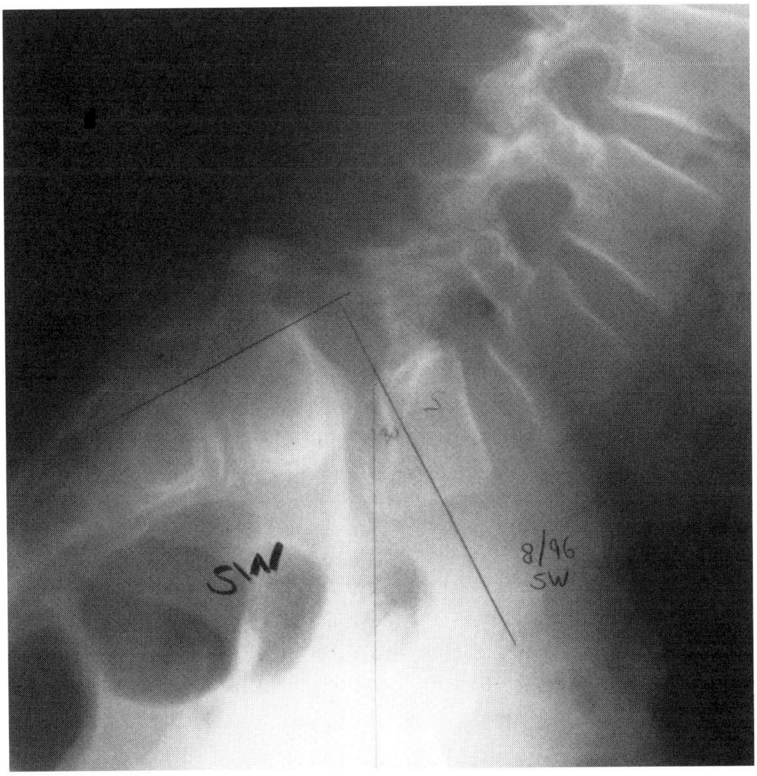

A

Figure 7.17. (A) This 11-year-old patient was successfully treated with reduction, instrumentation, and fusion of a high-grade isthmic spondylolisthesis. The procedure was monitored with intraoperative electromyography of the L4, L5, S1, and pudendal nerves. Bursts of motor unit potentials were observed in the external anal sphincter electrodes after the deformity was reduced by 50%, and no further attempts at reduction were performed.

evaluation carry a long list of differential diagnoses. Surgical indications and patient selection are the most critical factors that determine the success of lumbar spinal surgery. Psychological assessment and treatment of depression may identify those patients whose complaints of back and leg represent somatization of an underlying psychiatric disorder. Compensation, litigation, and issues of secondary gain have a profound negative effect on the outcome of surgery. More rarely, a lack of understanding of the surgical pathology may lead to a technically inadequate surgery with no improvement in symptoms. The patient shown in Figure 7.18 was treated elsewhere with lumbar laminectomy, but his radicular symptoms persisted. An isthmic L4 on L5 spondylolisthesis and the bony hook of the fractured pars interarticularis with resultant neuroforaminal compression of the exiting fourth root are clearly identified (see Figure 7.18A). Unfortunately, the surgeon performed a left-sided laminotomy with decompression of the fifth lumbar root underneath its named pedicle shown by the arrow in Figure 7.18B. This demonstrates a lack of understanding of the surgical neuropathology, as the fourth root should have been anticipated to be compressed. As anticipated, the left parasagittal MRI (see Figure 7.18C) demonstrates severe neuroforaminal compression of the L4 nerve root. The patient was returned to surgery for decompression of the left L4 nerve root. A new left-sided laminotomy tracing the course of the L4 root underneath its named pedicle is shown (see Figure 7.18D). The patient experienced complete relief of his radicular symptoms.

An additional example of the failure to perform an adequate neural decompression is outlined in Figure 7.19. This patient suffered paraparesis as the result of an L1 burst fracture. The patient underwent a left-sided thoracoabdominal approach to the anterior spine for decompression of the retropulsed bone fragments, but was worse neurologically after surgery. The preoperative CT scan (see Figure 7.19A) demonstrates the large retropulsed fragment of bone. The postoperative CT (see Figure 7.19B)

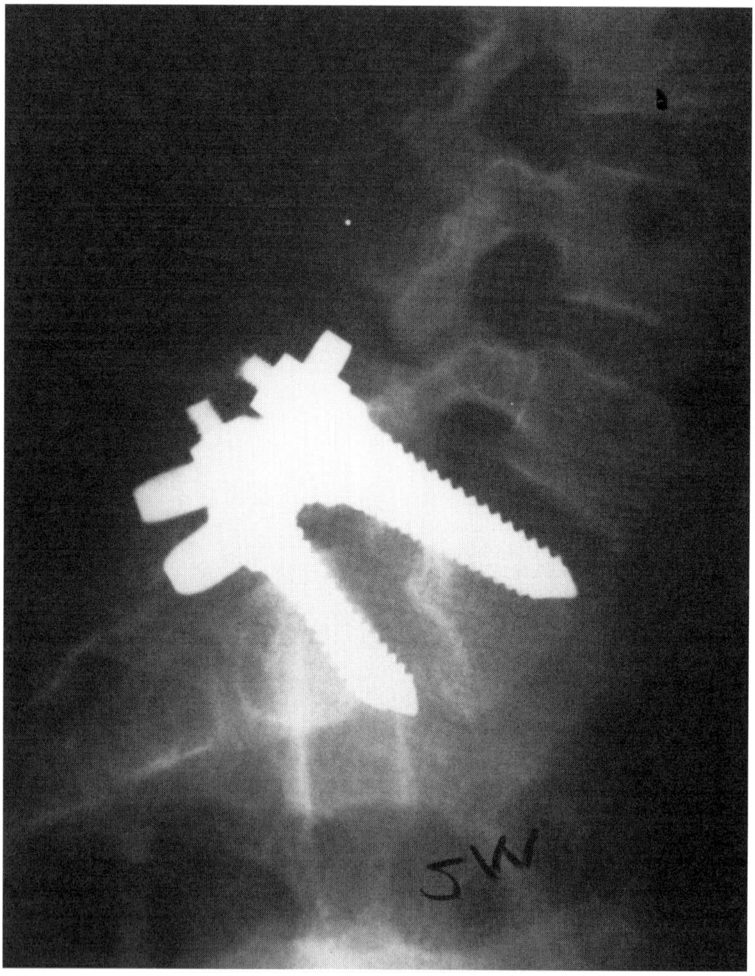

B

Figure 7.17. *continued.* (B) The postreduction radiographs are shown.

demonstrates an inadequate surgical decompression with a large fragment of bone causing continued compression of the conus medullaris.

The incidence of postlaminectomy iatrogenic instability with spondylolisthesis is reported to be from 2% to 10%.[224, 225] Patients who undergo laminectomy in the presence of preexisting degenerative or isthmic spondylolisthesis are at risk for further deformity and return of sciatica.[226] Wide laminectomy that sacrifices the facet joints or transects the pars interarticularis may predispose to postoperative spondylolisthesis. The patient shown in Figure 7.20 was a 62-year-old, obese, blind, diabetic patient with a cardiac arrhythmia controlled by a permanent pacemaker. However, the patient was a community ambulator. The patient had undergone a Gill-type lumbar laminectomy with resection of the loose posterior element associated with an isthmic lumbosacral spondylolysis. Lumbar fusion was initially considered because of the spondylolysis but was withheld because of the patient's overall ill health. Severe symptoms of neurogenic claudication and back pain reappeared within 6 months of surgery, and the patient became wheelchair bound. The myelogram (see Figure 7.20A) showed a complete block. The lateral radiograph (see Figure 7.20B) demonstrated radiographic osteopenia, a new spondylolisthesis of L5 on the sacrum, and retrolisthesis of L4 on L5. The patient was returned to surgery for a tech-

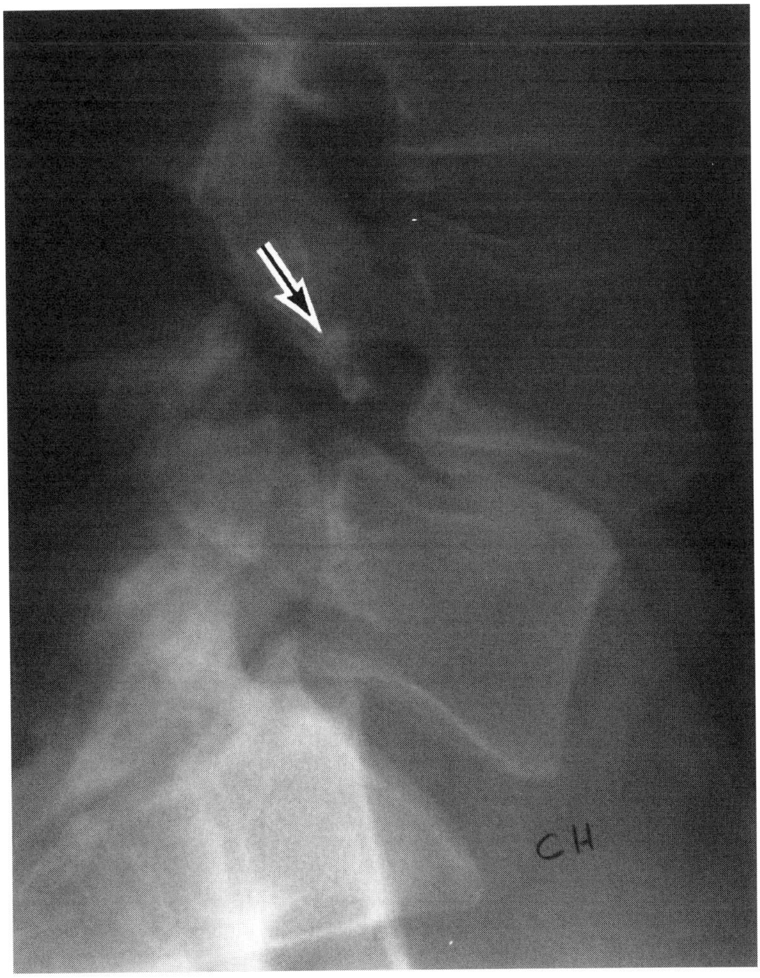

A

Figure 7.18. This patient was treated elsewhere with lumbar laminectomy, but his radicular symptoms persisted. (A) An isthmic L4 on L5 spondylolisthesis and the bony hook (arrow) of the fractured pars interarticularis with resultant neuroforaminal compression of the exiting fourth root are clearly identified.

nically difficult decompression and reconstruction (see Figures 7.20C and D). The patient now ambulates up to one-fourth of a mile without external aids.

Spinal instrumentation, including the use of pedicle screws, has rapidly evolved to a standard of care in North America for the treatment of spondylolisthesis, fractures, tumors, deformity, and selected degenerative conditions of the lumbar spine. The use of spinal pedicle screw implants is associated with a small but definite incidence of postoperative radiculopathy.[227–232] Techniques for pedicle screw insertion depend largely on individual surgeon preferences and training. Most surgeons, however, incorporate the techniques of intraoperative anatomic landmark localization with intraoperative radiographic or fluoroscopic assistance.[232, 233] Additional techniques that may be useful to help guide spinal pedicle screw insertion include direct nerve root inspection through laminotomy and electrophysiologic monitoring.[227, 229, 231, 234–236] Despite all these measures, pedicle screw insertion is essentially a blind technique. Several studies have demonstrated intraoperative radiography to be unreliable for confirmation of satisfactory pedicle screw placement.[232, 233] Laminotomy for direct root visualization may be useful for evaluation of a limited number of screws, especially if it is a planned part of the surgical procedure. Lami-

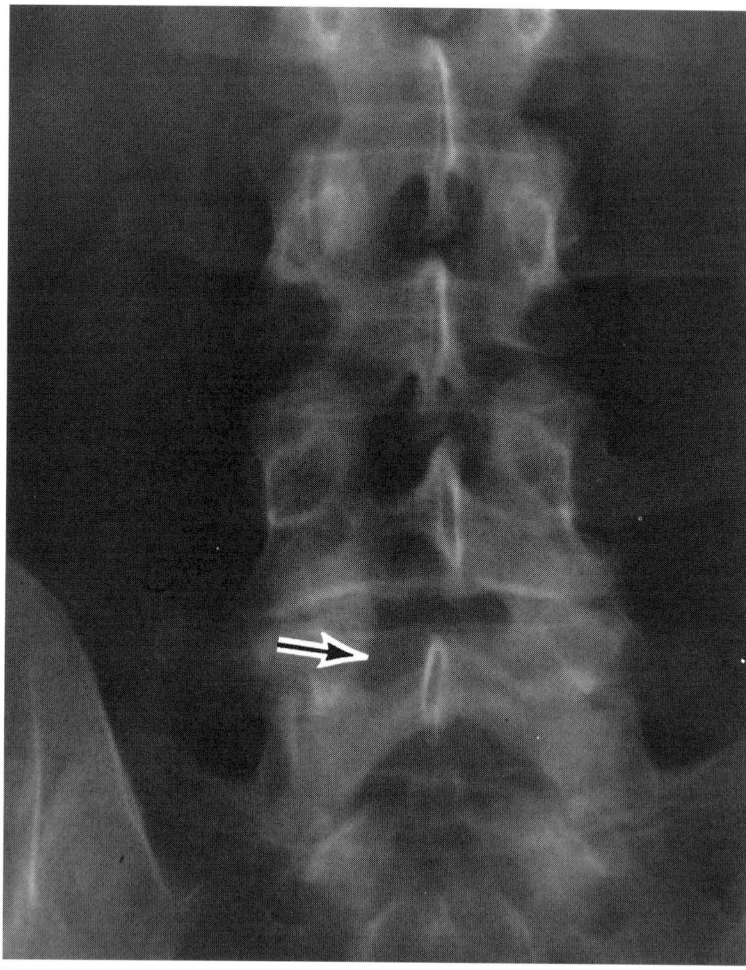

B

Figure 7.18. *continued.* (B) Unfortunately, the surgeon performed a left-sided laminotomy with decompression of the fifth lumbar root underneath its named pedicle shown by the arrow. This demonstrates a lack of understanding of the surgical neuropathology, as the fourth root should have been anticipated to be compressed. (C) As anticipated, the left parasagittal magnetic resonance imaging scan demonstrates severe neuroforaminal compression of the L4 nerve root (arrow). The patient was returned to surgery for decompression of the left L4 nerve root. (D) A new left-sided laminotomy (arrow) tracing the course of the L4 root underneath its named pedicle is shown. The patient experienced complete relief of his radicular symptoms.

notomy, however, is time consuming if neural decompression is not a necessary part of the procedure or if numerous screws will be placed.

The patient shown in Figure 7.21 complained bitterly of left leg pain after lumbar fusion with use of pedicle screw instrumentation. Both the myelogram and CT (see Figures 7.21A and B) demonstrate a screw that has penetrated the medial wall of the pedicle with resultant L4 root compression. For comparison, an MRI of a different patient (see Figure 7.21C) demonstrates ideal placement of a pedicle screw; the screw had been removed to allow imaging of local recurrence of metastatic disease.

Electrophysiologic monitoring techniques include mixed nerve SSEP, MEP, dermatome-specific SSEP, and intraoperative evoked EMG. Electrophysiologic monitoring techniques are effective as supplemental aids, alerting the surgeon to potentially avoidable or correctable spinal cord or nerve root injury.[112] SSEP and MEP are especially useful for monitoring of cord level function during placement of sublaminar hooks and wires within the spinal canal and during intraoperative manipulative reduction techniques for correction of deformity associated with spinal fractures, kyphosis, scoliosis, and spondylolisthesis.[102, 111–114] SSEP, however, is less effective for monitoring individual nerve root function during spinal pedicle screw insertion. Multiple nerve roots of the posterior tibial nerve contribute to the SSEP, and damage to an individual root may not be detected in the mixed nerve

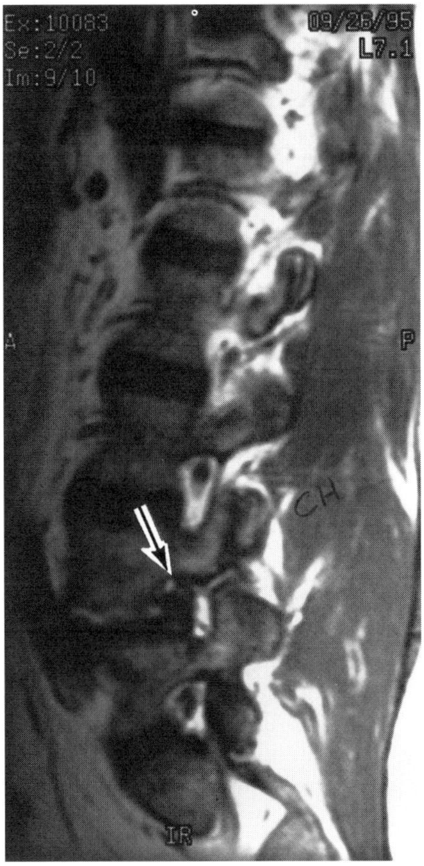

C

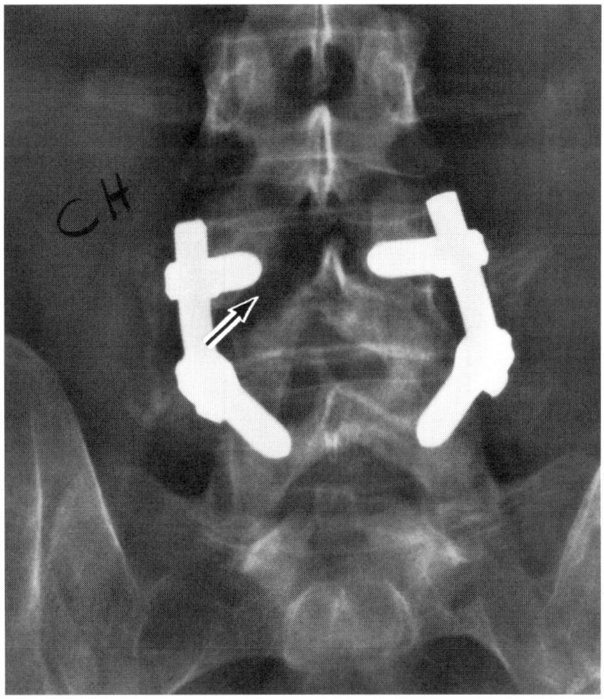

D

response.[234, 235, 237–239] Dermatome-specific SSEPs allow individual nerve root monitoring.[235, 238, 239] However, unless there is nerve root injury, this technique may not be sensitive to pedicle cortical wall breakthrough.[239] In addition, dermatomal SSEP responses are averaged and cannot provide instantaneous feedback to the surgeon. Dermatomal SSEPs are also sensitive to anesthetic variables and may therefore be unreliable during surgery.[239]

To address these concerns, intraoperative EMG techniques have been developed that allow monitoring of muscle groups innervated by individual nerve roots thought to be at risk during the surgical procedure. A correctly placed screw should be surrounded by bone, providing a high impedance to electrical current and resultant nerve root stimulation. However, if the pedicle cortical wall is disrupted, current could flow through the defect, leading to stimulation of the adjacent nerve root with a resultant evoked EMG response at a lower threshold.[234, 237, 240] Present electrophysiologic techniques are very sensitive for detection of pedicle wall cortical breakthrough. The stimulus threshold values suggesting adequate pedicle screw position have been established by several authors as ranging from 5 mA to 15 mA.[237, 240–245] Direct root stimulation occurs with an evoked response of 2.2 mA.[245] Two authors have described 7 and 6 mA, respectively,[237, 245] as an abnormally low threshold and recommend a careful reevaluation of such implanted screws that likely have broached the pedicle cortex and may endanger a lumbar root. Spinal screws that demonstrate a decreased threshold response to electrical stimulation do not necessarily require screw removal or repositioning, but they do alert the surgeon and electrophysiologist to potential postoperative nerve root irritation. Of more concern is the possibility of direct mechanical nerve root displacement by a

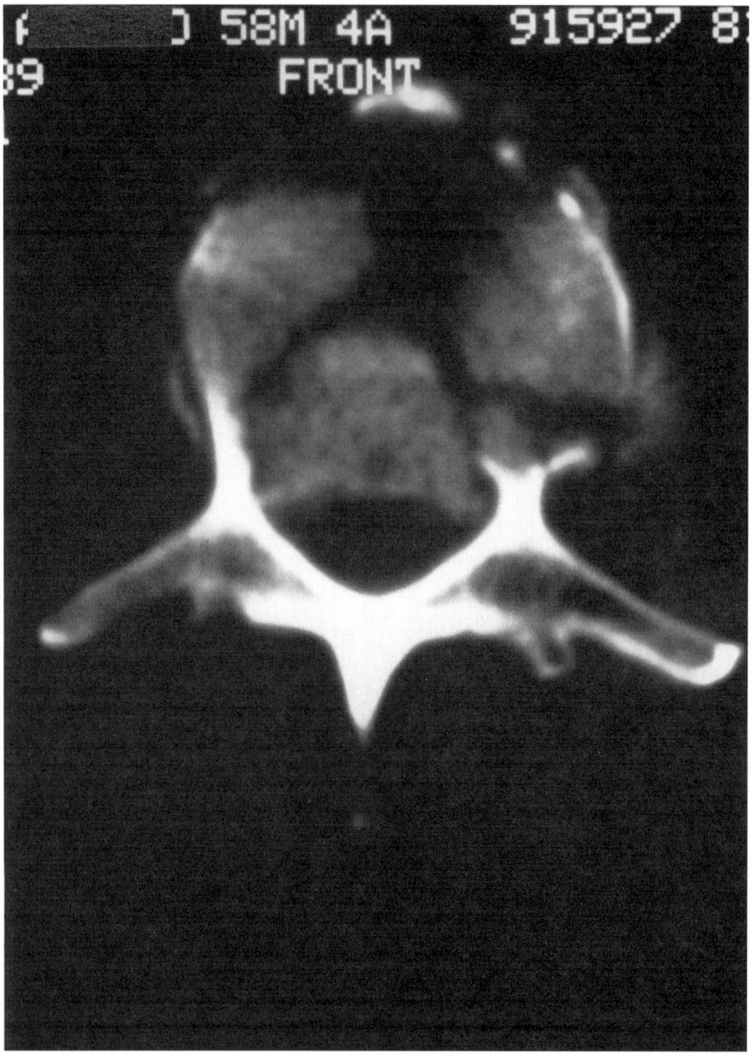

A

Figure 7.19. This patient suffered paraparesis as the result of an L1 burst fracture. The patient underwent a left-sided thoracoabdominal approach to the anterior spine for decompression of the retropulsed bone fragments, but was worse neurologically after surgery. (A) The preoperative computed tomography scan demonstrates the large retropulsed fragment of bone. (B) The postoperative computed tomography scan demonstrates an inadequate surgical decompression with a large fragment of bone (arrow) causing continued compression of the conus medullaris.

screw as indicated by bursts of motor unit potentials described by Owen et al.[239]

The patient identified by the intraoperative EMG tracing reproduced in Figure 7.22 underwent pedicle screw placement for scoliosis. EMG parameters included both spontaneous and constant current stimulus threshold EMG. Monitored muscle groups included the external abdominal oblique (T7–T12), the rectus abdominus (T11–T12), adductor longus (L2–L4), vastus lateralis and medialis (L2–L4), tibialis anterior (L4, L5), peroneus longus (L5, S1, S2), and medial gastrocnemius (S1, S2). Bursts of motor unit potentials were recorded during attempted insertion of a right-sided T10 pedicle screw monitored by the external abdominal oblique. The screw was removed, and an obvious medial and inferior bone defect was identified. Screw placement at this level was aborted. The patient suffered no postoperative evidence of neurologic deficit.

Spinal epidural abscess is a well-recognized complication of epidural anesthesia and epidural corticosteroid injections.[246–250] In addition, spinal epidural abscess is associated with patients infected with human immunodeficiency virus, intravenous drug abusers, immune-compromised

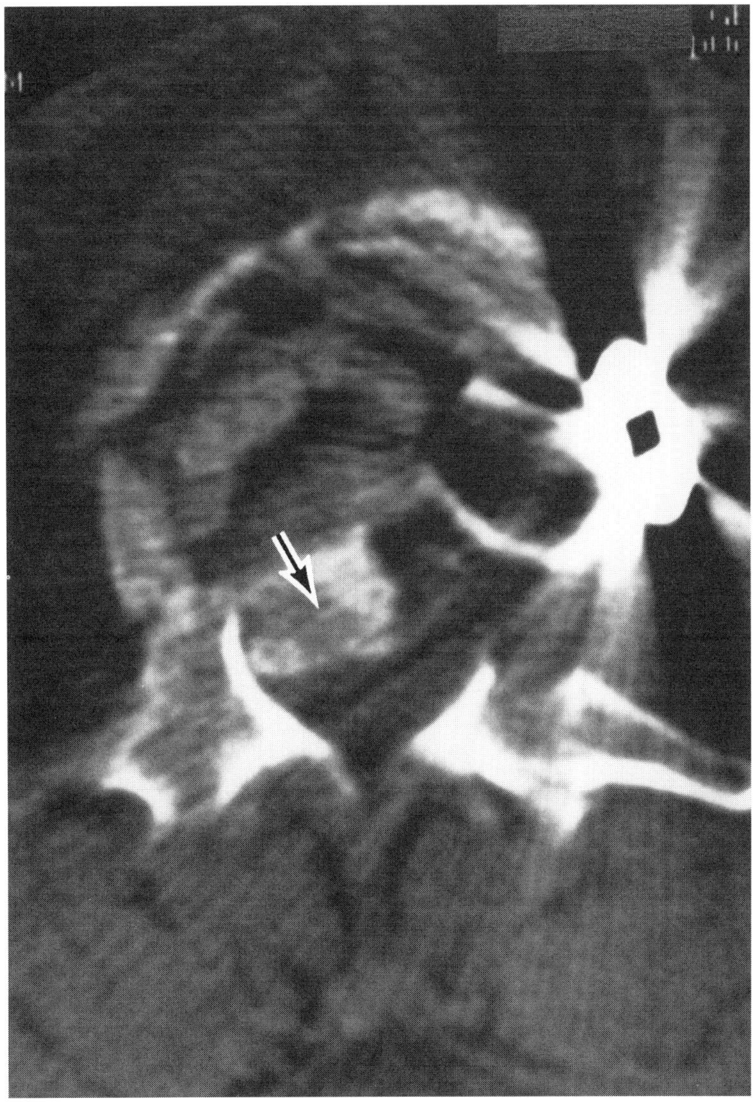

B

patients, spontaneous occurrence, and hematogenous seeding from surgery, abscess, or skin lesions at a distant site.[251–261] Epidural abscess has a mortality of 7–23%.[251, 252] Neurologic deficits may persist in 21–32% of such patients.[251, 252] Epidural abscess in the absence of diskitis or vertebral osteomyelitis is extremely rare following spine surgery. However, an epidural abscess may develop adjacent to and further complicate a postoperative diskitis or vertebral osteomyelitis.[251, 252, 255, 259–261] Curling et al. documented a history of recent spinal surgery in seven of 29 patients who presented with epidural abscess over a 14-year period.[251] Nussbaum et al. reported on 40 cases of spinal epidural abscess identified over a 22-year period; six patients had undergone spinal procedures.[255] Hlavin et al. identified 40 patients with spinal epidural abscess over a 10-year period and five were associated with spinal procedures.[252] Epidural abscess has been treated by both medical and surgical means.[258, 262] In summary of the previously men-

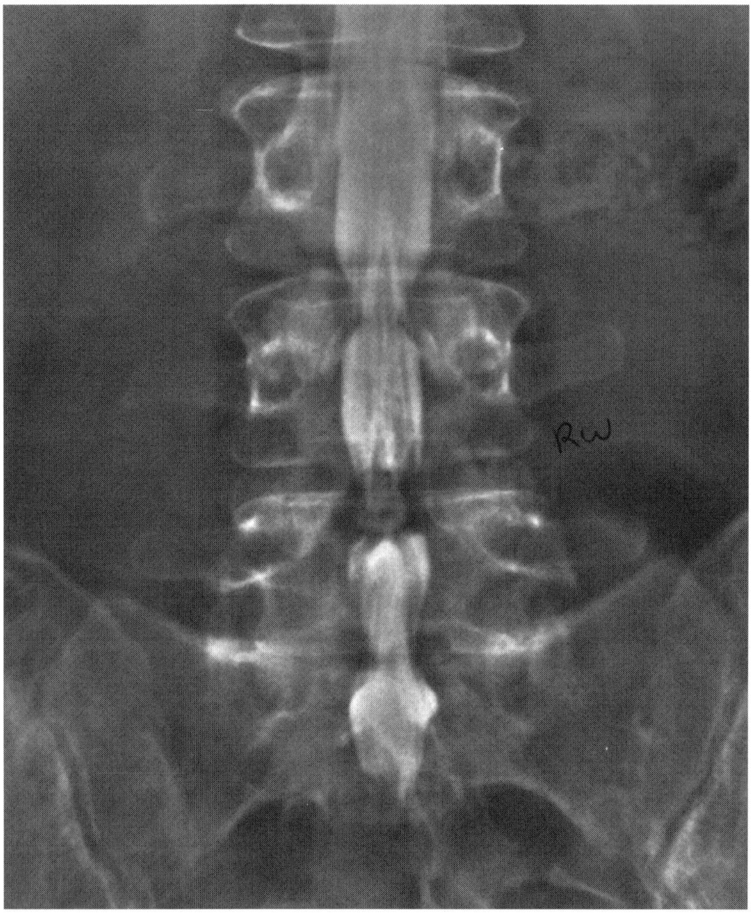

A

Figure 7.20. This patient is a 62-year-old, obese, blind, diabetic patient who has a cardiac arrhythmia controlled by a permanent pacemaker. However, the patient was a community ambulator. The patient had undergone a Gill-type lumbar laminectomy with resection of the loose posterior element associated with an isthmic lumbosacral spondylolysis. Lumbar fusion was initially considered because of the spondylolysis but was withheld because of the patient's overall ill health. Severe symptoms of neurogenic claudication and back pain reappeared within 6 months of surgery and the patient became wheelchair bound. (A) The myelogram showed a complete block. (B) The lateral radiograph demonstrated radiographic osteopenia, a new spondylolisthesis of L5 on the sacrum, and retrolisthesis of L4 on L5.

tioned studies, spinal epidural abscess occurred rarely but was associated with recent spinal surgery in 12–25% of patients.

Figure 7.23 identifies thoracic spine vertebral osteomyelitis with associated large prevertebral and epidural abscesses. This patient had undergone spinal needle placement and injection (discography) into the thoracic disk to elucidate the cause of chronic back pain. Paraparesis developed rapidly after 4 weeks. The paraspinous and epidural abscesses were drained via a costotransversectomy. The patient regained lower extremity function.

The clinical presentation of epidural abscess includes severe back pain, fever, and neurologic deficit. The differential diagnosis of worsening pain and neurologic deficit after spine surgery must include CES, large recurrent disk herniation, postoperative diskitis, vertebral osteomyelitis, epidural hematoma, and epidural abscess. The MRI, myelography, or CT, when correlated with the patient's physical examination, blood culture results, erythrocyte sedimentation rate, and white blood count, should be diagnostic. Following spine surgery, the erythrocyte sedimentation rate should return to normal within 2 weeks.[263] Persistent elevation is associated with postoperative infection.[251, 252, 254, 255, 257, 260, 261] The erythrocyte sedimentation rate is elevated in nearly 100% of patients with epidural abscess, diskitis, or vertebral osteomyelitis.[251, 252, 254, 255, 257]

The patient shown in Figure 7.24 suffered severe back pain and CES 6 weeks after lumbar laminectomy. The emergency MRI (see Figure 7.24A) revealed vertebral osteomyelitis and

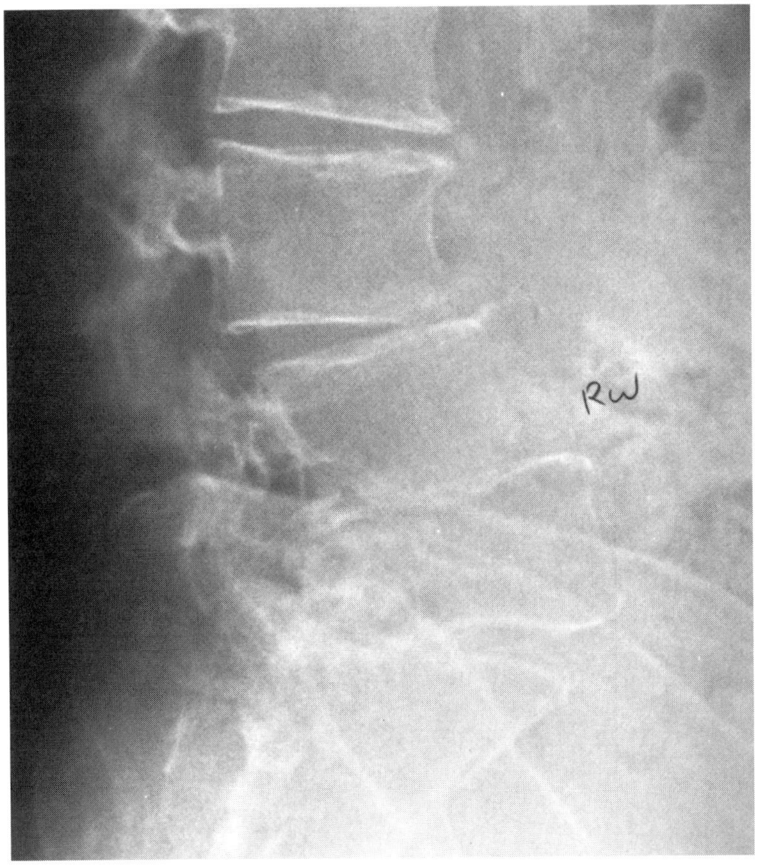

B

retropulsion of debris into the epidural space. Emergency laminectomy revealed friable granulation tissue that cultured positive for *Staphylococcus aureus*. The patient recovered bowel and bladder function. Staged reconstruction of the patient's lumbar spine (see Figure 7.24B) included anterior spine debridement through a flank incision, placement of a temporary allograft bone spacer, and posterior placement of an external spinal skeletal fixator. The external spinal skeletal fixator is placed percutaneously and lies posterior and external to the skin (see Figure 7.24C). The external spinal skeletal fixator allowed the patient to remain fully ambulatory and prevented spinal collapse and kyphosis while intravenous antibiotics were administered and the infection treated. After 6 weeks, the patient was returned to the operating room for a repeat anterior debridement, structural bone graft placement, and definitive reconstruction (see Figure 7.24D). At 18 months' follow-up, the patient has done remarkably well and has returned to most premorbid activities.

Conclusion

Recognizing that entire textbooks have been written on the subject of complications in spinal surgery, we have sharply focused this chapter and discussed only iatrogenic neurologic complications. Our goal is not to provide an exhaustive compilation of all possible problems. Rather, we choose to focus on the prevention of potentially avoidable neurologic complications.

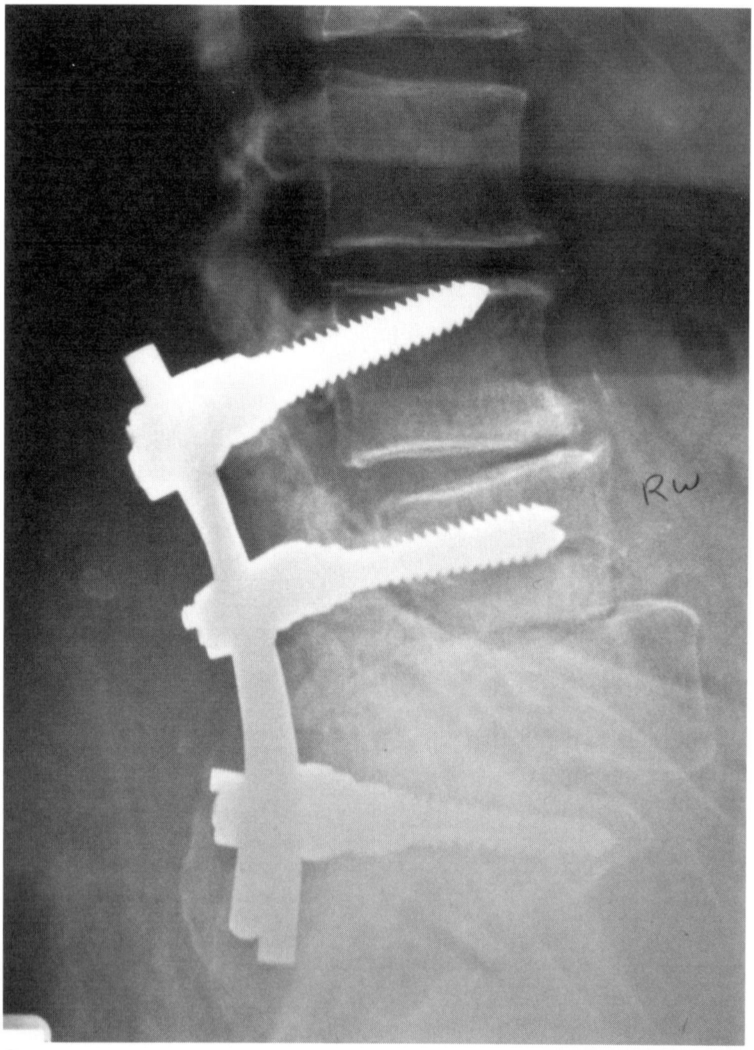

C

Figure 7.20. *continued.*
(C and D) The patient was returned to surgery for a technically difficult decompression and reconstruction. The patient now ambulates up to one-fourth of a mile without external aids.

In addition, for those problems that will inevitably occur, we have emphasized early recognition and treatment, thereby minimizing the impact and morbidity.

Acknowledgment

We would like to thank the medical photography section of the Department of Medical Illustration at the Indiana University Medical Center. One of their many talents is producing quality camera-ready photographs of often very marginal radiographs. Their expertise is well documented in this work.

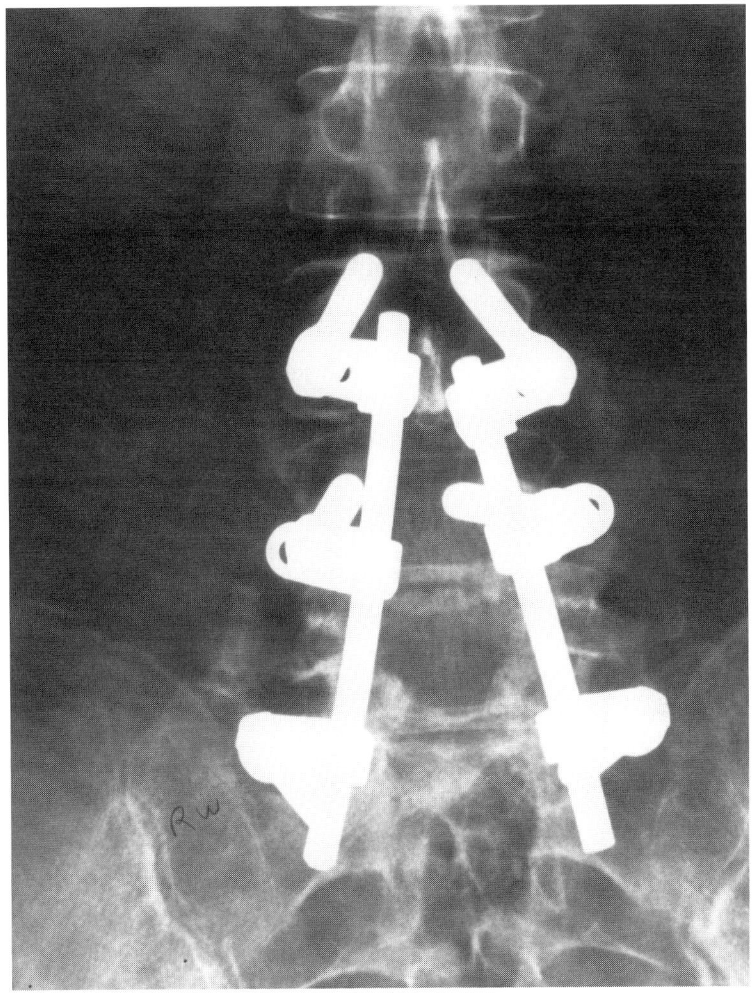

D

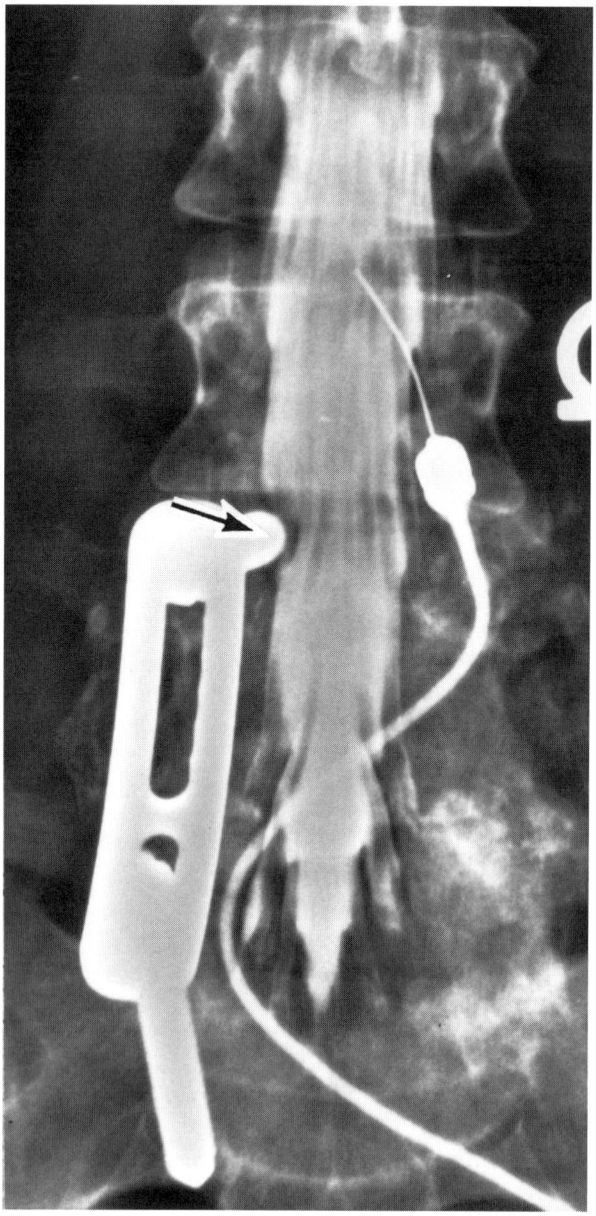

A

Figure 7.21. This patient complained bitterly of left leg pain after lumbar fusion with use of pedicle screw instrumentation. (A and B) Both the myelogram and computed tomography scan demonstrate a screw that has penetrated the medial wall of the pedicle (arrow) with resultant L4 root compression. (C) For comparison, a magnetic resonance imaging scan of a different patient demonstrates ideal placement (arrow) of a pedicle screw; the screw had been removed to allow imaging of local recurrence of metastatic disease.

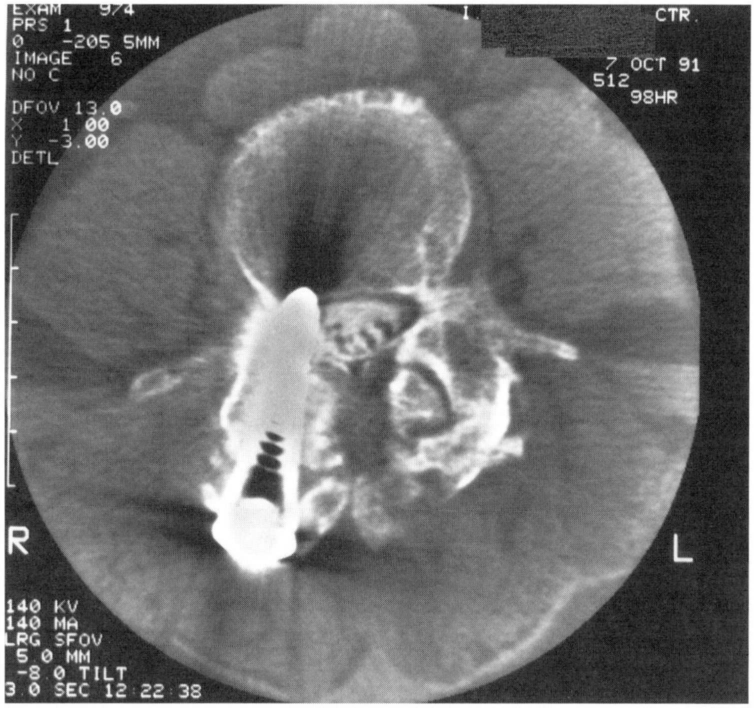
EXAM 974
PRS 1
0 -205 5MM
IMAGE 6
NO C
DFOV 13.0
X 1.00
Y -3.00
DETL
CTR.
7 OCT 91
512
98HR
R
L
140 KV
140 MA
LRG SFOV
5.0 MM
-8.0 TILT
3.0 SEC 12:22:38

B

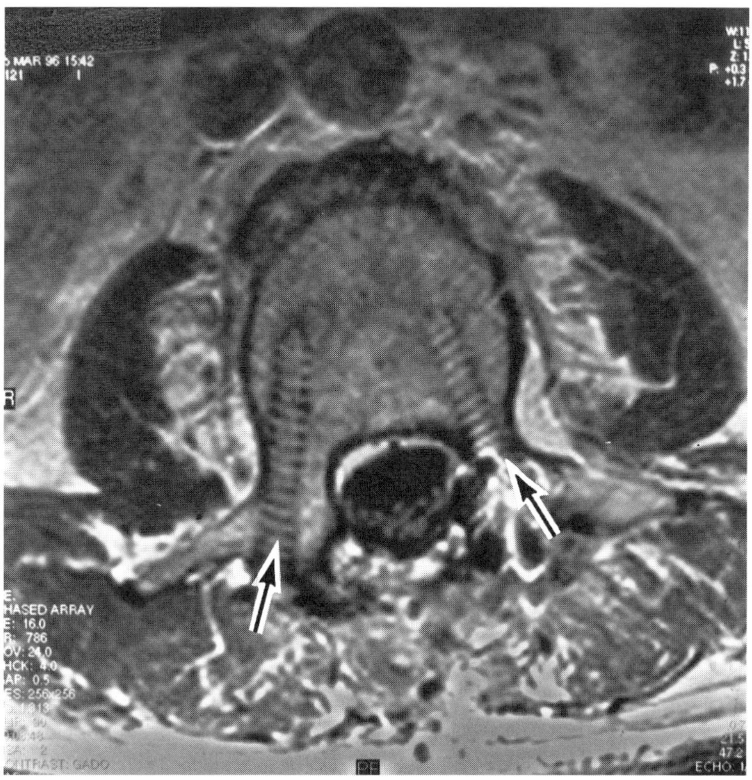
MAR 96 15:42
121
R
HASED ARRAY
E: 16.0
R: 786
OV: 24.0
HCK: 4.0
AP: 0.5
ES: 256×256
ONTRAST: GADO
PE

C

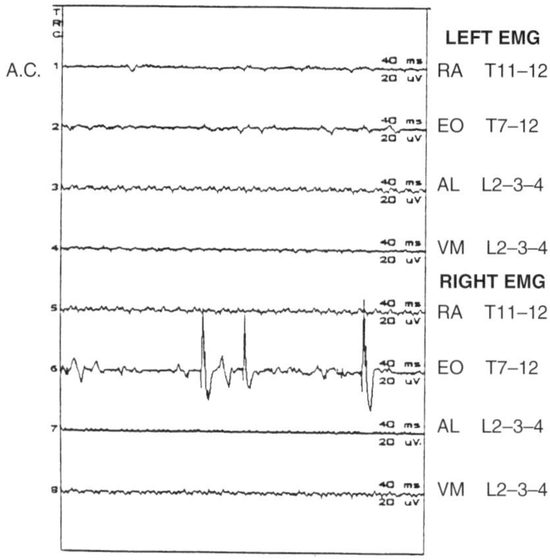

Figure 7.22. This intraoperative electromyographic (EMG) tracing demonstrates bursts of motor unit potentials in a patient treated with pedicle screw placement for scoliosis. EMG parameters included both spontaneous and constant current stimulus threshold electromyography. Monitored muscle groups included the rectus abdominus (T11–T12), external abdominal oblique (T7–T12), adductor longus (L2–L4), vastus lateralis and medialis (L2–L4), tibialis anterior (L4, L5), peroneus longus (L5, S1, S2), and medial gastrocnemius (S1, S2). Bursts of motor unit potentials were recorded during attempted insertion of a right-sided T10 pedicle screw monitored by the external abdominal oblique view. The screw was removed, and an obvious medial and inferior bone defect was identified. Screw placement at this level was aborted. The patient suffered no postoperative evidence of neurologic deficit.

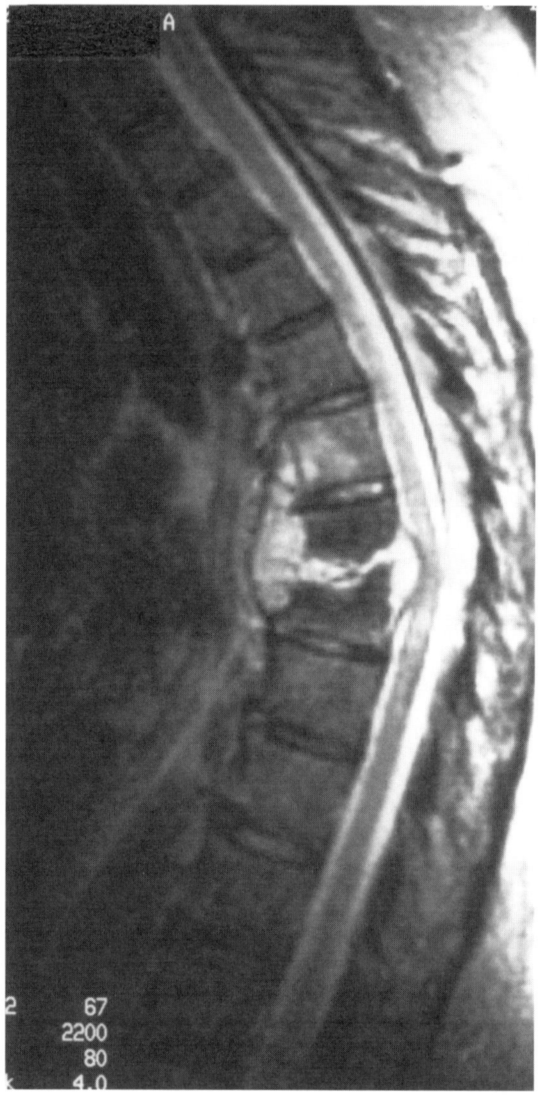

Figure 7.23. This patient had undergone spinal needle placement and injection (diskography) into the thoracic disk to elucidate the cause for chronic back pain. Paraparesis developed rapidly after 4 weeks. The thoracic spine vertebral osteomyelitis was associated with a large prevertebral and epidural abscess. The paraspinous and epidural abscess were drained via a costotransversectomy. The patient regained lower extremity function.

Figure 7.24. This patient suffered severe back pain and cauda equina syndrome 6 weeks after lumbar laminectomy. (A) The emergency magnetic resonance imaging scan revealed vertebral osteomyelitis and retropulsion of debris into the epidural space. Emergency laminectomy revealed friable granulation tissue that cultured positive for *Staphylococcus aureus*. The patient recovered bowel and bladder function. (B) Staged reconstruction of the patient's lumbar spine included anterior spine debridement through a flank incision, placement of a temporary allograft bone spacer, and posterior placement of an external spinal skeletal fixator.

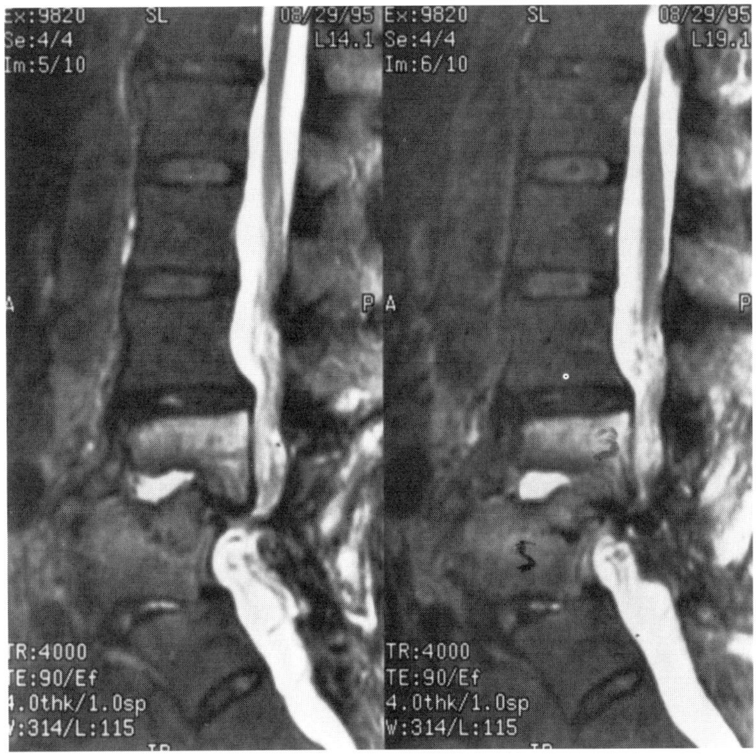

A

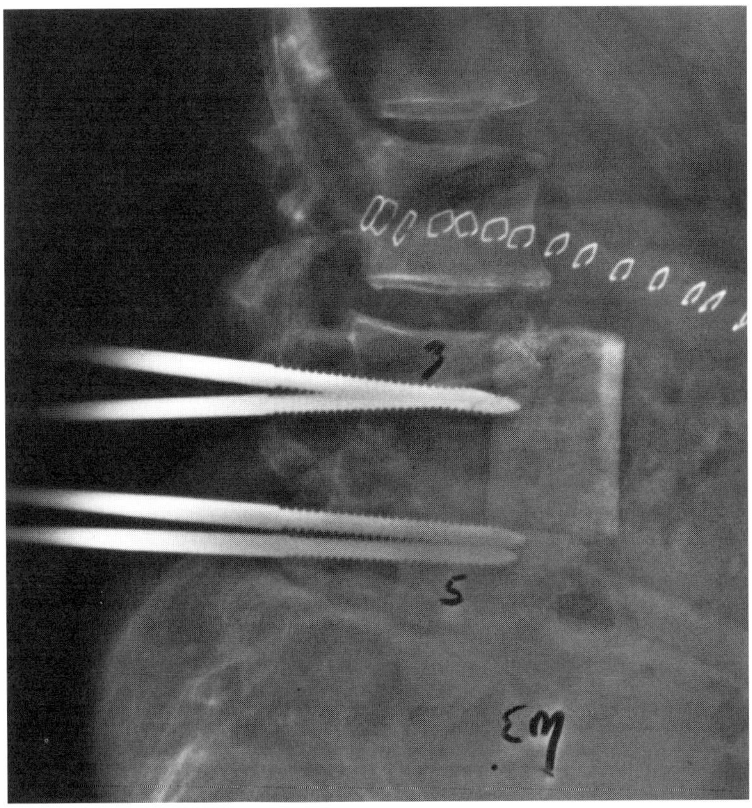

B

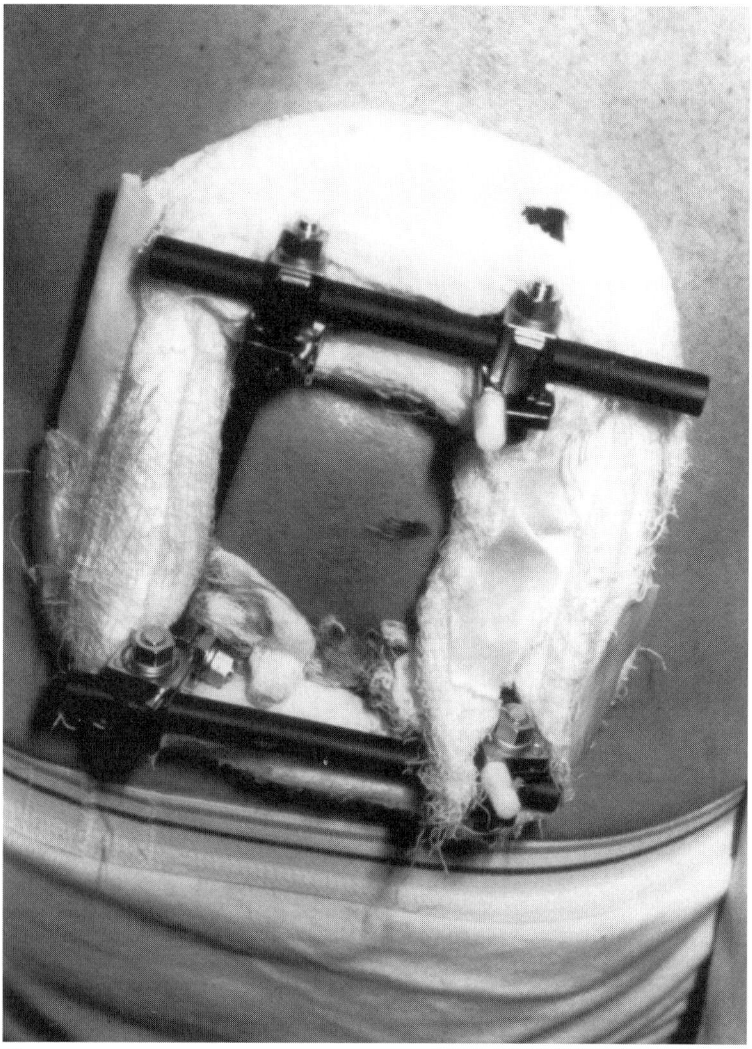

C

Figure 7.24. *continued.* (C) The external spinal skeletal fixator is placed percutaneously and lies posterior and external to the skin. The external spinal skeletal fixator allowed the patient to remain fully ambulatory and prevented spinal collapse and kyphosis while intravenous antibiotics were administered and the infection treated. (D) After 6 weeks, the patient was returned to the operating room for a repeat anterior debridement, structural bone graft placement, and definitive reconstruction. At 18 months' follow-up, the patient had done remarkably well and returned to most premorbid activities.

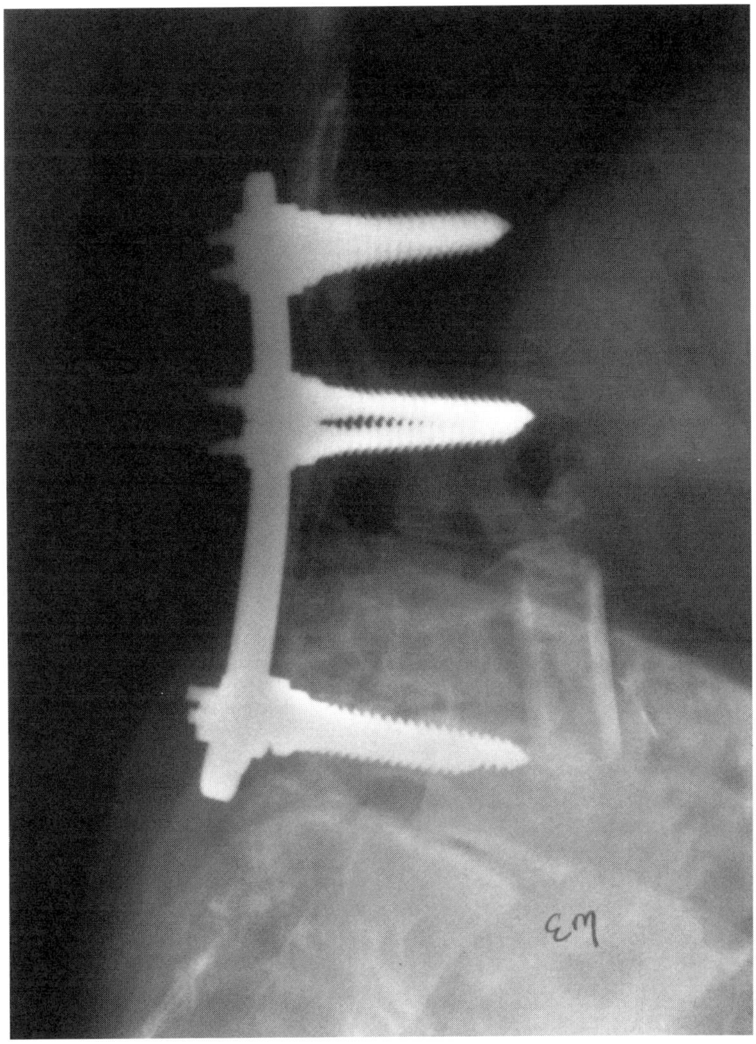

D

References

1. Cotler JM, Cotler HB. Complications of Injury and Treatment of the Spine. In CH Epps (ed), Complications in Orthopaedic Surgery (3rd ed). Philadelphia: Lippincott, 1994;723.
2. Kurz LT, Garfin SR, Booth RE. Harvesting autogenous iliac crest bone graft. A review of complications and techniques. Spine 1989;14:1324.
3. Papastefanou SL, Stevens K, Mulholland RC. Femoral nerve palsy. An unusual complication of anterior interbody fusion. Spine 1994;19:2842.
4. Chevalier X, Larget-Piet B. Femoral neuropathy due to psoas hematoma revisited. Report of three cases with serious outcomes. Spine 1992;17:724.
5. Graham JM. Rectus sheath hematoma after anterior lumbar fusion. Spine 1991;16:1377.
6. Albin MS, Caroll RG, Maroon JC. Clinical considerations concerning detection of venous air embolism. Neurosurgery 1978;3:380.
7. Buckland RW, Manners JM. Venous air embolism during neurosurgery: a comparison of various methods of detection in man. Anaesthesia 1976;31:633.
8. Clayton DG, Evans P, Williams C, et al. Paradoxical air emoblism during neurosurgery. Anaesthesia 1985;40:981.
9. Cucchiara RF. Safety of the sitting position. Anesthesiology 1984;61:790.
10. Perkins-Pearson NAK, Marshall WK, Bedford RF. Atrial pressures in the seated position: implication for paradoxical air embolism. Anesthesiology 1982;57:493.

11. Roberts MP. Complications of Positioning for Neurosurgical Operations on the Spine. In EC Tarlov (ed), Complications of Spinal Surgery. Park Ridge, IL: American Association of Neurological Surgeons, 1991;1.
12. Sato S, Toya S, Ohira T, et al. Echocardiographic detection and treatment of intraoperative air embolism. J Neurosurg 1986;64:440.
13. Young ML, Smith DS, Murtagh F, et al. Comparison of surgical and anesthetic complications in neurosurgical patients experiencing venous air embolism in the sitting position. Neurosurgery 1986;18:157.
14. Curtis BH. Air embolism as complication of spine fusion. J Bone Joint Surg Am 1972;54:201.
15. McCarthy RE, Lonstein JE, Mertz JD, Kuslich SD. Air embolism in spinal surgery. J Spine Disord 1990;3:1.
16. Gronert GA, Messick JM, Cucchiara RF, et al. Paradoxical air embolism from a patent foramen ovale. Anesthesiology 1979;50:548.
17. Lynch JJ, Schuchard GH, Gross CM, et al. Prevalence of right-to-left atrial shunting in a healthy population: detection by Valsalva maneuver contrast echocardiography. Am J Cardiol 1984;53:1478.
18. Stoelting RK, Dierdorf SF. Anesthesia and Co-Existing Disease (3rd ed). New York: Churchill Livingstone, 1993;194.
19. Myers MA, Hamilton SR, Bogosian AJ, et al. Visual loss as a complication of spine surgery. A review of 37 cases. Spine 1997;22:1325.
20. Grossman W, Ward WT. Central retinal artery occlusion after scoliosis surgery with a horseshoe headrest. Case report and literature review. Spine 1993;18:1226.
21. Sys J, Michielsen J, Mertens E, et al. Central retinal artery occlusion after spinal surgery. Eur Spine J 1996;5:74.
22. Stevens WR, Glazier PA, Lietman TM, et al. Ophthalmic complications after spinal surgery. Spine 1997;22:1319.
23. Langmayr JJ, Ortler M, Obsegeser A, Felber S. Quadriplegia after lumbar disc surgery. Spine 1996;21:1932.
24. Toole JF, Tucker SH. Influence of head position upon cerebral circulation: studies on blood flow in cadavers. Arch Neurol 1960;3:616.
25. Britt BA, Gordon RA. Peripheral nerve injuries associated with anesthesia. Can Anaesth Soc J 1964;11:514.
26. Dornette WHL. Compression neuropathies: medical aspects and legal implications. Int Anesthesiol Clin 1986;24:201.
27. Cameron MGP, Stewart OJ. Ulnar nerve injury associated with anesthesia. Can J Anaesth 1975;22:253.
28. Albanese S, Buterbaugh G, Palmer AK, et al. Incomplete anterior interosseus nerve palsy following spinal surgery. A report of two cases. Spine 1986;11:1037.
29. Gwinnutt CL. Injury to the axillary nerve. Anesthesia 1988;43:205.
30. Shaffer JW. Suprascapular nerve injury during spine surgery. A case report. Spine 1994;19:70.
31. Cooper DE, Jenkins RS, Bready L, et al. The prevention of injuries to the brachial plexus secondary to malposition of the patient during surgery. Clin Orthop 1988;228:31.
32. Kwaan JH, Rappaport I. Postoperative brachial plexus palsy. Arch Surg 1970;101:612.
33. Nambisan RN, Karakousis CP. Axillary compression syndrome with neuropraxia due to operative positioning. Surgery 1989;105:449.
34. Parks BJ. Postoperative peripheral neuropathies. Surgery 1973;74:348.
35. Herkowitz HN. A comparison of anterior cervical fusion, cervical laminectomy, and cervical laminoplasty for the surgical management of multiple level spondylotic radiculopathy. Spine 1988;13:774.
36. Flynn TB. Neurologic complications of anterior cervical interbody fusion. Spine 1982;7:536.
37. Bertalanffy H, Eggert HR. Complications of anterior cervical discectomy without fusion in 450 consecutive patients. Acta Neurochir (Wien) 1989;99:41.
38. Eperson JO, Buhl M, Eriksen EF, et al. Treatment of cervical disc disease using Cloward's technique. I: general results, effect of different operative methods and complications in 1,106 patients. Acta Neurochir (Wien) 1984;70:97.
39. Lesoin F, Bouasakao N, Clarisse J, et al. Results of surgical treatment of radiculomylopathy caused by cervical arthrosis based on 1000 operations. Surg Neurol 1985;23:350.
40. Lunsford LD, Bissonette DJ, Jannetta PJ, et al. Anterior surgery for cervical disc disease. I: treatment of lateral cervical disc herniation in 253 cases. J Neurosurg 1980;53:1.
41. Lunsford LD, Bissonette DJ, Zorub DS. Anterior surgery for cervical disc disease. II: treatment of cervical spondylotic myelopathy in 32 cases. J Neurosurg 1980;53:12.
42. Simmons EH, Bahalla SK. Anterior cervical discectomy and fusion. A clinical and biomechanical study with eight year follow-up. J Bone Joint Surg Br 1969;51:225.
43. Yonenobu K, Hosono N, Iwasaki M, et al. Neurologic complications of surgery for cervical compression myelopathy. Spine 1991;16:1277.
44. An HS, Simeone FA. Complications in Cervical Disc Disease Surgery. In HS An, RA Balderston (eds), Complications in Spinal Surgery. Philadelphia: Saunders, 1991;41.
45. Hardy RJ. Complications of Anterior Cervical Surgery. In EC Tarlov (ed), Complications of Spinal Surgery. Park Ridge, IL: American Association of Neurological Surgeons, 1991;85-94.
46. Kraus DR, Stauffer ES. Spinal cord injury as a complication of elective anterior cervical fusion. Clin Orthop 1975;112:130.
47. Sugar O. Spinal cord malfunction after anterior cervical discectomy. Surg Neurol 1981;15:4.
48. McAfee PC. Anterior Surgical Approaches to the

Lower and Upper Cervical Spine. In H Sherk (ed), The Cervical Spine: An Atlas of Surgical Procedures. Philadelphia: Lippincott, 1994;37.
49. McAfee PC, Bohlman HH, Riley LH, et al. Anterior Retropharyngeal Approach to the Upper Cervical Spine. In HH Sherk (ed), The Cervical Spine (2nd ed). Philadelphia: Lippincott, 1989;808.
50. Watkins RG. Surgical Approaches to the Spine. New York: Springer-Verlag, 1983.
51. Bulger RF, Rejowski JE, Beatty RA. Vocal cord paralysis associated with anterior cervical fusion: considerations for prevention and treatment. J Neurosurg 1985;62:657.
52. Sanders G, Uyeda RY, Karlan MS. Nonrecurrent inferior laryngeal nerves and their association with a recurrent branch. Am J Surg 1983;146:501.
53. Heeneman H. Vocal cord paralysis following approaches to the anterior cervical spine. Laryngoscope 1973;83:17.
54. McAfee PC, Bohlman HH, Riley LH, et al. The anterior retropharyngeal approach to the upper part of the cervical spine. J Bone Joint Surg Am 1987;69:1371.
55. Menezes AH. Complications of Surgery of the Craniovertebral Junction. In EC Tarlov (ed), Complications of Spinal Surgery. Park Ridge, IL: American Association of Neurological Surgeons, 1991;77.
56. Krieger AJ, Rosomoff HL. Sleep-induced apnea. Part 2. Respiratory failure after anterior spinal surgery. J Neurosurg. 1974;181.
57. Brust JC. Symptoms of Neurologic Disorders, Coma. In LP Rowland (ed), Merritt's Textbook of Neurology (9th ed, Vol 21). Baltimore: Williams & Wilkins, 1995;688.
58. Fielding JW. Complications of anterior cervical disk removal and fusion. Clin Orthop 1992;228:10.
59. Miyachi S, Okamura K, Watanabe M, et al. Cerebellar stroke due to vertebral artery occlusion after cervical spine trauma. Two case reports. Spine 1994;19:83.
60. Hoshino Y, Kurokawa T, Nakamura K, et al. A report on the safety of unilateral vertebral artery ligation during cervical spine surgery. Spine 1996;21:1454.
61. Epstein NE, Silvergleid R. Magnetic resonance angiographic diagnosis of ectatic vertebral artery. J Spinal Disord 1995;8:308.
62. Smith MD, Emery SE, Dudley A, et al. Vertebral artery injury during anterior decompression of the cervical spine. A retrospective review of ten patients. J Bone Joint Surg Br 1993;75:410.
63. Golfinos JG, Dickman CA, Zabran JM, et al. Repair of vertebral artery injury after anterior cervical decompression. Spine 1994;19:2552.
64. Pfeifer BA, Freidberg SR, Jewell ER. Repair of injured vertebral artery in anterior cervical procedures. Spine 1994;19:1471.
65. Oga M, Itaru Y, Terada K, et al. Tortuosity of the vertebral artery in patients with cervical spondylotic myelopathy. Risk factor for the vertebral artery injury during anterior cervical decompression. Spine 1996;21:1085.
66. Heary RF, Albert TJ, Ludwig SC, et al. Surgical anatomy of the vertebral arteries. Spine 1996;21:2074.
67. Arnold V, Lehrmann R, Kursawe HK, Luckel W. Hypoplasia of vertebrabasilar arteries. Neuroradiology 1991;33(Suppl):426.
68. Davis WL, Jacobs J. Cerebral Vasculature: Normal Anatomy and Pathology. In AG Osborn (ed), Diagnostic Neuroradiology. St. Louis: Mosby, 1994;117.
69. Brazis PW, Masdeu JC, Biller J. Localization in Clinical Neurology. Boston: Little, Brown, 1996;104, 347.
70. Heros RC. Cerebellar infarction resulting from traumatic occlusion of a vertebral artery. Case report. J Neurosurg 1979;51:111.
71. Mikawa Y, Shikata J, Yammamuro T. Spinal deformity and instability after multilevel cervical laminectomy. Spine 1987;12:6.
72. Callahan RA, Johnson RM, Margolis RN, et al. Cervical facet fusion for control of instablity following laminectomy. J Bone Joint Surg Am 1977;59:991.
73. Bell DF, Walker JL, O'Connor G, Tibshirani R. Spinal deformity after multiple-level cervical laminectomy in children. Spine 1994;19:406.
74. Francis WR Jr, Noble DP. Treatment of cervical kyphosis in children. Spine 1988;13:883.
75. Rizzolo SJ, Piazza MR, Cotler JM, et al. Intervertebral disc injury complicating cervical spine trauma. Spine 1991;16:S187.
76. Eismont FJ, Aruna MJ, Green BA. Extrusion of an intervertebral disc associated with traumatic subluxation or dislocation of cervical facets. J Bone Joint Surg Am 1991;73:1555.
77. Mahale YJ, Silver JR, Henderson NJ. Neurological complications of the reduction of cervical spine dislocations. J Bone Joint Surg Br 1993;75:403.
78. Graham JJ. Complications of Cervical Spine Surgery. In HH Sherk (ed), The Cervical Spine (2nd ed). Philadelphia: Lippincott, 1989;831.
79. Bracken MB, et al. A randomized, controlled trial of methyl-prednisolone or naloxone in the treatment of acute spinal cord injury: results of the second national acute spinal cord injury study. N Engl J Med 1990; 322:1405.
80. Costabile G, Husaag L, Probst C. Spinal epidural hematoma. Surg Neurol 1984;21:8.
81. Pan G, Kulkarni M, MacDougall DJ, Miner ME. Traumatic epidural hematoma of the cervical spine: diagnosis with magnetic resonance imaging. J Neurosurg 1988;68:798.
82. Scott BB, Quisling RG, Miller CA, Kindt GW. Spinal epidural hematoma. JAMA 1976;235:513.
83. Sang UH, Wilson CB. Postoperative epidural hematoma as a complication of anterior cervical discectomy. Report of three cases. J Neurosurg 1978;49:288.
84. Earman WA, Semba R. Postsurgical epidural hematoma reproducing a lumbar radiculopathy. Orthop Rev 1988;12:1201.
85. Mayfield FH. Cervical spondylosis: a comparison of the anterior and posterior approaches. Clin Neurosurg 1976;13:435.

86. Matsunaga S, Salou T, Imamura T, Morimoto N. Dissociated motor loss in the upper extremities. Clinical features and pathophysiology. Spine 1993;18:1964.
87. Tsuzuki N, Abe R, Siki K. Extradural tethering effect as one mechanism of radiculopathy complicating posterior decompression of the cervical spinal cord. Spine 1996;21:203.
88. Tsuzuki N, Abe R, Siki K, Okai K. Paralysis of the arm after posterior decompression of the cervical spinal cord. Eur Spine J 1993;2:197.
89. Saunders RL. Complications of Surgical Management. In RL Saunders, PM Bernini (eds), Cervical Spondylotic Myelopathy. Boston: Blackwell, 1992;203.
90. Saunders RL. Complications of Corpectomy. In EC Tarlov (ed), Complications of Spinal Surgery. Park Ridge, IL: American Association of Neurological Surgeons, 1991;111.
91. Shinomiya K, Yoshiroh K, Michiyuiki F, Furuya K. Clinical study of dissociated motor weakness following anterior cervical decompression surgery. Spine 1989;14:1211.
92. Shinomiya K, Ojawa A, Nakao K, et al. Morphology of C5 ventral nerve rootlets as part of dissociated motor loss of deltoid muscle. Spine 1994;19:2501.
93. Winter RB, Denis F, Lonstein JE, Garamella J. Techniques of Surgery. In JE Lonstein, DS Bradford, RB Winter, JW Ogilvie (eds), Moe's Textbook of Scoliosis and Other Spinal Deformities (3rd ed). Philadelphia: Saunders, 1995;133.
94. Haller GS, Shulman BJ, Taylor PD. Anesthesia for Surgery of the Spine. In JE Lonstein, DS Bradford, RB Winter, JW Ogilvie (eds), Moe's Textbook of Scoliosis and Other Spinal Deformities (3rd ed). Philadelphia: Saunders, 1995;595.
95. Lazorthes G, Gouaze A, Zadeh JO, et al. Arterial vascularization of the spinal cord: recent studies of the anastomotic substitution pathways. J Neurosurg 1971;35:253.
96. Dommisse GF. The blood supply of the spinal cord: a critical vascular zone in spinal surgery. J Bone Joint Surg Br 1974;56:225.
97. Ben-David B, Haller G, Taylor PD. Anterior spinal fusion complicated by paraplegia. Spine 1987;12:536.
98. Dwyer AF, Schafer MF. Anterior approaches to scoliosis: surgical results of 51 cases. J Bone Joint Surg Br 1974;56:218.
99. Faciszewski T, Winter RB, Lonstein JE, et al. The surgical and medical perioperative complications of anterior spinal fusion surgery in the thoracic and lumbar spine in adults. A review of 1223 procedures. Spine 1995;20:1592.
100. Riseborough EJ. The anterior approach to the spine for the correction of deformity of the axial skeleton. Clin Orthop 1973;93:207.
101. Winter RB, Lonstein JE, Denis F, et al. Paraplegia resulting from vessel ligation. Spine 1996;21:1232.
102. Bassett G, Johnson C, Stanley P. Comparison of preoperative selective spinal angiography and somatosensory evoked potential monitoring with temporary occlusion of segmental vessels during anterior spinal surgey. Spine 1996;21:1996.
103. Bradford DS, Boachie-Adjei O. One-stage anterior and posterior hemivertebrae resection and arthrodesis for congenital scoliosis. J Bone Joint Surg Am 1990;72:536.
104. Leatherman KD, Dickson RA. Two-stage corrective surgery for congenital deformities of the spine. J Bone Joint Surg Br 1979;61:324.
105. Montgomery SP, Hall JE. Congenital kyphosis. Spine 1982;7:360.
106. Sarwark JF. Complications in the Treatment of Kyphosis (Nonneuromuscular). In CH Epps, JR Bowen (eds), Complications in Pediatric Orthopedic Surgery. Philadelphia: Lippincott,1995;291.
107. Transfeldt EE. Complications of Treatment. In JE Lonstein, DS Bradford, RB Winter, JW Ogilvie (eds), Moe's Textbook of Scoliosis and Other Spinal Deformities (3rd ed). Philadelphia: Saunders, 1995;451.
108. Winter RB. Neurologic safety in spinal deformity surgery. Spine 1997;22:1527.
109. Winter RB. Complications of Treatment of the Congenital Spine. In CH Epps, JR Bowen (eds), Complications in Pediatric Orthopaedic Surgery. Philadelphia: Lippincott,1995;271.
110. Winter RB. Congenital Spinal Deformity. In JE Lonstein, DS Bradford, RB Winter, JW Ogilvie (eds), Moe's Textbook of Scoliosis and Other Spinal Deformities (3rd ed). Philadelphia: Saunders, 1995;257.
111. Apel DM, Marrero G, King J, et al. Avoiding paraplegia during anterior spinal surgery: the role of somatosensory evoked potential monitoring with temporary occlusion of segmental spinal arteries. Spine 1991;16S:S365.
112. Herdman J, Deletis V, Edmonds HL, Morota N. Spine update. Spinal cord and nerve root monitoring in spine surgery and related procedures. Spine 1996;21:879.
113. Kai Y, Owen JH, Allen BT, et al. Relationship between evoked potentials and clinical status in spinal cord ischemia. Spine 1995;20:291.
114. Yukihiro K, Owen JH, Allen BT, et al. Relationship between evoked potentials and clinical status in spinal cord ischemia. Spine 1995;20:291.
115. Berendes JN, Bredee JJ, Schipperheyn JJ, et al. Mechanism of spinal cord injury after cross-clamping of the descending thoracic aorta. Circulation 1982;66:1112.
116. Brewer LA, Fosburg RG, Mulder GA, Verska JJ. Spinal cord complications following surgery for coarctation of the aorta: a study of 66 cases. J Thorac Cardiovasc Surg 1972;64:368.
117. Coles JG, Wilson GJ, Sima AF, et al. Intraoperative detection of spinal cord ischemia using somatosensory cortical evoked potentials during thoracic occlusion. Ann Thorac Surg 1982;34:29.
118. Shallat RF, Klump TE. Paraplegia following thoracolumbar sympathectomy. J Neurosurg 1971;34:569.
119. Miller CA. Complications of Surgery of the Thoracic Spine. In EC Tarlov (ed), Neurosurgical Treatment of

Disorders of the Thoracic Spine. Park Ridge, IL: American Association of Neurological Surgeons, 1991;111.

120. Ridenour TR, Haddad SF, Hitchon PW, et al. Herniated thoracic disks: treatment and outcome. J Spinal Disord 1993;6:218.
121. Stillerman CB, Weiss MH. Principles of Surgical Approaches to the Thoracic Spine. In EC Tarlov (ed), Neurosurgical Treatment of Disorders of the Thoracic Spine. Park Ridge, IL: American Association of Neurological Surgeons, 1991;1.
122. Tarlov EC. Thoracic Disc Herniation. In EC Tarlov (ed), Neurosurgical Treatment of Disorders of the Thoracic Spine. Park Ridge, IL: American Association of Neurological Surgeons, 1991;53.
123. Simpson MJ, Silveri CP, Sim FA, et al. Thoracic disc herniation. Re-evaluation of the posterior approach using modified costotransversectomy. Spine 1993;18:1872.
124. Arce CA, Dohrmann GJ. Herniated thoracic disks: symposium on neurosurgery. Neurol Clin 1985;13:383.
125. Bennett MH, McCallum JE. Experimental decompression of the spinal cord. Surg Neurol 1977;8:63.
126. Doppman JL, Girton M. Angiographic study and the effect of laminectomy in the presence of acute anterior epidural masses. J Neurosurg 1976;45:195.
127. Lonstein JE. Patient Evaluation. In JE Lonstein, DS Bradford, RB Winter, JW Ogilvie (eds), Moe's Textbook of Scoliosis and Other Spinal Deformities (3rd ed). Philadelphia: Saunders, 1995;45.
128. Isu T, Chono Y, Iwasaki Y, et al. Scoliosis associated with syringomyelia presenting in children. Childs Nerv Syst 1992;8:97.
129. Isu T, Iwasaki Y, Akino M, Abe H. Hydrosyringomyelia associated with Chiari I malformation in children and adolescents. Neurosurgery 1990;26:591.
130. Depotter J, Rigault P, Pouliquen JC, et al. Syringomyelia and scoliosis in children and adolescents. Rev Chir Orthop 1987;73:203.
131. Huebert HT, Mackinnon WB. Syringomyelia and scoliosis. J Bone Joint Surg Am 1969;51:338.
132. Hugus JJ, Taylor T, McGee-Collett M, et al. Syringomyelia and scoliosis, a new view. J Bone Joint Surg Br 1990;72:1098.
133. Nokes SR, Murtaugh FR, Jones JD, et al. Childhood scoliosis: MR imaging. Pediatr Radiol 1987;164:791.
134. Arai S, Ohtsuka Y, Moriya H, et al. Scoliosis associated with syringomyelia. Spine 1993;18:1591.
135. Mejia EA, Hennrikus WL, Schwend RM, Emans JB. A prospective evaluation of idiopathic left thoracic scoliosis with magnetic resonance imaging. J Pediatr Orthop 1996;16:354.
136. Schwend RM, Hennrikus WL, Hall JE, Emans JB. Childhood scoliosis: clinical indications for magnetic resonance imaging. J Bone Joint Surg Am 1995;77:46.
137. Lewonowski K, King JD, Nelson MD. Routine use of magnetic resonance imaging in idiopathic scoliosis patients less than eleven years of age. Spine 1992;17:S10.
138. Nordvall A, Wikkelson C. A late neurologic complication of scoliosis surgery in connection with syringomyelia. Acta Orthop Scand 1979;50:407.
139. Williams BP. Orthopaedic features in the presentation of syringomyelia. J Bone Joint Surg Br 1979;61:324.
140. An HS, Balderston R. Complications in Scoliosis, Kyphosis, and Spondylolisthesis Surgery. In HS An, RA Balderston (eds), Complications in Spinal Surgery. Philadelphia: Saunders, 1991;5.
141. Been HD, Kalkman CJ, Traast HS, Ongerboer de Visser BW. Neurologic injury after insertion of laminar hooks during Cotrel-Dubousset instrumentation. Spine 1994;19:1402.
142. Byrd JA, Scoles PV, Winter RB, et al. Adult idiopathic scoliosis treated by anterior and posterior spinal fusion. J Bone Joint Surg Am 1987;69:843.
143. Court-Brown CM, Stoll JE, Gertzbein SD. Thoracic facetectomy and bone grafting in the surgical treatment of adult idiopathic scoliosis. Spine 1987;12:992.
144. Goldstein LA. Treatment of idiopathic scoliosis by Harrington instrumentation and fusion with fresh autogenous iliac bone grafts. J Bone Joint Surg Am 1969;51:209.
145. Harrington PR, Dickson JH. An eleven-year clinical investigation of Harrington instrumentation. A preliminary report on 578 cases. Clin Orthop 1973;93:113.
146. Herndon WA, Sullivan JA, Yngve DA, et al. Segmental spinal instrumentation with sublaminar wires. A critical appraisal. J Bone Joint Surg Am 1987;69:851.
147. Kostuik JP, Israel J, Hall JE. Scoliosis surgery in adults. Clin Orthop 1973;226:225.
148. Lonstein JE, Winter RB, Moe JH, et al. Neurologic deficits secondary to spinal deformity: a review of the literature and report of 43 cases. Spine 1980;5:331.
149. Lonstein JE, Akbarnia BA. Operative treatment of spinal deformities in patients with cerebral palsy or mental retardation. J Bone Joint Surg Am 1983;65:43.
150. Lovallo JL, Banta JV, Renshaw TS. Adolescent idiopathic scoliosis treated by Harrington-rod distraction and fusion. J Bone Joint Surg 1986;68A:1326.
151. Luque ER. Segmental spinal instrumentation for correction of scoliosis. Clin Orthop 1982;163:192.
152. Ponder RC, Dickson JH, Harrington PR, et al. Results of Harrington instrumentation and fusion in the adult idiopathic scoliosis patient. J Bone Joint Surg Am 1975;57:797.
153. Sponseller PD, Cohen MS, Nachemson AF, et al. Results of surgical treatment of adults with idiopathic scoliosis. J Bone Joint Surg Am 1987;69:667.
154. Swank S, Lonstein JE, Moe JH, et al. Surgical treatment of adult scoliosis. J Bone Joint Surg Am 1981;63:268.
155. Thompson GH, Wilber RG, Shaffer JW, et al. Segmental spinal instrumentation in idiopathic scoliosis. Spine 1985;10:623.
156. VanDam BE, Bradford DS, Lonstein JE, et al. Adult idiopathic scoliosis treated by posterior spinal fusion and Harrington instrumentation. Spine 1987;12:32.

157. Zindrick MR, Knight GW, Bunch WH, et al. Factors influencing the penetration of wires into the neural canal during segmental wiring. J Bone Joint Surg Am 1989;71:742.
158. MacEwen GD, Bunnell, Siram K. Acute neurologic complications in the treatment of scoliosis. J Bone Joint Surg Am 1975;57:404.
159. Scoliosis Research Society Morbidity and Mortality Committee 1987 report. Park Ridge, IL: American Academy of Orthopaedic Surgeons, 1987.
160. Scoliosis Research Society Morbidity and Mortality Committee 1995 report. Park Ridge, IL: American Academy of Orthopaedic Surgeons, 1995.
161. Johnston CE, Happel LT, Norris R, et al. Delayed paraplegia complicating sublaminar segmental instrumentation. J Bone Joint Surg Am 1986;68:556.
162. Letts RM, Hollinberg C. Delayed paresis following spinal fusion with Harrington instrumentation. Clin Orthop 1977;125:45.
163. Taylor BA, Webb PJ, Hetreed M, et al. Delayed postoperative paraplegia with hypotension in adult revision scoliosis surgery. Spine 1994;19:470.
164. Bell GR, Gurd AR, Orlowski JP, Andrish JT. The syndrome of inappropriate antidiuretic hormone secretion following spinal fusion. J Bone Joint Surg Am 1986;68:720.
165. Brazel PW, McPhee IB. Inappropriate secretion of antidiuretic hormone in postoperative scoliosis patients. The role of fluid management. Spine 1996;21:724.
166. Elster AD. Hyponatremia after spinal fusion caused by inappropriate anti-diuretic hormone (SIADH). Clin Orthop 1985;194:136.
167. Mason RJ, Betz RR, Orlowski JP, Bell GR. The syndrome of inappropriate antidiuretic hormone secretion and its effect on blood indices following spinal fusion. Spine 1989;14:722.
168. Cowley DM, Pabari M, Johnson S, et al. Pathogenesis of postoperative hyponatremia following correction of scoliosis in children. Aust N Z J Surg 1988;58:485.
169. Sterns RH, Riggs JE, Schochet SS. Osmotic demyelination syndrome following correction of hyponatremia. N Engl J Med 1986;314:1536.
170. Watkins RG. Anterior Surgical Approach to the Thoracolumbar, Lumbar, and Lumbosacral Spine. In SW Wiesel, JN Weinstein, H Herkowitz, et al. (eds), The Lumbar Spine (2nd ed). Philadelphia: Saunders,1996;1253.
171. Watkins RG. Anterior lumbar fusion complications. Clin Orthop 1992;284:47.
172. Tiusanen H, Seitsalo S, Osterman K, Soini J. Retrograde ejaculation after anterior interbody lumbar fusion. Eur Spine J 1995;4:339.
173. Faraj AA, Webb JK, Lemberger RJ. Urinary bladder dysfunction following anterior lumbosacral spine fusion: case report and review of the literature. Eur Spine J 1996;5:121.
174. Bell GR. Complications of Lumbar Spine Surgery. In SW Wiesel, JN Weinstein, H Herkowitz, et al. (eds), The Lumbar Spine (2nd ed). Philadelphia: Saunders, 1996;945.
175. Johnson RM, McGuire EJ. Urogenital complications of anterior approaches to the lumbar spine. Clin Orthop 1981;154:114.
176. Sacks S. Anterior interbody fusion of the lumbar spine: indications and results in 200 cases. Clin Orthop 1966;33:163.
177. Sacks S. Anterior interbody fusion of the lumbar spine. J Bone Joint Surg 1965;47B:211.
178. Garfin SR, Glover M, Booth RE, et al. Laminectomy: a review of the Pennsylvania hospial experience. J Spinal Disord 1988;1:116.
179. Rish BL. A critique of the surgical management of lumbar disc disease in a private neurological practice. Spine 1984;9:500.
180. Weir BKA, Jacobs GA. Reoperation rate following lumbar discectomy. An analysis of 662 lumbar discectomies. Spine 1980;5:366.
181. Williams RW. Microlumbar discectomy: a 12-year statistical review. Spine1986;11:851.
182. Herron L. Recurrent lumbar disc herniation: results of repeat laminectomy and discectomy. J Spinal Disord 1994;7:161.
183. McCulloch JA. Complications in Lumbar Microsurgery. In RW Williams, JA McCulloch, PH Young (eds), Microsurgery of the Lumbar Spine. Rockville, MD: Aspen, 1990;159.
184. Hueftle MG, Modic MT, Ross JS, et al. Lumbar spine: postoperative MR imaging with Gd-DTPA. Radiology 1988;167:817.
185. Tullberg T, Grane P, Isacson J. Gadolinium-enhanced magnetic resonance imaging of 36 patients one year after lumbar disc resection. Spine 1994;19:176.
186. Ramirez LF, Thisted R. Complications and demographic characteristics of patients undergoing lumbar discectomy in community hospitals. Neurosurgery 1989;25:226.
187. Nagata H, Schendel MJ, Transfeldt EE, Lewis JL. The effects of long segments of the spine on the adjacent and distal facet force and lumbosacral motion. Spine 1993;18:2471.
188. Brodsky AE. Post-laminectomy and post-fusion stenosis of the lumbar spine. Clin Orthop 1976;115:130.
189. Cochran T, Irstram L, Nachemson A. Long-term anatomic and functional changes in patients with adolescent idiopathic scoliosis treated by Harrington rod fusion. Spine 1983;8:576.
190. Connolly PJ, Von Schroeder HP, Johnson GE, Kostuik JP. Adolescent idiopathic scoliosis. Long term effect of instrumentation extending to the lumbar spine. J Bone Joint Surg Am 1995;77:1210.
191. Frymoyer JW, Hanley EN, Howe J, Kuhlmann D. The long-term effects of spinal fusion on the sacroiliac joints and ilium. Clin Orthop 1978;134:196.
192. Frymoyer JW, Hanley EN, Howe J, et al. A comparison of radiographic findings in fusion and nonfusion patients ten or more years following lumbar disc surgery. Spine 1979;4:435.

193. Ginsburg HH, Goldtein LA, Robinson SC, et al. Back pain in postoperative idiopathic scoliosis. Long-term follow-up study [abstract]. Spine 1979;4:518.
194. Hsu KY, Zucherman JF. The Long Term Effect of Lumbar Spine Fusion: Deterioration of Adjacent Motion Segments. In K Yonenobu, K Ono, Y Takemitsu (eds), Lumbar Spinal Fusion and Stabilization. Berlin: Springer-Verlag, 1993;54.
195. Lee CK, Langrana NA. Lumbosacral spinal fusion. A biomechanical study. Spine 1984;9:574.
196. Lehmann TR, Spratt KF, Tozzi JE, et al. Long-term follow-up of lower lumbar fusion patients. Spine 1987;12:97.
197. Rahm MD, Hall BB. Adjacent-segment degeneration after lumbar fusion with instrumentation: a retrospective study. J Spinal Disord 1996;9:392.
198. Lorenz M, Zindrick M, Schwaegler P, et al. A comparison of single-level fusions with and without hardware. Spine 1991;16:S455.
199. Moskowitz A, Moe JH, Winter RB, Binner H. Long-term follow-up of scoliosis fusion. J Bone Joint Surg Am 1980;62:365.
200. Zdeblick TA. A prospective, randomized study of lumbar fusion. Preliminary results. Spine 1993;18:983.
201. Hedman TP, Kostuik JP, Fernie GR, Hellier WG. Design of an intervertebral disc prosthesis. Spine 1991;16:S86.
202. Kostuik JP. Controversies in Cauda Equina Syndrome and Lumbar Disc Herniation. In SW Wiesel, JN Weinstein, H Herkowitz, et al. (eds), The Lumbar Spine (2nd ed). Philadelphia: Saunders, 1996;582.
203. Kostuik JP, Harrington I, Alexander D, et al. Cauda equina syndrome and lumbar disc herniation. J Bone Joint Surg Am 1986;68:386.
204. McLaren AC, Bailey SI. Cauda equina syndrome: a complication of lumbar discectomy. Clin Orthop 1986;204:143.
205. Ramirez LF, Thisted R. Using a national health care data base to determine surgical complications in community hospitals: lumbar discectomy as an example. Neurosurgery 1989;25:218.
206. Stromqvist B, Jonsson B, Annertz M, Holtas S. Cauda equina syndrome caused by migrating fat graft after lumbar spinal decompression. Spine 1991;16:100.
207. Prusick VR, Lint DS, Bruder WJ. Cauda equina syndrome as a complication of free epidural fat grafting. J Bone Joint Surg Am 1988;70:1256.
208. Spangfort EV. The lumbar disc herniation—a computer aided analysis of 2504 operations. Acta Orthop Scand (Suppl) 1971;1432:52.
209. Mayfield F. Complications of laminectomy. Clin Neurosurg 1975;23:435.
210. Ani N, Keppler L, Biscup RS, Steffee AD. Reduction of high-grade slips (Grades III–V) with VSPTM instrumentation: report of a series of 41 cases. Spine 1991;16:S302.
211. Dick WT, Schnebel B. Severe spondylolisthesis. Reduction and internal fixation. Clin Orthop 1988;232:70.
212. Collazo-Bonilla JA, Bowen JR. Complications in the Management of Spondylolisthesis. In CH Epps, JR Bowen (eds), Complications in Pediatric Orthopaedic Surgery. Philadelphia: Lippincott, 1995;301.
213. Freeman BL, Donati NL. Spinal arthrodesis for severe spondylolisthesis in children and adolescents. A long-term follow-up study. J Bone Joint Surg Am 1989;71:594.
214. Harris IE, Weinstein SL. Long-term follow-up of patients with grade III and IV spondylolisthesis. Treatment with and without fusion. J Bone Joint Surg Am 1987;69:960.
215. Hu SS, Bradford DS, Transfeldt EE, Cohen M. Reduction of high-grade spondylolisthesis using Edwards instrumentation. Spine 1996;21:367.
216. Matthiass HH, Heine J. The surgical reduction of spondylolisthesis. Clin Orthop 1994;203:34.
217. Maurice HD, Morley TR. Cauda equina lesions following fusion in situ and decompressive laminectomy for severe spondylolisthesis. Spine 1989;14:214.
218. O'Brien JP, Mehdian H, Jaffray D. Reduction of severe lumbosacral spondylolisthesis. A report of 22 cases with a 10-year follow-up period. Clin Orthop 1994;300:64.
219. Peek RD, Wiltse LL, Reynolds JB, et al. In situ arthrodesis without decompression for grade III or IV isthmic spondylolisthesis in adults who have severe sciatica. J Bone Joint Surg Am 1989;71:62.
220. Petraco DM, Spivak JM, Cappadona JG, et al. An anatomic evaluation of L5 nerve stretch in spondylolisthesis reduction. Spine 1996;21:1133.
221. Schoenecker PL, Cole HO, Herring JA, et al. Cauda equina syndrome after in situ arthrodesis for severe spondylolisthesis at the lumbosacral junction. J Bone Joint Surg Am 1990;72:164.
222. Transfeldt EE, Dendrinos GK, Bradford DS. Paresis of proximal lumbar roots after reduction of L5-S1 spondylolisthesis. Spine 1989;14:884.
223. Cohen BA, Major MR, Huizenga BA. Pudendal nerve evoked potential monitoring in procedures involving low sacral fixation. Spine 1991;16:S375.
224. Lee CK. Lumbar spinal instability (olisthesis) after extensive posterior spinal decompression. Spine 1983;8:429.
225. Shenkins HA, Hask CJ. Spondylolisthesis after multiple bilateral laminectomies and facetectomies for lumbar spondylosis. Follow-up review. J Neurosurg 1987;67:45.
226. Herkowitz HN, Kurz LT. Degenerative lumbar spondylolisthesis with spinal stenosis: a prospective study comparing decompression and decompression and intertransverse process arthrodesis. J Bone Joint Surg Am 1991;73:802.
227. Castro HM, Halm H, Jerosch J, et al. Accuracy of pedicle screw placement in lumbar vertebrae. Spine 1996;21:1320.
228. Esses SI, Sachs BL, Dreyzin V. Complications associated with the technique of pedicle screw fixation. Spine 1993;18:2231.
229. Gertzbein S, Robbins S. Accuracy of transpedicular screw placement in vivo. Spine 1990;15:11.
230. Marchesi DG, Aebi M. Pedicle devices in the treatment of adult lumbar scoliosis. Spine 1992;17:S304.

231. Matsuzaki H, Tokuhashi Y, Matsumoto F, et al. Problems and solutions of pedicle screw plate fixation of lumbar spine. Spine 1990;15:1159.
232. Weinstein JN, Spratt KF, Spengler D, et al. Spinal pedicle fixation: reliability and validity of roentgenogram-based assessment and surgical factors on successful screw placement. Spine 1988;13:1012.
233. Farber GL, Place HM, Mazur RA, et al. Accuracy of pedicle screw placement in lumbar fusions by plain radiographs and computed tomography. Spine 1995;20:1494.
234. Calancie B, Lebwohl N, Madsen P, Klose KJ. Intraoperative evoked EMG monitoring in an animal model: a new technique for evaluating pedicle screw placement. Spine 1992;17:1229.
235. Cohn BA, Major MR, Huizenga BA. Predictability of adequacy of spinal root decompression using evoked potentials. Spine 1991;16:S379.
236. Darden BV, Wood KE, Hatley MK, et al. Evaluation of pedicle screw insertion monitored by intraoperative evoked electromyography. J Spine Disord 1996;9:8.
237. Calancie B, Madsen P, Lebwohl N. Stimulus-evoked DMG monitoring during transpedicular lumbosacral spine instrumentation. Initial clinical results. Spine 1994;24:2780.
238. Keim HA, Hajdu M, Gonzalez EG, et al. Somatosensory evoked potentials as an aid in the diagnosis and intraoperative management of spinal stenosis. Spine 1985;10:338.
239. Owen JH, Padberg AM, Spahr-Hallond LL, et al. Clinical correlation between degenerative spine disease and dermatomal somatosensory evoked potentials in humans. Spine 1991;16:S201.
240. Owen JH, Kostuik JP, Gornet M, et al. The use of mechanically elicited electromyograms to protect nerve root during surgery for spinal degeneration. Spine 1994;19:1704.
241. Clements DH, Morledge DE, Martin WH, Betz RR. Evoked and spontaneous electromyography to evaluate lumbosacral pedicle screw placement. Spine 1996;21:600.
242. Glassman SD, Dimar JR, Puno RM, et al. A prospective analysis of intraoperative electromyographic monitoring of pedicle screw placement with computed tomographic scan confirmation. Spine 1995;20:1375.
243. Hamill CL, Lenke LG, Bridwell KH, et al. The use of pedicle screw fixation to improve correction in the lumbar spine of patients with idiopathic scoliosis: is it warranted? Spine 1996;21:1241.
244. Lenke LG, Padberg AM, Russo MH, et al. Triggered electromyographic threshold for accuracy of pedicle screw placement: an animal model and clinical correlation. Spine 1995;14:1585.
245. Maguire J, Wallace S, Madiga R, et al. Evaluation of intrapedicular screw position using intraoperative evoked electromyography. Spine 1995;20:1068.
246. Dawson P, Nitescu P, Sjoberg M, et al. Complications of intrathecal opioids and bupivacaine in the treatment of "refractory" cancer pain. Clin J Pain 1995;11:45.
247. Borum SE, McLeskey CH, Williamson JB, et al. Epidural abscess after obstetric epidural analgesia. Anesthesiology 1995;82:1523.
248. Strafford MA, Wilder RT, Berde CB. The risk of infection from epidural analgesia in children: a review of 1620 cases. Anesth Analg 1995;80:234.
249. Rosenfeld JV, Murphy MA, Hellyar AG. Epidural abscess associated with postoperative epidural analgesia. Anaesth Intensive Care 1991;19:569.
250. Mamourian AC, Dickman CA, Drayer BP, Sonntag VA. Spinal epidural abscess: three cases following spinal epidural injection demonstrated with magnetic resonance imaging. Anesthesiology 1993;78:204.
251. Curling OD, Gower DJ, McWhorter JM. Changing concepts in spinal epidural abscess: a report of 29 cases. Neurosurgery 1990;27:185.
252. Hlavin ML, Kaminski HJ, Ross JS, Ganz E. Spinal epidural abscess: a ten-year perspective. Neurosurgery 1990;27:177.
253. Koppel BS, Tuchman AJ, Mangiardi JR, et al. Epidural spinal infection in intravenous drug abusers. Arch Neurol 1988;45:1331.
254. Baker AS, Ojemann RG, Swartz MN, Richardson EP. Spinal epidural abscess. N Engl J Med 1975;293:463.
255. Nussbaum ES, Rigamonti D, Standiford H, et al. Spinal epidural abscess: a report of 40 cases and review. Surg Neurol 1992;38:225.
256. Lee HJ, Bach JR, White RE. Spinal epidural abscess complicating vertebral osteomyelitis: an insidious cause of deteriorating spinal cord function. J Am Para Soc 1992;15:18.
257. Leim LK, Rigamonti D, Wolf AL, et al. Thoracic epidural abscess. J Spinal Disord 1994;7:449.
258. Rea GL, McGregor JM, Miller CA, Miner ME. Surgical treatment of the spontaneous spinal epidural abscess. Surg Neurol 1992;37:274.
259. Ericsson M, Algers G, Schlimser SE. Spinal epidural abscess in adults: review and report of iatrogenic cases. Scand J Infect Dis 1990;22:249.
260. Hitchon PW, Osenbach RK, Yuh WTC, et al. Spinal infections. Clin Neurosurg 1992;38:373.
261. Osenbach RK, Hitchon PW, Menezes AH. Diagnosis and management of pyogenic vertebral osteomyelitis in adults. Surg Neurol 1990;33:266.
262. Wheeler D, Keiser P, Rigamonti D, Keay S. Medical management of spinal epidural abscesses: case report and review. Clin Infect Dis 1992;15:22.
263. Jonsson B, Soderholm R, Stromqvist B. Erythrocyte sedimentation rate after lumbar spine surgery. Spine 1991;16:1049.

Chapter 8

Neurologic Complications of Spinal Manipulation

Rajesh K. Bindal and Paul B. Nelson

Objectives

- To understand spinal manipulation and what it involves
- To review the literature on benefits of spinal manipulation and identify patients who might benefit the most
- To identify major and minor complications of cervical spinal manipulation and the estimated incidence
- To understand the pathogenesis, incidence, and sequelae of vertebral artery dissection
- To identify major and minor complications of lumbar spinal manipulation and the estimated incidence
- To identify "red flags" to alert practitioners to patients who might benefit from additional workup before receiving spinal manipulation

Low back and neck pain are among the most commonly encountered ailments in modern clinical practice, accounting for up to 4.5% of all physicians' office visits.[1] The estimated cost to society is from $8–16 billion annually in lost productivity and treatment.[2] Spinal manipulation is among the most common conservative treatments for low back and neck pain, and it is estimated that chiropractors treat 25% of all patients with low back pain.[3] Up to 75 million spinal manipulations are performed annually in North America, and approximately 5% of the population will visit a chiropractor in a given year.[4]

There is no standard definition of spinal manipulation therapy (SMT) or its techniques. There are, however, two main classifications of SMT: long-lever, low-velocity manipulation and short-lever, high-velocity manipulation.[5] Long-lever manipulation is also referred to as nonspecific manipulation and involves use of one of the long bones of the limb to amplify the load applied by the hands to one or more of the spinal joints. Short-lever manipulation, or specific manipulation, uses a short, forceful thrust on a specific vertebral transverse process, moving only a specific joint. Of these two main types of SMT, physical therapists and osteopaths most often use long-lever manipulation, whereas chiropractors are more likely to use short-lever manipulation.

Indications and Results of Spinal Manipulation

Meta-Analysis of the Literature

Despite the relatively common use of SMT in Western society for the treatment of back and neck pain, there are few high-quality blinded randomized trials to definitively determine indications and efficacy. Shekelle et al. in 1992 performed a detailed and thorough review and meta-analysis of 25 randomized trials of SMT compared with standard alternative therapy for low back pain.[6] This review is probably the highest regarded and most often quoted study on this subject. Subjects were subdivided into studies on patients with acute back pain without sciatica, those with chronic back pain, and those with back pain and sciatic nerve root irritation.

Shekelle et al. analyzed nine studies that examined patients with acute back pain, generally defined as 3 weeks or less in duration. The two studies with the highest quality scores both showed statistically significant improvement with SMT. Further detailed analysis of the components of the outcome indices were not given. The remaining seven trials did give more details. These seven trials were included in a meta-analysis. This analysis showed that at 2–3 weeks after the start of treatment, SMT resulted in a 0.17 increase in probability of improvement. Clinically, this means that if 50% of patients improve with non-SMT conservative treatment, which is roughly accurate, then 67% of patients treated with SMT will recover. Of interest, all nine of these studies indicated that the beneficial effects of SMT disappeared within a few weeks to months.

Shekelle et al. also reviewed five studies examining patients with chronic back pain, generally defined as 13 weeks or longer. Of these studies only two had data that could be evaluated in a meaningful way. One showed a benefit and one did not. Three trials evaluated patients with low back pain and sciatic nerve root irritation. Meta-analysis indicated that there was a 0.098 increase in probability of improvement with SMT compared with other treatments, which was not significant.

The highest quality study as rated by Shekelle et al. evaluated 741 patients with acute and chronic back pain without radicular symptoms who were randomized to receive either chiropractic or hospital-based treatments, which were at the discretion of the individual practitioner. Chiropractors were allowed to give a maximum of 10 treatments in the first year. This trial showed a statistically significant improvement in outcome with SMT even at 2 years after initiation of treatment with chiropractic treatment. Interestingly, this benefit was greatest in those patients with chronic or more severe pain.

Other Studies

In a more recent study 256 randomized patients with back, neck, or both kinds of pain of at least 6 weeks' duration were divided into four treatment groups: SMT, physiotherapy, treatment by general practitioners, and placebo.[7] Patients treated by general practitioners consisted of medication, advice about posture, home exercises, and rest. All treatments could last no longer than 3 months. When the SMT and physiotherapy groups were compared, patients in the SMT group had a statistically significant improvement in their main complaint as determined by a blinded research assistant. This benefit was present even after 12 months follow-up. There was a trend toward greater improvement in physical functioning with SMT, although this was not significant. When patients were questioned about their perceived benefit from treatment, however, there was no difference between SMT and physiotherapy at 12 months follow-up.

The methodology and quality of existing studies has been examined by other authors. In their meta-analysis, Shekelle et al. stratified and graded the studies using a quality score.[6] The score of SMT trials ranged from 22 to 62 out of a possible 100, indicating that the quality of studies was varied and often poor. Koes et al. reviewed the literature and concluded that most studies showed major methodologic flaws.[8] They thought that future studies should pay more attention to methodological quality.

Few studies have examined the efficacy of SMT specifically for neck pain. These studies are of poor quality and the results are mixed.[2] Thus, the efficacy of cervical manipulation has not been clearly defined.

Guidelines

The general consensus is that SMT appears to have some value in the treatment of acute low back pain, generally defined as back pain of less than 3 weeks' duration. There may also be some benefit for more chronic low back pain, although additional studies are required to prove this. The U.S. Department of Health and Human Services has issued guidelines on the management of acute low back pain in adults based on current evidence.[9] These guidelines recommend that manipulation may be of benefit in patients with acute low back pain of less than 4 weeks' duration without radiculopathy. With progressive or severe neurologic symptoms, appropriate diagnostic studies should be performed to rule out serious conditions before manipulation. Efficacy in patients with radiculopathy is unproven. A trial of manipulation with pain of more than 4 weeks' duration is probably safe but of unproven benefit. Finally, they recommended that if manipulation does not result in benefit after 1 month of treatment, treatments should be stopped and the patient reevaluated. More data are required to determine which patients, if any, with chronic pain are likely to benefit from SMT.

Complications of Cervical Manipulation

Cervical manipulation has been associated with the greatest number and most serious complications of SMT.[10] By far the most publicized complication is that of stroke. We review the incidence and pathogenesis of stroke in these patients and also review the many other less commonly associated complications.

Vertebrobasilar Territory Infarction

In 1947, Pratt-Thomas and Berger reported a case of vertebrobasilar stroke after chiropractic manipulation of the neck.[11] Since then, hundreds of similar cases have been reported.[12, 13] The incidence of stroke after cervical manipulation is not definitively known. Numerous studies have indirectly attempted to determine this risk, and most of them indicate an incidence of 1–3 per million manipulations, with patients often receiving 10–15 manipulations during treatment. Dvorak and Orelli conducted a mail survey among members of the Swiss Society for Manual Medicine.[14] The results of this survey indicated that slight neurologic complications occurred at a rate of 1 per 40,000 manipulations and serious complications occurred in 1 of 400,000 procedures. In a study of Australian chiropractors, it was estimated that approximately 5 in 100,000 patients receiving neck manipulation suffered stroke.[15] A major problem with estimating the incidence of vertebrobasilar territory distribution infarction after manipulation is that of underreporting. It is likely that the true incidence of the complication is higher than that discernible through literature reviews and surveys because a certain number of cases will simply not be reported.[16] Thus, the true incidence of stroke is likely to be higher than that estimated by some authors. The actual figure cannot be known without prospective studies with intensive follow-up.

The pathogenesis of vertebrobasilar infarction after cervical manipulation has not been fully elucidated, although various theories have been proposed. Simple head turning can be associated with a decrease in flow or occlusion of vertebral artery flow. Toole and Tucker examined the influence of head position on extracranial cerebral artery flow in 20 cadavers.[17] They found that turning the head in a certain manner resulted in cessation of flow through a single vertebral artery in 35% of cases, both vertebral arteries but not simultaneously in 25% of cases, and simultaneous bilateral occlusion in 30% of cases. Temporary flow blockage in the carotid ipsilateral to the side of rotation was noted in one carotid in 40% of cases and bilaterally but not simultaneously in 45% of cases. Extension and rotation can occlude the vertebral artery contralateral to the side of rotation in 5 of 41 cadavers.[18] This number increased to 18 of 41 with the use of traction. The site of occlusion is thought to be at the atlantoaxial joint where the artery changes from its vertical course to a horizontal one, because this is also the site of greatest total rotation in the neck.

Infarction is associated with arterial dissection in 82% of cases.[19] Simple occlusion with head turning is unlikely to directly cause arterial dissection. There are few autopsy data on victims of this complication, but a few reports do exist, allowing theories on pathogenesis. The most commonly accepted mechanism of vertebral artery dissection from spinal manipulation involves a series of events. It begins with injury to the tunica intima or media of a vertebral artery. This is thought to most likely occur at or around C1–C2. Evidence of injury in this region was found in 89% of cases in which lesion site was reported in one review.[19] This can occur subclinically with repeated manipulations. Resulting granulation tissue can predispose a patient to acute intramural hematoma with continued manipulations.[20] Another report details an interesting case in which a patient sought chiropractic manipulation for neck pain that in retrospect was thought to have been from an early dissection without neurologic deficits.[21] Immediately after manipulation, the patient progressed to a fatal vertebrobasilar dissection. Autopsy demonstrated both a new dissection and an old one dating to the onset of pain. Reports also indicate that patients often experience a transient prodrome of neurologic symptoms while receiving their manipulations, before developing a stroke.[22] It has been suggested that patients experiencing transient symptoms during cervical manipulation should not undergo further manipulations.

Vertebral artery dissection can result in wide variety of symptoms.[23] Symptoms generally result from infarction of the brain in the distribution of the posterior circulation, generally the vertebral and basilar arteries and their branches. The most common consequence is infarction of the lateral medulla. This can result in loss of pain and temperature sensation in the face and body; Horner's syndrome (miosis, ptosis, and decreased sweating); vertigo; nystagmus; nausea and vomiting; ataxia; and dysfunction of the ninth and tenth cranial nerves, resulting in hoarseness, dysphagia, and paralysis of one side of the vocal cords and palate. Infarction of the brain stem and cerebellum in other locations can also develop. In addition to the previously mentioned symptoms, patients can present with loss of light touch and proprioception and weakness. Occipital lobe infarctions can result in visual impairments. Infarction of the cerebellum can result in significant posterior fossa swelling and herniation, leading to death.

Sequelae of Strokes After Cervical Manipulation

In a survey of California neurologists, 42% of patients had moderate or severe residual deficits and 2% died.[13] Only 14% had no permanent deficits. In a review of the literature, of 159 patients whose outcomes were known, 29 died and 86 had residual handicap.[24] Clinical syndromes in another study included occipital lobe in 5%, cerebellar in 8%, "locked-in" in syndrome 8%, Wallenberg's syndrome in 28%, other brain stem with or without cerebellar signs in 49%, and unclassifiable in 2%.[19]

Other Complications of Cervical Manipulation

A variety of other complications have also been reported after cervical manipulations. The incidence of these complications is likely to be much rarer than that of stroke because significantly fewer cases have been reported. Numerous cases of atlantoaxial dislocation have been reported as early as 1925.[25] Cervical internal carotid artery aneurysms have also been reported following neck manipulation, as have anterior circulation infarcts.[26] Five percent of all strokes after cervical manipulation occur in the carotid distribution.[13] Additionally, patients have been reported to develop either herniated cervical disks or marked cervical myelopathy from a herniation that may already have been present.[27] Two cases of cervical epidural hematomas have been reported, both requiring surgical evacuation.[28, 29] A case of long thoracic nerve palsy has also been reported.[30] Cadaveric studies have demonstrated that by flexing and turning the head to the opposite side and raising the ipsilateral arm, the length of the nerve between its points of fixation can be doubled, resulting in injury. Finally, unilateral and bilateral phrenic nerve palsies have also been reported by a number of authors.[31, 32]

Cervical manipulation can be associated with a number of severe complications. Some of these complications are life threatening or can result in permanent neurologic sequelae. Practitioners should inform patients of the risks involved before receiving manipulation. Further studies are needed to fully define the role of cervical manipulation in treating neck pain.

Complications of Lumbar Manipulation

Cauda Equina Syndrome

The most important complication of spinal manipulation for back pain is the cauda equina syndrome.[33–36] Cauda equina syndrome is a feared complication of lumbar disk herniation that can result in permanent bowel and bladder incontinence, lower extremity weakness, numbness, and pain.[37] In a review of the literature, Assendeltf et al. found 56 cases in which spinal manipulation resulted in exacerbation of a disk herniation, 82% of which concerned progression to cauda equina symptoms.[24] Of the 39 cases with known sequelae, 54% had residual handicaps. Interestingly, half of

Table 8.1. Red Flags for Spinal Manipulation

Signs and Symptoms	Possible Underlying Pathology
Severe leg or arm pain	Severe nerve root compression
Myelopathy	Cervical or thoracic spinal cord compression
Bowel and bladder dysfunction	Cauda equina syndrome
Back pain associated with fever	Spinal epidural abscess
Back pain associated with severe spasms	Diskitis
Back pain associated with weight loss and fatigue	Metastatic cancer or multiple myeloma
Back pain in a child	Underlying tumor or developmental abnormality
Back pain with weakness and numbness	Spinal cord or cauda equina lesion
Back pain after trauma	Fracture or dislocation
Back pain in an osteopenic patient	Compression fracture
Night pain	Spinal tumors

the cases reported occurred during manipulation under anesthesia, a practice that has since been abandoned. Haldeman and Rubinstein reported three cases and reviewed the literature.[34] They believed the incidence of this complication was "one in many million treatments." Shekelle estimated the risk at 1 per 100 million manipulations from an extensive literature review.[5] Thus, the incidence of cauda equina syndrome with manipulation of the back, although small, should not be ignored.

Other Complications of Lumbar Manipulation

Other complications have been reported related to manipulation for back pain. Livingston in 1971 reported that 12 of 172 patients receiving spinal manipulation had suffered an injury.[4] The definition of injury in this study was broad. Reported injuries ranged from minor soft-tissue trauma, delay in diagnosis of a medical disorder, serious neurologic injury, and treatment of conditions that could not possibly benefit from manipulation. Two patients had exacerbations of radicular symptoms, and another patient with undiagnosed thoracic spine involvement by multiple myeloma developed significantly worsened myelopathy.

Other serious complications have also been reported. Most of these complications are extremely rare. A few cases of spinal compression fractures have been reported that may be related to spinal manipulation, especially in patients with neoplastic disease of the spine and osteoporosis. However, such cases are rare. In a 1991 review, Haldeman and Rubinstein presented four cases involving litigation in which chiropractic manipulation was believed to result in compression fractures in patients with osteoporosis.[38, 39] The authors thought only one case had merit, and in a review of the literature found only two additional cases reported, both in patients with neoplastic disease of the spine. A case of lumbar artery aneurysm with acute aortic occlusion has also been reported to have occurred after chiropractic manipulation.[40] Although these complications are all rare, they highlight that both the practitioner and patient must be aware that a variety of complications can occur.

Red Flags

There are a number of red flags that may indicate a serious underlying spinal problem in which SMT may be contraindicated. Some of these signs and symptoms and the underlying problem they may be manifestations of are presented in Table 8.1. These red flags in most cases should be evaluated further before starting SMT.

Conclusion

A significant percentage of the population of Western countries seek spinal manipulation at some point in their lives for treatment of back and neck pain. Except for acute low back pain, the efficacy of these treatments is not fully defined. Although numerous studies have been conducted on this topic, few of these studies are of good quality. Although the efficacy of spinal manipulation is not clear, a small but measurable percentage of patients undergoing spinal manipulation develop complications. In particular, cervical manipulation is most often associated with vertebral artery dissection, whereas lumbar manipulation is most often associated with cauda equina syndrome. Physicians and chiropractors should be aware of signs and symptoms associated with neck or back pain that can suggest more serious disease entities and deserve further evaluation.

References

1. Hart GL, Deyo RA, Cherkin DC. Physician office visits for low back pain: frequency, clinical evaluation and treatment patterns from a US national survey. Spine 1995;20:11.
2. Powell FC, Hanigan WC, Olivero WC. A risk/benefit analysis of spinal manipulation therapy for relief of lumbar or cervical pain. Neurosurgery 1993;33:73.
3. Carey TS, Evans A, Hadler N, et al. Care-seeking among individuals with chronic low back pain. Spine 1995;20:312.
4. Livingston MCP. Spinal manipulation causing injury: a three year study. Clin Orthop 1971;81:82.
5. Shekelle PG. Spine update: spinal manipulation. Spine 1994;19:858.
6. Shekelle PG, Adams AH, Chassin MR, et al. Spinal manipulation for low back pain. Ann Intern Med 1992;117:590.
7. Koes BW, Bouter LM, van Mameren H, et al. Randomized clinical trial of manipulative therapy and physiotherapy for persistent back and neck complaints: results of one year follow-up. BMJ 1992;304:601.
8. Koes BW, Assendelft WJJ, van der Heijden GJMG, et al. Spinal manipulation and mobilisation for back and neck pain: a blinded review. BMJ 1991;303:1298.
9. United States Department of Health and Human Services. Acute Low Back Problems in Adults. Clinical Practice Guideline, Quick Reference Guide Number 14. Rockville, MD: AHCPR Pub. No. 95-0643, December 1994;41.
10. Hosek RS, Schram SB, Verman HS, et al. Cervical manipulation. JAMA 1981;245:922.
11. Pratt-Thomas HR, Berger KE. Cerebellar and spinal injuries after chiropractic manipulation. JAMA 1947;133:600.
12. Biller J, Hingtgen WL, Adams HP, et al. Cervicocephalic arterial dissections: a ten-year experience. Arch Neurol 1986;43:1234.
13. Lee KP, Carlini WG, McCormick GF, et al. Neurologic complications following chiropractic manipulation: a survey of California neurologists. Neurology 1995;45:1213.
14. Dvorak J, Orelli F. How dangerous is manipulation to the cervical spine? J Manual Med 1985;2:1.
15. Haynes MJ. Stroke following cervical manipulation in Perth. Chiropractic J Aust 1994;24:42.
16. Haman G, Felber S, Haass A, et al. Cervicocephalic artery dissections due to chiropractic manipulations. Lancet 1993;341:764.
17. Toole JF, Tucker SH. Influence of head position upon cerebral circulation. Arch Neurol 1960;2:616.
18. Brown BSJ, Tatlow WFT. Radiographic studies of the vertebral arteries in cadavers: effects of position and traction of the head. Radiology 1963;81:80.
19. Frisoni GB, Anzola GP. Vertobrobasilar ischemia after neck motion. Stroke 1991;22:1452.
20. Sherman MR, Smialek JE, Zane WE. Pathogenesis of vertebral artery occlusion following cervical spine manipulation. Arch Pathol Lab Med 1987;111:851.
21. Mas JL, Henin D, Bousser MG, et al. Dissecting aneurysm of the vertebral artery and cervical manipulation: a case report with autopsy. Neurology 1989;39:512.
22. North CM. Vertebral artery injuries following chiropractic cervical spine manipulation: case reports. Angiology 1990;41:445.
23. Adams RD, Victor M. Principles of Neurology. New York: McGraw-Hill, 1993;688.
24. Assendelft WJ, Bouter LM, Knipschild PG. Complications of spinal manipulation: a comprehensive review of the literature. J Fam Pract 1996;42:475.
25. Blaine ES. Manipulative (chiropractic) dislocations of the atlas. JAMA 1925;85:1356.
26. Murthy JM, Naidu KV. Aneurysm of the cervical internal carotid artery following chiropractic manipulation. J Neurol Neurosurg Psychiatry 1988;51:1237.
27. Destee A, Lesoin F, Paola FD, et al. Intradural herniated cervical disc associated with chiropractic spinal manipulation. 1989;52:1113.
28. Segal DH, Lidov MW, Camins MB. Cervical epidural hematoma after chiropractic manipulation in a healthy young woman: case report. Neurosurgery 1996;39:1043.
29. Zupruk GM, Mehta Z. Brown-Séquard syndrome associated with posttraumatic cervical epidural hematoma: case report and review of the literature. Neurosurgery 1989;25:278.
30. Oware A, Herskovitz S, Berger AR. Long thoracic nerve palsy following cervical chiropractic manipulation. Muscle Nerve 1995;18:1351.
31. Pandit A, Kalra S, Woodcock A. An unusual case of bilateral diaphragmatic paralysis. Thorax 1992;47:201.
32. Sivakumaran P, Wilson M. Diaphragmatic palsy and chiropractic manipulation. N Z Med J 1995;108:279.
33. Gallinaro P, Cartesegna M. Three cases of lumbar disc rupture and one of cauda equina associated with spinal manipulation (chiropraxis). Lancet 1983;11:411.
34. Haldeman S, Rubinstein SM. Cauda equina syndrome

in patients undergoing manipulation of the lumbar spine. Spine 1992;17:1469.
35. Ryan MD. Massive disc sequestration after spinal manipulation. Med J Aust 1993;158:718.
36. Slater RN, Spencer JD. Central lumbar disc prolapse following spinal manipulation: a call for audit of "alternative practice." J R Soc Med 1993;86:637.
37. Shapiro S. Cauda equina syndrome secondary to lumbar disc herniation. Neurosurgery 1993;32:743.
38. Haldeman S, Rubinstein SM. Compression fractures in patients undergoing spinal manipulative therapy. J Manipulative Physiol Ther 1992;15:450.
39. Plaugher G. Compression fractures in patients undergoing spinal manipulative therapy. J Manipulative Physiol Ther 1992;15:450.
40. Kornberg E. Lumbar artery aneurysm with acute aortic occlusion resulting from chiropractic manipulation: a case report. Surgery 1988;103:122.

Chapter 9

Postoperative Infectious Complications in Neurosurgical Patients

Karen L. Roos

Objectives

- To recognize that the risk of infection in nonimplant neurosurgical procedures can be reduced by the use of perioperative prophylactic antimicrobial therapy
- To understand that the majority of cerebrospinal fluid (CSF) shunt infections are due to intraoperative wound and shunt component contamination from organisms on the patient's skin at the time of the procedure
- To increase familiarity with the antibiotics that are recommended for intraventricular use and their adverse effects
- To recognize that the prolonged preoperative use of broad-spectrum antibiotics, corticosteroid therapy, or both predispose neurosurgical patients to central nervous system (CNS) fungal infections
- To appreciate the risk of surgical instruments and human tissue and tissue products in the transmission of Creutzfeldt-Jakob disease (CJD)

The postneurosurgical patient who has undergone a clean nonimplant procedure is at risk for any of a number of infectious complications, including superficial and deep incisional wound infections, meningitis, osteomyelitis, subdural or epidural empyema, and stitch abscess.[1] The most common bacteria causing infection in these patients are the staphylococci and gram-negative bacilli. Postneurosurgical patients who have had an insertion of a ventriculoperitoneal shunt, an externalized device (i.e., externalized ventriculostomy or intracranial pressure monitor), or an implanted CSF reservoir have a greater risk of infection than postneurosurgical patients who have undergone a nonimplant procedure, and they are considered separately.[2] The increasing number of immunosuppressed patients has led to an increase in fungal infections in postneurosurgical patients. Perhaps the most dreaded infectious complication of a neurosurgical procedure is CJD, which has been reported following the placement of cadaveric dural grafts, corneal transplantation, and native human growth hormone therapy and from contaminated stereotactic electroencephalographic electrodes. The risk of iatrogenic CJD is reviewed. Postneurosurgical patients are also at risk of sepsis, pneumonia, urinary tract infections, and infections secondary to intravenous catheters.

Postoperative Meningitis

The risk of postoperative meningitis in a patient who has undergone a clean nonimplant neurosurgical procedure where perioperative prophylactic antibiotics have been used is low, in the range of 0.5–0.7%. The majority of cases of meningitis are caused by *Staphylococcus aureus*, coagulase-negative staphylococci, aerobic gram-negative bacilli, and streptococci.[3] Contamination of the operative area at the time of surgery is the most likely source of infection.[2] The risk of postoperative meningitis is slightly higher in clean, contaminated neurosurgical operations, which are those procedures that traverse an area of bacterial colonization, such as the frontal, sphenoidal, or mastoid air sinuses (e.g., a transsphenoidal approach to the pituitary fossa), the nasopharynx, or oropharynx.[2, 3] The causative organisms of meningitis in these patients include not only the staphylococci, but also a mixture of aerobic and anaerobic bacteria. The rate of postoperative meningitis is recorded to be 0.4–2.0% in clean, contaminated neurosurgical operations.[2]

The diagnosis of postoperative meningitis may be difficult and is confounded by the clinical difficulty in interpreting an altered level of consciousness in a patient who has undergone a neurosurgical procedure and is being treated with CNS depressant agents and in distinguishing this from an aseptic or chemical meningitis syndrome. The latter was initially termed the *posterior fossa syndrome*, but although it appears with greatest frequency after posterior fossa operations, it may occur after any intracranial operation, and the preferred term is *aseptic meningitis syndrome*. This syndrome is characterized by spiking fever, which may continue for many days or even weeks, and meningismus. Examination of the CSF reveals a pleocytosis that is typically of mononuclear cells, hypoglycorrhachia, and an increased protein concentration. CSF Gram's stain and culture results are negative. Patients receive no clinical benefit from the administration of antibiotics but do respond to large doses of corticosteroids.[4, 5] The proposed etiology is a chemical irritation of the meninges caused by the breakdown of blood introduced into the subarachnoid space during surgery, and corticosteroids are beneficial because they reduce meningeal inflammation.[2] In general, patients with aseptic meningitis syndrome do not appear as critically ill as patients with bacterial meningitis; specifically, the degree of alteration in the level of consciousness is mild, and there are no new or increased focal neurologic deficits.[4, 5] The diagnosis of bacterial meningitis should be considered in any neurosurgical patient who is febrile and who has a deterioration in the level of consciousness or evidence of new focal neurologic deficits. The definitive diagnosis of bacterial meningitis is based on the detection of bacteria, either by Gram's stain or in culture. Patients with bacterial meningitis have a predominance of polymorphonuclear leukocytes in CSF, and a decreased glucose concentration. The latex agglutination test and the limulus amebocyte lysate test are useful in making a rapid diagnosis of bacterial meningitis. The latex agglutination test detects bacterial antigens of group B *Streptococcus*, *Haemophilus influenzae* type b, *Streptococcus pneumoniae,* and *Neisseria meningitidis*. The limulus amebocyte lysate test detects gram-negative endotoxin in CSF.

Empiric therapy for postoperative meningitis should include a combination of vancomycin and a third-generation cephalosporin. Cefotaxime, ceftriaxone, and ceftazidime penetrate well into inflamed CSF and are highly active against gram-negative enteric bacilli with the exception of *Pseudomonas aeruginosa*. Ceftazidime is the only third-generation cephalosporin that is active against this organism in the CNS and is presently the recommended third-generation cephalosporin when infection with this organism is a possibility. An alternative choice is cefepime, a fourth-generation cephalosporin that has activity similar to that of ceftazidime against *P. aeruginosa* but has better in vitro activity than ceftazidime against *S. pneumoniae*. Table 9.1 lists the recommended antimicrobial agent to use when the etiologic organism has been identified.

General consensus favors antimicrobial prophylaxis in clean, nonimplant surgical procedures and clean, contaminated procedures (Table 9.2). Controversy exists as to the choice of antibiotic and the number of doses required for optimal prophylaxis. The choice of antibiotic for prophylaxis is left to the individual neurosurgeon and should be based on the incidence of methicillin-sensitive and methicillin-resistant staphylococci as well as the antimicrobial resistance patterns of gram-negative bacilli at the neurosurgeon's institution. A dose of antimicrobial therapy should be administered by the intravenous route at induction of anesthesia, and patients should receive intraoperative doses at 3-hour intervals throughout the procedure.[3] The decrease in the incidence of wound infections over the last 30 years has been attributed to present aseptic techniques that include perioperative parenteral antimicrobial prophylaxis, preparation of the field with povidone-iodine soap and solution, the use of adhesive plastic

Table 9.1. Antimicrobial Therapy in Neurosurgical Patients

Organism	Antibiotic	Dosage
Staphylococci		
Methicillin-sensitive	Nafcillin	Adult: 9–12 g/day in divided doses q4h; child: 200–300 mg/kg/day in divided doses q4h
Methicillin-resistant	Vancomycin	Parenteral: adult: 1 g q12h; child: 40 mg/kg/day. Intraventricular or intrathecal: adult: 20 mg qd; child: 10 mg qd
Gram-negative bacilli		
Escherichia coli	Cefotaxime	Adult: 8–12 g/day in divided doses q6h; child: 200 mg/kg/day in divided doses q6h
	Ceftriaxone	Adult: 2 g q12h; child: 80–100 mg/kg/day in divided doses q12h
Klebsiella sp.	Same as *E. coli*	
Pseudomonas sp.	Ceftazidime	Adult: 2 g q8h; child: 125–150 mg/kg/day in divided doses q8h
	Cefepime	2 g q12h
Streptococcus pneumoniae	Cefotaxime or ceftriaxone	Add vancomycin if cephalosporin resistance is a possibility (vancomycin: adult: 1 g q12h; child: 40 mg/kg/day)
Cryptococcus neoformans	Amphotericin B	0.5 mg/kg/day IV
	Flucytosine	25 mg qid PO
Coccidioides immitis	Amphotericin B	0.60–0.75 mg/kg/day IV
		0.5–1.0 mg/day 3 times per week (intrathecal)
Aspergillus sp.	Amphotericin B	0.8–1.0 mg/kg/day IV
	Flucytosine	25 mg qid PO
Candida sp.	Amphotericin B	0.5–0.7 mg/kg/day IV
	Flucytosine	25 mg qid PO

Sources: Adapted from KL Roos, AR Tunkel, WM Scheld. Acute Bacterial Meningitis in Children and Adults. In WM Scheld, RJ Whitley, DT Durack (eds), Infections of the Central Nervous System (2nd ed). Philadelphia: Lippincott–Raven, 1997;335; and L Christin, AM Sugar. Fungal Infections. In KL Roos (ed), Central Nervous System Infectious Diseases and Therapy. New York: Marcel Dekker, 1997;167.

drapes, double-gloving, and the irrigation of the surgical wound with saline and topical antibiotics.[6]

Cerebrospinal Fluid Leak

A CSF leak can develop in any instance where a fracture of the skull base is associated with a laceration of the dura and the formation of a fistula that allows for the exit of CSF and the entry of bacteria.[2] The most common etiology of a CSF leak is a basilar skull fracture from head trauma, but a CSF leak may also develop as a complication of a neurosurgical procedure (e.g., transsphenoidal resection of a pituitary tumor).[7] A fracture of the bone of the anterior fossa, the cribriform plate, may result in leakage of CSF into the nose or pharynx (rhinorrhea). Fracture of the bone in the middle or posterior fossa may result in leakage of CSF into the auditory canal (otorrhea).[2] A CSF leak can present immediately after a fracture of the bone or weeks to years later. The presence of a CSF leak greatly increases the risk of meningitis because it

Table 9.2. Efficacy of Prophylactic Antibiotics in Neurosurgical Procedures

Procedure	Efficacy
Clean, nonimplant procedure	Proven
Ventriculoperitoneal shunt	Unproven
Ventriculostomy	Unproven

allows for the ingress of micro-organisms into the subarachnoid space. The most common organisms causing meningitis in patients with CSF leaks complicating neurosurgical procedures are gram-negative bacilli and staphylococci. The presence of a CSF leak can be documented by injecting indium radionuclide intrathecally by a lumbar puncture and then determining the radioactivity count in cotton pledgets that have been placed in the nasopharynx.[8] Surgical exploration with dural closure is often required to repair the leak. Empiric antimicrobial therapy should include a combination of a third- or fourth-generation cephalosporin with vancomycin.

Craniotomy Flap Infection

Craniotomy bone flaps may become infected. An increased risk of infection is associated with reopening surgical wounds, prior irradiation of the scalp, the presence of a drain or foreign body, and immunosuppression. Local signs of bone flap infection include pain and tenderness, edema, erythema, and drainage of serous or purulent material. Fever may not be present. *S. aureus* is the most common infecting organism, but coagulase-negative staphylococci, *Streptococcus* spp., and gram-negative bacilli are also causative organisms of bone flap infections. The identification of a flap infection necessitates opening the wound with removal of all purulent material followed by mechanical debridement and irrigation. Systemic antimicrobial therapy is initiated with a third- or fourth-generation cephalosporin plus vancomycin. The infected bone flap is either removed and a subsequent cranioplasty planned for later on, or the closed irrigation-suction procedure introduced by Erickson et al. that uses a continuous infusion of a saline-antibiotic mixture at the site of infection combined with systemic antimicrobial therapy can be used to salvage the bone flap.[9, 10]

Osteomyelitis of the Skull

Osteomyelitis of the skull may develop as a complication of craniotomy wound infections. *S. aureus* and coagulase-negative staphylococci are the most common pathogens in osteomyelitis of the skull. The clinical signs of osteomyelitis are pain, low-grade fever, swelling, and erythema. The erythrocyte sedimentation rate, white blood cell count, or both may be elevated. Radionuclide bone scan, gallium scan, computed tomographic, and magnetic resonance imaging scans are the recommended imaging studies to confirm or localize the infection. Microbiologic diagnosis is made by aerobic and anaerobic culture of bone or biopsy specimen obtained from the site of infection. Treatment of osteomyelitis of the skull requires complete surgical debridement of necrotic bone and soft tissue in addition to at least 2 weeks of intravenous antimicrobial therapy, followed by 6–12 weeks of oral antimicrobial therapy.[9, 11] Sequestered dead bone may serve as a focus for persistent infection.[11]

Abscess and Empyema

Subdural or epidural abscess or empyema may develop as a postoperative infection. Subdural empyemas can result from direct infection of the subdural space during a neurosurgical procedure, such as drainage of a subdural hematoma. The staphylococci and aerobic microaerophilic streptococci are the causative organisms in the majority of cases of subdural empyema. An epidural abscess may develop as a complication of a craniotomy. *S. aureus* is the most common infecting organism. Early diagnosis of these infections is sometimes difficult because the intracranial or intraspinal postoperative abnormalities at a craniotomy site resembles these infections on neuroimaging.

Cerebrospinal Fluid Shunt Infections

There is general agreement that the majority of CSF shunt infections result from perioperative bacterial contamination from organisms on the patient's skin at the time of the procedure. The overall incidence of infection is reported to be 10%.[12] The majority of shunt infections are caused by coagulase-negative staphylococci, followed by *S. aureus* and gram-negative enteric organisms, usually *Escherichia coli* and *Klebsiella* species. *Proteus* and *Pseudomonas* species and streptococcal species are found in 8–10% of infections. Polymicrobial cultures are obtained in approximately 10–15% of shunt infections, and one of the organisms isolated is usually staphylococci or *E. coli*.[2, 12] The risk of infection has been associated with techniques of skin preparation and exposure of large areas of the patient's skin during the procedure, the length of the shunt procedure (the longer the procedure, the greater the risk), inherent properties of the staphylococci (including their ability to adhere to, grow, and proliferate on the inner and outer surfaces of catheters), the age of the patient (neonates and young children have a higher incidence of shunt infection than older patients), the duration of hospitalization, and antibiotic history immediately before the shunting procedure (prior antibiotic therapy increases the risk of skin colonization by multiresistant organisms).[2, 12, 13]

The majority of CSF shunts in use today are ventriculoperitoneal shunts. The most frequent symptoms of a ventriculoperitoneal shunt infection are the result of shunt malfunction and include headache, nausea, lethargy, or an alteration in the level of consciousness. Shunt malfunction is due to the development of inflammation in the tissue surrounding the distal end of the shunt, with subsequent failure of CSF absorption in the peritoneal space. The diagnosis of a ventriculoperitoneal shunt infection depends on the direct culturing of fluid from the shunt. CSF should be obtained from the shunt reservoir because the fluid in the lumbar space may not reveal the presence of infection. The reason for the latter is that there is usually an absence of communication between the infected ventricles and the CSF in the lumbar space, due either to the original reason for shunting or aqueductal stenosis acquired after ventricular shunting.[2] Blood culture results are almost universally negative in ventriculoperitoneal shunt infections, presumably due to lack of direct access of the organisms to the bloodstream.[12] Ventriculoperitoneal shunts are treated with systemic and intraventricular antibiotics and early shunt removal. The shunt can either be immediately replaced or an external ventricular drain can be used temporarily to treat hydrocephalus and for administration of intraventricular antibiotics.

Decreasing the skin bacterial density and minimizing intraoperative wound contamination and shunt component contamination during the procedure appear to be critical to reducing the incidence of shunt infection. Chlorhexidine shampoo before surgery has been shown to be effective in reducing skin bacterial density. In addition, the isolation of wound edges with antiseptic-soaked packs during surgery may also reduce the incidence of infection. It is recommended that the surgeon change gloves before handling the shunt.[13] Because there is no consensus of opinion about the use of prophylactic antibiotics in shunt surgery, a recommendation in favor of or against this practice cannot be made at this time.[14] It is anticipated that the development of a shunt impregnated with antibiotics may be resistant to colonization by microorganisms, and this may decrease the incidence of shunt infection.[14]

External Ventricular Devices

Ventriculostomy catheters are used to monitor intracranial pressure, drain CSF, and administer intraventricular antimicrobial agents. Infection has been cited as the most common complication of ventriculostomy. The risk of infection can be minimized by meticulous surgical technique during insertion of the ventriculostomy and with attention to the maintenance of a sterile closed system. CSF leakage is associated with an increased risk of infection. Previously, it was the consensus of opinion that the risk of infection increased with the duration that a ventriculostomy catheter was in place, leading to the practice of replacing the catheters at 5-day intervals. More recent clinical trials have suggested that there is no linear relationship between the duration of monitor placement and the daily infection rate.[15, 16] In addition, it is not clear if catheter flushes with antibiotics decrease or increase the risk of infection. Intraventricular hemorrhage does increase the risk of infection, most likely because bloody CSF and proteinaceous CSF necessitate frequent irrigation of the system to maintain system patency.[16]

The Ommaya reservoir is a subcutaneous reservoir connected to the frontal horn of the lateral ventricle by a catheter that is used for the administration of intrathecal chemotherapy. Staphylococ-

Table 9.3. Antibiotics for Intraventricular Use

Antibiotic	Dose	Toxicity
Vancomycin	10–20 mg/day	Pleocytosis, transient ventriculitis
Gentamicin	2–5 mg/day	Seizures, ototoxicity
Amphotericin B	0.1–0.5 mg/day	Headache
	0.5–1.0 mg three times per week	Back and leg pain, myelopathy, visual disturbance
Miconazole	20 mg/day	None known but clinical experience is limited

Source: Adapted from DY Wen, AG Bottini, WA Hall, SJ Haines. The intraventricular use of antibiotics. Neurosurg Clin North Am 1992;3:343.

cal meningitis may develop as a complication of the use of an Ommaya reservoir. Infection is the result of the natural colonization of the skin's surface with coagulase-negative staphylococci and the necessity of puncturing the reservoir twice weekly to administer chemotherapy. Meticulous attention to sterile technique before and during the procedure is critical to preventing infection.

The treatment of an infection of an external ventricular catheter requires removal of the device and antimicrobial therapy appropriate for the infecting organism. If the continuous use of the device is required, another device is inserted at a different location.[2]

Intraventricular Antibiotics

The use of either intrashunt or intraventricular vancomycin has become fairly standard therapy for the treatment of methicillin-resistant coagulase-negative staphylococci shunt infections. The toxicity of intraventricular vancomycin is fairly minimal and primarily based on anecdotal reports including rare cases of mental status changes, fever, headache, and tinnitus.[17, 18] The parenteral administration of vancomycin is well known for its association with the "red man syndrome," and there have been cases of CSF eosinophilia secondary to the intraventricular administration of vancomycin. Mast cells are believed to have a role in both the red man syndrome and the development of CSF eosinophilia.[19]

Gentamicin, amphotericin B, and miconazole are the other antimicrobial agents recommended for intraventricular use. The reported adverse effects from intraventricular gentamicin include seizures and ototoxicity. Back and leg pain, myelopathy, headache, visual disturbance, and meningismus have been reported after the intrathecal administration of amphotericin B. Miconazole is reported to have less toxicity than amphotericin B when administered into the intrathecal space, but clinical experience with this antifungal agent in the intrathecal space is limited.

Intrathecal penicillin has tremendous neurotoxicity including seizure activity, paraplegia, hemiplegia, and radiculitis. The intrathecal administration of cephalosporins has also been associated with seizure activity; presently penicillin and the cephalosporins are not used intrathecally, because vancomycin and gentamicin are efficacious and less toxic.[17] Table 9.3 lists the dose and toxicity of the antimicrobial agents that are presently recommended for intraventricular use.

Central Nervous System Fungal Infections

As a general rule, fungal infections occur in individuals who are immunosuppressed due to (1) cytotoxic chemotherapy; (2) chronic corticosteroid therapy; (3) organ transplantation; (4) chronic disease including renal failure, hepatic failure, diabetes mellitus, and alcoholism; and (5) acquired immunodeficiency syndrome. In the neurosurgical patient, the most frequently cited predisposing factor for the development of a fungal infection is the prolonged preoperative use of broad-spectrum antibiotics with or without corticosteroid therapy.[20, 21] *Candida* species infection of ventriculoperitoneal shunts in children have been reported primarily in premature infants. Shunt infections with this fungus may be the result of either direct contamination of the shunt at the time of surgery or result from disseminated candidiasis, a complication of the use of broad-spectrum antibiotics. Very low birth weight, prolonged broad-spectrum antimicrobial therapy, prolonged administration of total parenteral nutrition, and prolonged ventilation are all known risk factors for the development of neonatal disseminated candidiasis.[22]

The therapy for fungal infection of a ventriculoperitoneal shunt consists of externalization of the shunt, the administration of amphotericin B (0.5 mg per kg per day) and flucytosine (25 mg four times a day) for at least 3 weeks, and placement of a new shunt.[20–22]

Fungal aneurysm as a complication of intracranial aneurysmal clipping has also been reported, and the most common etiologic agent of fungal aneurysms is *Aspergillus*.[21, 23–34] Intracranial aspergillosis results from hematogenous dissemination from a primary focus in another organ (typically the lungs) or by direct extension from a contiguous infection in the ear, paranasal sinuses, or orbit. Intracranial aspergillosis may also complicate a neurosurgical procedure, and in this setting the prolonged preoperative use of broad-spectrum antibiotics or chronic corticosteroid therapy is typically cited as a risk factor.[21, 23, 24] Aspergillotic aneurysms are generally large and arise from the vessels of the circle of Willis or the trunk of major arteries (internal carotid artery, basilar artery, middle or anterior cerebral artery, vertebral artery, posterior cerebral artery, or posterior communicating artery [in contrast to bacterial aneurysms, which are typically small and usually situated in the peripheral branches of the middle cerebral artery]).[23] CNS aspergillosis may present as single or multiple ischemic infarctions or subarachnoid hemorrhage from a ruptured mycotic aneurysm or as a brain abscess or abscesses. The majority of patients with aspergillosis have unremitting fever, despite broad-spectrum antibiotics, and pulmonary infiltrates on chest radiography.[25] Diagnosis typically requires culture of the resected specimen.[23] The recommended antifungal therapy is intravenous amphotericin B (0.8–1.0 mg per kg per day) plus flucytosine (100 mg per day in four divided doses).

Iatrogenic Creutzfeldt-Jakob Disease

The first case of iatrogenic CJD, a transmissible spongiform encephalopathy, was reported in 1974 in a corneal transplant recipient whose symptoms began 18 months after surgery. The transplant donor was later found to have died of CJD.[26, 27] In 1977, CJD was reported in two patients after they had had stereotactic electroencephalographic depth recording; the same electrodes had previously been used in a patient with CJD in an attempt to localize the origin of her myoclonus. The electrodes had been sterilized by a procedure using 70% alcohol and formaldehyde vapor, which, although effective for conventional pathogens, does not inactivate the infective agent of CJD. One of the electrodes subsequently transmitted spongiform encephalopathy to a chimpanzee 18 months after implantation in the cerebral cortex, and inoculated brain tissue from both infected patients also transmitted spongiform encephalopathy to primates after incubation periods of 15–25 months.[26, 28] There have been a number of cases of CJD transmitted by cadaveric dura mater grafts. One was in a 28-year-old woman who developed gait ataxia 19 months after surgical resection of a cholesteatoma during which she received an imported, commercially prepared human dura mater graft.[29] The source of the graft in this case, as well as in a subsequent case of a 21-year-old woman who had received a cadaveric dural graft during surgery for a Chiari 1 malformation, and in a 31-year-old woman who received a cadaveric dura mater graft after removal of a giant pituitary adenoma, were all traced back to a single manufacturer (Lyodura).[30, 31] Based on the recommendations of Brown et al. for the decontamination of the infectious agent of CJD and scrapie, the Committee on Health Care Issues of the American Neurologic Association recommended 1 mol per liter NaOH for 1 hour or steam autoclaving for 1 hour at 132°C as standard sterilization procedures for CJD tissue or contaminated materials.[31–33] Lyodura implemented these recommendations in 1987, and since then no new cases of CJD after Lyodura grafting have been reported; however, some investigators have raised the concern that complete inactivation cannot be obtained using 1 mol per liter NaOH, and that such treatment merely extends the incubation period.[31, 34, 35] Iatrogenic CJD has also been reported in growth hormone recipients treated with growth hormone derived from pools of human cadaver pituitary glands.[36] In 1992, the risk of dying from CJD in the patient population that had received cadaver-derived human growth hormone was 1 in 200 patients.[26]

CJD is one of the human prion diseases also referred to as a transmissible spongiform encephalopathy. Kuru, Gerstmann-Sträussler-Scheinker disease, and fatal familial insomnia are also human prion diseases. Prion diseases also occur in animals, causing scrapie in sheep and goats and bovine spongiform encephalopathy in cattle. These diseases are caused by an infectious agent termed a *prion* to emphasize its proteinaceous and infectious nature.[37] The human prion diseases, whether sporadic, dominantly inherited, or acquired by infection all involve the aberrant metabolism of the prion protein. The prion protein is encoded by a gene on the short arm of chromosome 20.[37] A fundamental event in prion diseases is the conversion of the normal cellular prion protein into a scrapie isoform (PrPSc), a post-translational process that involves a conformational change in the protein. The normal cellular isoform (PrPC) of the protein is rich in alpha-helices and is virtually devoid of beta-sheet content. The scrapie isoform (PrPSc) differs physically from PrPC by its high beta-sheet content, insolubility in detergents, propensity to aggregate, and relative resistance to proteolysis.[37] Infectious prions are composed almost entirely of PrPSc. The conversion of PrPC into PrPSc appears to involve the unfolding of alpha-helices and their refolding into beta sheets.[37] CJD is characterized clinically by dementia, visual deterioration, incoordination and apraxia, and involuntary movements that are typically myoclonic jerks but may also be more complex and include choreoathetosis.[36] The classic neuropathologic features include spongiform degeneration, gliosis, and neuronal loss in the absence of an inflammatory reaction.[37]

It has been suggested that an individual's genetic makeup may render him or her susceptible to iatrogenic CJD. Homozygosity for the valine allele in the normally polymorphic valine-methionine codon 129 has been found in patients with iatrogenic CJD in the United Kingdom.[26] Homozygosity for the valine allele at codon 129 has also been associated with an accelerated pathogenesis (early age at onset and short duration of illness) in sporadic CJD and in familial forms of the disease. The genotype of codon 129 may be a predisposing factor for exogenous infection.[38]

Because there still is controversy regarding whether or not 1 mol per liter NaOH inactivates the infectious agent of CJD, a number of other recommendations have been made to prevent the transmission of this disease, including that (1) autologous graft material such as temporal fascia or tensor fascia lata should be used as an alternative to cadaveric dural grafts whenever possible[31]; (2) surgical instruments should be discarded after procedures that are performed on known or possible CJD patients[39]; (3) human tissue or tissue products should not be used from donors with dementing or cerebellar illnesses and those who have a family history of such illnesses[39]; and (4) a constant awareness by the medical community should be maintained of the potential infectivity of tissue and body fluids obtained from patients with CJD.[40]

References

1. Pons VG, Denlinger SL, Guglielmo BJ, et al. Ceftizoxime versus vancomycin and gentamicin in neurosurgical prophylaxis: a randomized, prospective, blinded clinical study. Neurosurgery 1993;33:416.
2. Kaufman BA, Tunkel AR, Pryor JC, Dacey RG. Meningitis in the neurosurgical patient. Infect Dis Clin North Am 1990;4:677.
3. Neurosurgery Working Party of the British Society for Antimicrobial Chemotherapy. Antimicrobial prophylaxis in neurosurgery and after head injury. Lancet 1994;344:1547.
4. Carmel PW, Greif LK. The aseptic meningitis syndrome: a complication of posterior fossa surgery. Pediatr Neurosurg 1993;19:276.
5. Ross D, Rosegay H, Pons V. Differentiation of aseptic and bacterial meningitis in postoperative neurosurgical patients. J Neurosurg 1988;69:669.
6. Savitz SI, Bottone EJ, Savitz MH, Malis LI. Investigations of the bacteriological factors in clean neurosurgical wounds. Neurosurgery 1994:34:417.
7. Haile-Mariam T, Laws E, Tuazon CU. Gram-negative meningitis associated with transsphenoidal surgery: case reports and review. Clin Infect Dis 1994;18:553.
8. Nguyen TT, Delashaw JB. Complications of skull base surgery. Clin Plast Surg 1995;22:573.
9. Sebring LA, Nussbaum ES, Haines SJ. Scalp and Skull Infections. In GT Tindall, PR Cooper, DL Barrow (eds), The Practice of Neurosurgery. Baltimore: Williams & Wilkins 1996;3377.
10. Erickson DL, Seljeskog EL, Chou SN. Suction-irrigation treatment of craniotomy infections. J Neurosurg 1974;41:265.
11. Gentry LO. Osteomyelitis and Other Infections of Bones and Joints. In KB Crossley, GL Archer (eds), The Staphylococci in Human Disease. New York: Churchill Livingstone, 1997;455.
12. Bayston R. Hydrocephalus shunt infections. J Antimicrob Chemother 1994;34(Suppl A):75.
13. Pople IK, Bayston R, Hayward RD. Infection of cerebrospinal fluid shunts in infants: a study of etiological factors. J Neurosurg 1992;77:29.

14. Brown EM. Antimicrobial prophylaxis in neurosurgery. J Antimicrob Chemother 1993;31(Suppl B):49.
15. Holloway KL, Barnes T, Choi S, et al. Ventriculostomy infections: the effect of monitoring duration and catheter exchange in 584 patients. J Neurosurg 1996;85:419.
16. Winfield JA, Rosenthal P, Kanter RK, Casella G. Duration of intracranial pressure monitoring does not predict daily risk of infectious complications. Neurosurgery 1993;33:424.
17. Wen DY, Bottini AG, Hall WA, Haines SJ. The intraventricular use of antibiotics. Neurosurg Clin North Am 1992;3:343.
18. Golledge CL, McKenzie T. Monitoring vancomycin concentrations in CSF after intraventricular administration. J Antimicrob Chemother 1988;21:262.
19. Grabb PA, Albright AL. Intraventricular vancomycin-induced cerebrospinal fluid eosinophilia: report of two patients. Neurosurgery 1992;30:630.
20. Nguyen MH, Yu VL. Meningitis caused by *Candida* species: an emerging problem in neurosurgical patients. Clin Infect Dis 1995;21:323.
21. Piotrowski WP, Pilz P, Chuang IH. Subarachnoid hemorrhage caused by a fungal aneurysm of the vertebral artery as a complication of intracranial aneurysm clipping. J Neurosurg 1990;73:962.
22. Chiou CC, Wong TT, Lin HH, et al. Fungal infection of ventriculoperitoneal shunts in children. Clin Infect Dis 1994;19:1049.
23. Takeshita M, Izawa M, Kubo O. Aspergillotic aneurysm formation of cerebral artery following neurosurgical operation. Surg Neurol 1992;38:146.
24. Ide W, Suematsu K, Matsuzaki T, et al. A case of newly formed mycotic *(Aspergillus)* aneurysm near the clipped middle cerebral artery aneurysm. Surg Cereb Stroke 1987;15:395.
25. Coleman JM, Hogg GG, Rosenfeld JV, Waters KD. Invasive central nervous system aspergillosis: cure with liposomal amphotericin B, itraconazole, and radical surgery—case report and review of the literature. Neurosurgery 1995;36:848.
26. Brown P, Preece MA, Will RG. "Friendly fire" in medicine: hormones, homografts, and Creutzfeldt-Jakob disease. Lancet 1992;340:24.
27. Duffy P, Wolf J, Collins G, et al. Possible person-to-person transmission of Creutzfeldt-Jakob disease. N Engl J Med 1974;290:692.
28. Bernoulli C, Siegfried J, Baumgartner G, et al. Danger of accidental person-to-person transmission of Creutzfeldt-Jakob disease by surgery. Lancet 1977;i:478.
29. Anon. Rapidly progressive dementia in a patient who received a cadaveric dura mater graft. JAMA 1987; 257:1036.
30. Lane KL, Brown P, Howell DN, et al. Creutzfeldt-Jakob disease in a pregnant woman with an implanted dura mater graft. Neurosurgery 1994;34:737.
31. Yamada S, Aiba T, Endo Y, et al. Creutzfeldt-Jakob disease transmitted by a cadaveric dura mater graft. Neurosurgery 1994;34:740.
32. Brown P, Rohwer RG, Gajdusek DC. Sodium hydroxide decontamination of Creutzfeldt-Jakob disease virus. N Engl J Med 1984;310:727.
33. Brown P, Rohwer RG, Gajdusek DC. New data on the inactivation of scrapie virus or Creutzfeldt-Jakob disease virus in brain tissue. J Infect Dis 1986;153:1145.
34. Tamai Y, Taguchi F, Miura S. Inactivation of the Creutzfeldt-Jakob disease agent [letter]. Ann Neurol 1988;24:466.
35. Tateishi J, Tashima T, Kitamoto T. Inactivation of the Creutzfeldt-Jakob disease agent [letter]. Ann Neurol 1988;24:466.
36. Brown P. The clinical neurology and epidemiology of Creutzfeldt-Jakob disease, with special reference to iatrogenic cases. Novel infectious agents and the central nervous system. Ciba Found Symp 1988;135:3.
37. Prusiner SB, Hsiao KK. Human prion diseases. Ann Neurol 1994;35:385.
38. Brown P, Cervenakova L, Goldfarb LG, McCombie WR. Iatrogenic Creutzfeldt-Jakob disease: an example of the interplay between ancient genes and modern medicine. Neurology 1994;44:291.
39. Brown P. Iatrogenic Creutzfeldt-Jakob disease. Aust N Z J Med 1990;20:633.
40. Rappaport EB. Iatrogenic Creutzfeldt-Jakob disease. Neurology 1987;37:1520.

Chapter 10

Iatrogenic Neurologic Problems in the Critical Care Unit

Marc D. Malkoff

Objectives

- To recognize the common types of iatrogenic neurologic problems seen in the critical care unit
- To understand the common types of iatrogenic neurologic problems caused by procedures in the critical care setting
- To appreciate the iatrogenic effects of sedative use in the critical care unit
- To learn the iatrogenic effects of neuromuscular blockade in the critical care setting
- To recognize the iatrogenic effects of common drugs used in the critical care unit
- To understand the iatrogenic effects of electrolyte disorders seen in the critical care unit

Neurologic problems are commonly encountered in the intensive care unit. It has been estimated that neurologic problems complicate more than 10% of all admissions to a medical intensive care unit and may more than double that in surgical and transplant units.[1,2] Patients with neurologic complications have a longer length of stay and a higher case-fatality ratio than their non-neurologic counterparts.[1] Nonetheless, many of these complications result from the illnesses that place people in the intensive care setting. These complications revolve around four main clinical disturbances: focal or generalized seizures, focal neurologic deficits, loss of consciousness, and muscle weakness.[2] Iatrogenic problems are a relatively infrequent cause of neurologic problems in the intensive care unit. This chapter takes a relatively narrow view of the term *iatrogenic*, in that it is implied that these are complications induced by physicians during the treatment of the patient's illness. This excludes, for example, many perioperative strokes from cardiopulmonary bypass because these occur intraoperatively or other neurologic complications that are reviewed in detail in other chapters.

Neurologic Problems

The most common causes of iatrogenic neurologic problems are complications occurring during procedures, during administration of medications, or after metabolic derangements. Problems with drug administration include both adverse reactions and side effects from changes in half-life and protein binding. Not surprisingly, these iatrogenic complications cause the same categories of problems as do the patient's primary illness.

Complications of Procedures

Air embolism is an infrequent complication of central venous cannulation. It has been reported in from 1 in 47 central venous catheterizations to 0 in 355 procedures.[3,4] Other authors have placed the incidence at approximately 2 in more than 1,500 catheterizations to 1 in 3,000.[5,6] Approximately one-third had a fatal outcome.[7] Air embolism has been reported both with insertion of central venous catheters as well as with pulmonary artery catheters. Air can enter the central veins during insertion or with careless maintenance during manometry or infusions.[8, 9] Pulmonary artery catheters have also been implicated in air embolism via the relative incompetence of the valves at the end of the introducer.[10, 11] An additional cause of air embolus is injection of air into a ruptured pulmonary artery balloon; however, this usually results in pulmonary complications and not systemic complications.[12] Air embolism may cause stroke via paradoxical embolus and may also cause cardiac arrest, producing secondary hypoxic ischemic neurologic damage.[9] Coppa et al., in a series of 14 cases of air embolization, noted that one-half had presenting signs of coma, although most patients in coma either had cardiac arrest or severe hypotension.[7] Generalized seizures and two cases of focal deficit were also recorded. Most of these patients, however, had respiratory presentations of apnea, hypoxia, cyanosis, or hypotension that most likely contributed to the neurologic symptoms.[7] Focal signs have also been noted from air embolism after subclavian venous catheterization.[13–15]

An additional complication of central venous catheterization (primarily jugular catheterization) is "carotid stick" (carotid artery puncture). This complication occurs in approximately 1% of all central lines.[16, 17] It can unfortunately lead to stroke from carotid dissection (by tearing of the intima), compression of the carotid artery by neck hematoma, dislodgment of an embolic plaque, or infusion of viscous substances.[17, 18] Nonetheless, there are only a few reported cases of stroke after inadvertent carotid puncture in line with the reported occurrence of stroke after direct carotid stick for angiography.[19] Brain stem infarction that occurs after inadvertent vertebral injury from an attempted jugular line placement is less frequent than hemispheric stroke.[20]

Intra-aortic balloon pumps are commonly used in the intensive care unit to augment blood flow and blood pressure in cases of cardiogenic shock. Fortunately, the incidence of neurologic complications associated with balloon pumps is relatively low.

There are reports of stroke resulting from both focal and global hypoperfusion with the use of balloon pumps, mostly from intraoperative use, but it is not clear whether this complication results from the use of or the need to use an intra-aortic balloon pump.[21–28] Stroke may result from air embolus after rupture of the balloon.[29] In a study of pure critical care unit use in complicated myocardial infarction, the pump group had fewer strokes than the controls.[27] Spinal cord ischemia has been reported to occur after intra-aortic balloon pump use.[30, 31]

Cholesterol embolization can lead to strokes after procedures in the aortic arch or carotid or vertebral arteries or after angiography.[19, 28, 32] External carotid artery manipulation has also been reported to produce cholesterol emboli, causing stroke.[33] Cholesterol emboli can occasionally lead to spinal cord as well as peripheral nerve infarction.[31, 34]

Positive end-expiratory pressure can cause adverse neurologic events by increasing intracranial pressure due to an increase in intrathoracic pressure and also by impeding venous return, which decreases cardiac output.[35, 36] This appears to be a problem only in the setting of elevated intracranial pressure or intracranial mass lesions. However, when used appropriately—that is, in the setting of stiff lungs—the increased intrathoracic pressure does not significantly impair venous return or cardiac output.[37, 38] Therefore, due to modern strategies of mechanical ventilation that seek to minimize intrathoracic pressure, positive end-expiratory pressure use, and barotrauma, this problem is rarely seen.

Intracranial pressure monitoring is another intensive care procedure used in the management of trauma, cerebrovascular disease, and hepatic coma. The primary neurologic comorbidities are central nervous system (CNS) infection and intracranial hemorrhage. The incidence of infection varies from 0% to 11%, depending on the series and the type of monitor used.[39–47] Fiberoptic monitoring devices tend to be associated with fewer infections (0–1%)[40, 41, 44, 45] than intraventricular catheters (4–11%),[39, 42, 43, 46, 47] but the reported infection rate has declined in the more recent case series (which use fiberoptic monitors). It is not clear if the duration of time a single monitoring device is left in place influences the infection rate.[42, 43, 46, 47] Intracranial hemorrhage tends to occur in coagulopathic settings and is less frequent than infectious complications.[41, 45, 48]

Drug Effects

Drug pharmacokinetics and pharmacodynamics are altered in critically ill patients.[49, 50] This is due to the effects of multiple drug interactions, decreased hepatic and renal function associated with critical illness, the interaction of critical illness on the CNS, which sensitizes it to drug effects, changes in protein binding, and alterations in drug half-life from prolonged administration.[49–51] This multiplicity of effects predisposes the critically ill patient to side effects of drug toxicity as well as prolonged duration of action of medication. The most common iatrogenic drug effects are encephalopathy (decreased level of consciousness or coma), seizures, and weakness.[49] Recent advances in pharmacology, including better knowledge of these effects as well as the use of agents with a shorter duration of action, has limited this problem, but has not entirely prevented it. Adverse drug events still complicate approximately 2% of all hospital admissions and increase costs and lengths of stay significantly.[52, 53]

Sedative Effects

The most common problem of drug interactions has been coma or stupor due to the prolonged duration of action of the medication. The most commonly used agents for sedation in the intensive care unit include benzodiazepines, opioids, neuroleptics, and propofol.[54, 55] Benzodiazepines are active at the gamma-aminobutyric acid (GABA) receptor, enhancing GABA-ergic transmission.[56] These drugs are also used to produce amnesia, muscle relaxation (centrally mediated), as well as seizure control.[54, 56]

Overdose of benzodiazepines can result from many etiologies. Most of the benzodiazepines except for oxazepam (rarely used in the intensive care unit) are hepatically metabolized. With changes in hepatic metabolism, half-life and sedative duration can be markedly prolonged.[49, 54] Benzodiazepines that are lipophilic, such as diazepam, are absorbed into fat and the brain, resulting in high tissue stores. With prolonged use, this leads to a prolonged sedative effect.[57] This is especially true with long-acting drugs, including drugs such as diazepam and chlordiazepoxide, which have a desmethyl-diazepam metabolite that also has a long half-life of approximately 96 hours.[49, 54] Finally, patients can develop tachyphylaxis that can lead to dose escalation, allowing higher tissue stores.[54, 58, 59]

Benzodiazepine overdose can result in prolonged coma and respiratory depression.[56, 58, 59] In addition, benzodiazepines decrease catecholamine release, causing arterial hypotension.[54, 60] Administration of a competitive benzodiazepine antagonist, flumazenil, may reverse the sedative effects of benzodiazepines.[54, 56, 61] Nonetheless, rapid antagonism of sedation carries its owns risks, including arterial hypertension, tachycardia, tachyarrhythmias, seizures, and increased intracranial pressure.[61, 62] Adverse events are more common with administration of large amounts of flumazenil with chronic benzodiazepine use.[61] Flumazenil also has a shorter duration of action than the drugs it antagonizes.[56, 61]

Opioids are another class of medications commonly used in the intensive care unit for analgesia and sedation. They are agonists of the opioid receptor sites located throughout the CNS and other tissues. Mu-1 agonism predicts and mediates most of their analgesic effect. Unfortunately, mu-2 receptor agonism produces respiratory depression.[54, 63, 64] Opioid overdose manifests with depressed level of consciousness, respiratory depression, and ileus.[63] An additional potential neurologic complication from opioids is an increase in intracranial pressure. Although most clinical studies show minimal changes in intracranial pressure with the use of opioids, there are a few reports suggesting that administration of fentanyl may precipitate increases in intracranial pressure in patients with mass lesions.[65, 66] This phenomenon is not entirely due to changes in carbon dioxide concentration. Meperidine has additional potential neurologic complications. First, meperidine has a tendency to cause histamine release that may lead to hypotension, a trait it shares with morphine.[54, 63] This can reduce cerebral perfusion pressure without affecting intracranial pressure. Second, the hepatic metabolite, normeperidine, may accumulate and is itself a neurotoxin, often causing encephalopathy or seizures. Finally, normeperidine may interact with the concomitant use of monoamine oxidase inhibitors, leading to the classic monoamine oxidase syndrome.[49, 54, 67]

All narcotics are hepatically metabolized, with prolongation of half-life in hepatic insufficiency.[49, 54, 63] Morphine also has significant renal excretion due to its active glucuronide metabolite.[49, 54] The commonly used short-acting narcotics—fentanyl, alfentanil, and sufentanil—are lipid soluble, and therefore may accumulate extensively in tissue stores, leading to a prolonged duration of action.[68]

Opioid withdrawal manifests with rhinorrhea, lacrimation, yawning, nausea, vomiting, gastrointestinal distress, diarrhea, and hypertension. Naloxone is a competitive opioid antagonist that can trigger abrupt withdrawal, leading to pain and hypertension.[54, 63] Naloxone appears to produce minor direct cerebral effects.[54] Unfortunately, this drug has a short duration of action and may require repeated boluses, especially when used in the setting of long-acting or tissue-stored narcotics.[63]

Neuroleptics are commonly used in the intensive care unit for sedation, as antipsychotic agents, and as antiemetics. Their primary mechanism of action is dopaminergic blockade in the limbic system and cortex.[54] Their common neurologic side effects are extrapyramidal symptoms and a reduction in seizure threshold.[54] In addition, the anticholinergic effects of several of these agents may lead to a psychosis if used in large doses.[44]

Neuroleptic malignant syndrome (NMS) is a syndrome of temperature dysregulation, accompanied by rhabdomyolysis and rigidity.[69] Not all temperature elevations from neuroleptics are NMS, because neuroleptics can cause temperature dysregulation without associated rhabdomyolysis.[69] Risperidone (Risperdal) appears less likely to cause temperature dysregulation.[69] In NMS, the serum creatine kinase level is usually elevated well over 1,000 units per dl and typically at least 5–10,000 units per dl. NMS is most often seen with dehydration, a medical reason for fever such as infection, and the use of long-acting neuroleptics.[70–72] Treatment of NMS consists of rehydration, treatment of any underlying infection, and administration of dopaminergic agents or muscle relaxants.[69, 70, 72] Dopaminergic agents used in this condition include bromocriptine and L-dopa/carbidopa; dantrolene sodium, administered intravenously or orally, is the muscle relaxant most commonly used.[69, 70, 72] Some authors recommend combination treatment.

There are relatively few reports of neurologic side effects from propofol, another commonly used sedative and hypnotic in the intensive care unit. Propofol appears to act on the GABA-receptor complex and appears to produce sedation with unfortunately significant hypotension and apnea.[54, 73] Its duration of action is relatively short, even when used for long periods.[58] The effects of propofol on intracranial pressure dynamics and cranial pressure are still not entirely understood. Propofol causes both decreases in intracranial pressure and blood pressure, but its overall effect on cerebral perfusion pressure is variable.[74–76] Propofol has been reported to cause myoclonus, but does not appear to be a direct proconvulsant; it may be used as an anticonvulsant at extremely high doses.[54, 77]

Neuromuscular Blockade

Several neuromuscular complications in the intensive care unit may be at least partially iatrogenic. These include a prolonged duration of action, critical illness polyneuropathy, critical illness myopathy, malignant hyperthermia, and inadvertent neuromuscular blockade.

The most common neuromuscular complication is prolonged duration of action of neuromuscular blockade.[78, 79] This occurs after prolonged administration of a nondepolarizing neuromuscular blocker. Nondepolarizing neuromuscular blocking agents are both hepatically and renally metabolized and excreted and can therefore accumulate in organ failure (atracurium does significantly accumulate in renal failure).[80, 81] Both pancuronium and vecuronium have active metabolites.[80, 81] Furthermore, with prolonged administration, tissue accumulation may occur.[81] Therefore, these agents may last longer than might otherwise be predicted. In addition, other drugs, such as aminoglycosides, can increase the duration of action of neuromuscular blocking agents, especially in patients with disorders of the neuromuscular junction (Table 10.1).[80] The increasing prevalence of nerve stimulators for monitoring in the intensive care unit allows for a more careful titration of neuromuscular blockade.[78, 81]

The second common neuromuscular problem in the intensive care unit is polyneuropathy of critical illness. This is an axonal neuropathy that develops in the setting of critical illness. Critical illness polyneuropathy manifests as weakness and an inability to wean from mechanical ventilation.[82–84] The most common risk factors for development of this entity include the presence of sepsis and multiorgan system failure. Several reports also have implicated the use of corticosteroids and corticosteroid-based neuromuscular blocking agents (vecuronium and pancuronium) as associated risk factors.[78, 83, 85] This is further supported by the relative lack of association with atracurium, a noncorticosteroid agent.[78] Recovery is prolonged (often more than 6 months) and overall outcome is generally good, if the patient survives.[78, 83, 85]

The myopathy of critical illness is an acute necrotizing myopathy seen in critically ill patients.[86–88] In its most severe form, patients develop a flaccid quadriparesis, often with severe but not complete facial paresis. Muscle biopsy has shown myonecrosis.[86–88] This entity is associated with sepsis, and most cases have been associated with glucocorticoid and vecuronium (a corticosteroid derivative) use.[78, 86–88] Both the polyneuropathy and myopathy of critical illness have a fair degree of morbidity from prolonged mechanical ventilation and rehabilitation. Recovery, although usually good, may be incomplete.[85–88]

Malignant hyperthermia is a genetic disorder that presents as hyperthermia and rigidity on anesthetic induction. It is most commonly seen in the operating room, but may occasionally be seen in the intensive care unit when neuromuscular blocking agents are used. Treatment consists of intravenous dantrolene sodium.[72]

Table 10.1. Drugs that Prolong the Duration of Action of Nondepolarizing Neuromuscular Blocking Agents and May Adversely Weaken Patients with Myasthenia Gravis

Antibiotics
Aminoglycosides (gentamicin, tobramycin, amikacin)
Polypeptides (polymyxin B)
Other antibiotics (clindamycin, tetracycline)
Local anesthetics and antiarrhythmics
Lidocaine
Procainamide
Quinidine
Magnesium
Calcium channel blockers
Beta-adrenergic blockers
Chemotherapeutic agents
Cyclophosphamide
Diuretics
Furosemide
Thiazides
Other
Lithium carbonate
Cyclosporine
Dantrolene

Source: Adapted from RC Prielipp, DB Coursin. Applied pharmacology of common neuromuscular blocking agents in critical care. New Horiz 1994;2:34.

Other Drugs

Many non-neurologic drugs have neurologic complications when used in the intensive care unit setting. Critically ill patients often have altered metabolism of these agents through a combination of protein binding, reduced excretion, and drug interactions, leading to CNS side effects. The most commonly described classes of agents are immunosuppressants, antiarrhythmics, respiratory care medications, H_2 blockers, and antibiotics.

Immunosuppressive therapy is commonly used in the critical care unit for organ transplantation. Neurologic complications from cyclosporine and FK506 are reported in more than 10% of all liver transplant recipients.[89, 90] These consist of a leukoencephalopathy manifesting with blindness, confusion, mutism, and seizures. In addition, a vasculopathy has also been described, manifesting with focal findings.[89–92] These effects usually abate, if the dose of the offending agent is reduced. Although corticosteroids are also commonly used, psychosis is not commonly attributed to their use.[89]

Neurologic side effects from medications used for respiratory care are also common. Theophylline and $beta_2$-agonists are both commonly used agents that have been implicated to cause tremor and in the case of theophylline, seizures.[93–95] Seizures are commonly seen when theophylline is either misused or misdosed. Hepatic dysfunction or drug interactions with medications, such as cimetidine or erythromycin, can acutely raise the concentration of theophylline beyond what is expected.[96]

H_2 blockers and antiarrhythmic agents are commonly employed in critical care units. Their ability to cause CNS side effects with toxicity is well known. Toxic levels of lidocaine can cause seizures and encephalopathy.[97, 98] At toxic levels, digoxin can cause hallucinations and mood disturbances.[99] Similar problems are seen with the effects of H_2 blockers. When used appropriately, there are minimal neurologic problems. However, these drugs, when overdosed, can induce an encephalopathy, especially in a setting of a multiple organ system failure and multiple drug interactions.[99, 100] This has been most commonly reported with cimetidine but has occasionally been reported with most of the other H_2 blockers except famotidine.[100]

The most common iatrogenic neurologic problem with antimicrobials is overdose of both aminoglycosides and beta-lactams (and related agents). Aminoglycosides are well known for their ototoxicity and vertigo.[101] Beta-lactams are used for experimental induction of seizures.[102, 103] This effect may occasionally be seen with maladministration of these medications in the critical care unit, especially in patients with renal failure. Imipenem is probably the most notorious of these antibiotics for inducing seizures, but this complication has been reported with most if not all of these medications.[101]

Metabolic Derangements

Metabolic derangements following procedures may also lead to neurologic complications. The most common is severe postoperative hyponatremia, which is most commonly noted after prostatic surgery but has been noted after a variety of procedures.[104–107] There are two distinct etiologies: the syndrome of inappropriate antidiuretic hormone release (often abetted by inappropriate fluid management) and direct absorption of hypotonic fluids used in surgery.[104–107] Although often asymptomatic, clinical manifestations include seizures, visual disturbances, and osmotic demyelination (myelinolysis).[104–107] The latter problem is usually seen in women and appears most commonly in the pons (central pontine myelinolysis).[104]

Disorders of magnesium are an infrequent cause of iatrogenic neurologic problems. Hypomagnesemia, which can be a side effect of diuretic use, can increase muscular and neuronal irritability, leading to fasciculations and seizures.[108] Hypermagnesemia, a complication of magnesium infusion for eclampsia, can cause muscular weakness and coma.[109, 110] Side effects of magnesium infusion, however, are rare with proper monitoring.[108, 110]

The final common iatrogenic electrolyte complication is hypophosphatemia. Although most commonly seen in septic, malnourished patients, hypophosphatemia can be seen as a result of poorly adjusted feedings or of refeeding syndrome, after massive blood transfusion, and with improper repletion.[111, 112] Clinical manifestations include muscular weakness (including diaphragmatic weakness and ventilatory dependence), seizures, and coma. These resolve with phosphate repletion.[111, 112]

Conclusion

Iatrogenic neurologic problems occur in the critical care unit on a relatively infrequent basis. Their manifestations are usually similar to the neurologic problems that may be caused by the underlying illness. Careful attention to drug dosing, drug interactions, and drug effects, as well as careful attention to expected complications of procedures, will help in prevention.

References

1. Bleck TP, Smith MC, Pierre-Louis SJ, et al. Neurologic complications of critical medical illnesses. Crit Care Med 1993;21:98.
2. Wijdicks EFM. Neurologic complications in critically ill patients. Anesth Analg 1996;83:411.
3. Doblar DD, Hinkle JC, Fay ML, et al. Air embolism associated with pulmonary artery catheter introducer kit. Anesthesiology 1982;56:307.
4. Ryan JA, Abel RM, Abbott WM, et al. Catheter complications in total parenteral nutrition. N Engl J Med 1974;290:757.
5. James PM, Myers RT. Central venous pressure monitoring. Ann Surg 1972;175:693.
6. Feliciano DV, Mattox KL, Graham JM, et al. Major complications of percutaneous subclavian vein catheters. Am J Surg 1979;138:869.
7. Coppa GF, Gouge TH, Hofstetter SF. Air embolism: a lethal but preventable complication of subclavian vein catheterization. J Parenter Enteral Nutr 1981;5:166.
8. Defalque RJ, Fletcher MV. Neurologic complications of central venous cannulation. J Parenter Enteral Nutr 1988;12:406.
9. Orebaugh SL. Venous air embolism. Clinical and experimental considerations. Crit Care Med 1992;20:1169.
10. Kondo K, O'Reilly LP, Chiota J. Air embolism associated with an introducer for pulmonary artery catheters. Anesth Analg 1984;63:871.
11. Cohen MB, Mark JB, Morris RW, et al. Introducer sheath malfunction producing insidious air embolism. Anesthesiology 1987;67:573.
12. Jastremski MS, Chelluri L. Air embolism and cardiac arrest in a patient with a pulmonary artery catheter: a possible association. Resuscitation 1986;14:113.
13. Acalovschi I, Corbaciu D, Paraianu I. Cortical blindness after subclavian vein catheterization. J Parenter Enteral Nutr 1988;12:526.

14. Jacobsen WK, Briggs BA, Mason LJ. Paradoxical air embolism associated with a central total parenteral nutrition catheter. Crit Care Med 1983;11:388.
15. Grace DM. Air embolism with neurologic complications: a potential hazard of central venous catheters. Can J Surg 1977;20:51.
16. Aghdami A, Ellis R. High oxygen saturation does not always indicate arterial placement of catheter during internal jugular venous cannulation. Anesthesiology 1985;62:72.
17. Todd MR. Barone JE. Recognition of accidental arterial cannulation after attempted central venipuncture. Crit Care Med 1991;19:1081.
18. Lynch JC, Shehabi Y. Stroke caused by inadvertent intra-arterial parenteral nutrition. Anaesth Intensive Care 1995;23:358.
19. Bauer J, Salazar JL, Sugar O, Pawl RP. Direct percutaneous cerebral angiography in neurosurgical practice. J Neurosurg 1980;52:525.
20. Sloan MA, Mueller JD, Adelman LS, Caplan LR. Fatal brainstem stroke following internal jugular vein catheterization. Neurology 1991;41:1092.
21. Safi HJ. Role of the BioMedicus pump and distal aortic perfusion in thoracoabdominal aortic aneurysm repair. Artificial Organs 1996;20:694.
22. Karalis DG, Quinn V, Victor MF, et al. Risk of catheter-related emboli in patients with atherosclerotic debris in the thoracic aorta. Am Heart J 1996;131:1149.
23. Edwards FH, Bellamy RF, Burge JR, et al. True emergency coronary artery bypass surgery. Ann Thorac Surg 1990;49:603.
24. Hedenmark J, Ahn H, Henze A, et al. Intra-aortic balloon counterpulsation with special reference to determinants of survival. Scand J Thorac Cardiovasc Surg 1989;23:57.
25. Elefteriades JA. Cardiac assist devices. Cardiol Clin 1988;6:449.
26. Lund O, Johansen G, Allermand H, et al. Intraaortic balloon pumping in the treatment of low cardiac output following open heart surgery—immediate results and long-term prognosis. Thorac Cardiovasc Surg 1988;36:332.
27. Ohman EM, George BS, White CJ, et al. Use of aortic counterpulsation to improve sustained coronary artery patency during acute myocardial infarction. Results of a randomized trial. The Randomized IABP Study Group. Circulation 1994;90:792.
28. Cohn LH, Rizzo RJ, Adams DH, et al. Reduced mortality and morbidity for ascending aortic aneurysm resection regardless of cause. Ann Thorac Surg 1996;62:463.
29. Myers GJ, Landymore RW, Leadon RB, Squires C. Fracture of the internal lumen of a Datascope Percor Stat-DL Balloon, resulting in stroke. Ann Thorac Surg 1994;57:1335.
30. Gottesman MH, Saraya I, Tenti F. Modified Brown-Séquard syndrome following coronary artery bypass graft: case report. Paraplegia 1992;30:178.
31. Harris RE, Reimer KA, Crain BJ, et al. Spinal cord infarction following intraaortic balloon support. Ann Thorac Surg 1986;42:206.
32. Fernandez-Samos R, Suarez D, Ortega JM, et al. Multiple cholesterol embolization syndrome: a lethal complication of vascular procedures. Report of two histologically proven cases. J Cardiovasc Surg 1995;36:87.
33. Khaffaf N, Karnik R, Winkler WB, et al. Embolic stroke by compression maneuver during transcranial Doppler sonography. Stroke 1994;25:1056.
34. Bendixen BH, Younger DS, Hair LS, et al. Cholesterol emboli neuropathy. Neurology 1992;42:428.
35. Burchiel KJ, Steege TD, Wyler AR. Intracranial pressure changes in brain-injured patients requiring positive end-expiratory pressure ventilation. Neurosurgery 1981;8:443.
36. Appuzzo MLJ, Weiss MH, Petersons V, et al. Effect of positive end-expiratory pressure ventilation on intracranial pressure in man. J Neurosurg 1977;46:227.
37. Cooper KR, Boswell PA, Choi SC. Safe use of PEEP in patients with severe head injury. J Neurosurg 1985;63:552.
38. Lodrini S, Montolivo M, Pluchino F, Borroni V. Positive end-expiratory pressure in supine and sitting positions: its effects on intrathoracic and intracranial pressures. Neurosurgery 1989;24:873.
39. Clark WC, Muhlbauer MS, Lowrey R, et al. Complications of intracranial pressure monitoring in trauma patients. Neurosurgery 1989;25:20.
40. Gambardella G, d'Avella D, Tomasello F. Monitoring of brain tissue pressure with a fiberoptic device. Neurosurgery 1992;31:918.
41. Jensen RL, Hahn YS, Ciro E. Risk factors of intracranial pressure monitoring in children with fiberoptic devices: a critical review. Surg Neurol 1997;47:16.
42. Mayhall CG, Archer NH, Lamb VA, et al. Ventriculostomy-related infections. A prospective epidemiologic study. N Engl J Med 1984;310:553.
43. Paramore CG, Turner DA. Relative risks of ventriculostomy infection and morbidity. Acta Neurochir 1994;127:79.
44. Pople IK, Muhlbauer MS, Sanford RA, Kirk E. Results and complications of intracranial pressure monitoring in 303 children. Pediatric Neurosurgery 1995;23:64.
45. Shapiro S, Bowman R, Callahan J, Wolfla C. The fiberoptic intraparenchymal cerebral pressure monitor in 244 patients. Surg Neurol 1996;45:278.
46. Sundbarg G, Nordstrom CH, Soderstrom S. Complications due to prolonged ventricular fluid pressure recording. Br J Neurosurg 1988;2:485.
47. Winfield JA, Rosenthal P, Kanter RK, Casella G. Duration of intracranial pressure monitoring does not predict daily risk of infectious complications. Neurosurgery 1993;33:424.
48. Blei AT, Olafsson S, Webster S, Levy R. Complications of intracranial pressure monitoring in fulminant hepatic failure. Lancet 1993;341:157.

49. Bodenham A, Shelly MP, Park GR. The altered pharmacokinetics and pharmacodynamics of drugs commonly used in critically ill patients. Clin Pharmacokinet 1988;14:347.
50. Rudy AC, Brater DC. Pharmacokinetics. In B Chernow (ed), The Pharmacologic Approach to the Critically Ill Patient. Baltimore: Williams & Wilkins, 1994;3.
51. Rudy AC, Brater DC. Drug Interactions. In B Chernow (ed), The Pharmacologic Approach to the Critically Ill Patient. Baltimore: Williams & Wilkins, 1994;18.
52. Bates DW, Spell N, Cullen DJ, et al. The costs of adverse drug events in hospitalized patients. JAMA 1997;277:307.
53. Classen DC, Pestotnik SL, Evans RS, et al. Adverse drug events in hospitalized patients. JAMA 1997;277:301.
54. Mirski MA, Muffelman B, Ulatowski JA, Hanley DF. Sedation for the critically ill neurologic patient. Crit Care Med 1995;23:2038.
55. Burns AM, Shelly MP, Park GR. The use of sedative agents in critically ill patients. Drugs 1992;43:507.
56. Höjer J. Management of benzodiazepine overdose. CNS Drugs 1994;2:7.
57. Greenblatt DJ, Ehrenberg BL, Gunderman J, et al. Kinetic and dynamic study of intravenous lorazepam: comparison with intravenous diazepam. Clin Pharmacol Ther 1989;45:356.
58. Barrientos-Vega R, Sánchez-Soria MM, Morales-Garcia C, et al. Prolonged sedation of critically ill patients with midazolam or propofol: impact on weaning and costs. Crit Care Med 1997;25:33.
59. Ritz R. Benzodiazepine sedation in adult ICU: 1992 patients. Intensive Care Med 1991;17(Suppl 2):73.
60. Durbin CG. Neuromuscular blocking and sedative drugs. Clinical uses and toxic effect in the critical unit. Crit Care Clin 1991;7:489.
61. Bodenham A. Reversal of prolonged sedation using flumazenil in critically ill patients. Anaesthesia 1989;44:603.
62. Chiolero RL, de Tribolet N. Sedatives and antagonists in the management of severely head-injured patients. Acta Neurochir 1992;55(Suppl):43.
63. Hung OL, Hoffman RS. Reversal of opioid intoxication. CNS Drugs 1991;3:176.
64. Ling GSF, Spiegel K, Lockhart SH, et al. Separation of opioid analgesia from respiratory depression. J Pharmacol Exp Ther 1985;232:149.
65. Albanese J, Durbec O, Viviand X, et al. Sufentanil increases intracranial pressure in patients with head trauma. Anesthesiology 1993;79:493.
66. Sperry RJ, Bailey PL, Reichman MV, et al. Fentanyl and sufentanil increase intracranial pressure in head trauma patients. Anesthesiology 1992;77:416.
67 Armstrong PJ, Berston A. Normeperidine toxicity. Anesth Analg 1986;65:536.
68. Mather LE. Clinical pharmacokinetics of fentanyl and its newer derivatives. Clin Pharmacokinet 1983;8:422.
69. Gratz SS, Simpson GM. Neuroleptic malignant syndrome. CNS Drugs 1994;2:429.
70. Caroff SN, Mann SC. Neuroleptic malignant syndrome. Med Clin North Am 1993;77:185.
71. Gurrera RJ. Diaphoresis and dehydration during neuroleptic malignant syndrome: preliminary findings. Psychiatry Res 1996;64:137.
72. Heiman-Patterson TD. Neuroleptic malignant syndrome and malignant hyperthermia. Important issues for the medical consultant. Med Clin North Am 1993;77:477.
73. Harris CE, Grounds RM, Murray AM, et al. Propofol for long-term sedation in the intensive care unit. Anaesthesia 1990;45:366.
74. Farling PA, Johnston JR, Coppel DL. Propofol infusion for sedation of patients with head injuries in intensive care. Anaesthesia 1989;44:22.
75. Herregods L, Verbeke J, Rolly G, et al. Effect of propofol on elevated intracranial pressure. Preliminary results. Anaesthesia 1988;43(Suppl):107.
76. Stephan S, Sonntag H, Schneck HD, et al. Effects of disoprivan on cerebral blood flow, oxygen consumption, and cerebrovascular reactivity. Anaesthetist 1987;36:60.
77. Mackenzie SJ, Kapadia F, Grant IS. Propofol infusion for control of status epilepticus. Anaesthesia 1990;45:1043.
78. Hoyt JW. Persistent paralysis in critically ill patients after the use of neuromuscular blocking agents. New Horiz 1994;2:48.
79. Prielipp RC, Coursin DB. Sedative and neuromuscular blocking drug use in critically ill patients with head injuries. New Horiz 1995;3:456.
80. Prielipp RC, Coursin DB. Applied pharmacology of common neuromuscular blocking agents in critical care. New Horiz 1994;2:34.
81. Isenstein DA, Venner DS, Duggan J. Neuromuscular blockade in the intensive care unit. Chest 1992;102:1258.
82. Bolton CF, Gilbert JJ, Hahn AF, Sibbald WJ. Polyneuropathy in critically ill patients. J Neurol Neurosurgery Psychiatry 1984;47:1223.
83. Wijdicks EFM, Litchy WJ, Harrison BA, Gracey DR. The clinical spectrum of critical illness polyneuropathy. Mayo Clin Proc 1994;69:955.
84. Zochodne DW, Bolton CF, Wells GA, et al. Critical illness polyneuropathy. Brain 1987;110:819.
85. Rudis MI, Guslits BJ, Peterson EL, et al. Economic impact of prolonged motor weakness complicating neuromuscular blockade in the intensive care unit. Crit Care Med 1996;24:1749.
86. Helliwell TR, Coakley JH, Wagenmakers AJM, et al. Necrotizing myopathy in critically-ill patients. J Pathol 1991;164:307.
87. Ramsay DA, Zochodne DW, Robertson DM, et al. A syndrome of acute severe muscle necrosis in intensive care unit patients. J Neuropathol Exp Neurol 1993;52:387.
88. Zochodne DW, Ramsay DA, Saly V, et al. Acute necrotizing myopathy of intensive care: electrophysiological studies. Muscle Nerve 1994;17:285.

89. Moreno E, Gomez SR, Gonzalez I, et al. Neurologic complications in liver transplantation. Acta Neurol Scand 1993;87:25.
90. Platz KP, Mueller AR, Jonas S, et al. Toxicity versus rejection—or why conversions between cyclosporine A and FK506 were performed after liver transplantation. Clin Transplant 1995;9:146.
91. Hauben M. Cyclosporine neurotoxicity. Pharmacotherapy 1996;16:576.
92. Wijdicks EF, Wiesner RH, Krom RA. Neurotoxicity in liver transplant recipients with cyclosporine immunosuppression. Neurology 1995;45:1962.
93. Melamed J, Beaucher WN. Minor symptoms are not predictive of elevated theophylline levels in adults on chronic therapy. Ann Allergy Asthma Immunol 1995;75:516.
94. O'Riordan JI, Hutchinson J, FitzGerald MX, Hutchinson M. Amnesic syndrome after theophylline associated seizures: iatrogenic brain injury. J Neurol Neurosurg Psychiatry 1994;57:643.
95. Rodrigo G, Rodrigo C. Metered dose inhaler salbutamol treatment of asthma in the ED: comparison of two doses with plasma levels. Am J Emerg Med 1996;14:144.
96. Pashko S, Simons WR, Sena MM, Stoddard ML. Rate of exposure to theophylline-drug interactions Clin Ther 1994;16:1068.
97. Siegmund JB, Wilson JH, Imhoff TE. Amiodarone interaction with lidocaine. J Cardiovasc Pharmacol 1993;21:513.
98. Wu FL, Razzaghi A, Souney PF. Seizure after lidocaine for bronchoscopy: case report and review of the use of lidocaine in airway anesthesia. Pharmacotherapy 1993;13:72.
99. Patten SB, Love EJ. Neuropsychiatric adverse drug reactions: passive reports to Health and Welfare Canada's adverse drug reaction database (1965–present). Int J Psychiatry Med 1994;24:45.
100. Dutta SK, Sood R. Clinical Pharmacology of Drugs Used in GI Disorders of Critically Ill Patients. In B Chernow (ed), The Pharmacologic Approach to the Critically Ill Patient. Baltimore: Williams & Wilkins, 1994;614.
101. Masur H. Antimicrobials. In B Chernow (ed), The Pharmacologic Approach to the Critically Ill Patient. Baltimore: Williams & Wilkins, 1994;685.
102. Fernandez-Guardiola A, Martinez A, Fernandez-Mas R. Repeated penicillin-induced amygdala epileptic focus in freely moving cats. EEG, polysomnographic (23-hr recording), and brain mapping study. Epilepsy Res 1995;22:127.
103. Grondahl TO, Langmoen IA. Epileptogenic effect of antibiotic drugs. J Neurosurg 1993;78:938.
104. Ayus JC, Arieff AI. Brain damage and postoperative hyponatremia: the role of gender. Neurology 1996; 46:323.
105. Barletta JP, Fanous MM, Hamed LM. Temporary blindness in the TUR syndrome. J Neuroophthalmol 1994;14:6.
106. Ekengren J, Conner P, Lindholm M, Hahn RG. Fluid absorption during transurethral bladder surgery. Scand J Urol Nephrol 1995;29:519.
107. Seidman DS, Goldenberg M, Mashiach S. Hyponatremic encephalopathy after endometrial ablation. JAMA 1994;271:345.
108. Durlach J, Durlach V, Bac P, et al. Magnesium and therapeutics. Magnes Res 1994;7:313.
109. Ben-Ami M, Giladi Y, Shalev E. The combination of magnesium sulphate and nifedipine: a cause of neuromuscular blockade. Br J Obstet Gynaecol 1994;101:262.
110. Lucas MJ, Leveno KJ, Cunningham FG. A comparison of magnesium sulfate with phenytoin for the prevention of eclampsia. N Engl J Med 1995;333:201.
111. Dwyer K, Barone JE, Rogers JF. Severe hypophosphatemia in postoperative patients. Nutr Clin Pract 1992;7:279.
112. Halevy J, Bulvik S. Severe hypophosphatemia in hospitalized patients. Arch Intern Med 1988;148:153.

Chapter 11

Drug-Induced Cognitive Impairment

Martin R. Farlow and Ann Marie Hake

Objectives

- To recognize those factors that increase risk for cognitive side effects with drug therapy
- To appreciate cholinergic side effects and recognize which drugs are most likely to cause them
- To recognize the potential neurologic complications of opioid therapy
- To learn the criteria that must be met to suggest that dementia or delirium are induced by drugs
- To appreciate which antiepileptic drugs (AEDs) are the most likely to cause cognitive impairment
- To be able to define the "serotonin syndrome" and which drugs are most likely to cause it

Adverse effects of drugs on the central nervous system (CNS) are the most common reversible cause of dementia or delirium in most hospital or clinic-based populations. Drug effects on cognition may be so subtle that they are not readily detectable on examination by the physician, but require more detailed neuropsychological testing for their recognition, as is sometimes seen in pediatric seizure patients taking AEDs on a long-term basis. At the other end of the spectrum, dementia or delirium in an elderly patient is usually much more apparent to the examining physician. Just 12% of the population in the United States is older than age 65, but this segment consumes more than 30% of all prescription drugs.[1] In addition, age-related changes in concentration and distribution of drugs occur in the elderly and are related to the following factors: reduced serum albumin, reduced glomerular filtration rate causing decreased urinary clearance, and reduced metabolism related to decreased hepatic function. All of these changes make this population more susceptible to adverse drug effects. Many elderly also have increased CNS sensitivity to drug effects.[2, 3] Given these vulnerabilities, it is not surprising that delirium has been estimated to be present in at least 10% of the elderly population at admission to the hospital for treatment of a medical illness, and another 15% of patients may develop it during their hospital stay.[4] A study of 325 elderly patients admitted to a teaching hospital found that 10% had delirium at admission and another 31% developed it during their hospitalization.[5] Only 4% of these patients totally resolved their delirious symptoms and signs during their inpatient stay, and only 18% had resolved all of their cognitive deficits within 6 months of discharge from the hospital. Preexisting dementia or cognitive impairment was a major risk factor for developing delirium in this study and in another large study of dementia and delirium involving 2,000 consecutive medical inpatients.[6] In this second study, it was estimated that 25% of newly diagnosed delirious patients had preexisting dementia. Delirium has been associated with longer durations of stay for patients in the hospital and correlated with an increased mortality, particularly in the elderly, although greater severity of coexisting medical illnesses in these patients may partially explain their increased death rate.[7]

Use of the diagnoses of dementia and delirium is often blurred in clinical practice, and some patients may be inappropriately labeled. The term *dementia* should be used to characterize a patient who has multiple cognitive deficits including memory impairment and at least one of the following: aphasia, apraxia, agnosia, or disturbance in executive functioning. These deficits usually develop slowly over weeks or months and impair occupational or social functioning.[4] Dementia, secondary to use of a medication, implies that the deficits persist well after withdrawal of the drug. When a drug is stopped, if the deficits immediately clear, the diagnosis should more appropriately be labeled as a substance intoxication.

In contrast, the term *delirium* refers to a more acute change in mental status, possibly fluctuating, that evolves over hours to days. Delirium also involves a disturbance of consciousness with reduced awareness and or impaired attention as well as cognitive deficits, including memory impairment, disorientation, language dysfunction, or perceptual disorders. There may be illusions, hallucinations, and or sleep-wake disturbances. For both drug-induced dementia and delirium, there should be evidence from the clinical history, physical examination, and laboratory studies to suggest that these conditions are etiologically related to one or more medications.[4] A history should be obtained from a friend or family member to document symptoms suggestive of cognitive impairment and whether the time course suggests it is drug-induced. Physical and neurologic examinations should be performed to document patients' impairment in cognitive functions, consciousness, and deficits in their ability to function in the activities of daily living. Laboratory studies should be undertaken to screen for other potential causes of impairment, such as infection or sepsis, metabolic disturbances, endocrine or other systemic diseases, decreased perfusion or hypoxia, and intracranial processes.

Dementia and delirium are often readily diagnosed, but the potential for multiple (often concurrent) etiologies provides a challenge to the treating physician who must sort through other probable causes for these conditions, including sepsis, metabolic disturbance, and environmental change (hospital psychosis), in order to provide optimal care.[4] Drug-induced delirium or dementia is suggested if the following criteria are met: (1) The drug in question has CNS effects; (2) the time course of the mental status change correlates with the period of drug administration; and (3) there is improvement with dosage reduction or cessation of use of the presumed offending drug.[7]

The major culprits and the relative frequency of adverse cognitive side effects for different classes of drugs are continuously changing as newer medications are introduced and older drugs fall out of favor in common clinical practice. What follows is a description of the major classes and some of the individual drugs that are often offenders.

Cardiovascular Drugs and Antihypertensive Agents

Most antihypertensive medications, in at least some patients, have been reported to cause cognitive side effects, including drowsiness, decreased memory, and impaired concentration or learning. Most available data are from case reports or small studies: There are few large randomized studies, and the overall cognitive impact of these medications is not well defined. Indeed, several meta-analyses of smaller studies have suggested no overall statistically significant impairment of cognitive function with any of the antihypertensive agents.[8,9] Clearly, however, some individuals have had adverse cognitive effects that have resolved after withdrawal of an antihypertensive drug. This occurs more frequently with centrally acting sympathomimetic drugs.[10]

Alpha-Adrenergic Receptor Blockers

Sedation and confusion are well recognized side effects of alpha-blockers, occurring in up to 60% of patients in some studies.[11] This is especially true with the centrally acting agents such as methyldopa, clonidine, and guanabenz. Confusion is also seen with the postganglionic agents reserpine and guanethidine. Reserpine has been reported to cause depression, which can sometimes be severe.[12]

Beta-Adrenergic Receptor Blockers

In patients treated with beta-blockers, complaints of somnolence and fatigue are common. Numerous case reports have noted confusion or memory problems, especially in elderly patients, that have improved after withdrawal of the beta-adrenergic blocking agent.[11] Some studies have suggested that mild cognitive impairment is more likely to occur in patients taking beta-blockers compared with other antihypertensives, particularly calcium channel blockers and angiotensin-converting enzyme inhibitors.[11, 13] However, no statistically significant differences in cognitive function were seen with the use of beta-blockers in a large longitudinal study of an aged population,[14] several double-blind placebo-controlled trials,[15–18] and meta-analysis of several smaller trials.[9] It has also been suggested that lipophilic beta-blockers, which cross the blood-brain barrier more readily than their hydrophilic counterparts, are more likely to cause cognitive side effects. This was not borne out, however, in a randomized double-blind crossover trial using atenolol and propranolol in 42 veterans[19] or in a review of 55 earlier studies.[20]

Calcium Channel Blockers

Adverse cognitive effects are not common in patients taking calcium channel blockers. Some studies have shown mild impairment in memory and learning detectable with neuropsychological testing in patients taking nifedipine but not with use of other calcium channel blockers.[18–21]

Diuretics

Treatment with diuretics may cause metabolic imbalances. The most common type of electrolyte disturbance to alter mental status is hyponatremia; patients may develop confusion when the plasma sodium levels decrease to 128 mEq per liter or less.[22] Hypokalemia is also common with diuretic use and may cause muscle weakness; however, CNS effects are uncommon, and their presence suggests a concomitant acid-base disturbance.[11]

Angiotensin-Converting Enzyme Inhibitors

Adverse cognitive effects from angiotensin-converting enzyme inhibitors are unusual. There is some evidence that these medications may mildly improve levels of alertness.[23]

Lidocaine

The class Ib antiarrhythmics, including lidocaine, mexiletine, tocainide, and aprindine, have all been reported to cause the following CNS side effects: nervousness, somnolence, hallucinations, and confusion. Similar adverse drug effects can also be seen with antiarrhythmics from other classes, including flecainide, bretylium, and amiodarone.[10]

Cardiac Glycosides

Digitalis and the other cardiac glycosides can occasionally cause delirium, which is more likely to occur under the following conditions: supratherapeutic blood levels, in elderly patients, and with hypokalemia, hypomagnesemia, hypercalcemia, or renal insufficiency.[10]

Quinidine

Toxicity of quinidine may produce difficulty speaking, confusion, and agitation or somnolence in some patients. Dementia has also been described. In one report, a woman who had been taking quinidine for 14 years developed a severe, progressive dementia over the course of several years. Her mental status returned to normal within a month of discontinuing the drug.[24]

Disopyramide

This antiarrhythmic has anticholinergic effects that may cause deficits in short-term memory in the elderly. This drug may also exacerbate Alzheimer's disease or unmask prodromal Alzheimer's disease in elderly patients who had not been previously symptomatic.[10]

Glucocorticoids

Up to 15% of patients on high dosages[3] (60 mg prednisone or equivalent per day) of corticosteroids may develop mental status changes ranging from hyperactivity and emotional lability to inattentiveness and confusion to frank psychosis. These symptoms are relieved by withdrawal of the corticosteroid medication, although complete resolution may take several weeks.[25] A separate syndrome of corticosteroid-induced dementia has also been described. In one report of six patients, significant disturbances of memory, attention, and occupational performance developed over a period of several weeks after initiation of corticosteroids. Two of these patients had recovered from an earlier corticosteroid psychosis; the other four had no previous cognitive or psychiatric symptoms. All recovered normal cognitive functions with discontinuation of the medication. A study of 24 women and one man taking low-dose chronic prednisone at dosages of 5–40 mg per day versus 25 matched controls revealed decrements in paragraph recall, a test of explicit memory.[26] Multiple regression analysis suggested that advanced age was a significant covariant that predicted greater dysfunction in memory for patients treated with prednisone.

Analgesics

Salicylates and Nonsteroidal Anti-Inflammatory Drugs

Ingestion of toxic doses of most drugs in this class can cause encephalopathy related to acid-base and or other metabolic imbalances. One case has been reported of a 72-year-old man who presented with encephalopathy and was ultimately found to have refractory hypoglycemia secondary to a topical salicylate.[27]

Opioids

These analgesic medications commonly affect mental status, even at therapeutic dosages. In this range, somnolence and psychomotor slowing commonly occur. With intoxication, the patient develops unresponsiveness, slow and shallow respirations, pinpoint pupils, bradycardia, and hypothermia. With severe intoxication, mydriasis may occur. Respiratory failure may result in death, and survivors may be left with an anoxic encephalopathy. Intoxication usually responds promptly and dramatically to the administration of naloxone: Failure of the patient to improve should raise doubts regarding the diagnosis of opioid intoxication. Opioid withdrawal, which can be precipitated by naloxone, produces restlessness and agitation in addition to sweating, shivering, yawning, piloerection, abdominal cramping, diarrhea, nausea, and vomiting.[28]

Antiepileptic Drugs

AEDs interact with cellular surface receptors or channels in the CNS to increase the threshold that must be crossed before seizures occur. Because the primary actions of AEDs are in the CNS, it is not surprising that many of these drugs produce subtle or occasionally more severe cognitive changes in treated patients. Most AEDs taken in their usual dosages cause little clinically apparent impairment of cognition in either children or adults.[29] However, some investigations using sensitive neuropsychological instruments do show decrements in cognitive function even for patients with AED blood levels in the therapeutic range. A study of 83 patients with chronic seizures on monotherapy using various AEDs used 12 computerized cognitive tests to evaluate for adverse effects of these medications. Patients were then taken off medication for at least 3 months and reevaluated. Changes in cognition were compared with testing in 83 matched controls. Overall, the epilepsy group on AEDs performed worse, but they did improve when taken off medication.[30] At higher blood levels all AEDs can produce global impairments in higher cortical function (encephalopathy), as well as cerebellar and brain stem signs.

Phenobarbital

This drug has been widely used to treat seizures for decades and is known to cause dose-related sedation. Three double-blind controlled trials have suggested that cognitive functions are mildly impaired by phenobarbital in epileptic children.[31–33] A double-blind, randomized crossover study with 59 healthy volunteers, comparing phenobarbital, diphenylhydantoin, and valproic acid, found that phenobarbital caused significantly greater impairment in cognitive functions as documented by poorer performance on 17 of 22 neuropsychological tests.[34] Phenobarbital has been shown to cause specific deficits in attention, reaction time, and short-term memory.[34, 35]

Diphenylhydantoin

Little disturbance of cognitive function is reported in most children and adults treated with diphenylhydantoin. In a study of 50 patients with seizures treated with diphenylhydantoin, however, neuropsychological testing demonstrated decreased motor and information processing speeds, but no differences in memory or attention.[36] Another study found that adult patients on diphenylhydantoin had impaired short-term memory, but normal functioning in other cognitive domains.[37] Diphenylhydantoin has been reported to cause encephalopathy or cause a clinical picture that mimics a neurodegenerative disorder.[38, 39]

Carbamazepine

Increased blood levels of carbamazepine have not been demonstrated to correlate with decreased cognitive functions.[40] Indeed, in an open parallel group trial of carbamazepine versus phenytoin monotherapy in 50 seizure patients, cognitive functions were consistently superior in patients treated with carbamazepine.[36] However, carbamazepine can cause hyponatremia, with Na^+ levels of less than 120 mEq per liter causing generalized impairment in cognitive function to frank encephalopathy.[41, 42]

Valproic Acid

With low doses of this drug, studies of normal volunteers have found slight sedation and impaired decision making, but improved vigilance.[43] Occasionally, valproic acid can cause marked sedation. Stupor has been reported to occur in patients treated with valproic acid associated with isolated increased levels of blood ammonia. A 21-year-old patient treated with valproate had documented declining cognitive abilities over 3 years and was diagnosed with dementia. Seven weeks after valproate was discontinued, there was dramatic improvement in all of this patient's cognitive functions.[44]

Vigabatrin, Lamotrigine, Gabapentin, and Felbamate

Vigabatrin, lamotrigine, gabapentin, and felbamate are newer AEDs that have been studied, for the most part, as add-on therapy to other AEDs in the treatment of refractory epilepsy. It is therefore difficult to know if there are specific therapy-related deficits in cognition with these drugs.[45] One double-blind, placebo-controlled crossover study of vigabatrin or placebo added to other AEDs demonstrated, using a neuropsychological test battery, no significant difference in cognitive function in patients between vigabatrin and placebo therapy.[46]

Sedatives and Hypnotics

Barbiturates

Although the use of barbiturates as sedative drugs has declined greatly in recent years, these medications are still commonly used for treatment of epilepsy, headache, spastic bowel disease, and general anesthesia. Ingestion of barbiturates produces varying degrees of somnolence, from mild drowsiness to coma, depending on the dose and patient tolerance. Intoxication with a barbiturate is similar clinically to alcohol intoxication: The patient's thinking is slowed, and he or she develops emotional lability, ataxia, incoordination, dysarthria, and nystagmus. Acute withdrawal can precipitate nervousness, insomnia, tremor, seizures, or delirium tremens indistinguishable from that seen with alcohol withdrawal.[28]

Long-term use of phenobarbital as an anticonvulsant in children has been associated with a mild reduction in intelligence quotient compared with children not receiving barbiturates,[33, 47] although other studies have shown no significant cognitive effect from phenobarbital in children.[48] Cognitive deficits have also been detected in adults on this medication compared with other anticonvulsants.[49, 50] These effects are generally reduced on withdrawal of the medication.[50]

Benzodiazepines

In a 1987 study, benzodiazepines were found to be the most common cause of cognitive impairment in a group of 300 elderly patients.[51] Similarly, a 1995 prospective study found that benzodiazepine use was the cause of delirium in 29% of patients who developed mental status changes in the hospital.[52] Like the barbiturates, benzodiazepines produce somnolence, confusion, and unsteady gait, although to a lesser degree than barbiturates. Memory loss is also frequently seen; this occurs for events occurring before or at the time of ingestion (anterograde amnesia) and is more likely in older patients, with intravenous administration, or in patients with hepatic dysfunction.[53] Triazolam and lorazepam are particularly prone to produce amnesia and are sometimes used for this purposely for painful or traumatic procedures.[28] Sedation can be reversed by the administration of flumazenil, but amnesia is less completely reversed.[54] Acute withdrawal of benzodiazepines may produce anxiety, tremor, or occasionally seizures, but true addiction or dependence is much less common for benzodiazepines than for alcohol, barbiturates, or opioids.[28]

Psychotropic Medications

Antidepressants

Cognitive changes, including memory deficits and delirium, have been reported with all of the antidepressants. Of the agents currently in common use, tricyclic antidepressants have the highest incidence of cognitive side effects.[55–57] This is related mainly to their anticholinergic effects.[10, 58] The memory and sedation effects of tricyclic antidepressants are, in general, dose related,[59–61] although there have been reports of delirium in dosages in the lower therapeutic range as well.[62] Hypnagogic and hypnopompic hallucinations in the absence of delirium have also been observed.[63] Monoamine oxidase (MAO) inhibitors, especially tranylcypromine, also can cause delirium.[10] In addition, precipitous withdrawal of MAO inhibitors can provoke delirium with severe anxiety, agitation, hallucinations, and paranoid delusions.[64] The newer antidepressants, including trazodone, bupropion, and the selective serotonin reuptake inhibitors, also produce sedation in some patients[65] but to a much lesser degree than the tricyclic antidepressants.[66, 67] Memory is not affected to a significant degree by these drugs.[68] There have been some reports of delirium in bulimic patients taking trazodone.[69] A potentially life-threatening side effect associated with the serotonergic antidepressants is the "serotonin syndrome." This is a clinical syndrome consisting of mental status changes, restlessness, myoclonus, hyperreflexia, hypertension, fever, chills, and diarrhea. It occurs most often during treatment with selective serotonin reuptake inhibitors and MAO inhibitors, administered either together or in close succession.[70–72] The serotonin syndrome has also been reported in patients taking amitriptyline, as well as with the combination of trazodone and buspirone.[73, 74]

Lithium

Delirium secondary to lithium therapy is most often due to toxic serum levels (more than 1.5–2.0 mEq per liter).[28] This can occur with overdose or concomitant administration of nonsteroidal anti-inflammatory drugs or neuroleptics.[75–78] Delirium has also been reported with therapeutic serum levels of lithium.[79] Lithium-induced hypothyroidism is also a potential cause for alteration of mental status.[80]

Antipsychotics

Delirium has been reported with all of the drugs in this class and is more likely to occur with the more sedating, anticholinergic drugs such as thioridazine and chlorpromazine.[10] Clozapine, a newer antipsychotic medication with fewer extrapyramidal side effects than the older antipsychotics, has relatively strong anticholinergic effects. In one case report, two patients on this drug required administration of physostigmine to reverse anticholinergic delirium.[81]

Anti-Parkinsonian Drug Therapy

Cognitive deficits and or delirium related to antiparkinsonian drug therapy occur much more commonly in the latter stages of this illness.[82] Patients are often treated with combinations of drugs given in escalating dosage regimens until adverse motor effects, disorientation, hallucinations, and cognitive deficits occur. All anti-parkinsonian drugs can cause delirium. Trihexyphenidyl, benztropine, diphenhydramine, and amantadine at therapeutic doses can all cause delirium (see the section on anticholinergic drugs). Levodopa and carbidopa, bromocriptine, and pergolide are dopaminergic agents that can impair cognition and cause hallucinations.[83] Infection, fever, dehydration, or electrolyte imbalance in combination with excessive intake of other centrally active drugs, including antidepressants, sedatives, and anxiolytics, can precipitate delirium.[84] The hallucinations associated with levodopa and carbidopa therapy can be treated with clozapine in low dosages (10–30 mg per day), but this does not improve cognitive decline or dementia.[85] During the 14 months of the DATATOP multicenter trial involving more than 800 patients with early Parkinson's disease, the group treated with selegiline (a selective MAO-B inhibitor) showed no change in cognition as measured during regular prospective assessments.[86] In patients with advanced Parkinson's disease selegiline can precipitate hallucinations and confusion.

Anticholinergics

Medications whose principal actions are anticholinergic as well as drugs in which anticholinergic effects are secondary and less prominent are both well recognized to cause deficits in memory, particularly in elderly patients with preexisting early amnestic syndromes or dementia. Additional clinical signs in these patients that suggest anticholinergic effects include dry mouth, urinary retention, pupillary dilation, restlessness, euphoria, irritability, confusion, delusions, or frank hallucinations.[87]

Typical scenarios in which anticholinergic adverse reactions may occur include oxybutynin in elderly men with urinary incontinence, benztropine in patients with Parkinson's disease, hydroxyzine or hyoscyamine (Levsin) in patients with gastrointestinal disturbances, and meclizine or scopolamine in patients with dizziness or motion sickness. The effects of scopolamine have been investigated in normal volunteers, and it was demonstrated using a battery of tests measuring various aspects of memory and information processing that the drug impairs immediate recall but not delayed recall.[88] Another placebo-controlled study of scopolamine in six elderly patients demonstrated that scopolamine impaired episodic but not autobiographical memory.[89]

Tricyclic antidepressants are now less commonly used for depression in elderly patients but may be used at higher dosages for headache or pain management. Amitriptyline, doxepin, and imipramine have prominent secondary anticholinergic effects and, in some patients, cause sedation and impair memory. Trihexyphenidyl and benztropine are often used in combination with antipsychotic drugs such as chlorpromazine and thioridazine to minimize akathisia. Additive anticholinergic effects often cause impairment in memory, particularly in the elderly and those with diseases that are already affecting the brain diffusely.

Recently, it has been reported that the use of selective serotonin reuptake inhibitors in conjunction with antipsychotics and benztropine appeared to cause delirium in five patients.[90] Multiple concomitant medications increase the likelihood that drugs with anticholinergic effects will cause memory impairment or delirium. In all cases of anticholinergic delirium, dosage reduction or cessation of the suspected drug is appropriate treatment.

H_2-Receptor Antagonists

All H_2 blockers have the potential to cause cognitive impairment and or delirium. Adverse effects generally occur within the first 2 weeks of therapy and resolve within 3 days after the drug is stopped. The incidence of clinically significant cognitive impairment has been estimated at 0.2% for outpatients to 1.6% or greater for medical inpatients.[91] Of this class, cimetidine is most frequently associated with delirium. The incidence of neuropsychiatric complications with ranitidine is probably substantially less than 1%.[92] Delirium is rare with famotidine but has been reported in six hospitalized patients whose symptoms cleared completely after the drug was stopped.[93] In a double-blind, randomized trial, 28 healthy volunteers were treated with placebo, cimetidine, or ranitidine, 150 mg given twice daily for 2 weeks. Subjects were then given single doses of the benzodiazepine midazolam at the end of the first and second weeks, after which they were evaluated with neuropsychological testing. The cimetidine group had significantly increased cognitive impairment ($P < .05$), suggesting an adverse interaction may exist between cimetidine and the benzodiazepines.[94]

Antibiotics

Most of the antibiotic drugs do not adversely affect the CNS. When cognitive side effects do occur with antibiotic therapy, they are often accompanied by headache or somnolence. Rifampin can cause headache, dizziness, drowsiness, inability to concentrate, and confusion.[95] Trimethoprim-sulfamethoxazole can cause confusion associated with antibiotic-induced aseptic meningitis.[96–98] Metronidazole can cause confusion, irritability, depression, and headache, as well as unusual metallic phantogeusia.[99] Clioquinol use has caused several cases of acute but completely reversible global amnestic syndrome.[100, 101]

Antineoplastics

Intrathecal administration of methotrexate on rare occasions causes a progressive encephalopathy that occurs within a few days after administration. However, encephalopathy accompanied by ataxia, drowsiness, and fever has been reported 2 weeks after intrathecal administration of methotrexate.[102] Late toxicity may develop 2–6 months after treatment. Patients present with lethargy and ataxia, followed by progressive dementia. Magnetic resonance imaging demonstrates leukoencephalopathy.[103] Children treated with methotrexate combined with radiation therapy have shown poor school performance, behavioral disturbance, and memory loss and on magnetic resonance imaging exhibit atrophy and or leukoencephalopathy.[104]

5-Fluorouracil, cytosine arabinoside, thymidine, asparaginase, mitotane, and fludarabine have been reported to cause diffuse encephalopathy.

Nitrogen mustard is still occasionally used in treatment regimens for Hodgkin's disease, other lymphomas, and lung or ovarian tumors. High-dose administration of this drug has caused encephalopathy with hallucinations accompanied by seizures and drowsiness.[105]

In high dosages, ifosfamide commonly causes acute but reversible encephalopathy, often accompanied by seizures and extrapyramidal features. Vincristine does not cross the blood-brain barrier but can cause syndrome of inappropriate antidiuretic hormone secretion and secondarily, encephalopathy.[106]

Treatment with alpha-interferons at high dosages can cause reversible encephalopathy.[107, 108]

Administered intravenously, interleukin 2 has caused acute fatal leukoencephalopathy.[109]

In general, many of the antineoplastic drugs given intrathecally at high dosage are more prone to cause an acute encephalopathy. Similarly, symptoms are occasionally seen with drugs that cross the blood-brain barrier when administered at high dosages intravenously. Cognitive declines are frequently transient and reversible. Dementia appears months or years after treatment, and magnetic resonance imaging shows atrophy or leukoencephalopathy. When dementia appears, it is most often irreversible.

Conclusion

Dementia or delirium are common complications occurring during treatment with several different classes of medications. These disorders are more prone to occur in elderly patients with multiple systemic illnesses and diffuse or degenerative brain diseases. Drugs suspected of altering mental status should be stopped if medically possible or reduced to the lowest possible therapeutic dosages.

In populations at risk for cognitive impairment, it is advisable to avoid anticholinergics, narcotics, and benzodiazepines. Drugs known to be centrally active should be initiated at the lowest dosage possible and increased cautiously to minimize the potential for adverse cognitive effects. Drugs with short half-lives should be used whenever possible to minimize drug accumulation. Polypharmacy should be avoided to decrease the potential for unexpected drug interactions. Drug schedules should be kept simple, particularly in elderly patients, to minimize the potential for accidental overdose. The treating physician should remain vigilant to the possibility of cognitive impairment during chronic therapy by periodically assessing cognitive status and, if there are deficits, adjusting therapy as necessary to minimize drug-related cognitive dysfunction.

References

1. Lowenthal DT, Nafdeau SE. Drug-induced dementia. South Med J 1991;84(Suppl 1):S24.
2. Dawling S, Crome P. Clinical pharmacokinetic considerations in the elderly: an update. Clin Pharmacokinet 1989;17:236.
3. Lipowski ZJ. Delirium in the elderly patient. N Engl J Med 1989;320:578.
4. American Psychiatric Association. Diagnostic and Statistical Manual of Mental Disorders (4th ed). Washington, DC: American Psychiatric Association, 1994;123.
5. Levkoff SE, Evans DA, Liptzin B, et al. Delirium: the occurrence and persistence of symptoms among elderly hospitalized patients. Arch Intern Med 1992;152:334.
6. Erkinjuntti T, Wikström J, Palo J, Autio L. Dementia among medical inpatients: evaluation of 2000 consecutive admissions. Arch Intern Med 1986;146:1923.
7. Francis J, Martin D, Kapoor WN. A prospective study of delirium in hospitalized elderly. JAMA 1990; 263:1097.
8. Muldoon MF, Manuck SB, Shapiro AP, Waldstein SR. Neurobehavioral effects of antihypertensive medications. J Hypertension 1991;9:549.
9. Beto JA, Bansal VK. Quality of life in treatment of hypertension. A metaanalysis of clinical trials. Am J Hypertension 1992;5:125.
10. Bowen JD, Larson EB. Drug-induced cognitive impairment: defining the problem and finding solutions. Drugs Aging 1993;3:349.
11. Markus HS. Cardiovascular Drugs. In FA Wolff (ed), Handbook of Clinical Neurology (Vol. 65). Amsterdam: Elsevier, 1995;433.
12. Webster J, Koch HF. Aspects of tolerability of centrally acting antihypertensive drugs. J Cardiovasc Pharmacol 1996;27(Suppl 3):S49.
13. Lichter I, Richardson PJ, Wyke MA. Differential effects of atenolol and enalapril on memory during treatment for essential hypertension. Br J Clin Pharmacol 1986;21:641.
14. Wurzelman J, Frishman WH, Aronson M, et al. Neuropsychological effects of antihypertensive drugs. Cardiol Clin 1987;5:689.
15. Steiner SS, Friedhoff AJ, Wilson BL, et al. Antihypertensive therapy and quality of life: a comparison of atenolol, captopril, enalapril and propranolol. J Hum Hypertension 1990;4:217.
16. Deary IJ, Capewell S, Hajducka C, Muir AL. The effects of captopril vs atenolol on memory, information processing and mood: a double-blind crossover study. Br J Clin Pharmacol 1991;23:347.
17. Dimsdale JE, Newton RP. Cognitive effects of beta blockers. J Psychosom Res 1992;36:229.
18. Skinner MH, Futterman A, Morrissette D, et al. Atenolol compared with nifedipine: effect on cognitive function and mood in elderly hypertensive patients. Ann Intern Med 1992;116:615.
19. Palac DM, Cornish RD, McDonald WJ, et al. Cognitive function in hypertensives treated with atenolol or propranolol. J Gen Intern Med 1990;5:310.
20. Dimsdale JE, Newton RP, Joist T. Neuropsychological side effects of beta blockers. Arch Intern Med 1989;149:514.
21. Fletcher AE, Bulpitt CJ. Quality of life in the treatment of hypertension. The effect of calcium antagonists. Drugs 1992;44(Suppl 1):135.
22. Arieff AI, Llach F, Massrey SG. Neurological manifestations and morbidity of hyponatremia: correlation with brain water and electrolytes. Medicine 1976;55:121.
23. Bulpitt CJ, Fletcher AE. Cognitive function and angiotensin-converting enzyme inhibitors in comparison to other antihypertensive drugs. J Cardiovasc Pharmacol 1992;19(Suppl 6):S100.
24. Gilbert GJ. Quinidine dementia. JAMA 1977;237:2093.
25. Varney NR, Alexander B, MacIndoe JH. Reversible steroid dementia in patients without steroid psychosis. Am J Psychiatry 1984;141:369.
26. Keenan PA, Jacobson MW, Soleymani MA, et al. The effect on memory of chronic prednisone treatment in patients with systemic disease. Neurology 1996;47:1396.
27. Raschke R, Arnold-Capell PA, Richeson R, et al. Refractory hypoglycemia secondary to topical salicylate intoxication. Arch Intern Med 1991;151:591.
28. Adams RD, Victor M, Ropper AH. Principles of Neurology (6th ed). New York: McGraw-Hill, 1997.
29. Aldenkamp AP, Alpherts WCJ, Blennow G, et al. Withdrawal of antiepileptic medication in children—effects on cognitive function: the multicenter Homfrid study. Neurology 1993;43:41.
30. Tonnby B, Nilsson HL, Aldenkamp AP, et al. Withdrawal of antiepileptic medication in children, correlation of cognitive function and plasma concentration—the multicentre "Holmfrid" study. Epilepsy Research 1994;19:141.
31. Camfield CS, Chaplin S, Doyle AB, et al. Side effects of phenobarbital in toddlers; behavioral and cognitive aspects. J Pediatr 1979;95:361.

32. Farwell JR, Lee YJ, Hirtz DG, et al. Phenobarbital for febrile seizures—effects on intelligence and seizure recurrence. N Engl J Med 1990;322:364.
33. Vining EPG, Mellits ED, Dorsen MM, et al. Psychological and behavioral effects of antiepileptic drugs in children: a double-blind comparison between phenobarbital and valproic acid. Pediatrics 1987;80:165.
34. Meador KJ, Loring DW, Nichols ME, et al. Comparative cognitive effects of phenobarbital, phenytoin, and valproate in healthy adults. Neurology 1994;44(Suppl 2):A322.
35. MacLeod CM, Dekaban AS, Hunt E. Memory impairment in epileptic patients: selective effects of phenobarbital concentration. Science 1978;202:1102.
36. Aldenkamp AP, Alpherts WCJ, Diepman L, et al. Cognitive side-effects of phenytoin compared with carbamazepine in patients with localization-related epilepsy. Epilepsy Research 1994;19:37.
37. Gillham RA, Williams N, Wiedmann KD, et al. Cognitive function in adult epileptics established on anticonvulsant monotherapy. Epilepsy Research 1990;7:219.
38. Vallharta JM, Bell DB, Reichert A. Progressive encephalopathy due to chronic hydantoin intoxication. Am J Dis Child 1974;128:27.
39. Logan WJ, Freeman JM. Pseudodegenerative disease due to diphenylhydantoin intoxication. Arch Neurol 1969;21:361.
40. Aman MG, Werry JS, Paxton JW, et al. Effects of carbamazepine on psychomotor performance in children as a function of drug concentration, seizure type, and time of medication. Epilepsia 1990;31:51.
41. Pendlebury SC, Moses DK, Eadie MJ. Hyponatraemia during oxcarbazepine therapy. Hum Toxicol 1989; 8:337.
42. Steinhoff BJ, Stoll KD, Stodieck SR, Paulus W. Hyponatraemic coma under oxcarbazepine therapy. Epilepsy Research 1992;11:67.
43. Betts TA, Crowe A, Alford C. Psychotropic effects of sodium valproate. Br J Clin Pract 1982;18(Suppl):145.
44. Zaret BS, Cohen RA. Reversible valproic acid-induced dementia: a case report. Epilepsia 1986;27:234.
45. Timmings PL, Richens A. Neurotoxicology of Antiepileptic Drugs. In FA Wolff (ed), Handbook of Clinical Neurology (Vol 65). Amsterdam: Elsevier, 1995;495.
46. Gillham RA, Blacklaw J, Mckee PJ, et al. Effect of vigabatrin on sedation and cognitive function in patients with refractory epilepsy. J Neurol Neurosurg Psychiatry 1993;56:1271.
47. Calandre EP, Domingue-Granados R, Gomez-Rubio M, Molina-Font JA. Cognitive effects of long-term treatment with phenobarbital and valproic acid in school children. Acta Neurologica Scand 1990;81:504.
48. Meador KJ, Loring DW, Huh K, et al. Comparative cognitive effects of anticonvulsants. Neurology 1990;40:391.
49. Wolf SM, Forsythe A, Stunden AA, et al. Long-term effect of phenobarbital on cognitive function in children with febrile convulsions. Pediatrics 1981;68:820.
50. Meador KJ, Loring DW, Nichols ME, et al. Comparative cognitive effects of phenobarbital, phenytoin, and valproate in healthy adults. Neurology 1995;45:1494.
51. Larson EB, Kukull WA, Buchner D, Reifler BV. Adverse drug reactions associated with global cognitive impairment in elderly persons. Ann Intern Med 1987;107:169.
52. Foy A, O'Connell D, Henry D, et al. Benzodiazepine use as a cause of cognitive impairment in elderly hospital inpatients. J Gerontology 1995;50A:M99.
53. Lader M. Hypnotics and Sedatives. In FA Wolff (ed), Handbook of Clinical Neurology (Vol. 65). Amsterdam: Elsevier, 1995;329.
54. Flumazenil in Intravenous Conscious Sedation Study Group I. Reversal of conscious sedation with midazolam: report of a multicenter clinical study. Clin Ther 1992;14:861.
55. Bye C, Clubley M, Peck AW. Drowsiness, impaired performance and tricyclic antidepressants drugs. Br J Clin Pharmacol 1978;6:155.
56. Branconnier RJ, Cole JO, Ghazvinian S, et al. Clinical pharmacology of bupropion and imipramine in elderly depressives. J Clin Psychiatry 1983;44:130.
57. Spring B, Gelenberg AJ, Garvin R, Thompson S. Amitriptyline, clovoxamine and cognitive function: a placebo-controlled comparison in depressed outpatients. Psychopharmacology 1992;108:327.
58. Oxman TE. Antidepressants and cognitive impairment in the elderly. J Clin Psychiatry 1996;57(Suppl 5):38.
59. Young RC, Mattis S, Alexopoulos GS, et al. Verbal memory and plasma drug concentrations in elderly depressives treated with nortriptyline. Psychopharm Bull 1991;27:291.
60. Lejoyeux M, Rouillon F, Ades J, Gorwood P. Neural symptoms induced by tricyclic antidepressants: phenomenology and pathophysiology. Acta Psychiatry Scand 1992;85:249.
61. Engel PA. Treatment of progressive supranuclear palsy with amitriptyline: therapeutic and toxic effects. J Am Geriatr Soc 1996;44:1072.
62. Godwin CD. Case report of tricyclic-induced delirium at a therapeutic drug concentration. Am J Psychiatry 1983;140:1517.
63. Hemmingsen R, Rafaelsen OJ. Hypnagogic and hypnopompic hallucinations during amitriptyline treatment. Acta Psychiatry Scand 1980;62:364.
64. Dilsaver SC. Monoamine oxidase inhibitor withdrawal phenomena: symptoms and pathophysiology. Acta Psychiatry Scand 1988;78:1.
65. Langemark M, Olesen J. Sulpiride and paroxetine in the treatment of chronic tension-type headache. An explanatory double-blind trial. Headache 1994;34:20.
66. Burns M, Moskowitz H, Jaffe J. A comparison of the effects of trazodone and amitriptyline on skills perfor-

mance by geriatric subjects. J Clin Psychiatry 1986;47:252.
67. Dunbar GC. Paroxetine in the elderly: a comparative meta-analysis against standard antidepressant pharmacotherapy. Pharmacology 1995;51:137.
68. Fudge JL, Perry PJ, Garvey MJ, Kelly MW. A comparison of the effect of fluoxetine and trazodone on the cognitive functioning of depressed outpatients. J Affect Disord 1990;18:275.
69. Damlouji NF, Ferguson JM. Trazodone-induced delerium in bulimic patients. Am J Psychiatry 1984; 141:434.
70. Feighner JP, Boyer WF, Tyler DL, Neborsky RJ. Adverse consequences of fluoxetine-MAOI combination therapy. J Clin Psychiatry 1990;51:222.
71. Sternbach H. The serotonin syndrome. Am J Psychiatry 1991;148:705.
72. Martin TG. Serotonin syndrome. Ann Emerg Med 1996;28:520.
73. Miyaoka H, Kamijima K. Encephalopathy during amitriptyline therapy: are neuroleptic malignant syndrome and serotonin syndrome spectrum disorders? Int Clin Psychopharmacol 1995;10:265.
74. Goldberg RJ, Huk M. Serotonin syndrome from trazodone and buspirone. Psychosomatics 1992;33:235.
75. Herschberg SN, Sierles FS. Indomethacin-induced lithium toxicity. Am Fam Physician 1983;28:155.
76. Spring GK. Neurotoxicity with combined use of lithium and thioridazine. J Clin Psychiatiatry 1979; 40:135.
77. Miller F, Menninger J, Whitcup SM. Lithium-neuroleptic neurotoxicity in the elderly bipolar patient. J Clin Psychopharmacol 1986;6:176.
78. Fuller MA, Sajatovic M. Neurotoxicity resulting from a combination of lithium and loxapine. J Clin Psychiatiatry 1989;50:187.
79. Brown AS, Rosen J. Lithium-induced delirium with therapeutic serum lithium levels: a case report. J Geriatr Psychiatr Neurol 1992;5:53.
80. Norris MS, Matthew RJ, Webb WW. Delirium associated with lithium-induced hypothyroidism: a case report. Am J Psychiatry 1983;140:355.
81. Schuster P, Gabriel E, Kufferle B, et al. Reversal by physostigmine of clozapine-induced delirium. Clin Toxicol 1977;10:437.
82. McDowell F, Cedarbaum JM. The extrapyramidal system and disorders of movement. Clin Neurol 1994;38:34.
83. Friedman A, Sienkiewcz J. Psychotic complications of long-term levodopa treatment of Parkinson's disease. Acta Neurol Scand 1991;84:111.
84. Drachman DA, Stahl S. Extrapyramidal dementia and levodopa. Lancet 1975;1:809.
85. Friedman JH, Lannon MC. Clozapine in the treatment of psychosis in Parkinson's disease. Neurology 1989;39:1219.
86. Kieburtz K, McDermott M, Como P, et al. The effect of deprenyl and tocopherol on cognitive performance in early untreated Parkinson's disease. Parkinson Study Group. Neurology 1994;44:1756.
87. Goetz CG, Cohen MM. Neurotoxic agents. Clin Neurol 1994;20:1.
88. Duka T, Redemann B, Voet B. Scopolamine and lorazepam exert different patterns of effects in a test battery assessing stages of information processing. Psychopharmacology 1995;119:315.
89. Litvan I, Sirigu A, Toothman J, Grafman J. What can preservation of autobiographic memory after muscarinic blockade tell us about the scopolamine model of dementia? Neurology 1995;45:387.
90. Roth A, Akyol S, Nelson JC. Delirium associated with the combination of a neuroleptic, an SSRI, and benztropine. J Clin Psychiatry 1995;56:537.
91. Cantu TG, Korek JS. Central nervous system reactions to histamine-2 receptor blockers. Ann Intern Med 1991;114:1027.
92. Vial T, Goubier C, Bergert A, et al. Side effects of ranitidine. Drug Saf 1991;6:94.
93. Cataloano G, Catalano MC, Alberts VA. Famotidine-associated delirium. A series of six cases. Psychosomatics 1996;37:349.
94. Sanders LD, Whitehead C, Gildersleve CD, et al. Interaction of H_2-receptor antagonists and benzodiazepine sedation. A double-blind placebo-controlled investigation of the effects of cimetidine and ranitidine on recovery after intravenous midazolam. Anaesthesia 1993;48:286.
95. Klawans HL, Weiner WJ. Textbook of Clinical Neuropharmacology. New York: Raven, 1981;341.
96. Koch-Weser J, Sidel VW, Dexter M, et al. Adverse reactions to sulfosoxazole, sulfamethoxazole, and nitrofurantoin. Manifestations and specific reaction rates during 2,118 courses of therapy. Arch Intern Med 1971;128:399.
97. Carrillo F, Cubero A, Hernandez GJ, et al. Recurrence of meningoencephalitis induced by cotrimoxazole. Rev Neurol 1995;23:142.
98. River Y, Averbuch-Heller L, Weinberger M, et al. Antibiotic induced meningitis. J Neurol Neurosurg Psychiatry 1994;57:705.
99. Ayyar DR, Dawes PJK, Hudgson P, et al. Neurotoxicity of metronidazole. Neurology 1979;29:533.
100. Ferrier TM, Schwieger AC, Eadie MJ. Delayed onset of partial epilepsy of temporal lobe origin following acute clioquinol encephalopathy. J Neurol Neurosug Psychiatry 1987;50:93.
101. Kaeser HE. Transient global amnesia due to clioquinol. Acta Neurol Scand 1984;100:175.
102. Boogerd W, v.d. Sande JJ, Moffie D. Acute fever and delayed leukoencephalopathy following low dose intraventricular methotrexate. J Neurol Neurosurg Psychiatry 1988;51:1277.
103. Asato R, Akiyama Y, Ito M, et al. Nuclear magnetic resonance abnormalities of the cerebral magnetic reso-

nance abnormalities of the cerebral white matter in children with acute lymphoblastic leukemia and malignant lymphoma during and after central nervous system prophylactic treatment with intrathecal methotrexate. Cancer 1992;70:1997.

104. Duffner PK, Cohen ME. The long-term effects of central nervous system therapy on children with brain tumours. Neurol Clin 1991;9:479.
105. Sullivan MP, Storb R, Shulman HM. Immediate and delayed neurotoxicity after mechlorethamine preparation for bone marrow transplantation. Ann Intern Med 1982;97:182.
106. Kaufman IA, Kung FH, Koenig HM. Overdosage with vincristine. J Pediatr 1976;89:671.
107. Yung WKA, Prados M, Levin VA, et al. Intravenous recombinant interferon beta in patients with recurrent malignant gliomas: a phase I/II study. J Clin Oncol 1991;9:1945.
108. Adams F, Fernandez F, Mavligit G. Interferon-induced organic mental disorders associated with unsuspected pre-existing neurological abnormalities. J Neurooncol 1988;6:355.
109. Vecht CJ, Keohane C, Menon RS, et al. Acute fatal leukoencephalopathy after interleukin-2 therapy [letter]. N Engl J Med 1990;323:1146.

Chapter 12

Drug-Induced Movement Disorders

Joanne Wojcieszek

Objectives

- To recognize that prescription drugs may cause tremor, parkinsonism, chorea, dystonia, myoclonus, or tics
- To emphasize the importance of reviewing all current and prior medications when evaluating patients with movement disorders
- To understand that the most common medicines that cause clinically significant and disabling movement disorders are those prescribed for psychiatric disorders such as psychosis and depression
- To gain familiarity with disorders caused by dopamine receptor–blocking agents (DRBAs), such as acute akathisia, acute dystonic reactions, neuroleptic malignant syndrome (NMS), neuroleptic-induced parkinsonism (NIP), and the tardive syndromes
- To appreciate that chronic levodopa therapy for Parkinson's disease (PD) frequently causes fluctuating chorea and dystonia
- To be aware that most drug-induced movement disorders are transient and remit with discontinuation of the offending agent; the main exceptions to this are the often permanent tardive syndromes

Abnormal, involuntary movements are a common side effect of many prescription drugs. It is imperative that the clinician review all current and prior medications when evaluating patients with movement disorders. The main categories of abnormal movements include tremor, parkinsonism, chorea, dystonia, myoclonus, and tics. Tremor is a rhythmic oscillation of a body part and may occur when the limb is at rest (resting tremor), when held in suspension (postural tremor), or when performing an action (action tremor). Parkinsonism consists of bradykinesia (slowness of movement), resting tremor, cogwheel rigidity (increase in muscle tone) and postural instability. Chorea involves brief, jerky, unpredictable movements that flit from one part of the body to another. Dystonia includes sustained muscle contractions that result in twisting repetitive movements or static abnormal postures. Myoclonus is a brief, lightning-like jerk that can involve active muscle contraction (positive myoclonus) or inhibition of ongoing muscle activity (negative myoclonus). Hiccups and sleep jerks are common examples of positive myoclonus, whereas asterixis represents negative myoclonus. Tics are brief, repetitive, stereotyped movements or sounds that occur randomly. Patients with tics often have a feeling of inner tension before a tic movement and a sense of relief once the movement has been completed. Unlike the previously described abnormal movements, which are involuntary, akathisia is a usually considered voluntary because the patient is compelled to move to relieve inner restlessness.

This chapter describes common culprits of drug-induced movement disorders. Most of the discussion

Table 12.1. Drugs that May Cause Tremor

Beta-adrenergic agonists
Theophylline
Caffeine
Nicotine
Lithium
Antiepileptic drugs (valproic acid, lamotrigine)
Tricyclic antidepressants
Monoamine oxidase inhibitors
Amphetamines
Dopamine receptor–blocking agents (antipsychotics, metoclopramide, prochlorperazine, droperidol, domperidone, promethazine)
Corticosteroids
Thyroid hormone
Cardiac antiarrhythmics (amiodarone, procainamide)
Calcium channel blockers (nimodipine, flunarizine)
Pindolol (see Chapter 20)
Cimetidine[139]
Ethanol

Source: Adapted from WC Koller. Treatment of Tremor Disorders. In R Kurlan (ed), Treatment of Movement Disorders. Philadelphia: Lippincott, 1995;407.

Table 12.3. Drugs that May Cause Chorea

Dopamine receptor–blocking agents (antipsychotics, metoclopramide, prochlorperazine, droperidol, domperidone, promethazine)
Levodopa
Antiepileptic drugs (phenytoin, carbamazepine, ethosuximide, valproate, gabapentin [in therapeutic range]; phenobarbital toxicity)
Anticholinergics[150]
Amphetamines (see Chapter 22)
Oral contraceptives
Tricyclic antidepressant
Selective serotonin reuptake inhibitors
Cimetidine[151]
Cyclosporin[152]
Theophylline[153]
Clebopride[154]
Oxymetholone (anabolic steroid)[155]
Lithium[156]

focuses on agents that alter brain dopamine activity such as neuroleptics and levodopa. The abnormal movements caused by antidepressants, especially the newer agents that alter serotonergic transmission, are also reviewed. Tables 12.1 through 12.6 summarize which drugs can potentially cause abnormal movements; however, not all of these drugs are discussed. Movement disorders caused by cardiovascular drugs are included in Chapter 20.

Table 12.2. Drugs that May Cause Parkinsonism

Dopamine receptor–blocking agents (antipsychotics, metoclopramide, prochlorperazine, droperidol, domperidone, promethazine)
Dopamine-depleting agents (tetrabenazine, reserpine)
Alpha-methyldopa
Meperidine[140]
Lithium
Calcium channel blockers[141–143]
Disulfiram[144]
Phenytoin
Selective serotonin reuptake inhibitors
Amiodarone (see Chapter 20)
Clebopride[145, 146]
Cephaloridine[147]
Amphotericin B (intraventricular)[148]
Manganese intoxication with parenteral nutrition[149]

Table 12.4. Drugs that May Cause Dystonia

Dopamine receptor–blocking agents (antipsychotics, metoclopramide, prochlorperazine, droperidol, promethazine, sulpiride[157] and domperidone[158])
Tetrabenazine[159]
Dopamine agonists (levodopa)
Antiepileptic drugs (phenytoin, carbamazepine, ethosuximide)
Selective serotonin reuptake inhibitors
Antimalarials (amodiaquine,[160] chloroquine[161])
Diphenhydramine[162]
Fentanyl[163]
Disulfiram[164]
Midazolam[165]
Ondansetron[166]

Dopamine Receptor–Blocking Agents

The medicines that have the most potential for causing uncomfortable, disabling, and often permanent movement disorders are the DRBAs, also referred to as neuroleptics (these terms may be used interchangeably). Although DRBA-induced neurologic dysfunction probably represents the most common iatrogenic disorder to result in liti-

Table 12.5. Drugs that May Cause Myoclonus

Antidepressants (tricyclics, monoamine oxidase inhibitors)
Levodopa
Lithium
Anti-infectious agents (penicillin, carbenicillin, ticarcillin, cephalosporins, antihelmintic agents)
Anesthetic drugs (amidate)
Bismuth subsalicylate (i.e., Pepto-Bismol)[167]
Chlorambucil
Antiepileptics (valproic acid, carbamazepine)
Sedative hypnotics (methaqualone, bromisovalum)
Fentanyl[163]
Antihistamine
Diclofenac
Water-soluble contrast media (metrizamide, myelografin, angiografin, isocarmate meglumine, iothalamate meglumine)
Nifedipine, verapamil (see Chapter 20)
Prednimustine[168]
Propafenone[169]

Source: Adapted from HL Klawans, PM Carvey, CM Tanner, et al. Drug-Induced Myoclonus. In S Fahn, CD Marsden, M Van Woert (eds), Advances in Neurology Series, Vol 43: Myoclonus. New York: Raven, 1986;251.

Table 12.6. Drugs that May Cause Tics

Stimulants
Levodopa
Dopamine receptor–blocking agents
Carbamazepine

Table 12.7. Neurologic Complications of Dopamine Receptor–Blocking Agents

Acute dystonic reactions
Acute akathisia
Neuroleptic malignant syndrome
Neuroleptic-induced parkinsonism (including "rabbit syndrome")
Tardive dyskinesia

gation, these agents remain one of the most widely used classes of drugs. The most common indication for prescribing DRBAs is for the primary treatment of psychosis and for the management of some affective and behavioral disorders. Although DRBAs are commonly prescribed for schizophrenia, these agents are often used to treat elderly demented patients with agitation, hallucinosis, or aggression. Some drugs used primarily for depression may have DRBA properties or may actually include a neuroleptic. Examples include Triavil, a combined preparation of amitriptyline and perphenazine (a neuroleptic), and amoxapine, a tricyclic with DRBA activity. Neuroleptics are often used by neurologists to treat tics and chorea. Other commonly used DRBAs include antiemetics such as metoclopramide (Reglan), prochlorperazine (Compazine), droperidol (Inapsine), and domperidone (Motilium), as well as the antivertigo agent, promethazine (Phenergan).

The abnormal involuntary movements caused by DRBAs are listed in Table 12.7. Acute dystonic reactions typically develop 23–28 hours after initiation of neuroleptic treatment,[1] with 85% of episodes occurring within 96 hours.[2] An increase in neuroleptic dose or discontinuation of anticholinergic drugs during ongoing neuroleptic treatment may also cause acute dystonia. The estimated incidence of neuroleptic-induced dystonia is approximately 10%,[3] but may vary depending on the patient population studied and the type of neuroleptic used. Risk factors for the development of acute dystonia include young age, male sex, use of high potency or depot neuroleptics (haloperidol [Haldol], fluphenazine [Prolixin]), prior vulnerability to acute dystonic reactions, recent cocaine abuse,[4] and concurrent medical conditions such as hyperthyroidism or hypoparathyroidism. The potency of a neuroleptic drug to cause extrapyramidal effects is related to its ability to bind to postsynaptic dopamine receptors in the striatum (caudate and putamen). The highest potency neuroleptics, in decreasing order of potency, are thiothixene (Navane), Prolixin, perphenazine (Trilafon), trifluoperazine (Stelazine), triflupromazine (Vesprin), and Haldol. Low-potency neuroleptics, in increasing order of potency, are clozapine (Clozaril), olanzapine (Zyprexa), risperidone (Risperdal), molindone (Moban), loxapine (Loxitane), thioridazine (Mellaril), and chlorpromazine (Thorazine). Clozapine, olanzapine, and risperidone are considered "atypical neuroleptics" because they have a weak propensity to bind dopamine receptors and probably exert antipsychotic effects by reducing serotonergic transmission.[5] Although clozapine (Clozaril) is more effective than standard neuroleptics in the treatment of refractory psychosis and has minimal DRBA activity, its use is often limited by an approximately 1% risk of agranulocytosis, requiring patients to have weekly monitoring of the complete blood cell count and differential.[6] Clozapine has been reported to cause oculogyric crisis[7] and acute dystonia,[8] although this should be considered rare.

Little is known about the pathophysiology of acute dystonic reactions, but alterations in cholinergic, dopaminergic, gamma-aminobutyric acid (GABA), and sigma opiate receptor activity have been suggested. It is generally accepted that cholinergic transmission is excessive, but it is unclear whether dopamine activity is too low or too high. On one hand, acute dystonia may result from a reduction of dopamine activity by postsynaptic receptor blockade. However, dopamine receptor supersensitivity occurs soon after the first dose of neuroleptic agent, suggesting increased dopamine transmission as causative.[9] Symptoms of acute dystonia may be mild and only include a sensation of tongue thickness with no dysarthria. More commonly, symptoms are more severe and include opening or closing of the jaw, protrusion of the tongue, grimacing, tightness in the throat, pulling of the head to the side or backward, posturing of the limbs or torso, or oculogyric crisis where the eyes are forced upward and often to one side. Most terrifying is the rare manifestation of extreme laryngeal spasm that can compromise airway function and lead to sudden death. Adults tend to have involvement of the eyes, face, neck, and throat, whereas children tend to develop generalized dystonia. Acute neuroleptic-induced dystonia resolves spontaneously if the drug is discontinued. Because symptoms are often frightening and uncomfortable, however, parenteral treatment is usually indicated and is uniformly successful. The most effective medications include anticholinergics such as benztropine (Cogentin) and biperiden (Akineton) or the anticholinergic and antihistaminic agent diphenhydramine (Benadryl). For acute dystonia in adults with intravenous access, benztropine, 1–2 mg over 2 minutes, or diphenhydramine, 10–50 mg, should be given. Symptoms usually resolve in 2–5 minutes. If dystonia persists, the dose should be repeated. If this is unsuccessful, give diazepam, 5–10 mg. In adults without intravenous access, benztropine, 1–2 mg, may be given intramuscularly, but the response will be delayed. For acute dystonia in children, give intravenous diphenhydramine, 1–2 mg per kg up to 50 mg over 2 minutes, with a maximum of 400 mg in 24 hours.[10] For patients who require continued neuroleptic treatment, oral anticholinergic treatment to prevent recurrence should be continued for 1–2 weeks or longer for patients receiving a depot preparation. Once the acute episode has resolved, the clinician may be faced with an angry (or litigious) patient if the possibility of acute dystonia was not mentioned before starting the DRBA. Sometimes, anticholinergic prophylaxis should be considered in patients who are at high risk of developing acute dystonia or in patients for whom such a reaction would be exceptionally disturbing. This category includes children, young adult men, patients with prior acute dystonic reactions, and paranoid patients who may have delusions of an outside force controlling their body that may be reinforced by the dystonia.

Akathisia is a subjective sensation of restlessness that is associated with difficulty remaining still. Movement temporarily relieves akathisia, only to return immediately once the patient is again resting. There is often a compulsion to move one's legs that results in pacing, rocking, tapping the foot, swinging one leg while sitting, or shifting from one foot to another while standing. When seated, akathisic patients appear fidgety, frequently shift position, and sometimes lift themselves off the chair. Prevalence estimates of acute akathisia range from 20% to 75%.[11] Although symptoms may begin within hours of initiating DRBA treatment, more commonly, akathisia develops after days or weeks and is more likely to occur with high-potency or depot agents. The physiologic disturbance in akathisia may be blockade of mesocortical dopamine receptors.[12] The subjective distress of akathisia is a major cause of noncompliance with antipsychotic medications and, when severe, can lead a patient to consider suicide. Treatment of akathisia includes DRBA discontinuation (if possible), dose reduction, change to a lower potency drug, or change to an atypical neuroleptic. When additional treatment of akathisia is required, beta-blockers are probably the drugs of choice (i.e., propranolol, 20–120 mg per day; metoprolol, 75–200 mg per day). When the patient has neuroleptic-induced parkinsonism (NIP) in addition to akathisia, amantadine (25–100 mg twice daily) or anticholinergics (benztropine, 1–2 mg three times per day; trihexyphenidyl, 2–5 mg three times per day; diphenhydramine, 25–50 mg three times per day; biperiden, 2–4 mg three times per day) should be used. The syrup preparation of amantadine (50 mg per teaspoon) allows the lowest therapeutic dosing. Patients resistant to these therapies may be given clonazepam or clonidine. Treatment of akathisia is usually continued for a few weeks and then stopped if possible. Even when the DRBA is discontinued, it may take 1–2 weeks for acute akathisia to resolve. A persistent form of akathisia is discussed later as tardive akathisia.

Neuroleptic malignant syndrome (NMS) is a rare but potentially fatal complication of DRBA treatment. Patients with PD are also at risk for NMS when dopaminergic drugs are drastically lowered or discontinued. Both situations reduce central dopaminergic transmission, especially in the hypothalamic temperature regulation area and striatum, which may lead to the development of the cardinal clinical features of NMS: (1) fever, (2) rigidity, (3) altered mental status, and (4) autonomic dysfunction. NMS occurs in approximately 1% of patients treated with standard neuroleptics.[13] Even the atypical neuroleptics, clozapine and risperidone, have on rare occasion, been reported to cause NMS,[14, 15] as has tetrabenazine, a dopamine-depletor with some DRBA activity.[16–18] Symptoms of NMS typically begin within 2 weeks of starting the DRBA but can occur hours after the first dose or after years of treatment. Patients who are dehydrated, exhausted, or severely agitated may be predisposed to developing NMS. Other risk factors include use of high-potency or depot neuroleptics. However, most patients with NMS have had prior uncomplicated exposure to neuroleptics. The diagnosis of NMS should always be considered in any patient taking a neuroleptic with new fever, confusion, and extrapyramidal symptoms. Fever is present in virtually all patients with NMS but may not appear until after the motor signs. Fever is usually in the range of 101–104°F but may be greater than 105°F.[19] Rigidity is present in approximately 90% of patients; tremor or dystonia are also common. Changes in mentation occur in 75% of patients and range from agitation to prominent reduction in consciousness. Autonomic disturbances include diaphoresis, cardiac arrhythmias, urinary incontinence, and labile blood pressure. Laboratory abnormalities that support the diagnosis of NMS include elevated creatine kinase, typically above 1,000 IU per liter, leukocytosis, elevated liver enzyme levels, low serum iron concentration, proteinuria, and myoglobinuria, although all of these are nonspecific.

Table 12.8. Differential Diagnosis of Neuroleptic Malignant Syndrome

Central nervous system infection (encephalitis, meningitis, rabies)
Acute dystonic reaction
Drug-induced parkinsonism
Heat stroke
Status epilepticus
Lethal catatonia
Drug allergy
Malignant hyperthermia
Serotonin syndrome
Diabetic ketoacidosis
Metabolic encephalopathy
Strychnine poisoning
Tetanus

The diagnosis of NMS is one of exclusion, requiring aggressive diagnostic studies to exclude other life-threatening conditions, most important, CNS infection or status epilepticus. Patients with heat stroke do not sweat, unlike patients with NMS who experience prominent diaphoresis. It is often difficult, if not impossible, to distinguish lethal catatonia from NMS; however, NMS develops over hours and days, whereas lethal catatonia often includes 1–2 weeks of prodromal symptoms of mood instability, insomnia, intense motor excitement, and confusion. Because an acute dystonic reaction may mimic NMS, a single dose of parenteral anticholinergic is often given to make this distinction. The differential diagnosis of NMS is summarized in Table 12.8.

Treatment of NMS includes rapid recognition of the diagnosis, immediate withdrawal of the DRBA, admission to an intensive care unit, and initiation of dantrolene sodium (50–100 mg every 6 hours per nasogastric tube or orally) and bromocriptine (2.5–10.0 mg three times per day).[20] When NMS is caused by reduction of Parkinson's medications, the previous doses should be restarted. NMS should be treated aggressively, given the mortality of 11%. Alkalinization of urine is recommended to prevent myoglobinuria. Symptoms should begin to resolve within 2–3 days. Treatment should be continued for

10 days if the DRBA was taken orally and for 2–3 weeks if a depot preparation was causative. Once NMS symptoms resolve, patients should not be challenged with standard neuroleptics for 2 weeks. Although clozapine, olanzapine, and risperidone may be the drugs of choice after NMS, it is also reasonable to introduce a lower potency standard neuroleptic and titrate slowly. Electroconvulsive therapy may be helpful in treating the psychosis in acute NMS during the time when neuroleptics are contraindicated.

NIP is caused by drugs that block striatal dopamine receptors (DRBAs) or by agents that function presynaptically by reducing dopamine stores (i.e., reserpine, tetrabenazine). NIP symptoms and signs include reduced facial expression, hypophonia, drooling, slowness of movement, rigidity, resting tremor, micrographia, reduced arm swing, flexed posture, and postural instability. NIP is clinically indistinguishable from PD, although signs are typically symmetric and bilateral in NIP compared with the asymmetric presentation and course of PD. The "rabbit syndrome" (perioral and perinasal rhythmic 4- to 6-Hz tremor that looks like a rabbit chewing) is most often a manifestation of NIP but can, on occasion, be seen in PD. The rabbit syndrome may be a restricted manifestation of NIP and, like NIP-induced tremor, responds well to anticholinergics. NIP generally occurs later than akathisia and acute dystonia, often developing weeks after initiation of neuroleptic therapy or after a dose increase during ongoing treatment. The main risk factors for development of NIP are high neuroleptic potency and high neuroleptic dose.

Treatment of NIP includes the following options: (1) withdrawal or dose reduction of the offending agent; (2) addition of antiparkinson drugs such as amantadine, anticholinergics, levodopa, or dopamine agonists; or (3) change to an atypical neuroleptic. NIP refractory to these measures may improve with electroconvulsive therapy. NIP usually resolves within a few weeks or months of stopping the DRBA but symptoms may persist for much longer. In general, the diagnosis of PD should not be given to anyone who has taken a DRBA within the past year unless there is clear evidence that the parkinsonism has worsened since the DRBA was stopped.

Whether treated or not, NIP is a transient phenomenon even during continued neuroleptic exposure. Antiparkinson drugs can usually be successfully stopped after a few weeks. On a final note, most patients with NIP receive the DRBA from their physician, and this is documented in the medical record. However, there are some patients who ingest medications belonging to a friend or relative without knowing the nature of the drug and may not admit this to their physicians. The clinician must sometimes be persistent in questioning such patients. There are rare but unusual reports of unsuspected, surreptitious neuroleptic exposure. As described by Albanese et al.,[21] three men with parkinsonism who repeatedly improved in the hospital but worsened at home were being given haloperidol by their wives. One man had the neuroleptic dissolved in his coffee. A clue that this was a drug-induced parkinsonism was the coexistence of akathisia.

Of all the drug-induced movement disorders, tardive dyskinesia (TD) is the most clinically significant and potentially disabling. TD refers to a variety of persistent (usually longer than 3 months in duration) abnormal involuntary movements caused by DRBAs. All of the standard neuroleptics have been implicated as culprits of TD. The prevalence of TD among patients on chronic neuroleptic therapy is approximately 20%.[22] Likely risk factors for the development of TD include advancing age[23] and, to a lesser extent, female sex[24] and duration of neuroleptic exposure. The risk of TD is fairly stable from ages 20 to 40 years but then increases dramatically. The risk of TD for a 20-year-old patient after 2 years of neuroleptic exposure is 10% and after 4 years is 18%. For a 40-year-old patient, the risk is 18% at 2 years and 30% at 4 years.[25] In patients older than age 45 years, the cumulative incidence of TD after neuroleptic exposure is 26%, 52%, and 60% after 1, 2, and 3 years, respectively.[26] Children and adolescents have an extremely low chance of developing persistent tardive syndromes.[27] Despite rare reports that the newer atypical neuroleptics risperidone and clozapine[28] may also cause TD, the risk with these agents is minimal compared with that of classic neuroleptics.[29] The three patients described with risperidone-associated TD all had prior exposure to standard neuroleptics, and one patient had a history of TD.[30–32]

TD typically begins insidiously after several years of ongoing DRBA treatment but can occur after only a few months (or even days) of exposure. Most strikingly, TD commonly appears acutely after DRBA discontinuation or dose reduction. It is generally accepted that a movement disorder should begin within 3 months of stopping a DRBA for a diagnosis of TD to be considered.[33] However, there is no absolute period of time between stopping a DRBA and onset of abnormal movements that excludes the diagnosis of TD. The TD syndromes behave predictably to DRBA manipulations, and this is often of diagnostic importance. For example, TD worsens on neuroleptic dose reduction or discontinuation and improves with neuroleptic dose increase. This clinical improvement is deceiving because the TD is being masked by higher doses of neuroleptics while the underlying physiologic disturbance persists or worsens with continued exposure to the offending agent. The cause of TD remains elusive but probably includes postsynaptic striatal dopamine supersensitivity due to upregulation in response to long-standing receptor blockade as well as D_1- and D_2-receptor imbalance. Changes in GABA, acetylcholine, serotonin, and sigma opiate receptors have also been implicated. In addition, neuroleptics may be toxic to neurons in the substantia nigra and striatum by generation of free radicals or lipid peroxidation.[34, 35]

The TD syndromes are listed in Table 12.9. "Classic TD" most often refers to the repetitive, rhythmic, purposeless movements (tardive stereotypies) or sounds that most physicians recognize as TD. Tardive stereotypies typically involve the oral-buccal-lingual region and include lip pursing or smacking, tongue protrusion ("fly-catcher's tongue"), rolling the tongue within the mouth, pressing the tongue against the cheek ("bon-bon sign"), chewing, blowing, teeth clenching, side-to-side jaw movements, and puffing out the cheeks. Examples of tardive stereotypies affecting the body are "piano-playing" movements of the fingers and pelvic rocking ("copulatory dyskinesia"). TD may be manifest as respiratory dyskinesia such as irregular breathing, panting, gasping, or as vocalizations such as moaning or humming. On occasion, patients with TD may develop true choreatic movements that flow from one muscle to another in random fashion unlike the repetitive movements of tardive stereotypy.

The withdrawal-emergent syndrome is the transient chorea that can occur after abrupt withdrawal of a DRBA. This most often affects children, and the chorea remits within 3 months. Tardive akathisia includes the same feeling of restlessness and need to move as does acute akathisia; however, tardive akathisia begins after many months or years of treatment with a DRBA and is a persistent disorder. Tardive akathisia often includes rubbing of the face, picking at clothes, rocking, side-to-side movement of the feet with legs crossed, pacing or marching in place, and alternating sitting and standing. There is a pharmacologic distinction between acute and tardive akathisia. DRBA discontinuation or dose reduction improves acute akathisia and exacerbates tardive akathisia. There is an overlap in the types of movements seen in akathisia and classic TD, such as body rocking or repetitive hand or foot movements. In general, patients with TD are moving and therefore restless, whereas patients with akathisia are restless and therefore moving.[36] When patients taking standard neuroleptics develop disabling akathisia, a change to clozapine appears to be helpful. Surprisingly, such patients often continue to experience restlessness albeit of lesser severity.[37] It is unclear whether clozapine is causing acute akathisia or whether it is masking tardive akathisia.[38]

Table 12.9. Tardive Dyskinesia Syndromes

Classic tardive dyskinesia
Tardive stereotypy
Tardive chorea
Withdrawal-emergent syndrome
Tardive akathisia
Tardive dystonia
Tardive myoclonus
Tardive tremor
Tardive tics
Painful oral and genital syndromes

Tardive dystonia appears to be clinically and pharmacologically distinct from the other tardive syndromes. This form of dystonia typically affects the face, neck, and trunk, with the abnormal postures becoming more prominent during actions such as walking. Patients often have retrocollis, back arching, anterior displacement of the shoulder, and arm extension. Patients with tardive dystonia or tardive akathisia often have associated oral-buccal-lingual TD. Unlike patients with classic TD, who may not be aware of their involuntary movements, patients with tardive dystonia are usually symptomatic and often have pain and disability from the dystonia. Myoclonus, tremor, and tics can be manifestations of TD but are relatively uncommon. Oral and genital tardive pain syndromes have also been described.[39]

The best treatment of classic TD is discontinuation of the DRBA if the psychiatric state allows. Anticholinergics should be stopped because they are thought to exacerbate oral-buccal-lingual dyskinesia, and, in fact, cholinergic agonists may be helpful in treating TD. During the period of DRBA withdrawal and for a short time thereafter, TD movement may temporarily worsen, sometimes requiring treatment with a benzodiazepine. After this transient worsening, the longer the patient is off neuroleptics, the greater is his or her chance of improvement. Glazer and Morgenstern reported that 40% of patients had reduction of TD signs after 6 months and 90% had improved at 1 year.[40] Some patients may continue to improve for up to 5 years.[41] Fahn reported complete remission in five of eight patients after 1.5–4.0 years of drug abstinence.[42] Unfortunately, TD is often permanent, despite DRBA discontinuation.

What is the natural history of TD when patients have had to continue standard neuroleptic treatment even though efforts are made to minimize drug exposure? Yagi and Itoh followed 20 such patients for 10 years and found that 45% experienced remission, 30% had persistent symptoms, and 25% had recurrence of TD.[43] Nowadays, patients with TD who require continued treatment for psychosis should be changed to an atypical neuroleptic or begin symptomatic TD therapy. Although the main reason to change from a standard to an atypical neuroleptic is to stop further dopamine-receptor blockade, some of these agents may have a therapeutic effect. Clozapine has been shown to improve TD symptoms in many patients, especially those with tardive dystonia.[44] Historically, treatment of TD has been difficult; however, the most effective agents have been the dopamine depletors. It is thought that reserpine masks TD symptoms while the underlying physiologic abnormality has a chance to reverse over time.[42] The reserpine dose is typically 0.75–6.00 mg per day. Theoretically, reserpine may be a better agent for TD than is tetrabenazine because although both drugs are presynaptic monoamine depletors, tetrabenazine also has DRBA properties. Although tetrabenazine may successfully mask TD symptoms, the continued postsynaptic dopamine blockade perpetuates the underlying disease process. Tetrabenazine is also more difficult to use because it is not commercially available in the United States. It is possible to get the drug by contacting the company that produces it, and the dose is typically 75–300 mg per day. The addition of alpha-methyltyrosine (metyrosine or Demser, 1–4 g per day) to either of these agents can sometimes be beneficial. The use of the dopamine depletors is often limited by side effects of depression, hypotension, and parkinsonism. Other drugs with possible efficacy in the treatment of TD include dopaminergic agents such as bromocriptine, levodopa, or apomorphine, although these may exacerbate psychosis and should be used with caution. Second-line treatment includes noradrenergic antagonists such as propranolol, the GABA agonist progabide, some calcium channel blockers (i.e., nifedipine, verapamil), vitamin E (1,600 IU per day), and clonidine. Last, when TD is refractory to other therapies and of disabling severity, reinstitution of standard neuroleptics improves TD in the majority of patients. However, patients need to be informed that such action virtually eliminates their chance for TD remission.

Tardive dystonia is usually more disabling and more difficult to treat than is classic TD; however, anticholinergics, dopamine-depleting agents,[45] clozapine,[46, 47] and local injections of botulinum toxin may be beneficial. The anticholinergic drugs often used are trihexyphenidyl (5–120 mg per day; average dose, 20 mg per day) or ethopropazine (50 mg per day). Benzodiazepines and baclofen may also be helpful. Tardive akathisia is best treated with dopamine-depleting agents and does not respond well to the drugs used to treat acute akathisia. The painful oral and genital tardive syndromes respond to dopamine depletors.

Prevention of DRBA-induced involuntary movements should be a priority for all clinicians. Unfortunately, these drugs are often used for inappropriate reasons or for longer than is medically necessary. For this reason, DRBAs should be prescribed only for conditions for which no alternative medicines are effective and should be used in the lowest therapeutic doses for the shortest required time. Informed consent should always be provided whenever a DRBA is prescribed, and this should be clearly documented in the medical record. Regarding the treatment of chronic psychosis, clinicians should consider preferential use of the atypical neuroleptics, given their lower incidence of neurologic complications, and routinely monitor patients for early signs of TD.

Dopaminergic Drugs for Parkinson's Disease

The abnormal movements that occur in untreated PD are resting tremor, dystonia, and akathisia. In particular, foot dystonia may be an early manifestation of the disease, especially in young patients. Once symptomatic treatment with levodopa is initiated, patients often develop a variety of new abnormal movements (dyskinesias) that were not present in the untreated condition, such as choreoathetosis, dystonia, stereotyped movements, myoclonus, or akathisia. Nearly one-half of PD patients develop dyskinesias after 5 years of levodopa treatment.[48] Young patients with PD (disease onset before age 40) are particularly vulnerable, with the incidence of dyskinesia being 54.9%, 74.5%, and 100% at 1, 3, and 6 years of treatment, respectively.[49] Although levodopa can produce dyskinesias in patients with other forms of parkinsonism such as multiple system atrophy (including striatonigral degeneration and olivopontocerebellar atrophy), a robust therapeutic response to levodopa and the induction of dyskinesias is highly suggestive of the diagnosis of PD. The physiologic requirement for the development of dyskinesia is repeated dosing of levodopa in the context of dopaminergic denervation. One of the main reasons to consider dopamine agonist monotherapy before use of levodopa in PD is that the agonists only rarely produce dyskinesia without prior or concurrent exposure to levodopa. In a study by Lees and Stern, only 3% of patients on bromocriptine monotherapy for more than 1 year developed peak dose chorea compared with 65% of comparable patients taking maximally tolerated doses of levodopa.[50]

Of the various levodopa-induced dyskinesias, chorea is the most common, often beginning as subtle truncal rocking, head nodding, facial grimacing, or worm-like movements of the hand or foot. Over time more severe generalized chorea or ballistic movements may develop. Although dystonia may affect any or all parts of the body, painful foot inversion, plantar flexion, and curling under of the toes (or toe extension) is a distinct pattern seen in patients treated with chronic levodopa. Stereotypic movements can include kicking or a tendency to lift one leg too high when walking, giving the appearance of a "hemi-goose-step march." These levodopa-induced dyskinesias classically begin on the side of the body first affected by PD symptoms, suggesting that disease severity may be a factor in the genesis of these movements.

In general, dyskinesias are not present all day but appear and disappear or fluctuate in severity in relation to clinical levodopa response. Levodopa response does not directly correlate with plasma levodopa level but rather with striatal dopamine concentration (which cannot be monitored). It is critical to determine when dyskinesia occurs in an individual patient and make medication adjustments accordingly. Patients and their spouses usually have to be taught how to make these observations so that they can report to the doctor the relationship between levodopa dosing and the onset and duration of the dyskinesia. When the patient feels that the levodopa has taken effect and PD symptoms and signs improve, he or she is having an "on" period. After a few hours of benefit, levodopa effect begins to lessen and the patient experiences "wearing off." When there is no levodopa effect, the patient is having an "off" period, with return of rest tremor and bradykinesia.

Most dyskinesias occur at the maximum of the on period (peak-dose dyskinesia) or during wearing off (wearing-off dyskinesia). The most difficult to treat are the dyskinesias that occur as levodopa is taking effect and again when the effect is wearing off (biphasic dyskinesia). For example, peak-dose chorea may be remedied by reducing the levodopa dose and giving less drug more often or by changing from a regular release to a controlled release preparation. If dystonia occurs during wearing off, a decrease in levodopa response should be prevented—for example, by giving the next scheduled dose sooner, increasing each dose of levodopa so that it will last longer, changing to a controlled release preparation, or adding a dopamine agonist such as amantadine or deprenyl. Off-period dystonia can be unbearably painful and may require use of dissolved levodopa, benzodiazepines, botulinum toxin injection, or clozapine, which appears to have an antidyskinetic effect.[51] When dyskinesia is severe, debilitating, and unresponsive to drug manipulations, consideration should be given to pallidotomy or thalamotomy.[52–54]

Levodopa-induced myoclonus is not as common as the other types of dyskinesia and is not linked to levodopa response fluctuations. Myoclonus in PD patients typically begins after 1 year of levodopa treatment. The myoclonic jerks are usually bilateral and symmetric but can be unilateral. Because the myoclonus occurs primarily during drowsiness or sleep, the main clinical complaint is sleep disruption of the patient or spouse. Myoclonus severity increases with higher doses of levodopa, and myoclonus improves when the levodopa dose is lowered. Anticholinergics, amantadine, and propranolol have no influence on the myoclonus whereas methysergide eliminates the myoclonus, suggesting that serotonergic mechanisms may be contributory.[55]

Akathisia may be a manifestation of either wearing off or as a peak-dose levodopa effect. This highlights the fact that levodopa fluctuations are not restricted to motor phenomena, but also include transient sensory (e.g., pain, numbness), autonomic (e.g., sweating, dyspnea, tachycardia, urinary frequency), and cognitive changes (e.g., depression, anxiety, panic, hypomania).[56]

Discussion of stimulant-induced movement disorders are covered in Chapter 22.

Tricyclic Antidepressants, Monoamine Oxidase Inhibitors, and Lithium

Tricyclic antidepressants commonly cause an action tremor that is related to plasma drug concentration.[57] This tremor disappears with dose reduction or drug discontinuation and lessens with propranolol.[58] Myoclonus occurs in up to 40% of patients taking therapeutic doses of tricyclics.[59] Although the movements are typically mild and not clinically significant, 9% of patients may have more severe myoclonus requiring drug withdrawal. Desipramine-induced jaw myoclonus and stuttering have been reported.[60] Prominent chorea and myoclonus can rarely occur in tricyclic overdose and may be temporarily relieved by physostigmine.[61] Amitriptyline and doxepin have been reported to cause dystonia or tardive-like movements; however, these are considered uncommon side effects of these drugs.[62, 63]

Tremor or myoclonus may be occasional complications of monoamine oxidase inhibitors.[64] The myoclonus is most pronounced during drowsiness or REM sleep and is frequently reported by the bed partner rather than by the patient.[65]

Lithium is a well-recognized cause of postural and action tremor, with a range of frequency of 3–15 Hz. Tremor lessens with dose reduction or with the addition of low doses of propranolol (10–20 mg three times a day). Generalized myoclonus commonly occurs as part of lithium toxicity in association with jerky eye movements and a reduced level of consciousness. The myoclonus typically remits when lithium levels return to normal. If temporary symptomatic relief is required, clonazepam or valproate may be considered. Lithium may rarely cause parkinsonism,[66] although the mechanism of this is uncertain.

Antidepressants with Potent Serotonin Agonist Properties

The selective serotonin reuptake inhibitors (SSRIs) differ from tricyclics because they block the reuptake of serotonin more than the reuptake of norepinephrine and dopamine. The SSRIs include fluoxetine (Prozac), sertraline (Zoloft), fluvoxamine (Luvox), paroxetine (Paxil), and citalopram. Of the tricyclics, clomipramine (Anafranil) is one of the more selective serotonin uptake inhibitors. However, the main metabolite of clomipramine, desmethyl-chlorimipramine, primarily blocks norepinephrine uptake, and its plasma level often exceeds that of the parent compound. For this reason, clomipramine is often referred to as a serotonin reuptake inhibitor. The SSRIs have become first-line agents for the treatment of depression given their equal efficacy to tricyclics and their favorable side-effect profile. There are many reports suggesting that the SSRIs may cause abnormal movements such as dystonia, chorea, parkinsonism, akathisia, and bruxism. Although it is clear that these agents do have the potential to cause a variety of dyskinesias, interpretation of the anecdotal reports is limited by polypharmacy, frequent absence of drug rechallenge, lack of medication compliance monitoring, and lack of a control group. Many of the patients had recent or concurrent exposure to neuroleptics when SSRIs were added. SSRIs appear to potentiate the effects of neuroleptics. Because SSRIs are often highly protein bound, they may displace neuroleptics from their binding in plasma and increase the physiologic activity of the neuroleptics. The physiologic mechanism of SSRI-induced abnormal movements is unknown; however, there is some evidence that the SSRIs reduce dopamine activity in the basal ganglia. Studies suggest that serotonergic pathways exert a tonic inhibition of the dopaminergic systems of the brain.[67, 68] Drugs that increase serotonin activity, such as fluoxetine, can inhibit dopamine synthesis in the corpus striatum, nucleus accumbens, and frontal cortex as well as reduce homovanillic acid in the cerebrospinal fluid.[69, 70] Increased serotonergic transmission may inhibit nigrostriatal, tuberoinfundibular, and ventral tegmental projection dopaminergic neurons.[70, 71] In addition to these indirect actions on dopamine pathways, clomipramine may possess mild dopamine receptor-blocking activity.[72]

Early experience with fluoxetine revealed that 10–15% of patients developed "anxiety, nervousness, and insomnia" as is written on the package insert. It has been suggested that many of these patients were actually experiencing akathisia, which is considered to occur in 0.2–3.5% of patients taking fluoxetine.[73, 74] Akathisia can occur with doses as low as 5 mg per day,[75] and symptoms typically begin 12 hours to 7 days after starting the drug. Many patients report that the sensation of restlessness and anxiety experienced with fluoxetine is identical to that experienced previously with neuroleptics, and this can be so intolerable as to make a patient suicidal. It is possible that the increased suicidal impulse observed in some patients taking fluoxetine may be due to akathisia.[76] The akathisia usually remits with drug discontinuation, dose reduction, or with the addition of lorazepam. Fluoxetine may also cause dystonia, parkinsonism, rabbit syndrome, blepharospasm, or bruxism.[77–83] The dystonia may be acute, appearing in the first days of therapy or subacute with onset after several weeks. Both types of dystonia respond to anticholinergics or diphenhydramine. TD-like movements such as oral facial dyskinesia can appear, especially when fluoxetine is added to a neuroleptic,[84–86] raising the question whether fluoxetine can cause latent TD to become clinically apparent. Although fluoxetine-induced dyskinesias usually remit within days of drug discontinuation, they may persist for up to 12 weeks in a manner suggestive of TD. Another contributory factor that may explain persistence of symptoms is the long physiologic effect of norfluoxetine, the active metabolite of fluoxetine that has a half-life of 7–15 days.

Sertraline has been reported to cause akathisia, even at low doses of 25 mg per day, with onset of symptoms within 3 days to 3.5 weeks.[87–92] Symptoms abate within 2 days to 1 week of stopping the drug. Interestingly, one patient did not have akathisia with fluoxetine but did so on subsequent exposure to sertraline. Fluvoxamine may cause reversible parkinsonism, jaw dystonia, oral-facial dyskinesia, akathisia, or myoclonus at a dose of 100–200 mg per day.[93–97] Paroxetine has been reported to cause parkinsonism when added to trifluoperazine.[98] There is one description of a TD-like syndrome occurring with clomipramine treatment.[99]

If SSRIs indirectly reduce brain dopamine activity, it is not surprising that they may cause increased motor disability in patients with PD who are treated for depression. The SSRIs are theoretically attractive agents for PD depression because serotonin deficiency may be involved in the pathogenesis of the disorder.[100] Although one retrospective study indicated that fluoxetine is well tolerated in patients with PD,[101] there are other reports that conclude that tremor, bradykinesia, and dexterity may worsen.[102] Deterioration of PD signs after the addition of serotonin precursors has been demonstrated.[103, 104]

Myoclonus has been described as a rare effect of buspirone.[105] The anxiolytic effects of buspirone are mediated through serotonergic pathways, and this agent binds to the 5-HT_{1A} receptor. Buspirone has a complex pharmacologic profile, possessing both partial antagonist and agonist effects at dopamine receptors, and is thought to modulate the extrapyramidal system.[106, 107] The rare reports of buspirone-associated dystonia,[108, 109] akathisia,[110] and orofacial dyskinesia[111] suggest that buspirone may possess atypical neuroleptic properties.[112] Buspirone may also improve neuroleptic-induced akathisia,[113] TD,[114] and levodopa-induced dyskinesia.[115, 116]

Trazodone (Desyrel) has been reported to cause atypical acute dystonia.[117]

Antiepileptic Drugs

Cerebellar ataxia is the most common movement disorder caused by antiepileptic drugs when blood levels are in the toxic range. A variety of hyperkinetic movements can occur in patients taking therapeutic or toxic doses of antiepileptics. Patients receiving chronic valproic acid therapy develop a 6- to 15-Hz postural or action tremor of the hands. There may be a resting component to the hand tremor; the head, neck, or trunk may also be affected. Valproate-induced tremor typically develops after 1–12 months of therapy when doses exceed 750 mg per day; however, there is no close correlation between tremor severity and plasma drug level.[118, 119] Tremor improves with dose reduction and resolves quickly on drug discontinuation. For patients who require continued treatment with valproate, propranolol (20–100 mg per day) usually reduces tremor. Valproate-related chorea has been described in three children, all of whom had severe brain damage.[120] Parkinsonism may be an uncommon side effect of valproate.[121, 122]

It is well documented that phenytoin can cause a variety of involuntary movements at any stage of treatment, although the mechanism is not understood.[123] Chorea is the most common manifestation and may be associated with orofacial dyskinesia, dystonia, ballism, or asterixis. Predisposing factors include static encephalopathy, prior dyskinesia (e.g., Sydenham's chorea, TD), structural brain abnormality, or neuroleptic treatment. If there is focal brain disease, the dyskinesia can be unilateral. More than half of the patients with phenytoin-induced dyskinesias have toxic drug levels. Free phenytoin levels are often elevated when the standard level is in the therapeutic range. The addition of phenobarbital, valproic acid, or ethosuximide can increase the relative free fraction of phenytoin in the serum, causing a predisposed individual to develop dyskinesia. Stopping the second agent results in resolution of dyskinesia, as will phenytoin dose reduction or withdrawal. The chorea or dystonia sometimes seen during parenteral loading with phenytoin for status epilepticus resolves as plasma levels drop. Phenytoin has been reported to cause parkinsonism on rare occasion.[124, 125]

Carbamazepine appears to have some dopaminergic properties that may explain why this drug may cause chorea, dystonia, asterixis, akathisia, tic disorder exacerbation, and de novo tics.[126–130] Ethosuximide may cause akathisia, limb chorea, orofacial dyskinesia, and tongue protrusion early in the course of therapy, often 12 hours after ingestion of the first dose, that is relieved by intravenous diphenhydramine. This is considered a rare idiosyncratic adverse effect of ethosuximide that remits with drug withdrawal.[131, 132] Chorea and dystonia may be rare manifestations of phenobarbital toxicity.[133] Gabapentin may cause muscle twitching, chorea, or oculogyric crisis.[134] Lamotrigine has been reported to cause severe tremor in three patients who were also taking valproate.[135]

Oral Contraceptives

Chorea occasionally appears in women when they are exposed to higher than normal levels of female sex hormones such as during pregnancy (chorea gravidarum) or when taking oral contraceptives. Although both progesterone and estrogen may be responsible for the emergence of chorea, it has been suggested that estrogen may be the more important culprit.[136] Contraceptive-induced chorea usually begins within 4 months of starting the agent but the onset can be delayed for up to 3 years.[137] Chorea can be bilateral or unilateral and always resolves within 1 month of drug discontinuation. In most instances, there is a history of prior Sydenham's chorea or rheumatic fever. It is generally believed that hormone-induced chorea occurs in women who have had prior striatal injury, even though this may not have been clinically apparent. All patients should be evaluated for rheumatic fever. However, serologic study results documenting exposure to beta-hemolytic streptococcus are positive only if the patient has had recent streptococcal infection. A cardiac examination is indicated to look for rheumatic valve disease, and echocardiography should be considered. Guidelines for the use of prophylactic penicillin in rheumatic fever have been clearly outlined.[138] New-onset chorea may be a manifestation of systemic lupus erythematosus or other collagen vascular disease, anticardiolipin-antibody syndrome, Huntington's disease, cerebral infarction, hyperthyroidism, and polycythemia rubra vera, all of which need to be excluded.

Conclusion

Prescription drugs can potentially cause a variety of involuntary movements such as tremor, parkinsonism, chorea, dystonia, myoclonus, and tics. The most important culprits of drug-induced movement disorders are the neuroleptics (DRBAs). Such agents should be used only after informed consent with full disclosure of the potential side effects (unless required for management of acute psychosis). The reversible side effects of neuroleptics include acute akathisia, acute dystonia, NMS, and parkinsonism. TD syndromes are often permanent sequelae of long-term neuroleptic exposure. The new atypical neuroleptics such as clozapine, olanzapine, and risperidone are significantly less likely to cause extrapyramidal effects.

Treatment of PD with dopaminergic drugs is frequently associated with development of choreatic movements that tend to occur at times of peak levodopa effect. Tricyclic antidepressants, MAO inhibitors, and lithium may cause a dose-related hand tremor. The myoclonus reported from tricyclics is usually not clinically bothersome. SSRIs may cause a variety of involuntary movements as well as akathisia. Because most patients with SSRI-associated abnormal movements have recent or concurrent neuroleptic exposure, it may be that neuroleptics increase striatal sensitivity to SSRI effects or that SSRIs displace neuroleptics from protein binding sites and thereby increase the physiologic effects of the neuroleptic agent. Buspirone has complex and poorly understood effects on the dopaminergic system and can sometimes cause dystonia, chorea, or akathisia. Of the antiepileptic agents, phenytoin, carbamazepine, ethosuximide, and possibly gabapentin may cause chorea, especially in patients with prior brain injury or in patients taking more than one antiepileptic drug. Valproate frequently causes a postural and action hand tremor that remits with dose reduction or by the addition of low-dose propranolol. Higher than normal levels of female sex hormone (especially estrogen) may cause chorea, especially in women with prior striatal insult.

The vast majority of drug-induced movement disorders remit with dose reduction or drug discontinuation, with the exception of some of the permanent tardive syndromes. A thorough drug history should be performed on all patients who present with abnormal movements. Even if the abnormal movement is not a documented adverse effect, one needs to be open minded to such a possibility. When there exists a temporal relationship between drug exposure and onset of new symptoms, one should attempt dose reduction and if necessary drug withdrawal (and even drug rechallenge when it is safe to do so) to determine if such a relationship exists. In addition to referencing well-recognized drug-induced movement disorders, a number of case reports were included. Although single case reports often lack scientific rigor and are not peer reviewed, they may alert physicians to possible drug effects not previously recognized and may prompt prospective controlled studies to determine the validity of such observations.

References

1. Garver DL, Davis JM, Dekirmenjian H, et al. Dystonic reactions following neuroleptics: time course and proposed mechanisms. Psychopharmacology 1976;47:199.
2. Keepers GA, Clappison VJ, Casey DE. Initial anticholinergic prophylaxis for neuroleptic-induced extrapyramidal syndromes. Arch Gen Psychiatry 1983; 40:1113.
3. Swett C. Drug-induced dystonia. Am J Psychiatry 1975;132:532.
4. Hegarty AM, Lipton RB, Merriam AE, et al. Cocaine as a risk factor for acute dystonic reactions. Neurology 1991;41:1670.
5. Meltzer HY. Pre-clinical pharmacology of atypical antipsychotic drugs: a selective review. Br J Psychiatry 1996;168(Suppl 29):23.
6. Alvir JMJ, Lieberman JA, Safferman AZ, et al. Clozapine-induced agranulocytosis. N Engl J Med 1993; 329:162.
7. Dave M. Tardive oculogyric crisis with clozapine [letter]. J Clin Psychiatry 1994;55:264.
8. Kastrup O, Gastpar M, Schwarz M. Acute dystonia due to clozapine [letter]. J Neurol Neurosurg Psychiatry 1994;57:119.
9. Christensen AV, Fjalland B, Møller Nielsen I. On the supersensitivity of dopamine receptors induced by neuroleptics. Psychopharmacology 1976;48:1.
10. Burg FD, Ingelfinger JR, Wald ER (eds). Gellis and

Kagen's Current Pediatric Therapy (14th ed). Philadelphia: Saunders, 1993;706.
11. Van Putten T, May PRA, Marder SR. Akathisia with haloperidol and thiothixine. Arch Gen Psychiatry 1984;41:1036.
12. Marsden CD, Jenner P. The pathophysiology of extrapyramidal side-effects of neuroleptic drugs. Psychol Med 1980;10:55.
13. Pope HG Jr, Keck PE Jr, McElroy SL. Frequency and presentation of neuroleptic malignant syndrome in a large psychiatric hospital. Am J Psychiatry 1986;143:1227.
14. Weller M, Kornhuber J. Does clozapine cause neuroleptic malignant syndrome [letter]? J Clin Psychiatry 1993;54:2:70.
15. Webster P, Wijeratne C. Risperidone-induced neuroleptic malignant syndrome [letter]. Lancet 1994;344:1228.
16. Burke RE, Fahn S, Mayeux R, et al. Neuroleptic malignant syndrome caused by dopamine-depleting drugs in a patient with Huntington disease. Neurology 1981;31:1022.
17. Mateo D, Muñoz-Blanco JL, Giménez-Roldán S. Neuroleptic malignant syndrome related to tetrabenazine introduction and haloperidol discontinuation in Huntington's disease. Clin Neuropharmacol 1992;15:63.
18. Ossemann M, Sindic CJM, Laterre C. Tetrabenazine as a cause of neuroleptic malignant syndrome [communication]. Mov Disord 1996;11:95.
19. Addonizio G, Susman VL, Roth SD. Neuroleptic malignant syndrome: review and analysis of 115 cases. Biol Psychiatry 1987;22:1004.
20. Granato JE, Stern BJ, Ringel A, et al. Neuroleptic malignant syndrome: successful treatment with dantrolene and bromocriptine. Ann Neurol 1983;14:89.
21. Albanese A, Colosimo C, Bentivoglio AR, et al. Unsuspected, surreptitious drug-induced parkinsonism. Neurology 1992;42:459.
22. Kane JM, Smith JM. Tardive dyskinesia. Arch Gen Psychiatry 1982;39:473.
23. Saltz BL, Woerner MG, Kane JM, et al. Prospective study of tardive dyskinesia incidence in the elderly. JAMA 1991;266:2402.
24. Yassa R, Jeste DV. Gender differences in tardive dyskinesia: a critical review of the literature. Schizophr Bull 1992;18:701.
25. Kane JM, Woerner M, Borenstein M, et al. Integrating incidence and prevalence of tardive dyskinesia. Psychopharmacol Bull 1986;22:254.
26. Jeste DV, Caligiuri MP, Paulsen JS, et al. Risk of tardive dyskinesia in older patients. Arch Gen Psychatry 1995;52:756.
27. Wolf DV, Wagner KD. Tardive dyskinesia, tardive dystonia, and tardive Tourette's syndrome in children and adolescents. J Child Adolesc Psychopharmacol 1993;3:175.
28. de Leon J, Moral L, Camuñas C. Clozapine and jaw dyskinesia: a case report. J Clin Psychiatry 1991;52:12:494.
29. Kane JM, Woerner MG, Pollack S, et al. Does clozapine cause tardive dyskinesia? J Clin Psychiatry 1993;54:327.
30. Addington DE, Toews JA, Addington JM. Risperidone and tardive dyskinesia: a case report [letter]. J Clin Psychiatry 1995;56:484.
31. Woerner MG, Sheitman BB, Lieberman JA, et al. Tardive dyskinesia induced by risperidone [letter]? Am J Psychiatry 1996;153:843.
32. Wijeratne C, Webster P. Risperidone-induced tardive dyskinesia [letter]. Am J Psychiatry 1996;153:734.
33. Fahn S. The tardive syndromes: phenomenology, concepts on pathophysiology, and treatment. Mov Disord 1992;7(Suppl 1):7.
34. Lohr JB, Kuczenski R, Bracha HS, et al. Increased indices of free radical activity in the cerebrospinal fluid of patients with tardive dyskinesia. Biol Psychiatry 1990;28:535.
35. Pall HS, Williams AC, Blake DR, et al. Evidence of enhanced lipid peroxidation in the cerebrospinal fluid of patients taking phenothiazines. Lancet 1987;2:596.
36. Munetz MR. Akathisia variants and tardive dyskinesia [letter]. Arch Gen Psychiatry 1986;43:1015.
37. Chengappa KNR, Shelton MD, Baker RW, et al. The prevalence of akathisia in patients receiving stable doses of clozapine. J Clin Psychiatry 1994;55:142.
38. Safferman AZ, Lieberman JA, Pollack S, et al. Clozapine and akathisia [letter]. Biol Psychiatry 1992;31:753.
39. Ford B, Greene P, Fahn S. Oral and genital tardive pain syndromes. Neurology 1994;44:2115.
40. Glazer WM, Morgenstern H. Predictors of occurrence, severity, and course of tardive dyskinesia in an outpatient population. J Clin Psychopharmacol 1988;8;(Suppl):10S.
41. Klawans HL, Tanner CM, Barr A. The reversibility of "permanent" tardive dyskinesia. Clin Neuropharmacol 1984;7:153.
42. Fahn S. A therapeutic approach to tardive dyskinesia. J Clin Psychiatry 1985;46:19.
43. Yagi G, Itoh H. A 10-year follow-up study of tardive dyskinesia—with special reference to the influence of neuroleptic administration on the long-term prognosis. Keio J Med 1985;34:211.
44. Small JG, Milstein V, Marhenke JD, et al. Treatment outcome with clozapine in tardive dyskinesia, neuroleptic sensitivity, and treatment-resistant psychosis. J Clin Psychiatry 1987;48:263.
45. Kang UJ, Burke RE, Fahn S. Natural history and treatment of tardive dystonia. Mov Disord 1986;1:193.
46. Friedman JH. Clozapine treatment of psychosis in patients with tardive dystonia: report of three cases. Mov Disord 1994;9:321.
47. Lamberti JS, Bellnier T. Clozapine and tardive dystonia [letter]. J Nerv Ment Dis 1993;181:137.
48. Sweet RD, McDowell FH. Five years' treatment of Parkinson's disease with levodopa: therapeutic results and survival of 100 patients. Ann Intern Med 1975;83:456.
49. Quinn N, Critchley P, Marsden CD. Young onset Parkinson's disease. Mov Disord 1987;2:73.
50. Lees AJ, Stern GM. Sustained bromocriptine therapy in

previously untreated patients with Parkinson's disease. J Neurol Neurosurg Psychiatry 1981;44:1020.
51. Bennett JP, Landow ER, Schuh LA. Suppression of dyskinesias in advanced Parkinson's disease. Neurology 1993;43:1551.
52. Laitinen LV, Bergenheim AT, Hariz MI. Leksell's posteroventral pallidotomy in the treatment of Parkinson's disease. J Neurosurg 1992;76:53.
53. Dogali M, Fazzini E, Kolodny E, et al. Stereotactic ventral pallidotomy for Parkinson's disease. Neurology 1995;45:753.
54. Narabayashi H, Yokochi F, Nakajima Y. Levodopa-induced dyskinesia and thalamotomy. J Neurol Neurosurg Psychiatry 1984;47:831.
55. Klawans HL, Carvey PM, Tanner CM, et al. Drug-Induced Myoclonus. In S Fahn, CD Marsden, Van M Woert (eds), Advances in Neurology Series, Vol 43: Myoclonus. New York: Raven, 1986;251.
56. Riley DE, Lang AE. The spectrum of levodopa-related fluctuations in Parkinson's disease. Neurology 1993;43:1459.
57. Nelson JC, Jatlow PI, Quinlan DM. Subjective complaints during desipramine treatment. Arch Gen Psychiatry 1984;41:55.
58. Kronfol Z, Greden JF, Athanasios PZ. Imipramine-induced tremor: effects of a beta-adrenergic blocking agent. J Clin Psychiatry 1983;44:225.
59. Garvey MJ, Tollefson GD. Occurrence of myoclonus in patients treated with cyclic antidepressants. Arch Gen Psychiatry 1987;44:269.
60. Masand P. Desipramine-induced oral-pharyngeal disturbances: stuttering and jaw myoclonus [letter]. J Clin Psychopharmacol 1992;12:444.
61. Burks JS, Walker JE, Rumack BH, Ott JE. Tricyclic antidepressant poisoning; reversal of coma, choreoathetosis, and myoclonus by physostigmine. JAMA 1974;230:1405.
62. Lee HK. Dystonic reactions to amitriptyline and doxepin [letter]. Am J Psychiatry 1988;145:649.
63. Yassa R, Camille Y, Belzile L. Tardive dyskinesia in the course of antidepressant therapy: a prevalence study and review of the literature. J Clin Psychopharmacology 1987;7:243.
64. Goldberg LI. Monoamine oxidase inhibitors. JAMA 1964;190:456.
65. Lieberman JA, Kane JM, Reife R. Neuromuscular Effects of Monoamine Oxidase Inhibitors. In S Fahn, CD Marsden, M Van Woert (eds), Advances in Neurology Series, Vol 43: Myoclonus. New York: Raven, 1986;231.
66. Lang AE. Lithium and parkinsonism [letter]. Ann Neurol 1984;15:214.
67. Costall B, Fortune DH, Naylor RJ, et al. Serotonergic involvement with neuroleptic catalepsy. Neuropharmacology 1975;14;859.
68. Carter CJ, Pycock CJ. Possible importance of 5-hydroxytryptamine in neuroleptic-induced catalepsy in rats. Br J Pharmacol 1977;60:267P.
69. Baldessarini RJ, Marsh E. Fluoxetine and side effects [letter]. Arch Gen Psychiatry 1990;47:191.
70. Meltzer HY, Young M, Metz J, et al. Extrapyramidal side effects and increased serum prolactin following fluoxetine, a new antidepressant. J Neural Transm 1979;45:165.
71. Lipinski JF, Mallya G, Zimmerman P, et al. Fluoxetine-induced akathisia: clinical and theoretical implications. J Clin Psychiatry 1989;50:339.
72. Austin LS, Lydiard RB, Ballenger JC, et al. Dopamine blocking activity of clomipramine in patients with obsessive-compulsive disorder. Biol Psychiatry 1991;30:225.
73. Teicher MH, Glod C, Cole JO. Emergence of intense suicidal preoccupation during fluoxetine treatment. Am J Psychiatry 1990;147:207.
74. Rothschild AJ, Locke CA. Reexposure to fluoxetine after serious suicide attempts by three patients: the role of akathisia. J Clin Psychiatry 1991;52:491.
75. Hamilton MS, Opler LA. Akathisia, suicidality and fluoxetine. J Clin Psychiatry 1992;53:401.
76. Wirshing WC, Putten TV, Rosenberg J, et al. Fluoxetine, akathisia, and suicidality: is there a causal connection [letter]? Arch Gen Psychiatry 1992;49:580.
77. Tate JL. Extrapyramidal symptoms in a patient taking haloperidol and fluoxetine [letter]. Am J Psychiatry 1989;146:399.
78. Bouchard RH, Pourcher E, Vincent P. Fluoxetine and extrapyramidal side effects [letter]. Am J Psychiatry 1989;146:1352.
79. Brod TM. Fluoxetine and extrapyramidal side effects [letter]. Am J Psychiatry 1989;146:1353.
80. Reccoppa L, Welch WA, Ware MR. Acute dystonia and fluoxetine [letter]. J Clin Psychiatry 1990;51:487.
81. Black B, Uhde TW. Acute dystonia and fluoxetine [letter]. J Clin Psychiatry 1992;53:327.
82. Dave M. Fluoxetine-associated dystonia [letter]. Am J Psychiatry 1994;151:149.
83. Fallon BA, Liebowitz MR. Fluoxetine and extrapyramidal symptoms in CNS lupus [letter]. J Clin Psychopharmacol 1991;11:147.
84. Stein MH. Tardive dyskinesia in a patient taking haloperidol and fluoxetine [letter]. Am J Psychiatry 1991;148:683.
85. Budman CL, Bruun RD. Persistent dyskinesia in a patient receiving fluoxetine [letter]. Am J Psychiatry 1991;148:1403.
86. Stoukides JA, Stoukides CA. Extrapyramidal symptoms upon discontinuation of fluoxetine [letter]. Am J Psychiatry 1991;148:1263.
87. LaPorta LD. Sertraline-induced akathisia [letter]. J Clin Psychopharmacol 1993;13:219.
88. Klee B, Kronig MH. Case report of probable sertraline-induced akathisia [letter]. Am J Psychiatry 1993;150:986.
89. Settle EC. Akathisia and sertraline [letter]. J Clin Psychiatry 1993;54:321.

90. Shihabuddin L, Rapport D. Sertraline and extrapyramidal side effects [letter]. Am J Psychiatry 1994;151:288.
91. Opler LA. Sertraline and akathisia [letter]. Am J Psychiatry 1994;151:620.
92. Altshuler LL, Pierre JM, Wirshing WS, et al. Sertraline and akathisia [letter]. J Clin Psychopharmacol 1994;14:278.
93. Wils V. Extrapyramidal symptoms in a patient treated with fluvoxamine [letter]. J Neurol Neurosurg Psychiatry 1992;55:330.
94. George MS, Trimble MR. Dystonic reaction associated with fluvoxamine [letter]. J Clin Psychopharmacol 1993;13:220.
95. Arya DK, Szabadi E. Dyskinesia associated with fluvoxamine [letter]. J Clin Psychopharmacol 1993;13:365.
96. Baldwin D, Fineberg N, Montgomery S. Fluoxetine, fluvoxamine and extrapyramidal tract disorders. Int Clin Psychopharmacol 1991;6:51.
97. Bauer M. Severe myoclonus produced by fluvoxamine [letter]. Am J Psychiatry 1995;56:589.
98. Nicholson SD. Extra pyramidal side effects associated with paroxetine. West of England Medical Journal 1992;7:90.
99. Gersten SP. Tardive dyskinesia-like syndromes with clomipramine. Am J Psychiatry 1993;150:165.
100. Mayeux R, Stern Y, Williams JBW, et al. Clinical and biochemical features of depression in Parkinson's disease. Am J Psychiatry 1986;143:756.
101. Caley CF, Friedman JH. Does fluoxetine exacerbate Parkinson's disease? J Clin Psychiatry 1992;53:278.
102. Jansen Steur ENH. Increase in Parkinson disability after fluoxetine medication. Neurology 1993;43:211.
103. Chase TN, Ng LKY, Watanabe AM. Parkinson's disease modification by 5-hydroxtryptophan. Neurology 1972;22:479.
104. Hall CD, Weiss EA, Morris CE, et al. Rapid deterioration in patients with parkinsonism following tryptophan-pyridoxine administration. Neurology 1972;22:231.
105. Ritchie EC, Bridenbaugh RH, Jabbari B. Acute generalized myoclonus following buspirone administration. J Clin Psychiatry 1988;49:242.
106. McMillan BA. Comparative chronic effects of buspirone or neuroleptics on rat brain dopaminergic neurotransmission. J Neural Transm 1985;64:1.
107. Cimino M, Ponzio F, Achilli G, et al. Dopaminergic effects of buspirone, a novel anxiolytic agent. Biochem Pharmacol 1983;32:1069.
108. Boylan K. Persistent dystonia associated with buspirone. Neurology 1990;40:1904.
109. LeWitt PA, Walters A, Hening W, et al. Persistent movement disorders induced by buspirone. Mov Disord 1993;8:331.
110. Patterson JF. Akathisia associated with buspirone [letter]. J Clin Psychopharmacol 1988;8:296.
111. Strauss A. Oral dyskinesia associated with buspirone use in an elderly woman. J Clin Psychiatry 1988;49:322.
112. Wood PL, Nair NPV, Lal S, et al. Buspirone: a potential atypical neuroleptic. Life Sci 1983;33:269.
113. D'Mello DA, McNeil JA, Harris W. Buspirone suppression of neuroleptic-induced akathisia: multiple case reports [letter]. J Clin Psychopharmacol 1989;9:151.
114. Moss LE, Neppe VM, Drevets WC. Buspirone in the treatment of tardive dyskinesia. J Clin Psychopharmacol 1993;13:204.
115. Bonifati V, Fabrizio E, Cipriani R, et al. Buspirone in levodopa-induced dyskinesias. Clin Neuropharmacol 1994;17:73.
116. Kleedorfer B, Lees AJ, Stern GM. Buspirone in the treatment of levodopa induced dyskinesias [letter]. J Neurol Neurosurg Psychiatry 1991;54:376.
117. Kramer MS, Marcus DJ, DiFerdinando J, et al. Atypical acute dystonia associated with trazodone treatment [letter]. J Clin Psychopharmacol 1986;6:117.
118. Karas BJ, Wilder BJ, Hammond EJ, et al. Valproate tremors. Neurology 1982;32:428.
119. Hyman NM, Dennis PD, Sinclair KGA. Tremor due to sodium valproate. Neurology 1979;29:1117.
120. Lancman ME, Asconapé JJ, Penry JK. Choreiform movements associated with the use of valproate. Arch Neurol 1994;51:702.
121. Armon C, Shin C, Miller P, et al. Reversible parkinsonism and cognitive impairment with chronic valproate use. Neurology 1996;47:626.
122. Alvarez-Gómez MJ, Vaamonde J, Narbona J, et al. Parkinsonian syndrome in childhood after sodium valproate administration. Clin Neuropharmacol 1993;16:451.
123. Harrison MB, Lyons GR, Landow ER. Phenytoin and dyskinesias: a report of two cases and review of the literature. Mov Disord 1993;8:19.
124. Goñi M, Jimenez M, Feijoo M. Parkinsonism induced by phenytoin [letter]. Clin Neuropharmacol 1985;8:383.
125. Prensky AL, DeVivo DC, Palkes H. Severe bradykinesia as a manifestation of toxicity to antiepileptic medications. J Pediatr 1971;78:700.
126. Bimpong-Buta K, Froescher W. Carbamazepine-induced choreoathetoid dyskinesias [letter]. J Neurol Neurosurg Psychiatry 1982;45:560.
127. Critchley EMR, Phillips M. Unusual idiosyncratic reactions to carbamazepine [letter]. J Neurol Neurosurg Psychiatry 1988;51:1238.
128. Joyce RP, Gunderson CH. Carbamazepine-induced orofacial dyskinesia. Neurology 1980;30;1333.
129. Jacome DJ. Movement disorder induced by carbamazepine [letter]. Neurology 1981;31:1059.
130. Kurlan R, Kersun J, Behr J, et al. Carbamazepine-induced tics. Clin Neuropharmacol 1989;12:298.
131. Ehyai A, Kilroy AW, Fenichel GM. Dyskinesia and akathisia induced by ethosuximide [letter]. Am J Dis Child 1978;132:527.
132. Kirschberg GJ. Dyskinesia-an unusual reaction to ethosuximide. Arch Neurol 1975;32:137.
133. Lightman SL. Phenobarbital dyskinesia. Postgrad Med J 1978;54:114.

134. Reeves AL, So EL, Sharbrough FW, et al. Movement disorders associated with the use of gabapentin. Epilepsia 1996;37:988.
135. Reutens DC, Duncan JS, Patsalos PN. Disabling tremor after lamotrigine with valproate [letter]. Lancet 1993;342:185.
136. Pulsinelli WA, Hamill RW. Chorea complicating oral contraceptive therapy: case report and review of the literature. Am J Med 1978;65:557.
137. Leys D, Destée A, Petit H, et al. Chorea associated with oral contraception. J Neurol 1987;235:46.
138. Dajani A, Taubert K, Ferrieri P, et al. Treatment of acute streptococcal pharyngitis and prevention of rheumatic fever: a statement for health professionals. Pediatrics 1995;96:758.
139. Bateman DN, Bevan P, Longley BP, et al. Cimetidine induced postural and action tremor [letter]. J Neurol Neurosurg Psychiatry 1981;44:94.
140. Olivé JM, Masana L, González J. Meperidine and reversible parkinsonism [communication]. Mov Disord 1994;9:115.
141. Daniel JR, Mauro VF. Extrapyramidal symptoms associated with calcium channel blockers. Ann Pharmacother 1995;29:73.
142. Nakashima K, Shimoda M, Kuno N, et al. Temporary symptom worsening caused by manidipine hydrochloride in two patients with Parkinson's disease [communication]. Mov Disord 1994;9:106.
143. Sampere AP, Duarte J, Cabezas C, et al. Parkinsonism induced by amlodipine [communication]. Mov Disord 1995;10:115.
144. Krauss JK, Mohadjer M, Wakhloo AK, et al. Dystonia and akinesia due to pallidoputaminal lesions after disulfiram intoxication. Mov Disord 1991;6:166.
145. Montagna P, Gabellini AS, Monari L, et al. Parkinsonian syndrome after long-term treatment with clebopride [communication]. Mov Disord 1992;7:89.
146. Sampere AP, Duarte J, Palomares JM, et al. Parkinsonism and tardive dyskinesia after chronic use of clebopride [communication]. Mov Disord 1994;9:114.
147. Mintz U, Liberman UA, de Vries A. Parkinsonian syndrome due to cephaloridine [letter]. JAMA 1971;216:1200.
148. Fisher JF, Dewald J. Parkinsonism associated with intraventricular amphotericin B. J Antimicrobial Chemother 1983;12:97.
149. Ejima A, Imamura T, Nakamura S. Manganese intoxication during total parenteral nutrition [letter]. Lancet 1992;339:426.
150. Nomoto M, Thompson PD, Sheehy MP, et al. Anticholinergic-induced chorea in the treatment of focal dystonia. Mov Disord 1987;2:53.
151. Kushner MJ. Chorea and cimetidine [letter]. Ann Intern Med 1982;96:126.
152. Cambarros O, Fábrega E, Polo JM, et al. Cyclosporin-induced chorea after liver transplantation for Wilson's disease. Ann Neurol 1993;33:108.
153. Stuart AM, Worley LM, Spillane J. Choreiform movements observed in an 8-year-old child following use of an oral theophylline preparation. Clin Pediatr 1992;31:692.
154. Martínez-Martín P. Transient dyskinesia induced by clebopride [communication]. Mov Disord 1993;8:125.
155. Tilzey A, Heptonstall J, Hamblin T. Toxic confusional state and choreiform movements after treatment with anabolic steroids. BMJ 1981;283:349.
156. Peters HA. Lithium intoxication producing chorea athetosis with recovery. Wis Med J 1949;December:1075.
157. Linazasoro G, Martí Massó JF, Olasagasti B. Acute dystonia induced by sulpiride. Clin Neuropharmacol 1991;14:463.
158. Bonuccelli U, Nocchiero A, Napolitano A, et al. Domperidone-induced acute dystonia and polycystic ovary syndrome. Mov Disord 1991;6:79.
159. Burke RE, Reches A, Traub MM, et al. Tetrabenazine induces acute dystonic reactions. Ann Neurol 1985;17:200.
160. Olabode Akindele M, Odejide AO. Amodiaquine-induced involuntary movements. BMJ 1976;24:214.
161. Umez-Eronini EM, Eronini EA. Chloroquine induced involuntary movements. BMJ 1977;9:945.
162. Etzel JV. Diphenhydramine-induced acute dystonia. Pharmacotherapy 1994;14:492.
163. Petzinger G, Mayer SA, Przedborski S. Fentanyl-induced dyskinesias [communication]. Mov Disord 1995;10:679.
164. de Mari M, De Blasi R, Lamberti P, et al. Unilateral pallidal lesion after acute disulfiram intoxication: a clinical and magnetic resonance study [communication]. Mov Disord 1993;8:247.
165. Stolarek IH, Ford MJ. Acute dystonia induced by midazolam and abolished by flumazenil [letter]. BMJ 1990;300:614.
166. Halperin JR, Murphy B. Extrapyramidal reaction to ondansetron. Cancer 1992;69:1275.
167. Gordon MF, Abrams RI, Rubin DB, et al. Bismuth subsalicyclate toxicity as a cause of prolonged encephalopathy with myoclonus. Mov Disord 1995; 10:220.
168. Martin M, Diaz-Rubio E, Casado A, et al. Prednimustine-induced myoclonus—a report of three cases [letter]. Acta Oncologica 1994;33:81.
169. Chua TP, Farrell T, Lipkin DP. Myoclonus associated with propafenone [letter]. BMJ 1994;308:113.

Chapter 13

Drug- and Toxin-Induced Optic Neuropathies

Marie Di Nome Acierno and James J. Corbett

Objectives

- To be aware that agents associated with toxic effects on the optic nerve may be encountered in the workplace, at home, as therapeutic agents, as commonly prescribed drugs, and as a result of alcohol or tobacco use
- To appreciate that drugs and various other substances with a toxic effect on the optic nerves can produce visual loss that may be irreversible despite withdrawal of the offending agent
- To recognize that certain drugs, even in recommended dosages, may produce toxic insult to the optic nerves
- To appreciate that a deficiency of a vital substance (e.g., vitamin B_{12}) or overindulgence of other agents may result in toxic optic neuropathies
- To understand that toxic optic neuropathies are often bilateral and produce painless visual loss, dyschromatopsia, or central or cecocentral scotomas
- To understand that the tempo of visual loss depends on the causative agent
- To understand that ocular adverse effects may be an inevitable consequence of using a systemic agent

Antimicrobial Drugs (Antitubercular Drugs and Other Antibiotics)

Ethambutol Hydrochloride (Myambutol)

Ethambutol is a tuberculostatic antibacterial agent introduced in 1961 for treatment of tuberculosis. The drug received wide clinical application as an oral agent against *Mycobacterium tuberculosis*. Shortly after its introduction, a significant number of patients receiving ethambutol presented with central or peripheral reduction of vision.[1] A bilateral retrobulbar optic neuropathy is the most common insult to the optic nerves due to ethambutol. Patients typically develop blurred vision, dyschromatopsia, and cecocentral scotomas.[2] In the original report of ethambutol toxicity, most ocular symptoms reversed with cessation of the drug.[3] Barron et al. reported two of 304 patients receiving ethambutol had documented visual changes clearly not due to other causes.[4] Visual changes reversed when the drug was stopped. Since the initial descriptions of ethambutol toxic optic neuropathy, it has been recognized that ethambutol retrobulbar optic neuropathy is a dose-related, cumulative condition.

Ethambutol was originally made as a mixture of dextro- and levo-isomers. Early studies of ethambutol ocular toxicity and its relation to dose showed that the chemical properties of the DL-racemic mixture was more severely toxic than the D-isomer. Only the D-isomer is called *ethambutol*. It is unclear but highly possible that generic forms of this compound used in different parts of the world may contain a racemic mixture.[1, 5]

Early reports described two types of ethambutol bilateral retrobulbar optic neuropathy. Patients had either axial toxicity with central visual loss or periaxial toxicity with peripheral visual loss. Patients with central visual field defects have reduced visual acuity and loss of red-green color vision. Patients with peripheral field constriction usually have spared visual acuity.[6] The funduscopic examination is typically normal, although some hyperemia of the optic nerves or disk edema is occasionally seen. Visual acuity may be reduced to hand motion vision, but is usually 20/100 or better. Visual recovery occurs in most patients within 2 months of discontinuing the drug.[7]

Ethambutol optic neuropathy occurs in 15% of patients receiving 50 mg per kg per day, in 5% of patients receiving 25 mg per kg per day, and in less than 1% of patients taking 15 mg per kg per day.[8] The recommended dose of ethambutol is 15 mg per kg per day. Some patients develop irreversible visual failure despite administration of ethambutol at its recommended dose. Chatterjee et al. described a patient who had progressive irreversible visual failure 3 days after starting treatment with ethambutol at the recommended clinically safe dose.[5] Ethambutol was stopped on the sixth day of therapy. Despite its discontinuation, the patient's vision continued to deteriorate and visual fields were peripherally constricted. Visual evoked responses were abnormal, and funduscopy showed normal-appearing optic nerves. Treatment with prednisolone and hydroxycobalamin at first produced transient improvement in vision followed by progressive reduction in vision to no light perception bilaterally. One year later, the patient remained bilaterally blind with bilateral optic atrophy. Despite prompt discontinuation of ethambutol in three patients, once visual changes were observed, two patients remained permanently legally blind, and one patient had vision return to 20/20 in one eye and 20/40 in the other eye.[9]

The precise mechanism by which the drug produces ethambutol optic neuropathy is unknown. Drug studies in dogs and cats demonstrated that ethambutol causes discoloration of the tapetum lucidum due to its ability to chelate zinc and other metals. The tapetum lucidum is retinal pigment epithelium with a high zinc content. The tapetum lucidum is pigmented in the nontapetal portion and unpigmented in the tapetal portion, and therefore not clinically observed on funduscopy.[10] Ethambutol causes loss of color in the tapetum lucidum by removal of its zinc content. This may be one explanation of ethambutol ocular toxicity. Other studies postulate that the optic neuropathy may relate to a direct retinal effect due to chelation of zinc by ethambutol.

Decreased renal clearance and diabetes mellitus increase the susceptibility to ethambutol toxicity, even at recommended daily doses.[1] Ethambutol is actively excreted by the kidneys. Patients with renal tuberculosis may not be suitable for ethambutol therapy due to compromise of renal function resulting in elevation of serum ethambutol concentrations, thus placing the patient at risk for optic neuropathy.[11]

The most characteristic disturbance of vision from ethambutol is bilateral reduction of visual acuity due to the development of central scotomas. Patients on ethambutol should have a baseline ophthalmologic examination before therapy is initiated, and visual acuity should be tested every 6 months thereafter. If vision declines or other visual disturbances develop, the drug should be discontinued immediately. Hydroxocobalamin, a derivative of vitamin B_{12}, has been advocated by some for ethambutol-induced optic neuropathy. Parenteral vitamin B_{12} administration may help to neutralize the chelating action of ethambutol on the optic nerve. Despite treatment with hydroxocobalamin, vision may recover spontaneously due to prompt withdrawal of the drug alone.[12, 13]

Isoniazid

Isoniazid, the hydrazide of isonicotinic acid, is the preferred primary drug for the treatment of tuberculosis. Isoniazid binds with vitamin B_6 (pyridoxine); thus, isoniazid may cause a peripheral neuropathy if pyridoxine is not given concurrently. Prophylactic administration of pyridoxine also helps prevent other neurotoxicity such as seizures and encephalopathy. A daily dose of 25–100 mg of pyridoxine is recommended to prevent peripheral neuropathy from isoniazid, and this dose is also recommended to prevent insult to the optic nerves.[14]

Optic neuropathy and the later development of optic atrophy have been observed with isoniazid therapy. The recommended daily dose for adults is 5 mg per kg, with a maximum of 300 mg, or 10 mg per kg, with a maximum of 600 mg in severely ill adults, and 10 mg per kg in children younger than 4 years of age.[7, 8]

Isoniazid-related optic neuropathy is unusual. Like ethambutol, isoniazid may produce both an anterior and retrobulbar optic neuropathy. The effect of isoniazid may be synergistic with ethambutol, yet in some cases, optic neuropathy developed solely with the use of isoniazid.[1] Several patients have been observed with bilateral optic disk swelling after starting isoniazid for pulmonary tuberculosis; visual failure ensued and isoniazid was discontinued. When pyridoxine was started for presumed isoniazid-induced optic neuropathy, visual acuity improved.[2]

Isoniazid and ethambutol are frequently used in combination for the treatment of tuberculosis; therefore, one must not overlook the potential optic nerve toxicity caused by either drug alone.[15–18] Thus, physicians should note that if vision does not improve after one drug is stopped, then any other antitubercular agent being used as part of the treatment regimen must also be stopped.

Several mechanisms have been proposed as being responsible for the optic neuropathy that develops during isoniazid therapy. Low serum zinc, pyridoxine deficiency, or slow acetylation of isoniazid resulting in high serum levels alone or in combination may be the cause of isoniazid optic neuropathy.[19] Patients on isoniazid therapy should have a baseline ophthalmologic examination and be tested every 6 months while on therapy. If visual dysfunction occurs, isoniazid should be immediately discontinued.[20]

Streptomycin

Streptomycin is an aminoglycoside antibiotic. Aminoglycosides are prone to produce both reversible and irreversible vestibular, cochlear, and renal toxicity. Bilateral retrobulbar optic neuropathy occurred in a patient treated with streptomycin for pyelonephritis.[2] The patient experienced bilateral blurred vision 9 days after streptomycin therapy was begun. Ophthalmologic examination showed sluggish pupils, 20/70 vision in each eye, bilateral central scotomas, and a normal ophthalmoscopic examination. Streptomycin was immediately stopped and thiamine was started. Complete visual recovery occurred 4 months after withdrawal of streptomycin. Several cases of blindness or optic atrophy following intrathecal injection of streptomycin have been reported.[1]

Rifampin

There have been no clinical reports of visual disturbances from the use of rifampin. Although animal experiments have shown selective effects of rifampin on uveal melanin in mice and rats and on pigment epithelial cells in sheep, optic nerve damage was not found to occur in rats treated with rifampin.[1]

Chloramphenicol

Chloramphenicol is primarily a bacteriostatic antibiotic produced by *Streptomyces venezuelae.* Chloramphenicol is currently seldom used because of bone marrow depression and fatal aplastic anemia. Optic neuropathy is reported in 3–5% of children treated chronically with chloramphenicol for cystic fibrosis. The optic neuropathy causes symmetrical loss of ganglion cells and atrophy of optic nerve fibers.[8] Optic nerve changes tend to occur in patients receiving large doses of the drug for long periods of time. One study of 98 children with cystic fibrosis receiving chloramphenicol demonstrated visual disturbances in 5.2%.[21] Patients had marked bilateral reduction in visual acuity and bilateral central scotomas, some patients had bilateral disk edema, and others had normal-appearing optic disks. Most patients had prompt visual recovery after drug discontinuation. Autopsies performed in three patients who had visual disturbances showed bilateral optic atrophy mainly involving papillomacular nerve fibers, loss of retinal ganglion cells, and gliosis of the nerve fiber layer. In this study, chloramphenicol was strongly believed to be the agent responsible for a toxic optic neuropathy because only two patients did not have improved vision after discontinuation of the drug and ocular symptoms recurred when patients were rechallenged with the drug. Three other cases of patients with cystic fibrosis treated with chloramphenicol were reported with visual disturbances.[22] Each patient had bilateral visual loss, visual field defects, dyschromatopsia, and hyperemic, swollen optic nerves. Interestingly, all three patients exhibited Uhthoff's phenomenon. Visual acuity was incomplete in all three, and bilateral optic atrophy developed despite withdrawal of chloramphenicol.

Metronidazole (Flagyl)

Metronidazole is used against infections due to trichomoniasis, amebiasis, giardiasis, and anaerobic organisms. One report documents seven patients who suffered decreased vision, dyschromatopsia, visual field defects, and bilateral optic nerve involvement.[23] Patients with visual symptoms received 750 mg to 1 g daily over a period of 1 week to 1 year. Two patients had residual visual deficits after the drug was discontinued.

Sulfonamides

Sulfonamides cause visual disturbances due to their effects on the optic nerve or retina. Patients have visual loss, central scotomas, and disk edema. After stopping sulfonamides, vision returns to normal. Optic atrophy is a known sequela.[1, 2]

Amantadine Hydrochloride (Symmetrel)

One patient receiving amantadine for essential tremor developed sudden bilateral visual loss 3 weeks after initiation of therapy.[24] Ophthalmoscopy showed normal appearing optic nerves. The patient had complete recovery of visual acuity after drug discontinuation.

Cardiac Drugs

Amiodarone Hydrochloride

Amiodarone is an iodinated benzofurane derivative used to control refractory ventricular dysrhythmias. Amiodarone can cause optic neuropathy.[25–28] Most patients present with reduced visual acuity and bilateral optic disk swelling. The overall incidence of optic neuropathy is greater in patients taking amiodarone as compared with age-matched populations not on the drug. No randomized study has assessed the risk of ischemic optic neuropathy in cardiac patients with ventricular arrhythmias because of the great risk to life entailed in withholding proper drug therapy in patients with intractable arrhythmias. The optic neuropathy seen in patients on amiodarone therapy differs in several ways from nonarteritic ischemic optic neuropathy. Most patients with amiodarone-induced optic neuropathy have substantial vision loss. Yet, visual recovery as well as resolution of optic nerve changes are observed in contrast to patients with nonarteritic ischemic optic neuropathies. Also, patients with optic neuropathy presumed to be due to amiodarone have increased cup-to-disk ratios unlike the "crowding phenomenon" with absent cups or small physiologic cups found in patients with ischemic optic neuropathy.[26] There are several reports of pseudotumor cerebri associated with administration of amiodarone.[25, 27] These reports are speculative because many patients did not have lumbar punctures performed to determine if cerebrospinal fluid pressure was elevated. Improvement in vision and resolution of optic disk changes follows discontinuation of the drug.[28]

Amiodarone is a cationic amphophilic drug with adjacent hydrophilic and hydrophobic moieties, allowing the drug to bind to polar lipids and accumulate within lysosomes. These properties are the basis for the formation of verticillate keratopathy (whorl-like deposits in the corneal epithelium). The corneal epithelial whorls seen by biomicroscopic examination are generally reversible when amiodarone treatment is stopped. Less than 10% of patients with verticillate keratopathy have visual symptoms. Histopathologic study from an asymptomatic patient on amiodarone therapy revealed accumulation of intracytoplasmic lamellar inclusions in the large axons of the optic nerve.[28, 29] These intracytoplasmic inclusions accumulate at the prelaminar level of the optic nerve and cause axonal swelling, resulting in axonal compression and impaired axoplasmic flow.

The presence of optic neuropathy due to amiodarone therapy is only a relative indication for withdrawal of the agent because many of these patients have potentially fatal, otherwise intractable cardiac arrhythmias that have not responded to other drugs. Nonarteritic or arteritic ischemic optic neuropathy should be excluded in these severely disabled cardiac patients on amiodarone therapy.[30]

Perhexiline Maleate (Pexid)

Perhexiline maleate is a coronary vasodilator that is used for treatment of severe angina pectoris. Serious side effects associated with this drug are hypoglycemia, peripheral neuropathy, hepatic dysfunction, and increased intracranial pressure. Gibson et al. reported a case of visual loss secondary to increased intracranial pressure and chronic papilledema associated with perhexiline toxicity.[31] In other case reports of bilateral disk edema in patients on perhexiline therapy, the intracranial pressure was either normal or not measured. It is not fully understood why perhexiline occasionally causes increased intracranial pressure and papilledema. Due to the amphophilic nature of perhexiline, the presence of a vortex keratopathy (whorl-like deposits in the corneal epithelium) should alert the physician to look for other potential side effects including optic neuropathy.[32–34]

Amoproxan

Amoproxan is a coronary artery dilator and antiarrhythmic drug that has been withdrawn from production. Bilateral optic neuropathies with visual loss and central scotomas have been reported with the use of amoproxan.[1, 2]

Digitalis

Digitalis causes a number of reversible visual disturbances such as flickering, dazzling, illusions of color, blue-colored borders on objects, or yellow, orange, or green discoloration. Some patients experience temporary blindness.[2] Reduced visual acuity is due to bilateral central scotomas. It is believed that the color vision disturbances associated with digitalis originate from a toxic effect on the cerebral cortex. The reduction of vision associated with central scotomas is due to a retrobulbar optic neuropathy.[35, 36] Others believe that the central scotomas are due to the influence of digitalis on the photoreceptor cells of the retina.[1]

Oral Hypoglycemic Agents: Chlorpropamide (Diabinese) and Tolbutamide (Orinase)

Chlorpropamide (Diabinese) is a sulfonylurea hypoglycemic that may cause a reversible optic neuropathy.[37] Tolbutamide (Orinase) is another sulfonylurea hypoglycemic capable of causing bilateral optic neuropathies.[1, 2]

Antimalarials

Chloroquine Sulfate (Nivaquine) and Hydroxychloroquine Sulfate (Plaquenil)

Chloroquine and hydroxychloroquine are quinoline derivatives used as antimalarials and as treatment for rheumatoid arthritis and systemic lupus erythematosus. These drugs are not toxic to the optic nerve, but cause retinal toxicity. Retinal damage occurs less frequently with hydroxychloroquine and is uncommon if the total daily dose does not exceed 400 mg. The recommended daily dosage of chloroquine should not exceed 250 mg. The major hazard with use of these drugs is that retinal changes may be irreversible or even progress in spite of the drug being discontinued.[1, 34]

In chloroquine retinopathy, the first and earliest retinal disturbance is a mottled pigmentary change around the macula. Later, concentric rings of hyperpigmentation and hypopigmentation appear around the macula, producing "bull's-eye" maculopathy (Figure 13.1). This configuration is not pathognomonic of chloroquine toxicity because it is also seen in cone dystrophy, Stargardt's flavimaculatus, Spielmeyer-Vogt-Batten-Mayou disease, and age-related macular degeneration. Ophthalmoscopic examination alone is often unreliable in detecting these macular changes. Stereoscopic fundus photographs are necessary to determine early signs of retinopathy. Visual field examination may show a pericentral scotoma to a red target. Unfortunately,

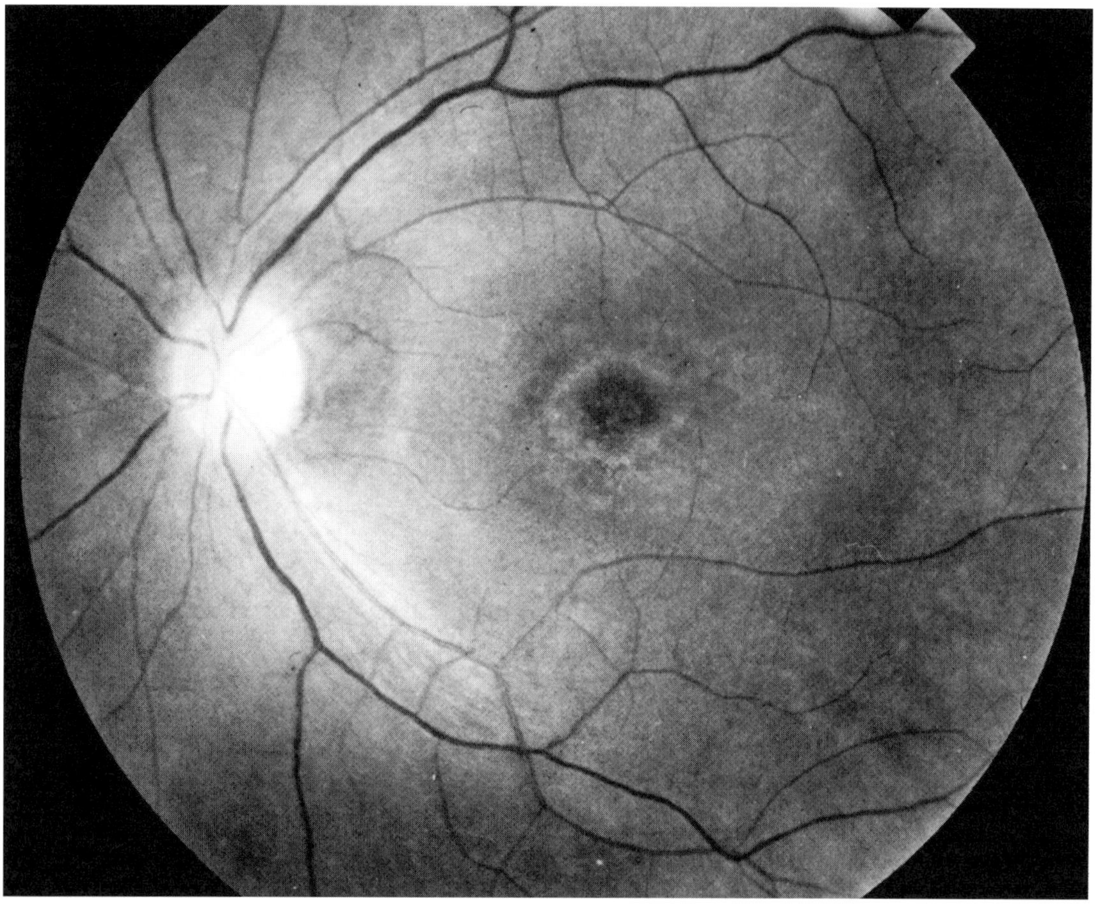

Figure 13.1. "Bull's-eye" maculopathy.

there is no reliable means of diagnosing chloroquine toxicity before serious visual disturbances occur. In extremely advanced cases of chloroquine toxicity, there is retinal arteriolar attenuation, optic disk pallor, and diffuse pigmentary changes in the retinal pigment epithelium.[38, 39]

Quinine

Quinine is the chief alkaloid found in the bark of the cinchona tree indigenous to regions of South America. Quinine is used to treat malaria and to relieve nocturnal leg cramps. It is found in low concentrations in tonic water. Quinine toxicity is due to overdose or hypersensitivity. Quinine toxicity produces tinnitus, headaches, nausea, and disturbed vision.[8]

Visual disturbances associated with quinine ingestion include visual flickering, alterations in color vision, photophobia, night blindness, visual field defects, and abnormal pupillary reactions.[40] Quinine poisoning with acute visual loss and varying degrees of visual recovery has been commonly reported. Both afferent and efferent pupillary defects have been reported with quinine poisoning. Ophthalmoscopic features include retinal edema and swollen optic nerves in some patients, whereas others have normal fundi or disk pallor. In animal experiments, severely poisoned dogs failed to recover vision; histopathologically, canine optic nerves were atrophic. Histopathologic study of human eyes after quinine poisoning shows degeneration of retinal ganglion cells and axons with atrophic rods and cones. Acute quinine damage appears to affect the outer layers of the retina and pigment epithelium early. There is also a direct toxic effect on retinal ganglion cells producing disk pallor and secondary narrowing of retinal arteries that continues despite improving vision. Fortunately, the clinical course in quinine overdose in human beings results in spontaneous visual recovery when quinine is discontinued.[1]

Gastrointestinal Drugs: Halogenated Hydroquinolines

The hydroquinolines are drugs used for a variety of gastrointestinal disorders. They comprise four groups: iodochlorhydroxyquin (clioquinol), diiodohydroxyquin (Diodoquin), broxyquinoline (Colipar), and chlorquinaldol (Steroxin). Clioquinol was formerly used as an antiamebic in the treatment of diarrhea. It has selective optic nerve and spinal cord toxicity that was discovered after patients received long-term therapy.[1]

An epidemic of 10,000 cases of a new gastrointestinal neurologic syndrome in Japan was first observed in 1956. This syndrome was named *subacute myelo-optic neuropathy* (SMON). The clinical syndrome was characterized by a symmetric sensory motor polyneuropathy of the lower limbs, ataxia, bilateral pyramidal signs, sphincteric dysfunction, and optic neuropathy. The responsible agent was the halogenated hydroxyquinoline, clioquinol. In September 1970, the Japanese government halted the sale of halogenated hydroxyquinolines, and the epidemic ended.[41] A wide spectrum of visual disturbances were described with SMON, including impaired color vision, central scotomas, and impairment of visual acuity from slight loss to blindness. Some patients had undetected visual loss until a severe optic atrophy ensued. At this point withdrawal of the drug did not result in visual recovery. In most patients, visual improvement occurred several months after withdrawal of clioquinol.[1,2]

Although clioquinol is used in a variety of pharmaceutical preparations, SMON has been rarely reported outside Japan. There have been other adult cases with a typical optic nerve and spinal cord syndrome reported throughout the world in which clioquinol has been the culprit. A report of 220 cases occurring outside Japan of possible neurotoxic reactions to hydroxyquinolines appeared in 1979.[42] In 42 patients, symptoms were directly related to use of clioquinol, and 69 patients had symptoms possibly related to its use. The most common manifestation, isolated optic atrophy, occurred in 15 patients. Others had a combination of myelopathy, visual disturbances, and peripheral neuropathy. Older patients were more symptomatic, and more women than men displayed the complete syndrome of SMON because they used the drug for longer periods of time.

Autopsy study of a patient diagnosed with SMON showed retinal and optic nerve degeneration and mixed motor and sensory neuropathy. The visual loss appeared to be due to degeneration of optic nerve axons and ganglion cell loss. Histopathologic studies demonstrated thinning of the retinal ganglion cell layer and subsequent demyelination of the optic nerves, chiasm, optic tracts, and occipital lobes. The lateral geniculate bodies showed transsynaptic degeneration. Histopathology demonstrated the loss of neurons and myelin with gliosis of the optic pathways, spinal cord, and peripheral nerves. The greatest abnormality in the visual pathway was due to loss of the retinal ganglion cell layer thickness in the retina.[43] The same clinical disabilities and neuropathology found in humans have been reproduced in dogs and cats, demonstrating the rather site-specific neurotoxic effects of clioquinol.[41]

A heritable fatal disease of zinc deficiency, acrodermatitis enteropathica, was formerly treated only with dihaloquinolinol drugs. Children who were treated for long periods with large doses developed varying degrees of visual loss and optic atrophy. The optic atrophy was initially attributed to use of hydroquinolines. Ultimately, the visual disturbances encountered in children with acrodermatitis enteropathica were attributed to zinc deficiency and not to the use of a hydroquinoline agent. Zinc is an essential element for nucleic acid synthesis, retinol oxidation, and brain tissue development. Therefore, treatment of childhood acrodermatitis enteropathica is aimed at treating the zinc deficiency rather than using clioquinol.[44]

Chemotherapeutic Drugs (Antineoplastic Drugs)

Vincristine

Vincristine is a *Vinca* alkaloid derived from the periwinkle plant, a species of myrtle. Vincristine acts as an inhibitor of mitosis in the treatment of leukemias and other malignancies. Vincristine is well known for its neurotoxic effects, causing a mainly sensory motor polyneuropathy and cranial neuropathies resulting in diplopia and facial palsies.[8] Optic neuropathy due to vincristine is rare.[45, 46] Retinal injury can occur from intravenous and intravitreal injection of vincristine.[1] Teichmann and Dabbagh described a case of vision loss following a single dose of vincristine for treatment of a grade II spinal cord astrocytoma in an 11-year-old patient.[47] The child received a total dose of 1.275 mg of vincristine. Six weeks later, the patient's visual acuity was hand motion in each eye with a left relative afferent pupillary defect. Ophthalmoscopic examination showed slight disk edema and bilateral temporal disk pallor. The patient never recovered vision and subsequently died. No autopsy was performed. This case points out that vincristine may cause severe visual loss on exposure to the drug alone. However, patients treated with vincristine have leukemia or other disorders that may cause optic nerve infiltration resulting in visual loss. This makes it doubly difficult to distinguish between loss of vision due to the disease process itself or due to the chosen antineoplastic agent. The 11-year-old child reported by Teichmann and Dabbagh had an extracranial grade II spinal cord astrocytoma tumor with a low likelihood of intracranial metastasis. Therefore, vincristine was the most probable cause of the severe, irreversible visual loss.

Sanderson et al. reported a patient with Hodgkin's disease treated with combination chemotherapy including vincristine.[45] During treatment, vision was reduced to 20/40 in each eye, and bilateral disk pallor developed. The patient died from a massive gastrointestinal hemorrhage. Autopsy of the visual system demonstrated loss of ganglion cells in the macula bilaterally and demyelination of the retrobulbar portion of the optic nerves. Vincristine was singled out as the possible culprit.

Unilateral optic neuropathy in children with acute lymphocytic leukemia following vincristine administration has been reported.[46] Patients reported severe ocular pain 6 days following intravenous administration of vincristine. Patients reported decreased visual acuity that improved after vincristine was discontinued following the onset of ocular pain.

Carmustine (BCNU)

Carmustine is a nitrosourea capable of crossing the blood-brain barrier. Nitrosoureas are toxic to bone marrow, lymphoid tissue, kidneys, lung, liver, and the gastrointestinal tract. Shingleton et al. reviewed 50 patients receiving high-dose intravenous carmustine and 10 patients receiving internal carotid artery administration of carmustine.[48] Delayed ocular toxicity after high-dose intravenous therapy with carmustine developed in two patients. One patient was asymptomatic; the second patient had bilateral visual field defects with subnormal visual acuity in each eye. Both patients had bilateral nerve fiber layer infarcts. Seven of 10 patients who received internal carotid artery carmustine injections complained of ocular problems 2–14 weeks after administration. Ocular changes occurred on the side ipsilateral to the carmustine infusion. After internal carotid artery carmustine administration, one patient had multiple nerve fiber–layer infarcts; one patient had a disk hemorrhage and nerve fiber layer infarcts; two patients had retinal hemorrhages and nerve fiber layer infarcts; one patient had peripapillary and posterior pole hemorrhages; one patient had retinal arteriolar narrowing and nerve fiber layer infarcts; and one patient had retinal hemorrhages, nerve fiber layer infarcts, and retinal arteriolar narrowing. The ocular findings in each of these patients are related to the dose and rate at which carmustine was administered. Carmustine is most effective for tumor therapy when given in high doses over a short period of time. Therefore, this chemotherapeutic agent may cause delayed ocular toxic effects.

Ocular toxicity is thought to be due to segmental intraretinal vasculitis or vascular obstruction. Intracarotid administration of carmustine allows a higher concentration of drug to reach the tumor and has fewer systemic side effects, but intracarotid infusion subjects the eye and its adnexa to a four times greater concentration of BCNU as compared with intravenous administration. One patient with a gemistocytic astrocytoma treated with intracarotid carmustine infusion presented with pallid unilateral disk swelling and an altitudinal visual field defect after a second infusion.[49] Intra-arterial administration of carmustine or cisplatin alone produced retinal or optic nerve abnormalities, depending on whether the agent was administered distal or proximal to the ophthalmic artery.[50] Carmustine and cisplatin are both toxic to retinal-neural tissue, and both cause vascular occlusive disease. Supraophthalmic intra-arterial carotid infusion of carmustine or cisplatin does not cause clinical retinal or optic nerve abnormalities. Infraophthalmic intra-arterial infusions of either agent, however, resulted in ophthalmoscopic changes. Another patient was reported to have acute bilateral optic neuropathies with disk edema after chemotherapy with carmustine, procarbazine, and cyclophosphamide.[51] Eight days after therapy, this patient rapidly progressed to no light perception vision. It is speculated that carmustine and procarbazine are the cause of the toxic optic neuropathy in this patient because both drugs are capable of crossing the blood-brain barrier.

Nitrosourea compounds soluble in both water and oil, such as hydoxyethyl-CNU (HeCNU), are associated with less severe ocular complications. No ocular toxicity was noted after a single course of HeCNU. This suggests that the vascular toxicity is due to a cumulative dose effect compared with BCNU, which may cause retinal or optic toxicity following a single infusion.[52]

Cisplatinum

Cisplatinum is an effective chemotherapeutic agent for both systemic and central nervous system (CNS) malignancies. It is nephrotoxic and ototoxic and has been reported to cause retrobulbar optic neuropathies, optic disk edema, retinopathy, and cortical blindness.[1] The mechanism of damage of intra-arterial cisplatinum toxicity is not well understood. Maiese et al. studied six patients exposed to this antineoplastic agent.[53] Four patients developed optic nerve damage ipsilateral to the side of intra-arterial injection. After further treatment, all patients had bilateral optic nerve toxicity. In contrast to other studies, administration of cisplatinum above or below the ophthalmic artery damaged the optic nerves.[50]

Tamoxifen Citrate (Nolvadex)

Tamoxifen is a nonsteroidal estrogen antagonist. White refractile retinal changes may be seen in the nerve fiber and inner plexiform layers, mainly in the macular area as a result of tamoxifen therapy. Tamoxifen retinopathy is usually dose related. One case report documented optic nerve toxicity due to low-dose tamoxifen therapy.[54] One patient developed bilateral consecutive optic disk edema with marked reduction in visual acuity while taking tamoxifen.[55] Visual recovery occurs after discontinuation of tamoxifen. Patients receiving tamoxifen therapy may warrant periodic eye examinations.

Methotrexate

Methotrexate is a folic acid analogue. Retinal pigment epithelium changes have been noted with methotrexate.[56] Axonal degeneration and demyelination of the optic nerves, brain stem, and spinal cord have also been reported with the administration of intrathecal methotrexate.[57]

Immunosuppressive Agents: Cyclosporine

Cyclosporine is a potent immunosuppressive agent used in transplant patients. Its major toxic effect is on the kidneys.[8] Cyclosporine is also neurotoxic, producing headaches, seizures, encephalopathy, hallucinations, coma, cortical blindness, and increased intracranial pressure.[58] Avery et al. studied eight patients with optic nerve edema attributed to cyclosporine treatment after bone marrow transplantation.[59] Optic disk edema improved when the immunosuppressant was discontinued or significantly reduced.

Drugs Associated with the Pseudotumor Cerebri Syndrome

Pseudotumor cerebri is defined by the modified Dandy criteria, consisting of increased intracranial pressure, normal brain imaging study results with the exception of small ventricles or an empty sella, normal cerebrospinal fluid formula, and no focal neurologic signs. Pseudotumor cerebri may occur with or without a precipitating cause. It is overwhelmingly more common in obese women of childbearing age. The syndrome is self-limited in patients in whom a causal relationship between drug intake and increased intracranial pressure is established. Pseudotumor cerebri, especially in the pediatric population, has been associated with withdrawal of corticosteroid treatment.[60, 61] Systemic corticosteroid treatment has been suggested as a cause of pseudotumor cerebri. Dees and McKay presented two patients with asthma who received systemic corticosteroids for 15 months and subsequently developed headache, vomiting, neck stiffness, abducens nerve palsy, and papilledema.[62] Ventriculography results were normal, and the cerebrospinal fluid pressure was elevated with normal fluid components. There appear to be more cases of pseudotumor cerebri consequent to reduction or cessation of corticosteroid treatment. When corticosteroid therapy is reduced or stopped, the signs of pseudotumor cerebri may become evident within a few days.[63]

Several antibiotics have been associated with increased intracranial pressure. Nalidixic acid and tetracyclines are among the antibiotics commonly implicated in pseudotumor cerebri. Minocycline (semisynthetic tetracycline)-induced pseudotumor cerebri is often reversible when the drug is stopped.[64]

Drugs used to treat acne such as vitamin A and isotretinoin may produce pseudotumor cerebri. Daily intake of 10,000 U or more of vitamin A over several months may produce increased intracranial pressure. Ocular side effects of isotretinoin include corneal opacities and papilledema. Isotretinoin-induced pseudotumor cerebri is probably due to hypervitaminosis A. Papilledema is reversible if the drug is discontinued.[65]

Many other drugs cause increased intracranial pressure and papilledema, including perhexiline maleate,[31] danazol, lithium, amiodarone,[25, 27] sulfamethoxazole, nitrofurantoin, and penicillin.[60] Drug-induced pseudotumor cerebri has a good outcome if recognized early and if the offending agent is promptly stopped. Diagnostic studies are often unnecessary if pseudotumor cerebri is presumed to be associated with the use of a particular drug. If no clinical improvement is observed after the presumed offending agent is discontinued, however, then neuroimaging studies and a lumbar puncture are required.

Chronic Alcoholism Treatment: Disulfiram (Antabuse)

Disulfiram was initially used as an antioxidant in the rubber industry. Factory workers exposed to this agent developed a hypersensitivity reaction to ethanol. Two Danish physicians who tried disulfiram as an antihelmintic became extremely ill at a cocktail party, and they soon realized that the disulfiram had altered their response to the alcohol.[8] Disulfiram given alone has few side effects. Ethanol is normally oxidized by alcohol dehydrogenase to acetaldehyde and then converted to acetyl coenzyme A. The later reaction requires the presence of the coenzyme nicotinamide adenine dinucleotide. The toxic effect of disulfiram on the optic nerve is speculated to be due to the accumulated by-products produced in the presence of alcohol by the enzyme blocking or to a direct toxic effect of the drug. Disulfiram competes with nicotinamide adenine dinucleotide for alcohol dehydrogenase, thus blocking the oxidation of acetaldehyde and increasing its serum levels. Acetaldehyde intoxication results in the so-called acetaldehyde syndrome. Patients with the acetaldehyde syndrome become flushed, with intense head and neck throbbing. They may also experience respiratory difficulties, nausea, vomiting, sweating, extreme thirst, chest pain, hypotension, weakness, vertigo, blurred vision, and confusion.[1, 8]

Numerous reports describe the ocular effects due to a disulfiram-induced reaction to alcohol. Disulfiram produces bilateral optic neuropathies. One patient had a retrobulbar optic neuropathy with decreased visual acuity and a cecocentral scotoma while using disulfiram.[66] Once the drug was stopped, however, visual symptoms improved. Symptoms reappeared when the drug was restarted, and on withdrawal of the drug a second time, visual recovery occurred. In another case report, a person developed blurred vision after stopping alcohol and starting a daily regimen of disulfiram.[67] The patient was a former cigar and cigarette smoker with adequate dietary intake. Visual acuity was $20/50^{-1}$ in the right eye and 20/50 in the left eye. The patient had bilateral cecocentral scotomas and disk pallor. The patient was instructed to discontinue disulfiram, and 1 month later his visual acuity had improved to 20/30 in the right eye and $20/20^{-3}$ in the left eye. Visual fields were unchanged. Several months later, the patient had no further visual improvement. Ophthalmoscopic examination was unchanged; however, the scotoma in the right eye was smaller, and the visual field was normal in the left eye. This case illustrates that visual recovery is usually complete within several weeks after withdrawal of disulfiram.

Visual recovery may occur after discontinuing disulfiram in patients who have stopped drinking but continue to smoke tobacco. Often, optic neuropathies in alcoholic patients are attributed to nutritional deficiencies. If a patient is using disulfiram and develops visual symptoms that do not respond to improved diet or vitamin supplements, withdrawal of disulfiram is recommended.

Monoamine Oxidase Inhibitors

Monoamine oxidase inhibitors block the oxidative deamination of monoamines, transiently elevating the cytoplasmic and vesicular concentrations of norepinephrine and serotonin. Retrobulbar optic neuropathies have been reported with the use of octamoxin and pheniprazine. Octamoxin has been associated with reduced central visual acuity, dyschromatopsia, bilateral central scotomas, and normal-appearing optic disks. Visual recovery is often incomplete with discontinuation of octamoxin. Pheniprazine previously used in the treatment of hypertension and depression caused visual disturbances in 1% of those receiving the drug. Patients experienced blurred vision, dyschromatopsia, and central scotomas. In some patients, the decreased visual acuity and central scotomas persisted, with the development of optic atrophy despite discontinuing the drug. Histopathologic studies showed loss of myelin in both the optic nerves and the optic tracts.[1, 2]

Other Drugs

Corticosteroids (Glucocorticoids)

Cessation or reduction in corticosteroid treatment may cause pseudotumor cerebri.[61] Teus et al. reported a single case of reversible, bilateral toxic optic neuropathy in a patient with bullous epidermolysis treated with fluprednisolone.[68] The cutaneous lesions improved within 1 month of corticosteroid treatment, but the patient noticed vision loss. The corticosteroid therapy was discontinued, and vision returned. The same patient was diagnosed at a later date with multiple myeloma and secondary amyloidosis. Once again, the patient was treated with systemic corticosteroids and had visual loss. Ophthalmologic examination demonstrated a vision of 20/20 in the right eye and 20/40 in the left eye, with a left relative afferent pupillary defect, dyschromatopsia, and an enlarged blind spot. Ophthalmoscopic examination was normal. Corticosteroid therapy was discontinued, and 9 days later vision was 20/20 in the right eye and 20/25 in the left eye, with no relative afferent pupillary defect.

Sumatriptan Succinate (Imitrex)

Sumatriptan succinate is a selective 5-hydroxytryptamine 1 receptor subtype agonist. When the drug binds to its receptor, it exerts its antimigrainous effect by causing vasoconstriction. A patient took 100 mg of sumatriptan during a severe headache episode associated with a visual aura.[69] Thirty minutes after ingestion of the tablet, the patient had blurred central vision in the left eye. Vision was reduced to 20/25 with reduced color vision. The left eye had a superior arcuate visual field defect. Funduscopy was normal. The patient was diagnosed with ischemic optic neuropathy associated with classic migraine. One month later, vision returned to 20/20 in the left eye with no residual field defect. The ischemic, reversible insult to the optic nerve that began 30 minutes after ingestion of sumatriptan may have been caused by the vasoconstrictive effect of sumatriptan on the posterior ciliary artery circulation. This case remains speculative.

Cocaine

Intranasal cocaine abuse has been associated with septal perforation and chronic osteolytic sinusitis. Unilateral and bilateral optic neuropathy due to chronic sinusitis has been reported after intranasal cocaine abuse.[70, 71]

Ibuprofen

Ibuprofen is a phenylpropionic acid derivative with analgesic, anti-inflammatory, and antipyretic actions. Ibuprofen overdose results in dizziness, nystagmus, apnea, unconsciousness, and hypotension. In 1971, 40 patients receiving ibuprofen were surveyed and examined for any visual disturbances.[72] Two patients developed cecocentral scotomas with reduced visual acuity. In both cases visual improvement occurred once the drug was withdrawn. In 1972 another case of ibuprofen-induced toxic optic neuropathy was reported.[73] After 6 months of ibuprofen therapy, the patient had reduced visual acuity and dyschromatopsia. Several months after discontinuation of ibuprofen, the patient had improved visual acuity and color vision. Ibuprofen-induced optic neuropathy is a rare and probably idiosyncratic reaction to a widely used drug.

Deferoxamine

Deferoxamine is a weak base, with a specific affinity for iron, used as a chelating agent for systemic siderosis. The mechanism of deferoxamine toxicity on the optic nerve and retina is not completely understood. Deferoxamine has the ability to translocate copper across cell membranes and also chelate other trace metals, including iron, nickel, copper, zinc, and cobalt. Toxic optic neuropathy due to deferoxamine may be caused by chelation of zinc. Metalloenzyme function may be decreased because these metals are necessary for enzyme activation. Decreased enzyme function may result in neurotoxicity.[1, 8, 34]

The most common reported side effect, albeit rare, with long-term therapy of deferoxamine is cataract formation. Toxic effects of deferoxamine include sudden visual loss, dyschromatopsia, visual field defects, optic neuropathy, and retinal pigmentary changes after intravenous administration of the agent.[74] Visual function improves when the drug is stopped. Pigmentary retinal degeneration resembles those seen with chloroquine retinopathy. Visual and auditory neurotoxicity has also been found in patients who had received subcutaneous deferoxamine infusions.[75] Patients had either visual loss, disk pallor, or abnormal pigmentary changes in the macula. The doses of deferoxamine administered to patients with visual symptoms were generally higher than those received by the asymptomatic group. Most symptomatic patients, however, were receiving standard doses. Many of the symptomatic patients were young and had low ferritin levels compared with the unaffected group. Patients receiving deferoxamine should be monitored for visual and auditory neurotoxicity with routine ophthalmoscopic examinations and auditory testing.[76–78] If patients become symptomatic, the drug should be immediately withdrawn, and the patients should be closely followed for improvement. When symptoms have improved and vision has stabilized, lower dose therapy may be considered if needed.

Alcohols

Isopropyl Alcohol

Isopropyl alcohol, or isopropanol, is a clear, colorless, volatile liquid with a characteristic odor and bitter taste. Rubbing alcohol, a common source of isopropanol exposure, contains either ethanol or isopropanol in a 70–91% concentration. Dermal absorption is not particularly hazardous, but inhalation may result in significant toxicity. Isopropanol produces gastrointestinal and CNS toxicity.[79] There are no reported cases of isopropanol-induced optic nerve toxicity. Systemic administration of isopropyl alcohol as a 70% concentration does not injure the eyes or affect the vision.[80] Ingestion of isopropyl alcohol often produces coma associated with miotic, sluggish pupils.[81] Hemodialysis is often needed to treat patients with isopropanol intoxication.[1, 79]

Ethylene Glycol (Antifreeze)

Ethylene glycol is an odorless, water-soluble solvent found in antifreeze and coolants. Although colorless, often a blue or green tint is seen in the liquid, which is an indicator dye. It has a pleasant, bittersweet, warm flavor. Once ingested it is rapidly absorbed, with peak serum levels reached within 1–4 hours after ingestion. Patients with ethylene glycol poisoning appear inebriated, but lack the odor of alcohol on their breath. An anion gap metabolic acidosis usually is found within 4–8 hours after ingestion.

Ethylene glycol is converted to glycoaldehyde by the enzyme alcohol dehydrogenase. Glycoaldehyde is oxidized to glycolate and then metabolized to glyoxylic acid, producing oxalic acid as a byproduct. Calcium oxalate crystals may precipitate in the urine. The systemic accumulation of these organic acids results in severe metabolic acidosis.

Most cases of ethylene glycol toxicity are associated with bilateral optic disk swelling. Death has been reported in adults following ingestion of approximately 75–100 g of ethylene glycol.[82] One person who drank a total of 8 oz of antifreeze over a 48-hour period had blurred vision and eventually went totally blind, with bilateral optic nerve swelling.[2] Over the next several months, visual acuity improved to 20/300 in the right eye and finger count vision in the left eye. The ophthalmoscopic examination then revealed bilateral optic atrophy. Another patient who ingested 120 ml of ethylene glycol developed progressive renal failure and several days later had deterioration of vision and bilateral disk edema.[2] Within 6 weeks, visual acuity began to improve, but the optic nerves remained mildly swollen, and hemodialysis was necessary due to persistent renal dysfunction.[2]

Once the diagnosis of ethylene glycol toxicity has been established, treatment should begin immediately. The stomach should be pumped once airway protection is secured. It is necessary to control the anion gap acidosis. If high blood levels of ethylene glycol persist, then hemodialysis is necessary.[79, 83]

Methyl Alcohol (Methanol, Wood Alcohol)

Methanol is found in solvents, paint thinners, duplicator fluid, carburetor fluids, dry gas, model engine fuels, and canned heat (Sterno). Bootlegged whiskey may be accidentally or intentionally contaminated with methanol. Methanol may be used by some individuals as an ethanol substitute. Methanol, or wood alcohol, is a by-product of destructive distillation of wood. In its crude form, the wood alcohol has an unpleasant taste and odor. If it is further distilled, it becomes odorless.

Small amounts of wood alcohol ingestion suffice in producing toxic optic nerve injury. Visual blurring occurs within several hours after ingestion. The dose of methanol needed to cause visual loss varies from a few milliliters to as much as a pint. The amount of food eaten and the amount of ethanol ingested prior to methanol consumption modify the amount of methanol absorbed. Visual impairment has resulted from ingestion of 10–15 ml of wood alcohol, and death has occurred after ingesting only 20 ml of wood alcohol. Some have survived ingesting more than 100 ml of methanol.

Initially, the ophthalmoscopic features include hyperemic optic nerves, shortly after which the optic nerves become edematous with adjacent retinal edema. As retinal edema develops, the retinal veins become engorged, and flame-shaped hemorrhages may be seen. At first, patients have central or cecocentral scotomas. Depending on the severity of the methanol poisoning and the effectiveness of treatment, vision may completely recover and there may either be resolution of the funduscopic changes or the optic nerve edema and retinal edema may persist with no visual recovery.[1, 2, 79]

Methyl alcohol intoxication produces a severe anion gap metabolic acidosis. Methanol is oxidized to formaldehyde by the enzyme alcohol dehydrogenase and then is converted to formic acid. The ocular toxicity of methanol is due to these two metabolic by-products. As with ethylene glycol, ethanol and methanol are metabolized by alcohol dehydrogenase. If the methanol serum concentrations are high, and there is severe metabolic acidosis, hemodialysis is necessary, in addition to ethanol administration.[83]

The Atlanta catastrophe in October 1951 resulted in 320 people being intoxicated with methanol. Ninety gallons of bootleg whiskey containing 35% methanol and 15% ethanol produced 41 fatalities.[84] In May 1979, 46 inmates had methanol poisoning when methyl alcohol from duplicating machines was used as homemade spirits in a Michigan prison. Three inmates died as a result.[85]

The mechanism of selective methanol toxicity on the optic nerve is not fully understood. A patient who ingested a liquor containing 80% methanol had bilateral optic disk and retinal edema before death.[86] Postmortem examination of the optic nerves showed central axonal necrosis, beginning 1–2 mm behind the lamina cribrosa and extending along the intraorbital portion of the optic nerve. Retinal examination demonstrated ganglion cell degeneration.

In methanol or ethylene glycol poisoning, the onset of systemic toxicity may be delayed. CNS toxicity is the predominant feature of isopropyl alcohol toxicity. Renal failure is more common with ethylene glycol poisoning. Ocular toxicity is more com-

Table 13.1. Clinical Manifestations that Differentiate Toxicity in Alcohol Substitutes

Type of Alcohol	Delayed Onset of Toxicity Depression	Central Nervous System	Renal Failure	Ophthalmoscopic Changes	Ketotic Breath	Severe Metabolic Acidosis	Anion Gap
Isopropanol	–	++	–	–	+	+	+
Ethylene glycol	+	+	++	+	–	++	++
Methanol	+	+	+	++	–	++	++

– = not present; + = present; ++ = markedly present.

mon with methanol toxicity. The odor of the breath may assist in determining the type of alcohol toxicity. Isopropanol produces a sweet ketotic breath. Ethylene glycol and methanol are odorless in their purified forms. The anion gap is smallest with isopropanol intoxication and greatest with methanol and ethylene glycol ingestion (Table 13.1).[79]

Lead

Lead can produce an anterior or retrobulbar optic neuropathy. Monkeys held in captivity have developed acute amaurotic epilepsy from lead paint chewed from bars on the zoo cages. One rhesus monkey, accidentally poisoned with lead, developed convulsions, loss of coordination, and blindness. Recovery was complete once the lead source was removed. Lead poisoning in children often produces increased intracranial pressure and cranial neuropathies. The optic nerves suffer injury due to increased intracranial pressure or due to a toxic effect of lead. Children may develop strabismus due to abducens nerve palsies caused by increased intracranial pressure. Bilateral disk edema or papilledema from increased intracranial pressure is then identified on ophthalmoscopy.[1]

Other cases of optic nerve damage due to lead poisoning do not result from increased intracranial pressure.[2] Lead may have either a direct toxic effect on the optic nerves or perhaps primary vascular disturbances result in optic nerve damage. Chronic lead exposure in developing mice produces a toxic effect on the optic nerve with hypomyelination and reactive gliosis.[87] The end result is optic atrophy due to increased intracranial pressure or a retrobulbar optic neuropathy. Other ophthalmoscopic findings in patients with chronic lead exposure include gliosis of the blood vessels of the optic nerve head, glistening gray spots on the disk, and a stippling pattern in the peripapillary area.[1]

Lead poisoning can be treated with calcium edetate or penicillamine. Large amounts of lead accumulate in the bones, and serum lead concentrations decrease slowly, even with effective chelation therapy.[1]

Insecticides

Dichlorodiphenyltrichloroethane

Dichlorodiphenyltrichloroethane (DDT) is a widely used insecticide throughout the world. Silverman and Laval reported a patient with bilateral papillitis thought to be secondary to exposure to DDT.[88] However, a study of 35 men with chronic exposure to DDT who had body fat concentrations of DDT and its isomers in concentrations 5–80 times greater than the general population had no ocular complaints. Other employees in the plant not included in the study also had no clinical signs of ocular toxicity.[1]

Organophosphates

Organophosphate pesticides produce a delayed distal axonopathy. Patients with chronic organophosphate intoxication developed bilateral optic neuropathies with bilateral visual loss, visual field defects, dyschromatopsia, and disk edema.[89] Later, these same patients developed optic atrophy and pigmentary retinopathy. The mechanism responsible for organophosphate ocular toxicity is unknown.[1, 2] Beagle dogs exposed to organophosphate pesticides for 2 years showed reduced numbers of nerve fibers in the optic nerves, with partial necrosis of retinal pigment epithelial cells and Müller cells; the retinal ganglion cells remained intact.[89a]

Cleaning Solvents

Carbon Tetrachloride

Carbon tetrachloride is a volatile, nonflammable organic solvent used for cleaning and degreasing. Toxic reactions occur through inhalation, skin absorption, and ingestion. There is no convincing evidence that carbon tetrachloride causes injury to the optic nerves or retina. Several cases have been reported, but a clear association is not easily identified.[1,2]

Trichloroethylene

Trichloroethylene is a nonflammable, colorless liquid used for degreasing and dry cleaning. In the past it has been used as an inhalational anesthetic and analgesic. Trichloroethylene toxicity is mainly caused by its decomposition products or impurities. Optic neuropathy and optic atrophy may occur. Visual disturbance from optic nerve damage due to trichloroethylene is less common than the trigeminal, facial, and oculomotor nerve cranial neuropathies that may develop with the use of this agent.[1,2]

Toxic Gases

Hydrogen Sulfide

Inhalation of high concentrations of hydrogen sulfide may cause coma and death from respiratory failure within seconds of exposure. The evidence for optic nerve toxicity is weak. A shipyard worker exposed to high concentrations of hydrogen sulfide for 15–20 minutes before rescue had delayed ocular symptoms.[90] After 2 days in a coma, the patient regained consciousness, but had impaired memory, hearing, and vision. His visual condition deteriorated until he became blind. However, no formal visual acuity was documented and the fundus examination was not reported.

Temporary damage by hydrogen sulfide to the corneal epithelium has been demonstrated in dogs, cats, and rabbits. One reported case documents an abnormal fundus as well as keratitis in a patient with acute exposure to hydrogen sulfide.[1] The first day after exposure, the patient developed engorged retinal veins. On the second day, bilateral disk edema with peripapillary hemorrhages was observed. The corneal epithelial defects healed after 5 days, but the funduscopic examination remained unchanged. The optic disk swelling was attributed to hydrogen sulfide exposure. Shortly thereafter, the fundus returned to normal.

Carbon Monoxide

Carbon monoxide competes with oxygen and binds to hemoglobin. Patients with low levels of carboxyhemoglobin often experience dyspnea on exertion and/or head tightness. As the levels of carboxyhemoglobin increase, nausea, dizziness, headaches, fatigue, and dimmed vision develop. Higher levels of carboxyhemoglobin produce vomiting, syncope, and confusion. Eventually, there is loss of consciousness, seizures, and respiratory arrest.[83]

Amaurosis, constricted visual fields, and optic neuropathies have been reported with carbon monoxide exposure. A patient had marked reduction in vision, binasal hemianopia, and bilateral disk edema after exposure to carbon monoxide fumes from dynamite blasting. Eventually, optic atrophy developed. A young child thought to have been exposed to carbon monoxide over a long period of time due to fumes escaping from a coal furnace was found to have visual disturbances with paracentral scotomas.[1] In carbon monoxide poisoning, no specific treatment is recommended for eye involvement other than removing the patient from exposure to the fumes and providing oxygen therapy.

Catha edulis (Kat, Khat, or Qat Leaves)

The main active principle in *Catha edulis* is cathione, which has sympathomimetic properties. *Catha edulis* is a member of the family Gelastraceae and is grown in parts of eastern Africa and southern Arabia. Khat-chewing is a main part of social gatherings in these areas. Inhabitants of these areas chew the fleshy khat leaves to produce euphoria and combat fatigue. The potency of the leaf is lost with drying and it must be chewed fresh. Two case reports showed decreased visual acuity and optic atrophy after an unusually high dose of khat alkaloids. One patient had bilateral central scotomas with hand motion vision in the right eye and finger count vision in the left eye. Ophthalmoscopic examination showed bilateral optic disk atrophy. Both patients had minimal alcohol intake at the time of their visual symptoms. The first patient was a moderate cigarette smoker and the second did not smoke. Chewing of khat leaves also causes a reduction in intraocular pressure in normal and glaucomatous patients.[91, 92]

Tobacco-Alcohol Amblyopia

Tobacco-alcohol amblyopia has become rare. Most patients with tobacco-alcohol amblyopia are men who develop a bilateral, symmetric, primarily retrobulbar optic neuropathy. The visual failure is gradual and is associated with bilateral cecocentral scotomas. The optic nerves are slightly swollen, are normal, or show temporal pallor. The etiology of tobacco-alcohol amblyopia has undergone much scrutiny. Many people who consume both tobacco and alcohol do not develop optic neuropathy. It is difficult to decipher whether tobacco, alcohol, or both have a direct toxic effect on the optic nerves. Tobacco-alcohol amblyopia may be a nutritional disorder because many people who also consume alcohol or tobacco have a deficiency of vitamin B_{12}, folic acid, or thiamine.[93–97] Alcohol reduces the absorption of vitamin B_{12}, but whether this condition results from vitamin B_{12}, thiamine, or folic acid deficiencies individually or collectively is unknown.[2]

Rizzo and Simmons studied two patients with tobacco-alcohol amblyopia.[98] Both patients smoked cigars; had no signs of malnutrition, no exposure to other toxic substances, and no substantial alcohol consumption; and were not deficient in vitamin B_{12}. One patient recovered vision with smoking cessation and administration of intramuscular hydroxocobalamin. The other patient had visual improvement after intramuscular hydroxocobalamin despite his usual consumption of cigars and 4–5 oz of alcohol daily. Bilateral visual loss due to smoking alone is rare, yet hydroxycobalamin and cessation of smoking can help with visual recovery.

Cyanide intoxication has been postulated as the agent responsible for tobacco-alcohol amblyopia. Thiocyanate is a detoxification product of cyanide by a ubiquitous hepatic enzyme, rhodanese. Smokers who develop tobacco-alcohol optic neuropathy have been found to exhale less thiocyanate than unaffected smokers.[99] This suggests that these patients may lack the ability to detoxify cyanide. Cyanide intoxication in smokers with tobacco-alcohol amblyopia has been postulated to be due to poor dietary habits resulting in low levels of vitamin B_{12}, folic acid, pyridoxine, or sulfur-containing amino acids, all of which play a vital role in the cyanide-detoxification process. Heaton et al. found that tobacco-alcohol amblyopia responded to treatment with vitamin B_{12}, even if the person continued to smoke.[100] Hydroxocobalamin is more effective in restoring visual loss than cyanocobalamin. Hydroxocobalamin has the ability to bind to cyanide, whereas cyanocobalamin cannot bind cyanide. Victor produced CNS lesions in rats with the chronic administration of cyanide in doses far larger than that consumed by the average smoker.[101] Lessell also produced bilateral retrobulbar optic neuropathy in 25% of rats injected with large, but sublethal doses of cyanide.[102] These experimental studies led these authors to argue against cyanide's role in tobacco-alcohol amblyopia. Of interest, patients with mitochondrial DNA mutations associated with Leber's hereditary optic neuropathy may be more susceptible to the effects of tobacco and alcohol, developing visual disturbances and a bilateral optic neuropathy, often mistaken for tobacco-alcohol amblyopia.[103, 104]

Tropical Ataxic Neuropathy and Konzo

The root of the cassava (*Manihot esculenta*), is part of a tropical plant that contains a cyanogenetic glycoside, linamarin, from which hydrocyanic acid is released during hydrolysis. Cassava is the fifth largest staple crop in the world and it is ingested by at least 500 million people. Natural cyanogens in the root crop cassava are removed by soaking, fermenting, or drying the plant before ingestion.

Often, insufficient processing of the plant, especially during a food shortage, results in high levels of cyanohydrins in the cassava. Cyanohydrins found in cassava flour are converted to cyanides in the alkaline environment of the small intestine. Cassava ingestion produces a slow decrease in visual acuity with constricted visual fields, optic atrophy, deafness, ataxia, weakness of the legs, and proprioceptive sensory loss secondary to dorsal column involvement. Patients have been shown to clinically improve when their hospital diet contains cassava only twice a week. Symptoms recur when patients returned to their usual daily diet of cassava.[1, 105]

Populations affected with Konzo share a history of high dietary intake of cassava and a lack of dietary proteins.[105] Two Tanzanian patients with Konzo also had specific visual symptoms.[106] One patient had bilateral central visual field defects with temporal disk pallor and dyschromatopsia, and the second patient had white spots in the macula with arteriolar sheathing.

Jamaican Optic Neuropathy

Jamaican optic neuropathy is thought to be caused by toxic products in bush teas. Bush teas are prepared from a variety of plants and are the beverage of many West Indian natives. Loss of visual acuity, central visual field defects, and temporal disk pallor have been attributed to bush tea ingestion.[2] Carroll examined 22 patients with visual symptoms thought to be due to exposure to bush teas and speculated on a number of genetic, infectious (treponemal), toxic, and nutritional factors in Jamaican optic neuropathy.[107] However, the actual cause of bush tea's effect on visual symptoms remains uncertain. More recently, nutritional deficiencies are believed to be the inciting toxic insult to the optic nerves.

Conclusion

Toxic optic neuropathies are often bilateral and produce painless visual loss, dyschromatopsia, and central or cecocentral scotomas. Swelling of the optic disks is not a universal occurrence. The visual loss may be irreversible despite withdrawal of the offending agent(s) and may occur despite administration of recommended dosages. Even though the drug is discontinued, vision may still continue to deteriorate, as sometimes occurs with ethambutol toxicity.

Physicians should have a high suspicion that drug exposure may be the contributing factor to visual failure in a patient. Patients should be warned of potential visual risks of drug treatment. Visual acuity at both distance and near, color vision testing, visual field testing, and anterior and posterior segment examination to observe for either optic nerve or retinal changes should be done at each ophthalmic examination. Patients receiving hydroxychloroquine also require stereoscopic fundus photographs to determine early signs of retinal toxicity. Fundus photographs allow for more precise detection of subtle interval changes of the optic nerve and retina. Patients should be informed that any visual disturbances be reported to the ophthalmologist immediately so that repeat ophthalmic testing can be performed. If vision has declined, the drug should be discontinued immediately.

References

1. Grant WM, Schuman JS. Toxicology of the Eye (4th ed). Springfield, IL: Charles C Thomas, 1993;135.
2. Miller NR. Walsh and Hoyt's Clinical Neuro-Ophthalmology (4th ed). Baltimore: Williams & Wilkins, 1982;254.
3. Carr RE, Henkind P. Ocular manifestations of ethambutol. Arch Ophthalmol 1962;67:566.
4. Barron GJ, Tepper L, Iovine G. Ocular toxicity from ethambutol. Am J Ophthalmol 1974;77:256.
5. Chatterjee VKK, Buchanan DR, Friedmann AI, Green M. Ocular toxicity following ethambutol in standard dosage. Br J Dis Chest 1986;80:288.
6. Leibold JE. The ocular toxicity of ethambutol and its relation to dose. Ann NY Acad Sci 1966;135:904.
7. Burde RM, Savino PJ, Trobe JD. Clinical Decisions in Neuro-Ophthalmology (2nd ed). St. Louis: Mosby-Year Book, 1992;60.
8. Gilman AG, Goodman LS, Rall TW, Murad F. Goodman and Gilman's The Pharmacological Basis of Therapeutics (7th ed). New York: MacMillan, 1985;382.
9. Smith JL. Should ethambutol be barred? J Clin Neuro-Ophthalmol 1987;7:84.
10. Slatter D. Fundamentals of Veterinary Ophthalmology (2nd ed). Philadelphia: Saunders, 1990;400.
11. DeVita EG, Miao M, Sadun AA. Optic neuropathy in ethambutol-treated renal tuberculosis. J Clin Neuro-Ophthalmol 1987;7:77.
12. Guerra R, Casu L. Hydroxycobalamin for ethambutol-induced optic neuropathy. Lancet 1981;2:1176.

13. Woung L-C, Jou J-R, Liaw S-L. Visual function in recovered ethambutol optic neuropathy. J Ocul Pharmacol Ther 1995;11:411.
14. Dixon GJ, Roberts GBS, Tyrrell WF. The relationship of neuropathy to the treatment of tuberculosis with isoniazid. Scott Med J 1956;1:350.
15. Jimenez-Lucho VE, del Busto R, Odel J. Isoniazid and ethambutol as a cause of optic neuropathy. Eur J Respir Dis 1987;71:42.
16. Renard G, Morax PV. Néurite optique au cours des traitements anti-tuberculeux. Ann Oculist (Paris) 1977;210:53.
17. Karmon G, Savir H, Zevin D, Levi J. Bilateral optic atrophy due to combined ethambutol and isoniazid treatment. Ann Ophthalmol 1979;11:1013.
18. Garret CR. Optic neuritis in a patient on ethambutol and isoniazid evaluated by visual evoked potentials. Case report. Mil Med 1985;150:43.
19. Leppert D, Waiske W. Neurotoxicity of antituberculous drugs in a patient without active tuberculosis. Neuro-Ophthalmology 1988;8:95.
20. Trobe JD. The Physician's Guide to Eye Care. San Francisco: American Academy of Ophthalmology, 1993;119.
21. Harley RD, Huang NN, Macri CH, Green WR. Optic neuritis and optic atrophy following chloramphenicol in cystic fibrosis patients. Trans Am Acad Ophthalmol Otol 1970;74:1011.
22. Godel V, Nemet P, Lazar M. Chloramphenicol optic neuropathy. Arch Ophthalmol 1980;98:1417.
23. Putnam D, Fraunfelder FT, Dreis M. Metronidazole and optic neuritis. Am J Ophthalmol 1991;112:737.
24. Pearlman JT, Kadish AH, Ramseyer JC. Vision loss associated with amantadine hydrochloride use. JAMA 1977;237:1200.
25. Gittinger JW Jr, Asdourian GK. Papillopathy caused by amiodarone. Arch Ophthalmol 1987;105:349.
26. Feiner LA, Younge BR, Kazmier FJ, et al. Optic neuropathy and amiodarone therapy. Mayo Clin Proc 1987;62:702.
27. Nazarian SM, Jay WM. Bilateral optic neuropathy associated with amiodarone therapy. J Clin Neuro-Ophthalmol 1988;8:25.
28. Garrett SN, Kearney JJ, Schiffman JS. Amiodarone optic neuropathy. J Clin Neuro-Ophthalmol 1988;8:105.
29. Mansour AM, Puklin JE, O'Grady R. Optic nerve ultrastructure following amiodarone therapy. J Clin Neuro-Ophthalmol 1988;8:231.
30. Sedwick LA. Getting to the heart of visual loss: when cardiac medication may be dangerous to the optic nerves. Surv Ophthalmol 1992;36:366.
31. Gibson JM, Fielder AR, Garner A, Millac P. Severe ocular side effects of perhexilene maleate: case report. Br J Ophthalmol 1984;68:553.
32. Stephens WP, Eddy JD, Parsons LM, et al. Raised intracranial pressure due to perhexiline maleate. BMJ 1978;1:21.
33. Hutchinson WM, Williams J, Gawler J. Papilloedema in patients taking perhexiline maleate. BMJ 1978; 1:305.
34. Rennie IG. Clinically important ocular reactions to systemic drug therapy. Drug Saf 1993;9:196.
35. Gillette DF. Visual disturbances due to digitalis. Trans Am Ophthalmol Soc 1946;44:156.
36. Wagener HP, Smith HL, Nickeson RW. Retrobulbar neuritis and complete heart block caused by digitalis poisoning: a report of a case. Arch Ophthalmol 1946; 36:478.
37. Wymore J, Carter JE. Chlorpropamide-induced optic neuropathy. Arch Intern Med 1982;142:381.
38. Brinkley JR Jr, Dubois EL, Ryan S. Long-term course of chloroquine retinopathy after cessation of medication. Am J Ophthalmol 1979;88:1.
39. Marks JS. Chloroquine retinopathy: is there a safe daily dose? Ann Rheum Dis 1982;41:2.
40. Gangitano JL, Keltner JL. Abnormalities of the pupil and visual-evoked potential in quinine amblyopia. Am J Ophthalmol 1980;89:425.
41. Otte G, de Coster W, Thiery E, et al. Ultrastructural study of a muscle biopsy from a patient with subacute myelo-optic neuropathy. J Neurol 1977;215:91.
42. Baumgartner G, Gawel MJ, Kaeser HE, et al. Neurotoxicity of halogenated hydroxyquinolines: clinical analysis of cases reported outside Japan. J Neurol Neurosurg Psychiatry 1979;42:1073.
43. Ricoy JR, Ortega A, Cabello A. Subacute myelo-optic neuropathy (SMON). J Neurol Sci 1982;53:241.
44. Sturtevant FM. Zinc deficiency, acrodermatitis enteropathica, optic atrophy, subacute myelo-optic neuropathy, and 5,7-dihalo-8-quinolinols. Pediatrics 1980; 65:610.
45. Sanderson PA, Kuwabara T, Cogan DG. Optic neuropathy presumably caused by vincristine therapy. Am J Ophthalmol 1976;81:146.
46. Norton SW, Stockman JA III. Unilateral optic neuropathy following vincristine chemotherapy. J Pediatr Ophthalmol Strabismus 1979;16:190.
47. Teichmann KD, Dabbagh N. Severe visual loss after a single dose of vincristine in a patient with spinal cord astrocytoma. J Ocul Pharmacol 1988;4:117.
48. Shingleton BJ, Bienfang DC, Albert DM, et al. Ocular toxicity associated with high-dose carmustine. Arch Ophthalmol 1982;100:1766.
49. Pickerell L, Purvin V. Ischemic optic neuropathy secondary to intracarotid infusion of BCNU. J Clin Neuro-Ophthalmol 1987;7:87.
50. Kupersmith MJ, Frohman LP, Choi IS, et al. Visual system toxicity following intra-arterial chemotherapy. Neurology 1988;38:284.
51. McLennan R, Taylor HR. Optic neuroretinitis in association with BCNU and procarbazine therapy. Med Pediatr Oncol 1978;4:43.
52. Defer G, Fauchon F, Schaison M, et al. Visual toxicity following intra-arterial chemotherapy with hydroxy-

ethyl-CNU in patients with malignant gliomas. Neuroradiology 1991;33:432.
53. Maiese K, Walker RW, Gargan R, Victor JD. Intra-arterial cisplatin-associated optic and otic toxicity. Arch Neurol 1992;49:83.
54. Ashford AR, Donev I, Tiwari RP, Garrett TJ. Reversible ocular toxicity related to tamoxifen therapy. Cancer 1988;61:33.
55. Torleif P, Von Eyben FE. Bilateral optic neuritis evolved during tamoxifen treatment. Cancer 1986;58:383.
56. Millay RH, Klein ML, Shults T, et al. Maculopathy associated with combination chemotherapy and osmotic opening of the blood-brain barrier. Am J Ophthalmol 1986;102:626.
57. Boogerd W, Moffie D, Smets LA. Early blindness and coma during intrathecal chemotherapy for meningeal carcinomatosis. Cancer 1990;65:452.
58. Wilson SE, de Groen PC, Aksamit AJ, et al. Cyclosporin A-induced reversible cortical blindness. J Clin Neuro-Ophthalmol 1988;8:215.
59. Avery R, Jabs DA, Wingard JR, et al. Optic disc edema after bone marrow transplantation. Ophthalmology 1991;98:1294.
60. Corbett JJ, Thompson S. The rational management of idiopathic intracranial hypertension. Arch Neurol 1989;46:1049.
61. Lessell S. Pediatric pseudotumor cerebri (idiopathic intracranial hypertension). Surv Ophthalmol 1992; 37:155.
62. Dees SC, McKay HW Jr. Occurrence of pseudotumor cerebri during treatment of children with asthma by adrenal steroids. Pediatrics 1959;23:1143.
63. Walker AE, Adamkiewicz JJ. Pseudotumor cerebri associated with prolonged corticosteroid therapy. JAMA 1964;188:779.
64. Monaco F, Agnetti V, Mutani R. Benign intracranial hypertension after minocycline therapy. Eur Neurol 1978;17:48.
65. Fraunfelder FT, LaBraico JM, Meyer SM. Adverse ocular reactions possibly associated with isotretinoin. Am J Ophthalmol 1985;100:534.
66. Perdriel G, Chevaleraud J. A propos d'un nouveau cas de néurite optique due au sulfirame. Bull Soc Ophtalmol Fr 1966;66:159.
67. Norton AL, Walsh FB. Disulfiram-induced optic neuritis. Trans Acad Ophthalmol Otol 1972;76:1263.
68. Teus MA, Teruel JL, Pascual J, Martin-Escobar E. Corticosteroid-induced toxic optic neuropathy. Am J Ophthalmol 1991;112:605.
69. Chiari M, Manzoni GC, van de Geijn EJ. Ischemic optic neuropathy after sumatriptan in a migraine with aura patient. Headache 1994;34:237.
70. Goldberg RA, Weisman JS, McFarland JE, et al. Orbital inflammation and optic neuropathies associated with chronic sinusitis of intranasal cocaine abuse. Arch Ophthalmol 1989;107:831.
71. Newman NM, DiLoretto DA, Ho JT, et al. Bilateral optic neuropathy and osteolytic sinusitis: complications of cocaine abuse. JAMA 1988;259:72.
72. Collum LMT, Bowen DI. Ocular side-effects of ibuprofen. Br J Ophthalmol 1971;55:472.
73. Palmer CAL. Toxic amblyopia from ibuprofen. BMJ 1972;3:765.
74. Lakhanpal V, Schocket SS, Jiji R. Deferoxamine (Desferal)-induced toxic retinal pigmentary degeneration and presumed optic neuropathy. Ophthalmology 1984;91:443.
75. Olivieri NF, Buncic JR, Chew E, et al. Visual and auditory neurotoxicity in patients receiving subcutaneous deferoxamine infusions. N Engl J Med 1986;314:869.
76. Orton RB, de Veber LL, Sulh HMB. Ocular and auditory toxicity of long-term, high-dose subcutaneous deferoxamine therapy. Can J Ophthalmol 1985;20:153.
77. Blake DR, Winyard P, Lunec J, et al. Cerebral and ocular toxicity induced by desferrioxamine. Q J Med 1985;56:345.
78. Freedman MH, Boyden M, Taylor M, Skarf B. Neurotoxicity associated with deferoxamine therapy. Toxicology 1988;49:283.
79. Litovitz T. The alcohols: ethanol, methanol, isopropanol, ethylene glycol. Pediatr Clin North Am 1986;33:311.
80. Wills JH, Jamesom EM, Coulston F. Effects on man of daily ingestion of small doses of isopropyl alcohol. Toxicol Appl Pharmacol 1969;15:560.
81. Lacoutoure PG, Wason S, Abrams A, Lovejoy FH Jr. Acute isopropyl alcohol intoxication diagnosis and management. Am J Med 1983;75:680.
82. Friedman EA, Greenberg JB, Merrill JP, Dammin GJ. Consequences of ethylene glycol poisoning. Am J Med 1962;32:891.
83. Wilkins EW Jr. Emergency Medicine (3rd ed). Baltimore: Williams & Wilkins, 1989;184.
84. Benton CD, Calhoun FP. The ocular effects of methyl alcohol poisoning. Report of a catastrophe involving 320 persons. Ophthalmology 1980;56:875.
85. Swartz RD, Millman RP, Billi JE, et al. Epidemic methanol poisoning: clinical and biochemical analysis of a recent episode. Medicine 1981;60:373.
86. Naeser P. Optic nerve involvement in a case of methanol poisoning. Br J Ophthalmol 1988;72:778.
87. Tenneloon G, Aitchison CS, Frangia J, et al. Chronic lead intoxication: effects on developing optic nerve. Ann Neurol 1979;5:558.
88. Silverman SM, Laval J. Bilateral simultaneous retrobulbar neuritis. Am J Ophthalmol 1963;55:1020.
89. Ishikawa S, Inaba K, Naito M, Oto K. Eye disease induced by organophosphate insecticide. Acta Soc Ophthalmol Jpn 1971;75:841.
89a. Uga S, Ishidawa S, Mukuno K. Histopathological study of canine optic nerve and retina treated by organophosphate pesticide. Invest Ophthalmol 1977;16:877.
90. Tvedt B, Edland A, Skyberg K, Forberg O. Delayed neuropsychiatric sequelae after acute hydrogen sulfide

poisoning: affection of motor function, memory, vision and hearing. Acta Neurol Scand 1991;84:348.
91. Roper JP. The presumed neurotoxic effects of *Catha edulis*—an exotic plant now available in the United Kingdom. Br J Ophthalmol 1986;70:779.
92. Drake PH. Khat-chewing in the near east. Lancet 1988;1:532.
93. Carroll FD. The etiology and treatment of tobacco-alcohol amblyopia. Part I. Am J Ophthalmol 1944;27:713.
94. Victor M, Dreyfus PM. Tobacco-alcohol amblyopia. Arch Ophthalmol 1965;74:649.
95. Potts AM. Tobacco amblyopia. Surv Ophthalmol 1973;17:313.
96. Stambolian D, Behrens M. Optic neuropathy associated with vitamin B_{12} deficiency. Am J Ophthalmol 1977;83:465.
97. Samples JR, Younge BR. Tobacco-alcohol amblyopia. J Clin Neuro-Ophthalmol 1981;1:213.
98. Rizzo JF III, Simmons L. Tobacco amblyopia. Am J Ophthalmol 1993;116:84.
99. Foulds WS, Chisholm IA, Pettigrew AR. The toxic optic neuropathies. Br J Ophthalmol 1974;58:386.
100. Heaton JM, McCormick AJA, Freeman AG. Tobacco amblyopia: a clinical manifestation of vitamin B_{12} deficiency. Lancet 1958;2:286.
101. Victor M. Neuro-Ophthalmic Defects Due to Alcoholism and Malnutrition. In JL Smith (ed), Neuro-Ophthalmology Focus. New York: Masson, 1979;357.
102. Lessell S. Experimental cyanide optic neuropathy. Arch Ophthalmol 1971;86:194.
103. Golnik KC, Schaible ER. Folate-responsive optic neuropathy. J Neuro-Ophthalmol 1994;14:163.
104. Cullom ME, Heher KL, Miller NM, et al. Leber's hereditary optic neuropathy masquerading as a tobacco-alcohol amblyopia. Arch Ophthalmol 1993;111:1482.
105. Tylleskar T, Banea M, Bikangi N, et al. Cassava cyanogens and konzo, an upper motoneuron disease found in Africa. Lancet 1992;339:208.
106. Tylleskar T, Howlett WP, Rwiza HT, et al. Konzo: a distinct disease entity with selective upper motor neuron damage. J Neurol Neurosurg Psychiatry 1993;56:638.
107. Carroll FD. Jamaican optic neuropathy in immigrants to the United States. Am J Ophthalmol 1971;71:261.

Chapter 14

Drug-Induced Vestibulocochlear Toxicity

B. Todd Troost and Melissa A. Waller

Objectives

- To increase familiarity with drugs causing cochlear and vestibular toxicity
- To understand the values and pitfalls of aminoglycoside monitoring
- To gain familiarity with the ototoxicity of topical agents
- To understand the therapeutic use of gentamicin in Ménière's disease
- To acquire information about the ototoxicity of chemotherapeutic agents
- To increase familiarity with mechanisms of drug-induced vestibulocochlear toxicity

A variety of drugs and topical agents have the potential of causing vestibulocochlear toxicity. It is a topic that generates significant interest and controversy among physicians and basic scientists. Neurologists need to be aware that drugs ranging from the well-known aminoglycosides to nonsteroidal anti-inflammatory drugs can have effects on the balance and hearing systems. Ototoxicity from topical preparations is an area of interest and concern for otolaryngologists using drops in the presence of perforated tympanic membranes; however, neurologists need to be aware as well of the potential damage to hearing. Vestibular damage from drugs can be put to efficacious use in the treatment of Ménière's disease as is discussed. As pointed out by Rybak, ototoxicity monitoring is in a constant state of flux, and information is presented on monitoring of drug levels as well as auditory function.[1] It is the intention of this brief review to present the effects of agents commonly used on the cochlear and vestibular system so that neurologists may recognize and understand the potential for imbalance and hearing disorders caused by ototoxic drugs.

Aminoglycoside Cochlear Toxicity

The aminoglycoside antibiotics streptomycin, kanamycin, neomycin, gentamicin, tobramycin, amikacin, and netilmicin all contain an amino acid sugar linked to an aminocyclitol ring by glycoside bonds.[2] In ordinary use, such antibiotics have been used for treating infections produced by aerobic gram-negative bacteria. The drugs are poorly absorbed with oral administration and are not transported into the cerebrospinal fluid readily. Ordinarily, they are excreted rapidly by the kidneys, with enhancement of toxicity in patients with decreased renal function. The majority of the toxicity comes from parenteral administration; however, toxicity from oral absorption has been reported, especially with neomycin, the toxicity being magnified in patients with gastrointestinal disease.

Aminoglycoside antibiotics interact with polyphosphoinositides in the hair cell membranes. The aminoglycosides increase the permeability of the membranes, causing the cells to lose magnesium, which is normally present in high concentrations in the mitochondria. It is believed that the loss of magnesium ions blocks enzymatic reactions, especially oxidative phosphorylation, in which magnesium is used as a cofactor, and leads to cell death. Studies on aminoglycoside toxicity in animals showed that giving a loop diuretic followed by an aminoglycoside does not affect cochlear toxicity any more than any drug singly. If the order is reversed, however, with an aminoglycoside antibiotic first and then a loop diuretic, the drugs act synergistically to produce toxicity, and the organ of Corti is severely damaged.[3]

Different definitions of cochlear toxicity have been employed while monitoring a large number of patients. The usual definition is a hearing loss of 10 dB bilaterally, or in some patients a 20-dB hearing loss. Matz and Lerner have shown in a number of studies that the rates of toxicity were similar for gentamicin, tobramycin, and amikacin, with netilmicin resulting in the lower incidence of cochlear toxicity.[4]

Neomycin and kanamycin are exquisitely toxic to the cochlea, and therefore, the parenteral use of such drugs should be limited. On a personal note (from B.T.T.), my first experience with iatrogeny with aminoglycosides came in a patient who was entirely paralyzed with Guillain-Barré syndrome and went on ventilatory support for a year. At that point, the patient was the longest survivor on total ventilatory support. She eventually returned to an ambulatory status, but was totally and bilaterally deaf because of the use of kanamycin to treat a gram-negative infection. Gentamicin affects the vestibular system twice as frequently as the cochlear system. At particular risk are patients with chronic osteomyelitis who are treated with gentamicin because of the long duration of therapy and the high doses required for treatment.[5] It should be emphasized that due to the extremely long half-life of gentamicin in the endolymph, vestibulotoxicity is probably equally dependent on dose as well as the length of therapy and can occur even with normal peak and trough levels. There is some evidence that there is an inherited mitochondrial DNA susceptibility for aminoglycoside toxicity. It is believed that the cochlear toxicity of gentamicin may be reversible in approximately 50% of the patients affected, with a recovery time ranging from 1 week to 6 months after discontinuation of therapy. As pointed out by Matz[6] and Kahlmeter and Dahlager,[7] investigators have attempted to determine whether once-daily versus continuous aminoglycoside dosage results in reduced ototoxicity. Some believe that intermittent dosage with an aminoglycoside antibiotic causes infrequent high maximum serum concentrations. This may be less toxic but as efficacious as a more frequent dosage. Kahlmeter and Dahlager reviewed reports of aminoglycoside toxicity in more than 10,000 patients, focusing particularly on prospective trials.[7] The authors found the incidence of ototoxicity to be 8.6% for gentamicin, 6.1% for tobramycin, 13.9% for amikacin, and 2.4% for netilmicin. Of interest is the fact that cochlear toxicity from aminoglycoside antibiotics is less common in neonates and children.

Monitoring of Aminoglycosides

Patients treated with aminoglycosides are monitored for two reasons: (1) to ensure that levels are adequate for therapy, and (2) to detect elevated levels that may be associated with a greater risk of ototoxicity and nephrotoxicity, with the belief that the dose can be altered appropriately. Matz states that there are no data showing that occasionally elevated peak and trough levels result in cochlear toxicity.[6] Toxicity can occur even in patients whose serum levels remain within an acceptable range.

Table 14.1 presents the suggested dose of aminoglycosides in adults with normal and impaired renal function. These peak levels may be modified according to the nature of the infection and the pathogen, according to Matz.[6] Relatively resistant organisms may require peak aminoglycoside levels above the recommended range for cure to be achieved. This is particularly true with severe infections such as endocarditis caused by *Pseudomonas*. If renal function is normal, the trough level generally decreases below the indicated ranges. An increasing trough level usually indicates a decline in renal function, although errors in timing of the sampling relative to administration of the dose must first be ruled out. As Matz again points out, peak and trough levels are obtained because of the convenience in relating them to the dose.[6] However, it is not clear whether

Table 14.1. Dose of Aminoglycosides in Adults with Normal and Impaired Renal Function

	Desirable Serum Level (μg/ml)			Maintenance Dose[a, d]		
Aminoglycoside	**Peak[a]**	**Trough[b]**	**Initial Dose[a, c]**	**Normal Renal Function**	**Impaired Renal Function[e]**	**After Each Hemodialysis**
Gentamycin and tobramycin	4–8	<2.5	2.0–3.0 mg/kg	1.7–2.0 mg/kg q8h	0.8–1.0 mg/kg at intervals (hr) approximately 4× serum creatinine level (mg/100 ml)	50% of the initial dose
Kanamycin and amikacin	15–30	<7.5	6.0–9.0 mg/kg	5.0–6.0 mg/kg q8h or 7.5 mg/kg q12h	2.5–3.0 mg/kg at intervals (hr) approximately 4× serum creatinine level (mg/100 ml)	50% of the initial dose

[a]Some infections may require higher dosage and serum levels.
[b]Patients with impaired renal function may have higher trough levels.
[c]An initial loading dose higher than the maintenance dose is given to patients with impaired renal function or for whom rapid onset of maximum therapy is essential (e.g., septic shock). Most patients with normal renal function receive the lower maintenance dose for the initiation of therapy.
[d]For obese patients, the appropriate dosage may be less than that indicated on a body weight basis.
[e]For example, if the serum creatinine level is 3.0 mg/100 ml, the maintenance dose would be given every 12 hours.
Source: Modified with permission from GJ Matz. Aminoglycoside cochlear ototoxicity. Otolaryngol Clin North Am 1993;26:705.

the risk of ototoxicity is related to either the peak level or the trough level; it is probably related to more complex pharmacokinetic function, such as the area under the curve, which is approximated by determining the peak and trough levels. The following is quoted from Matz[6] as a suggested schedule for determination of serum levels:

1. For patients with normal renal function, the peak level is determined within the first 1–2 days of therapy, the trough level within 1 week, and both peak and trough levels approximately weekly thereafter.

2. For patients with impaired but stable renal function, the peak level is determined within the first 1–2 days of therapy, the trough level and another peak level within 1 week, and peak and trough levels approximately twice a week from then on.

3. In the case of impaired and unstable renal function, peak and trough levels are determined within the first 1–2 days of therapy. Determination of serum levels may have to be made as often as daily thereafter while renal function remains unstable.

4. After any adjustments of dosage, the peak and trough levels should be determined within 1–2 days.

When monitoring renal function and serum levels, the incidence and severity of aminoglycoside ototoxicity is reduced. Unfortunately, once ototoxicity occurs, it may be irreversible and can even progress after the cessation of therapy. Once ototoxicity is detected, unless there is a compelling reason to continue aminoglycoside therapy, it should be stopped. In patients for whom even subtle additional inner ear damage would be catastrophic or who are at high risk for ototoxicity, such as those patients with impaired renal function, one should consider testing vestibular and auditory function.[6] Because this is rarely done, the benefits of such early detection are not completely known.

Vestibular Ototoxicity

Vestibular ototoxicity is defined as a chemical substance's having a destructive or damaging effect on the structure and function of the labyrinthine hair cells and their connections through the eighth nerve to the central nervous system (CNS). Vestibular toxicity can vary from minimal damage to complete loss of auditory and vestibular function. Such losses may be temporary or permanent. Vestibular toxicity, in particular, can be devastating.[8–10] The historic aspects of ototoxicity are well reviewed elsewhere.[11] With vestibular toxicity, the initial and most extensive hair cell damage occurs in the apex of the cristae and the striolar regions of the maculae. Next, there is further hair cell loss extending toward the periphery of the vestibular receptor and additional damage to the otoconial membrane and the otolith structures themselves. As pointed out by Black and Pesznecker, we may not understand the true incidence of ototoxicity because the initial ototoxic destruction of hair cells occurs well outside the speech range for the auditory system and outside the normal active and passive head movement frequency range for the vestibular system.[11–13] And even though the goal is always to use the most effective drug, depending on the pathogen, the use of specific antibiotics may, in fact, be mandated by clinical factors beyond the physician's control, such as the patterns of bacterial resistance or susceptibility. Costs may also be a factor, because gentamicin is vestibulotoxic but continues to be widely used because it is relatively inexpensive.[11, 14]

Prospective studies by Black et al. and others strongly suggest that vestibular ototoxicity occurs precipitously and without warning.[13] Vestibular toxicity may be associated with and follow signs and symptoms of cochleotoxicity. Tinnitus is often the initial symptomatic manifestation of cochleotoxicity and is usually high pitched and continuous, reflecting the cochlear hair cell damage in the basilar turn. If the tinnitus is subtle and the patient is very ill, the patient may not complain of tinnitus, becoming aware of it later only when he or she is well.[11] A majority of patients who receive potentially ototoxic antibiotics because of life-threatening infection are those who spend long periods hospitalized or at bed rest. It is only when the patient becomes well enough to be up and about that vestibular symptoms are first noted. The symptoms are often attributed incorrectly to the patient's general debility. Unfortunately, an accurate diagnosis of toxicity may be delayed or even overlooked. If the patient is ambulatory, the disequilibration becomes readily apparent. The patient may have an ataxic gait, lose his or her balance when turning quickly, or need to hold onto the wall while ambulating. Patients may complain of transient positional vertigo, but mainly complain of disequilibration. As the vestibular toxicity progresses, the patient may begin to complain of movement of the external environment or oscillopsia. The patient is no longer able to sense head movements and make compensatory ocular movements within the orbit. The symptom of jiggling or bouncing of the external environment, oscillopsia, is caused by the loss of the vestibulo-ocular reflex. With progressive loss of vestibular function, a patient may have to rely entirely on visual and proprioceptive input to control ambulation and becomes a "vestibular cripple," being totally unable to ambulate without the danger of falling. The patient then needs to be confined to a wheelchair.

Congenital ototoxicity can occur when a pregnant woman receives an ototoxic agent. If an ototoxic agent passes through the placenta to the developing embryo or fetus, damage to the auditory or vestibular system may occur, often with catastrophic results. Cleft lip and palate, skeletal malformations, ocular defects, and abnormalities of the cardiovascular, genitourinary, and gastrointestinal systems have been identified besides permanent deafness or balance impairment. When these conditions are present in an infant, it may be prudent to thoroughly query the mother's medication history during pregnancy and to follow up with the appropriate auditory or vestibular screening tests. The first trimester, especially the sixth to eighth weeks, appears to be the most vulnerable period. Quinine, salicylates, streptomycin, and dihydrostreptomycin have been among the drugs implicated.

In arriving at the proper diagnosis, a careful history is most important. The symptoms may have remained unnoticed when the patient was bedridden. For patients who complain of balance problems after hospitalization for a severe illness, it is clear that medical records need to be reviewed carefully for the drugs administered and cumulative doses. A recent prototypic case is presented.

A 68-year-old woman was readmitted to the hospital with complaints of dizziness, nausea, and vomiting. Neurology was consulted for the possibility of new brain stem infarction. The patient had recently been discharged from the urology service, where she had been treated more than 4 years for multiple urinary tract infections. The most recent admission was for another urethral infection. The initial evaluation included pelvic magnetic resonance imaging and ultrasound studies, which produced negative results. The patient was discharged on enteric-coated aspirin and seen as an outpatient 3 weeks later. She then complained bitterly of "blurry vision." On further questioning, she reported that things "jump around" as she looked at them. On examination, the patient had a greatly impaired vestibulo-ocular reflex, being unable to fixate on a target as her head was gently moved from side to side. Review of her recent admission showed that she had been treated with gentamicin for 4 days. She was asymptomatic until 4 days after discharge. A single trough level of 4.2 was noted during her hospitalization. Our impression was that the patient, whose renal function was not impaired, had an idiosyncratic sensitivity to gentamicin and a delayed vestibular toxicity. Unfortunately, she was totally unable to ambulate and had a major reduction in vestibular function, demonstrated by no response to caloric testing and standard electronystagmography.

Vestibular testing has been discussed in detail by Black and Pesznecker.[11] Figure 14.1 shows serial responses for the vestibular ocular reflex at baseline, when a patient was ototoxic, and during recovery.[13] Electrocochleography has been shown to demonstrate an immediate reduction in action potential and cochlear microphonic within minutes after an intravenous dose of aminoglycoside.[15] Such testing is not routinely done, but may have a role as a screening tool in patients that are particularly susceptible to ototoxic drugs. In general, such drugs should be avoided in patients with risk factors or those predisposed to ototoxicity such as those with end-stage renal or hepatic impairment or a previous history of hearing or balance disorders.

Whether there will be recovery is unknown. If ototoxic damage is incomplete, and this may be difficult to tell clinically, the chances of some reversible damage has been quoted at 10–15%, depending on the agent involved and the risk factors.[11] If damage is severe, in all likelihood the damage will be permanent, and a subject must be prepared for this eventuality.[11, 16] In our experience, however, significant recovery can occur in even the most severely vestibulotoxic patients. One patient with impaired renal function received gentamicin because of a shunt infection. She was inadvertently given the full dose rather than the renal dose. Severe oscillopsia and total imbalance persisted for a year, but over the next 24 months gradual improvement ensued. She was able to move from a wheelchair, to a walker, to two canes, and eventually to ambulation with the use of a single cane, at which time she no longer complained of oscillopsia. The recovery in this patient was unique in our experience.

After the induced loss of vestibular function from aminoglycosides the patient becomes "visually dependent," relying exclusively on vision and proprioception to compensate for the loss of control.[11] Such patients should be advised not to attempt to navigate in situations of reduced illumination and, because they are dependent on proprioceptive cues, must be extremely careful when moving on uneven surfaces. Black and colleagues indicate that they have never seen an ototoxic patient completely adapt or compensate.[11] Because of visual dependence and oscillopsia, ototoxic patients should not climb on chairs or step stools, ladders, roofs, or other high places from which they could fall and be injured. They should also not operate dangerous machinery (e.g., power lawn mowers, construction equipment) and should not drive until balance and coordination have stabilized and until they can pass the driver's license test. Patients should avoid swimming underwater, as the perceived loss of gravity induced by the water's buoyancy could cause a loss of orientation, so they are unable to locate the surface; in preparation for this eventuality, patients should be trained to blow out a bubble and follow it upward.[11]

It is difficult to monitor for potential vestibular ototoxicity because of the expense and time-consuming nature of vestibular testing. Most patients receiving potentially ototoxic drugs are confined to bed and are unable to cooperate fully and maintain alertness for the testing. If any vestibular toxicity is suspected, the decision should be made to discontinue the aminoglycoside drug unless there is no other way to treat the infection. Serum trough levels are not uniformly useful in determining whether there will be vestibular toxicity. According to Black

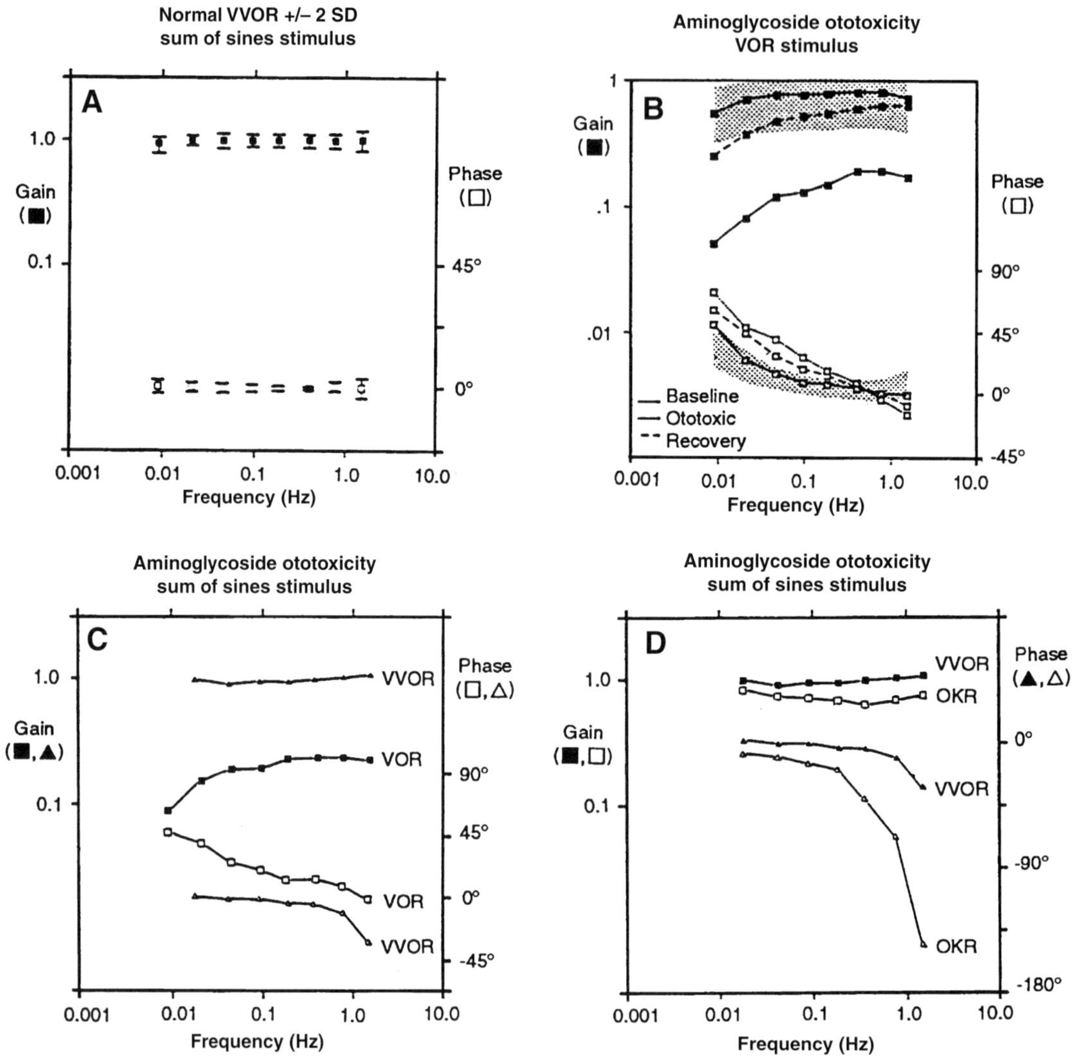

Figure 14.1. Serial responses on one ototoxic patient (typical) shown with respect to population data for vestibulo-ocular reflex (VOR) and visual VOR (VVOR) responses as a function of frequency and recovery (compensation). In order to see clearly during head movement, it is necessary to achieve a gain of unity and zero phase (i.e., head/eye velocity) at all frequencies of active or passive head movement. (A) The VVOR gain (left ordinate) and phase (right ordinate) of 10 normal subjects as a function of frequency (abscissa) indicating unity gain and zero (compensatory) phase (velocity) during passive head rotations with the subjects' eyes open and viewing an earth-fixed, full-field visual surround. Rotational stimulus was sum of sines 0.01–1.50 Hz. Nystagmus recorded with electro-oculography. Error bars indicate 2 standard deviations. (B) Plot of baseline and serial test results of VOR response to same rotational stimulus, plotted with respect to a normal population (shaded).[13] Note recovery of responses above 0.1 Hz to low normal range during compensation. Response phases did not return to normal below approximately 0.8 Hz. (C) Both VVOR and VOR responses of this patient following compensation. VVOR gain returned to normal; however, a high-frequency phase lag persists with eyes open (VVOR) but not with eyes closed (VOR), indicating increased dependence on vision to stabilize eyes, with respect to visual surrounds, with loss of vestibular function. (D) Comparison of VOR and optokinetic responses (OKR) from the same patient. The OKR phase begins to lag above 0.1 Hz (normal). The VOR, and consequently, the VVOR, phase lags occur at higher frequencies, demonstrating OKR contribution to the VVOR, which is especially important for compensation of low-frequency head movements when vestibular function is compromised. Higher frequency head movements cannot be compensated for by the ototoxic subjects. This patient's compensatory strategy must limit head movements to frequencies below approximately 1 Hz to avoid oscillopsia. (Reprinted with permission from FO Black, RJ Perterka, SE Elardo. Vestibular reflex changes following aminoglycoside induced ototoxicity. Laryngoscope 1987;97:582.)

and Pesznecker, on the basis of their studies, there was no correlation between serum levels and vestibular ototoxicity.[11] They remarked that "serum levels can be useful in guiding clinicians to use a systemic dose that achieves a minimum effective blood level while avoiding and reducing additional risk of ototoxicity related to excessive dosage."[11]

The following high-risk groups should be periodically monitored[16]: (1) patients with impaired renal function, evident either before or during therapy; (2) patients with elevated peak and trough serum levels; (3) patients with preexisting sensorineural hearing loss; (4) patients receiving more than one ototoxic drug (particularly an aminoglycoside and a loop diuretic); (5) patients with a history of receiving ototoxic drugs; (6) patients who are expected to receive ototoxic agents for more than 14 days; (7) patients with symptoms of cochlear or vestibular toxicity that become obvious during treatment; and (8) patients older than age 65. Dose and monitoring guidelines for individual drugs listed in the *Physician's Desk Reference* should be followed.[17]

Therapeutic Use of Aminoglycosides in Ménière's Disease

Although there has been iatrogenic injury to the peripheral vestibular apparatus due to ototoxicity, this can be put to use in the therapy of Ménière's disease. Ménière's disease, a condition of unknown etiology, has the clinical spectrum of sudden attacks of severe vertigo, progressive hearing loss, roaring in the ears or tinnitus, and a sensation of fullness in the ears. Although medical therapy can be beneficial to some people in the form of vestibular suppressant medication and diuretics, eventually 10% or more of those suffering from Ménière's disease become so disabled that surgery is considered. Destructive procedures such as labyrinthectomy have been proposed for the control of Ménière's disease. However, aminoglycosides may be used to treat Ménière's disease because of the differential effect on vestibular hair cells as opposed to cochlear hair cells.[18–21] Therefore, selective end-organ lesion may be achieved with a relative preservation of hearing. Initially, intramuscular streptomycin was used.[18, 22, 23] More recently, aminoglycosides have been applied to the middle ear in unilateral Ménière's disease. Schuknecht initially developed a technique to administer streptomycin solution to the middle ear via catheter tubing.[24] More recently, different protocols have been employed with gentamicin to reduce the incidence of hearing loss.[25–27] Currently, a standard technique is to inject gentamicin through the tympanic membrane. In one series of 20 patients, with at least 2 years' follow-up, vertigo was controlled in 90%.[27] Injections into the lateral semicircular canal have also been employed; however, these cause hearing loss in a high proportion of patients.[28] It is believed that intratympanic administration may be the most promising for future development and treatment.[29, 30] The effects can be titrated by giving smaller doses over a period of time, which, it is hoped, will result in effective therapy for Ménière's disease with preservation of hearing.

Other Drug-Related Sources of Ototoxicity

Chemotherapeutic Agents and Ototoxicity

An excellent review of the ototoxicity of chemotherapeutic agents is presented by Schweitzer.[31] The most commonly reported ototoxic chemotherapeutic agents include the following:

1. Platinum compounds
   a. *cis*-diamminedichloraplatinum II: permanent dose-related, cumulative cochlear toxicity
   b. *cis*-diammine-1,1-cyclobutaine decar boxylate platinum II: minimal clinical cochlear toxicity
2. Nitrogen mustard: cochlear toxicity
3. 6-Amino nicotinamide: neurotoxic and cochlear toxic (dose-related, cumulative, irreversible sensorineural hearing loss); not in current clinical use
4. Vincristine and vinblastine sulfate: dose-related peripheral and autonomic neuropathy; rare reports of cochlear toxicity
5. Misonidazole: cochlear toxic, neurotoxic (paresthesias); not marketed in the United States
6. α-Diflouromethylornithine: transient or permanent dose-related toxicity

7. Dichloromethotrexate: permanent cochleovestibular toxicity; not marketed in the United States
8. Lonidamine: questionable reversible ototoxicity; not approved for marketing in the United States or Europe

The most commonly used chemotherapeutic agent and a major ototoxic agent among these compounds is cisplatin. Figure 14.2 shows a progressive hearing loss in a patient receiving cisplatin. Cisplatin is a divalent platinum compound that produces a dose-limiting, permanent, high-frequency sensorineural hearing loss and peripheral neuropathy as well as a dose-related cumulative renal insufficiency with tubular necrosis and interstitial nephritis. The potential for dose-limiting and permanent cochlear (neuro) toxicity remains despite present methods of hypertonic saline, prehydration, and mannitol diuresis before drug administration. As pointed out by Schweitzer, the biochemistry, pharmacokinetics, biodistribution, and immunologic mechanisms of platinum complexes are still undefined.[31] There is significant variability in presentation and susceptibility to cisplatin-mediated ototoxicity. Ototoxicity resulting from treatment may be subjectively experienced as hearing loss and tinnitus. The tinnitus may be transient or permanent.[32] Tinnitus may accompany hearing loss, particularly at high frequencies, or may be present without any sign of hearing impairment. The overall early incidence of tinnitus, where clearly specified in clinical trials, is approximately 7% (range of 2–36%). The tinnitus is commonly transient, disappearing a few hours to weeks after discontinuation of treatment.

Hearing loss due to cisplatin is well documented. The high-frequency hearing loss may cause difficulties in speech discrimination with background noise and may also involve middle-frequency ranges, with inhibition of speech communication even in quiet surroundings.[32, 33] The hearing loss in most cases is permanent, but recovery has been described.[33]

Although the cochlear toxicity of cisplatin is well documented histologically and functionally, there are still a few reports confirming cisplatin-induced vestibular toxicity.[34, 35]

Nitrogen mustard, the first clinically useful chemotherapeutic agent, has limited modern application owing to severe toxicity. The toxicity has been characterized by irreversible sensorineural hearing loss and tinnitus.

Vincristine sulfate induces a dose-related peripheral and autonomic neuropathy, and there are few reported cases of vincristine-induced ototoxicity.[36, 37]

Anti-Inflammatory Drugs and Ototoxicity

A side effect of salicylates and many nonsteroidal anti-inflammatory drugs is ototoxicity manifesting as mild to moderate, reversible hearing loss and tinnitus. Aspirin ototoxicity occurs in 11 per 1,000 patients, with a much higher incidence reported for the long-acting aspirins.[38, 39] Elderly patients are at a significantly high risk of salicylate toxicity even at lower salicylate doses.[40] Quinine ototoxicity is quite similar to salicylate clinical manifestations and has a mechanism distinct from that of salicylates. The increasing popularity of quinine for treatment of nocturnal leg cramps makes quinine ototoxicity a relevant clinical problem. The manifestations of salicylate ototoxicity are quite well known: nausea, vomiting, tinnitus, hearing loss, headache, mental changes, and increased respiration.[41] The hearing loss is typically mild to moderate and bilaterally symmetric. It may be flat or just in the high frequencies. Recovery usually occurs 24–72 hours after cessation of the drug. Temporary high-frequency hearing loss with tinnitus after aspirin treatment has occurred in normal volunteers.[42] Tinnitus also occurs with salicylates with the usual frequency of tinnitus being in the 7- to 9-kHz range.[42] Tinnitus may be used as an initial sign of salicylate ototoxicity and may be used as a baseline in patients with initially normal hearing.[43] It is believed that the mechanism of salicylate ototoxicity is related to reversible biochemical or metabolic changes in the cochlear, rather than any permanent morphologic abnormality. Nonsteroidal anti-inflammatory drugs are a heterogeneous group of compounds that share therapeutic actions and side effects of salicylates.[41] In one study, five patients suffered hearing loss while receiving naproxen, and only two recovered their hearing after discontinuing the drug.[44] Rarely, there may a significant and permanent loss of hearing shortly after the start of a nonsteroidal agent (Figure 14.3).

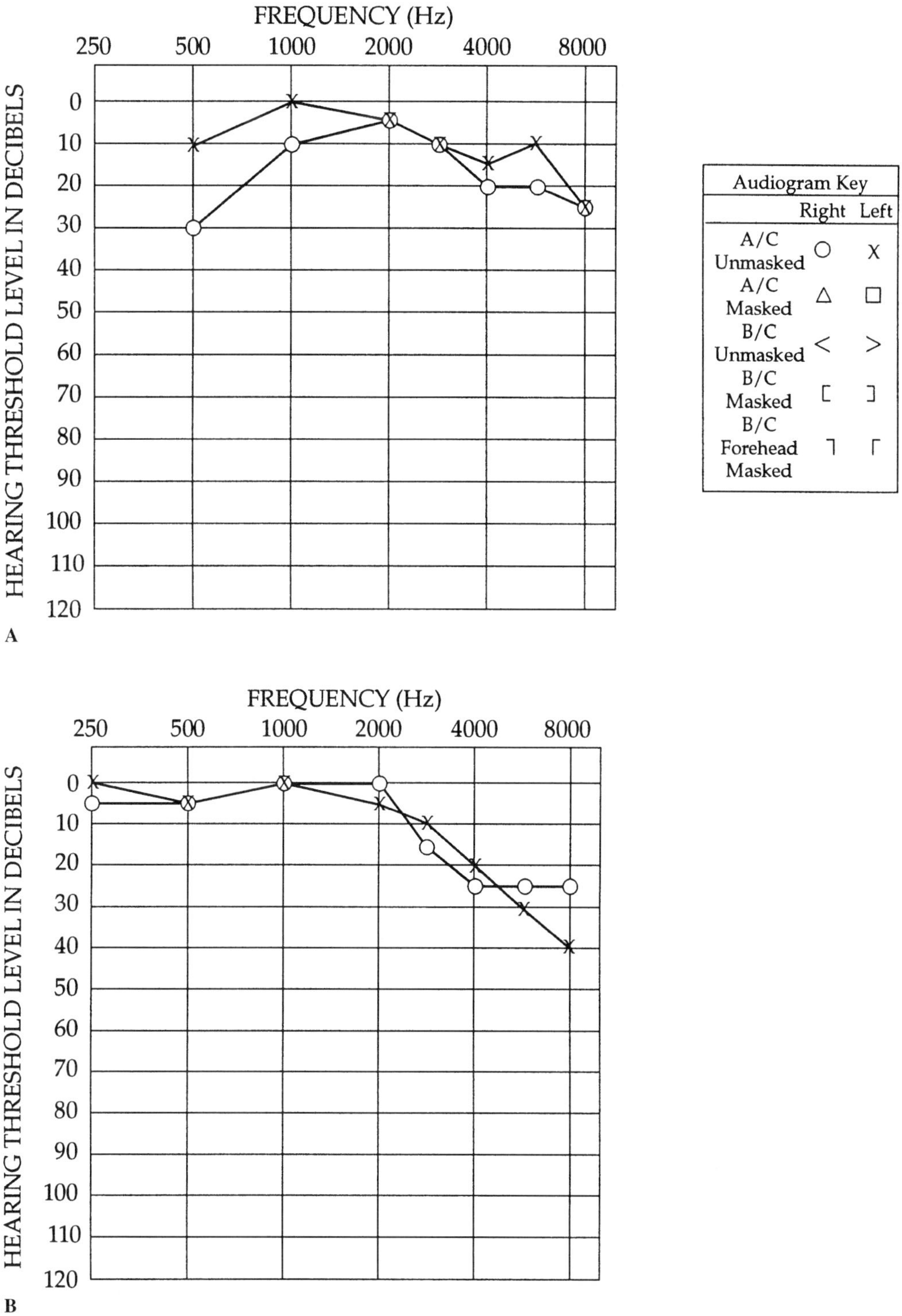

Figure 14.2. Progressive hearing loss in a patient receiving cisplatin. (A) Baseline. (B) One month later.

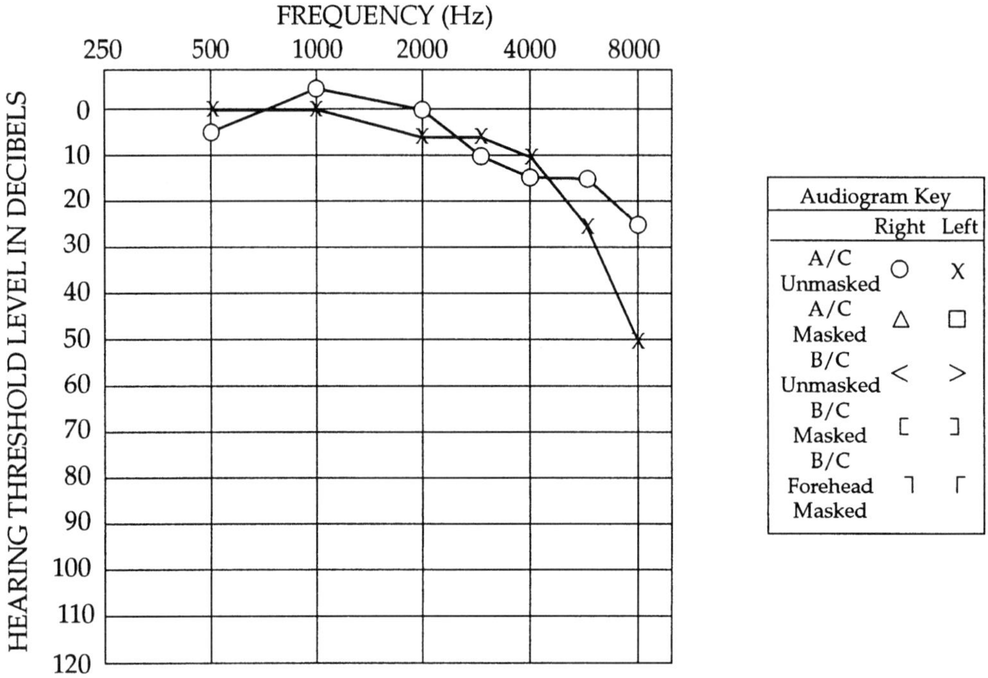

C

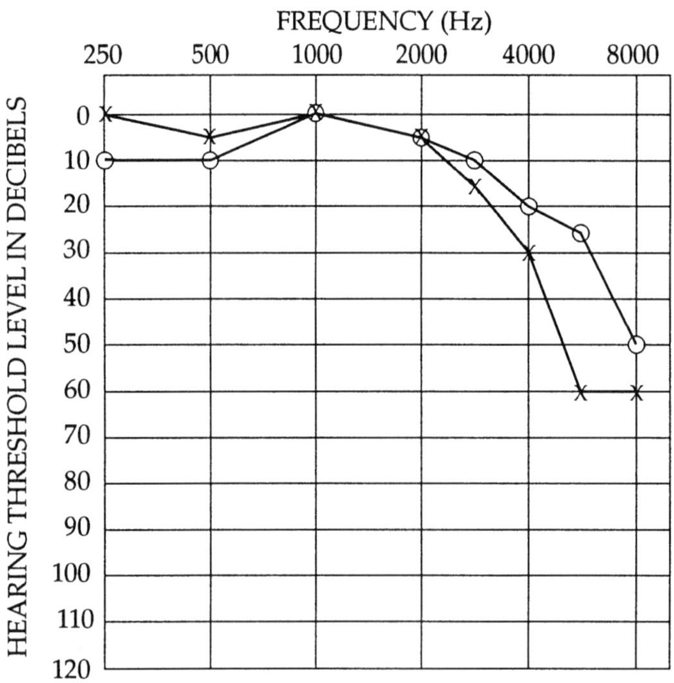

D

Figure 14.2 *continued.* (C) Two months after baseline. (D) Three months after baseline. Progressive hearing loss is seen at the high frequencies.

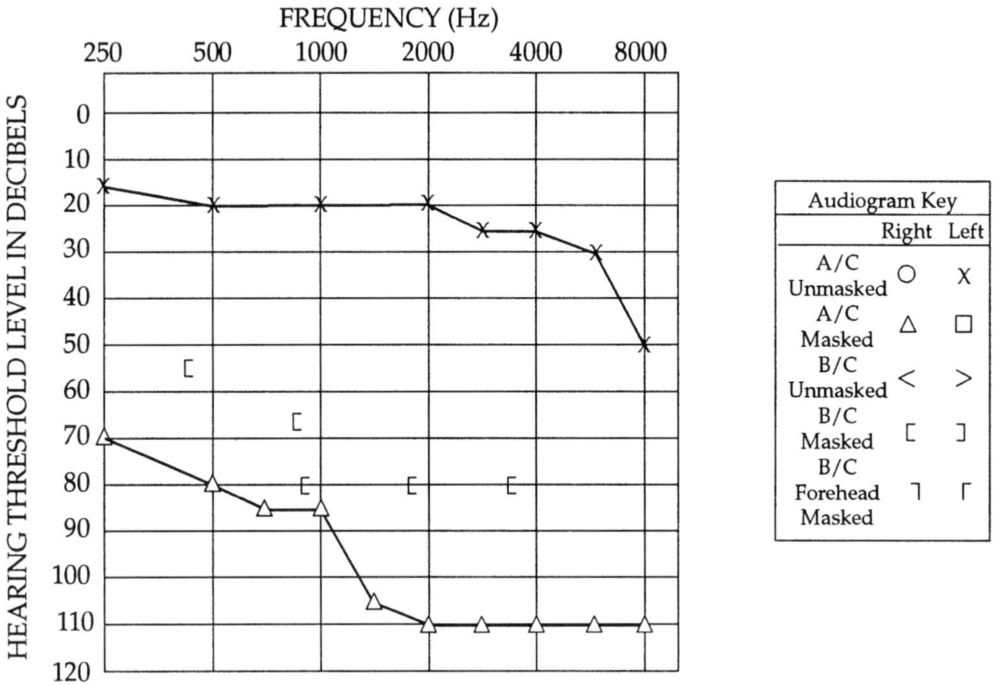

SPEECH TESTS

TESTS		R	L
Sp. Reception Threshold (SRT)		80 db	25 db
Sp. Discrim. Scores	100 dB SL	12%	96%

Figure 14.3. Audiogram of a patient who suffered the sudden onset of unilateral hearing loss while receiving high-dose nonsteroidal therapy for tendinitis.

Quinine ototoxicity is manifested both by auditory and vestibular dysfunction. Toxicity is called *cinchonism* and presents as deafness, vertigo, tinnitus, headache, nausea, and visual loss. Transient hearing loss, usually the first side effect, occurs a few hours after initiating high-dose therapy—for example, in the treatment of malaria. With prolonged treatment for malaria, 20% of patients can be expected to suffer hearing loss.[45] The sensorineural hearing loss is usually reversible bilaterally and symmetric, particularly affecting the high frequencies first. Tinnitus similar to that caused by quinine is caused by salicylates. Vestibular effects of quinine are also recognized. Low serum quinine concentrations, which may occur among tonic beverage drinkers, may lead to clinically significant vestibular changes. Blood quinine levels of 0.2 mg per ml found in pilots who died in aviation accidents suggested that quinine toxicity may have played a causative role.[46] Prolonged administration of high-dose quinine in many patients leads to loss of outer hair cells. There may also be an effect on cochlear blood flow.[47]

Erythromycin Ototoxicity

Although erythromycin was first introduced in 1952, it has been only since the mid-1970s that ototoxicity has been recognized as a potential complication.[48] An extensive number of cases transient and rarely permanent hearing loss, secondary to erythromycin, have been reported by Brummett.[49] There are two newer similar antibiotics, clarithromycin and azithromycin, that have the potential for ototoxicity.[50, 51] Brummett suggests that when parenteral forms of these agents become available ototoxicity may be manifest.[49] The ototoxicity due to erythromycin and its analogues is related to dosage. Of note is the fact that the hearing losses due to erythromycin appear to occur in speech frequencies at the same time the deficit occurs at higher frequencies. For this reason, the patient can easily recognize a change in hearing, a significant difference from the hearing loss resulting from aminoglycoside antibiotics, which begins at the very high frequencies and can go unnoticed for some period of time.

Vancomycin Ototoxicity

Vancomycin, originally introduced in the late 1950s and still used for partial resistance to *Staphylococcus aureus* infection, was initially replaced by methicillin, but reintroduced in the early 1980s because of its effect against methicillin-resistance *S. aureus* infections. Because of its *-mycin* suffix, vancomycin was, and still is, often mistakenly identified as an aminoglycoside antibiotic. The first case of ototoxicity due to vancomycin was reported by Geraci and colleagues.[52] Other reports are catalogued by Brummett.[49] It is clearly less toxic than an aminoglycoside, so the initial concern may have been because of the incorrect belief that vancomycin was an aminoglycoside. In most cases of reported permanent ototoxicity, the patients were treated before or during vancomycin therapy with erythromycin or an aminoglycoside antibiotic. It may well be that permanent ototoxicity could be the result of a vancomycin-induced augmentation of aminoglycoside ototoxicity.

Loop Diuretic Ototoxicity

As reported by Rybak, loop diuretics are organic compounds that exert potential saluretic effects by acting on the epithelial cells in the loop of Henle of the kidney.[53] Unfortunately, many of the loop diuretics are ototoxic, both in clinical reports and experimental studies. Ethacrynic acid, a potent loop diuretic, is recognized as causing acute and sometimes permanent hearing loss.[54] One of the most widely used loop diuretics, furosemide (Lasix), has a significant potential for hearing loss. Heidland and Wigand found that infusion of furosemide at a constant rate of 25 mg per minute caused noticeable hearing loss in two-thirds of patients.[55] Although most cases of furosemide ototoxicity have been reversible, a number of reports describe patients with permanent deficits.[56, 57] Other loop diuretics also have potential ototoxicity. One of its most significant problems is the potentiation of aminoglycoside ototoxicity by the concurrent use of loop diuretics, as previously noted. As Rybak points out, perhaps the kidney and the cochlea have some common receptors for the loop diuretics, and it appears that all loop diuretics are ototoxic to some degree.[53]

Topical Agent Ototoxicity

Local preparations for the ear, namely ear drops, are often the prescribed treatment for ear infections such as chronic otitis media, particularly those with a tympanic membrane perforation. It has been pointed out, however, that in patients with tympanotomy tubes or perforated tympanic membranes such preparations enter the inner ear when applied to the external auditory canal.[58] Hearing loss and vestibular loss through this route are virtually unknown to neurologists. In a 1992 survey of otolaryngologists, 80% believed that the risk of sensorineural hearing loss due to otitis media was greater than the risk of loss from ear drops. Only a small percentage (3.4%) believed that they had witnessed irreversible inner ear damage secondary to ototopical agents.[59] The usual topical agent preparations currently available consist of combinations of various acids, solvents, antiseptics, corticosteroids, antifungals, and four antibiotics (polymyxin B, polymyxin E [Colistin], chloramphenicol, and neomycin), as pointed out by Rohn et al.[60] These authors have done extensive studies on the solvents, antiseptics, anti-inflammatory agents, and antifungals. Antibiotic preparations mentioned previously are the ones most likely to cause iatrogenic injury to the inner ear. The otolaryngologic literature has well documented that there is potential ototoxicity of these topical agents in experimental animals. However, it is difficult to relate the animal research to human clinical applications.[61] It is believed that some inner ear injury follows the chronic application of ear drops to the middle ear. It should be realized that even though there may not be an obvious hole through the eardrum, such as a perforation or a tympanotomy tube, the chances are that an inflamed tympanic membrane permits transport of ototoxic agents directly to the sensitive inner ear. As pointed out by Rohn et al., additional well-controlled studies are needed to investigate further the potential clinical implications of the use of ototopical agents.[60]

Other Agents that May Cause Ototoxicity

Other agents may cause cochleovestibular toxicity. Inhaled toxic agents also cause disturbances in the peripheral and central parts of the vestibulo-ocular motor system.[62] A number of studies have looked prospectively and retrospectively at risk factors for hearing loss and show that periods of neonatal apnea and hypoxia are strongly predisposed to subsequent hearing loss.[63] In addition to the normal environmental chemicals found in modern society, there exists the possibility that otologic surgery can expose the inner ear to ototoxic chemicals. Scrub solutions used to sterilize the external ear may reach the middle ear through tympanic perforations and from there these substances can be absorbed into the inner ear via the round window.[64] Povidone-iodine preparations and chlorhexidine have both been proven to be toxic to the cochlea and vestibular sensory neuroepithelium in the inner ear after reaching the middle ear space.[65–68] Therefore, surgeons should be alerted to this possibility.

Mechanisms of Ototoxicity

The aminoglycoside antibiotics are the first ototoxic agents that highlighted the problem of drug-induced hearing and vestibular loss. They are highly water-soluble compounds, and their charge prevents entry into cells via diffusion across the plasma membrane. The incidence of clinical and functional hearing loss due to aminoglycosides has been significantly diminished because some of the newer derivatives have lower ototoxic potential and perhaps efficient monitoring of serum levels of drugs have allowed for better dosing schedules. The problem is significant, however, because aminoglycosides are still widely used in the treatment of serious gram-negative infections as pointed out by Schacht.[69] The concentration of aminoglycoside in plasma produced by the initial or loading dose is dependent only on the volume of the distribution of the drug. Because the elimination of aminoglycosides is almost entirely dependent on the kidney, a linear relationship exists between the concentration of creatinine in plasma and the half-life of all aminoglycosides in patients with moderately compromised renal function. In anephric patients, the half-life varies from 20 to 40 times that determined in normal individuals. Because the incidence of nephrotoxicity and ototoxicity is related to the concentration to which an aminoglycoside accumulates, it is critical to reduce the maintenance dosage of these drugs in patients with impaired renal function.[2]

The mechanism of ototoxicity and vestibular toxicity has been elusive. Mechanisms for acute and chronic toxicity may be different. It appears that there is an antagonistic relationship between aminoglycosides and calcium, which can block the acute aminoglycoside-induced depression of microphonic potentials experimentally.[70] A number of potential synaptic mechanisms are postulated.[69] For example, streptomycin blocks the postsynaptic actions of excitatory amino acids on primary afferents in the vestibular system, blocks the glutamate-gated ionophore at the crayfish neuromuscular junction, and antagonizes quisqualate-induced excitation of cortical neurons. The chronic toxicity of aminoglycosides appears to target exclusively the kidney, cochlea, and the vestibular system. Aminoglycosides have been reported to affect a wide variety of intracellular reactions that are probably responsible for the permanent deficits of chronic toxicity. DNA, RNA, protein synthesis, energy metabolism, and ion transport are affected, as well as synthesis or degradation of prostaglandins, gangliosides, mucopolysaccharides, and lipids. An important feature is the delayed onset of auditory and vestibular damage in almost all cases of chronic glycoside toxicity, both in experimental animals and in patients. Early studies of aminoglycoside pharmacokinetics gave rise to the hypothesis that the toxicity of these drugs was based on their accumulation in inner ear fluids. This early hypothesis has been questioned.[69,71] It may well be that a metabolite of the aminoglycoside is involved in the toxic action of such drugs. This hypothesis is reviewed in detail by Schacht.[69] Drug metabolism may also explain the selective toxicity toward kidney and the inner ear, as well as why some aminoglycosides preferentially damage the cochlea and others the vestibular system. For example, although the vestibular system may have a preference to metabolize vestibulotoxic drugs, it may conversely have a greater capacity to detoxify those aminoglycosides that spare the vestibular system.

Conclusion

In summary, the acute effects of such drugs are primarily based on calcium antagonism and blocking of ion channels. Chronic cochlear vestibular toxicity requires metabolism. The expression of tissue-specific toxicity is a balance between synthesis of a toxic metabolite and its detoxification. Only through a detailed knowledge of the molecular basis of toxicity can rational approaches be pursued in the development of new aminoglycosides as well as other drugs with less potential for serious cochlear vestibular toxicity.

References

1. Rybak LP (Guest Editor). Ototoxicity. Otolaryngol Clin North Am 1993;26(5).
2. Chambers HF, Sande MA. Antimicrobial Agents (Continued). In JG Hardman, LE Limbird, Molinoff TB, et al. (eds), Goodman & Gilman's: The Pharmacological Basis of Therapeutics (9th ed). New York: McGraw-Hill, 1996;1103.
3. Brummett RE. Drug-induced ototoxicity. Drugs 1980;19:412.
4. Matz GJ, Lerner SA. Aminoglycoside ototoxicity. Am J Otol 1980;1:169.
5. Esterhal JL, Bednar J, Kimmelman CP. Gentamicin induced ototoxicity complicating treatment of chronic osteomyelitis. Clin Orthopaed Res 1986;209:186.
6. Matz GJ. Aminoglycoside cochlear ototoxicity. Otolaryngol Clin North Am 1993;26:705.
7. Kahlmeter G, Dahlager J. Aminoglycoside toxicity and review of medical studies published between 1975 and 1982. J Antimicrob Chemother 1984;13:9.
8. Crawford J. Living without a balancing mechanism. N Engl J Med 1952;246:458.
9. Lerner SA, Schmitt BA, Seligsoh R, et al. Comparative study of ototoxicity and nephrotoxicity in patients randomly assigned to treatment with amikacin or gentamicin. Am J Med 1986;80:98.
10. Rybak LP, Matz GJ. Auditory and Vestibular Effects of Toxins. In CW Cummings, JM Frederickson, LA Harker (eds), Otolaryngology—Head and Neck Surgery. St. Louis: Mosby, 1986;3161.
11. Black FO, Pesznecker SC. Vestibular ototoxicity: clinical considerations. Otolaryngol Clin North Am 1993;26:713.
12. Baloh RW, Honrubia V, Yee RD, et al. Changes in the vestibulo-ocular reflex after loss of peripheral sensitivity. Ann Neurol 1984;16:222.
13. Black FO, Peterka RJ, Elardo SE. Vestibular reflex changes following aminoglycoside induced ototoxicity. Laryngoscope 1987;97:582.
14. Matz GJ. Clinical perspectives on ototoxic drugs. Ann Otol Rhinol Laryngol 1990;99:39.
15. Keene M, Graham JM. Clinical monitoring of the effects of gentamicin by electrocochleography. J Laryngol Otol 1984;98:11.
16. Rybak LP, Matz GJ. Ototoxicity. In PW Alberti, RJ Ruben (eds), Otologic Medicine and Surgery. New York: Churchill Livingstone, 1988;1605.
17. Physician's Desk Reference (51st ed). Montvale, NJ: Medical Economics Co., 1997.
18. Fowler EP. Streptomycin treatment of vertigo. Trans Am Acad Ophthalmol Otolaryngol 1948;52:239.
19. Hanson HV. The treatment of endolymphatic hydrops (Ménière's disease) with streptomycin. Ann Otol Rhinol Laryngol 1951;60:676.
20. Monsell EM, Cass SP, Rybak LP. Aminoglycoside treatment for vertigo: development and current status. Adv Otolaryngol Head Neck Surg 1993;7:7.
21. Monsell EM, Cass SP, Rybak LP. Chemical Labyrinthectomy. In Brackmann DE (ed), Otologic Surgery. Philadelphia: Saunders, 1993.
22. Hamberger CA, Hyden H, Koch H. Streptomycin bei der Menierschen Krankheit. Arch Ohren-Nasen Kehlkopth 1949;155:667.
23. Ruedi L. Therapeutic and toxic effects of streptomycin in otology. Laryngoscope 1951;61:613.
24. Schuknecht HF. Albation therapy in the management of Ménière's disease. Acta Otolaryngol 1957;132:1.
25. Beck C, Schmidt CL. Ten years of experience with intratympanically applied streptomycin (gentamicin) in the therapy of morbus Ménière. Arch Otolaryngol 1978;21:149.
26. Magnusson M, Padoan S. Delayed onset of ototoxic effects of gentamicin in treatment of Ménière's disease. Acta Otolaryngol 1991;111:67.
27. Nedzelski J, Schessel D, Bryce G, Pfleiderer A. Chemical labyrinthectomy: local application for the treatment of unilateral Ménière's disease. Am J Otolaryngol 1992;13:18.
28. Van Deinse F. Medical treatment for Ménière's disease. Ned Tijdschr Geneeskd 1949;31:2619.
29. Hirsch BE, Kamerer DB. Intratympanic gentamicin therapy for Ménière's disease. Am J Otology 1997;18:44.
30. Murofushi T, Halmagyi GM, Yavor RA. Intraympanic gentamicin in Ménière's disease: results of therapy. Am J Otol 1997;18:52.

31. Schweitzer VG. Ototoxicity of chemotherapeutic agents. Otolaryngol Clin North Am 1993;26:759.
32. Hayes DM, Cvitkovic E, Golbey RB, et al. High dose *cis*-platinum diammine dichloride: amelioration of renal toxicity by mannitol diuresis. Cancer 1977;39:1372.
33. Aguilar-Markulis NV, Beckley S, Priore R, Mattlin C. Auditory ototoxicity effects on long-term *cis*-dichlorodiammine platinum II therapy in genitourinary cancer patients. J Surg Oncol 1981;16:111.
34. Black F, Myers E, Schramm V, et al. Cisplatinum vestibular ototoxicity: preliminary report. Laryngoscope 1982;92:1363.
35. Schaefer SD, Wright CG, Post JD, et al. Cisplatinum vestibular therapy toxicity. Cancer 1981;47:857.
36. Mahajan SL. Acute acoustic nerve palsy associated with vincristine therapy. Cancer 1981;47:2404.
37. Lugassy G. Sensorineural hearing loss associated with vincristine treatment. Blutalkohol 1990;61:320.
38. Anonymous. Boston Collaborative Drug Surveillance Program: drug induced deafness. JAMA 1973;224:515.
39. Miller RR. Deafness due to plain and long-acting aspirin tablets. J Clin Pharmacol 1978;18:468.
40. Grigor RR, Spitz PW, Furst DE. Salicylate toxicity in elderly patients with rheumatoid arthritis. J Rheumatol 1987;14:60.
41. Insel PA. Analgesic-Antipyretics and Antiinflammatory Agents; Drugs Employed in the Treatment of Rheumatoid Arthritis and Gout. In AG Gilman, LS Goodman, TW Rall, et al. (eds), Goodman and Gilman's: The Pharmacological Basis of Therapeutics (8th ed). New York: Pergamon, 1990;638.
42. McCabe PA, Dey DL. The effect of aspirin upon auditory sensitivity. Ann Otol Rhinol Laryngol 1965;74:312.
43. Mongan E, Kelly P, Nies K, et al. Tinnitus as an indication of therapeutic serum salicylate levels. JAMA 1973;226:142.
44. Chapman P. Naproxen and sudden hearing loss. J Laryngol Otol 1982;96:163.
45. Anonymous. Antimalarial Drugs. In RR Miller (ed), CRC Handbook of Ototoxicity. Boca Raton, FL: CRC Press, 1985;9.
46. Balfour AJC. The bite of Jesuits' bark. Aviation, Space, Environmental Medicine 1989;60:7:A4.
47. Lee CS, Heinrich J, Jung TTK. Quinine-induced ototoxicity: alterations in cochlear blood flow. Otolaryngol Head Neck Surg 1992;107:233.
48. Mintz U, Amir J, Pinkhas J, et al. Transient perceptive deafness due to erythromycin lactobionate. JAMA 1983;255:1122.
49. Brummett RE. Ototoxic liability of erythromycin and analogues. Otolaryngol Clin North Am 1993;26:811.
50. Dabernat H, Delmas C, Seguy M, et al. The activity of clarithromycin and its 14-hydroxy metabolite against *Haemophilus influenzae*, determined by in-vitro and serum bactericidal tests. J Antimicrob Chemother 1991;27:19.
51. Hopkins S. Clinical toleration and safety of azithromycin. Am J Med 1991;91:40S.
52. Geraci JR, Heilman FR, Nichols DR, et al. Antibiotic therapy of bacterial endocarditis. VII: vancomycin for acute micrococcal endocarditis. Staff Meet Mayo Clin 1958;April:172.
53. Rybak LP. Ototoxicity of loop diuretics. Otolaryngol Clin North Am 1993;26:829.
54. Rybak LP. Totoxicity of ethacrynic acid (a persistent clinical problem). J Laryngol Otol 1988;102:518.
55. Heidland H, Wigand ME. The effect of furosemide at high doses on auditory sensitivity in patients with uremia. Klin Wochenschr 1978;87:32.
56. Brown CG, Ogg CS, Cameron JS, et al. High dose furosemide in acute reversible intrinsic renal failure. Scott Med J 1974;19:35.
57. Rifkin SI, DeQuesada AM, Pickering MJ, et al. Deafness associated with oral furosemide. South Med J 1978;71:86.
58. Meyerhoff WL, Morizono T, Wright CG, et al. Tympanostomy tubes and otic drops. Laryngoscope 1983;93:1022.
59. Lundy LB, Graham MD. Ototoxicity and ototopical medications: a survey of otolaryngologists [abstract]. Presented at the Ninth Shambaugh-Shea Weekend of Otology, Chicago, IL, March 6–8, 1992.
60. Rohn GN, Meyerhoff WL, Wright CG. Ototoxicity of topical agents. Otolaryngol Clin North Am 1993;26:747.
61. Brummett RE, Harris RF, Lindgren JA. Detection of ototoxicity from drugs applied topically to the middle ear space. Laryngoscope 1976;86:1177.
62. Odkvist LM, Moller C, Thuomas K. Otoneurologic disturbances caused by solvent pollution. Otolaryngol Head Neck Surg 1992;106:687.
63. Scott PMJ, Griffiths MV. A clinical review of ototoxicity. Clin Otolaryngol 1994;19:3.
64. Norris CH. Drugs affecting the inner ear: a review of their clinical efficacy, mechanisms of action, toxicity and place in therapy. Drugs 1988;36:754.
65. Aursnes J. Ototoxic effect of iodine disinfectants. Acta Otolaryngol 1982;93:219.
66. Morizono T, Sikora M. The ototoxicity of topically applied providone-iodine solutions. Arch Otolaryngol 1982;108:210.
67. Aursnes J. Vestibular damage from chlorhexidine in guinea pigs. Acta Otolaryngol 1981;92:89.
68. Igarashi Y, Suzuki U. Cochlear ototoxicity of chlorhexidine gluconate in cats. Arch Otolaryngol Rhinol Laryngol 1985;242:167.
69. Schacht J. Biochemical basis of aminoglycoside ototoxicity. Otolaryngol Clin North Am 1993;26:845.
70. Takada A, Schacht J. Calcium antagonism and reversibility of gentamicin-induced loss of cochlear microphonics in the guinea pig. Hear Res 1982;8:179b.
71. Tran Ba Huy P, Bernard P, Schacht J. Kinetics of gentamicin uptake and release in the rat: comparison of inner ear tissues and fluids with other organs. J Clin Invest 1986;77:1492.

Chapter 15

Drug-Induced Peripheral Neuropathies

Margaret A. Laycock

Objectives

- To know that the differential diagnosis of peripheral neuropathies must include possible iatrogenic sources
- To realize that most drug-induced neuropathies are axonopathies
- To understand that most drug-induced neuropathies improve after drug withdrawal, that permanent neurologic sequelae may result, and that early drug withdrawal increases the chances for favorable outcome
- To realize that recovery from axonal injury may take months to years, and that recovery in patients with neuronopathies (injury at the level of the nerve cell body) is often incomplete
- To recognize that some drug-induced peripheral neuropathies may progress for weeks to months after discontinuation of the etiologic drug
- To understand that the risk of drug-induced nerve injury may be dose dependent and may be altered by the mode of drug administration or by use of concurrent neurotoxins

The vast array of drugs used to treat specific diseases not only brings more effective treatments for patients, but also a formidable task of recognizing drug-associated toxicities for clinicians. Drugs, or their metabolites, may cause peripheral nervous system dysfunction. They may be directly or indirectly toxic to the nerve cell, axon, or myelin by interfering with normal cellular function, interfering with local blood supply, or producing local or systemic conditions that affect normal cellular functioning. Drug-induced immunomodulation may also play a role in the development of some peripheral neuropathies.

Clinicians must maintain a high index of suspicion of medications as potential causes of peripheral neuropathies. Historic information from patients, families, pharmacies, and involved physicians are critical in identifying the etiologic agent. Favorable neurologic outcome, in many cases, is dependent on early withdrawal of the suspected toxin. Devastating and often avoidable neurologic consequences are too frequently the result of the clinician's failure to recognize iatrogenic sources of neuropathy.

Most toxic neuropathies are characterized by predominantly axonal injury, although most biopsy specimens show some evidence of demyelination as well. Pure demyelinating toxic neuropathies are unusual. These neuropathies may involve sensory or motor fibers alone or in combination.

The mechanism of injury in most drug-induced neuropathies remains speculative. Neurologic examination and biopsy abnormalities frequently vary between patients treated with the same drug and may reflect more than one mechanism of drug-induced nerve injury. Attempts to understand these

Table 15.1. Drug-Induced Peripheral Neuropathies

Anti-inflammatory and antirheumatic drugs
Allopurinol
Colchicine
Gold
Antimicrobial drugs
Chloramphenicol
Chloroquine
Dapsone
Didanosine
Ethambutol
Isoniazid
Metronidazole
Nitrofurantoin
Nucleoside and pyrimidine analogues
Podophyllum
Stavudine
Sulfonamides
Zalcitabine
Antineoplastic and immunomodulating drugs
Cisplatin
Cytarabine
Interferon
Interleukin 2
Taxol (Taxotere, investigational)
Vincristine
Vindesine
Cardiovascular drugs
Other
Antiepileptic drugs
Disulfiram
Amitriptyline
Etretinate
Lithium
Pyridoxine (vitamin B_6)

mechanisms are further complicated by the prevalence of anecdotal reports and the lack of large, controlled studies. The lack of uniform standards for identification and evaluation of peripheral nerve dysfunction also hampers our understanding of drug-induced nerve toxicity.

The following discussion includes a partial listing of drugs that are commonly recognized or suspected in causing peripheral neuropathies (Table 15.1). Drugs that are not widely used in North America or are not available for commercial use are not discussed. Drug information centers, pharmaceutical texts, and pharmaceutical companies are valuable sources of information for drug investigation and may provide clinicians with information on published, unpublished, or sporadic reports of drugs suspected of inducing peripheral neuropathies.

Anti-Inflammatory and Antirheumatic Drugs

Allopurinol

Allopurinol, commonly used for the treatment of hyperuricemia, may rarely induce an axonal sensory motor polyneuropathy.[1, 2] According to these reports, patients present with distal limb dysesthesias and weakness. Neurologic examination shows a stocking-and-glove distribution of sensory loss and diminished or absent muscle stretch reflexes. Electromyographic (EMG) and nerve conduction studies (NCSs) are consistent with an axonal sensory motor polyneuropathy. Sural nerve biopsy shows both axonal degeneration and segmental demyelination.[1] The neuropathy occurs after 2–15 years of treatment, and symptoms improve over several months after allopurinol is discontinued.[1, 2]

Colchicine

Colchicine has been used for the treatment of gout for more than 200 years. Although well known for its etiologic role in producing a toxic myopathy, colchicine may also produce an axonal sensory motor peripheral neuropathy. Researchers speculate that impaired microtubule assembly, with resultant impairment in axonal transport, may result in neuronal damage. Sural nerve biopsy specimens show axonal degeneration.[3] Signs and symptoms of colchicine-induced peripheral neuropathy consist of distal paresthesias and diminished muscle stretch reflexes, and the stocking-and-glove distribution of sensory loss may be overshadowed by the proximal weakness of concurrent myopathy.[3] Symptoms usually begin after several weeks to years of treatment with colchicine and improve over a period of weeks to months after drug withdrawal.[3–5] NCSs show predominantly sensory nerve abnormalities, although there may be minor motor nerve abnormalities as well. EMG may show distal denervation and reinnervation, in addition to small polyphasic motor unit potentials in proximal muscles.[5–7]

Prevention and treatment of colchicine-induced myoneuropathy is achieved by avoiding this drug in patients with impaired renal function and by withdrawing the drug at the first sign of otherwise unexplained weakness or paresthesias. The lack of inflammatory infiltrates and the presence of vacuolar degeneration in muscle fibers helps to distinguish colchicine-induced myopathy from polymyositis.[6]

Gold (Gold Sodium Thiomalate, Gold Sodium Aurothioglucose, and Gold Sodium Thioglucose)

Gold salts, used in the treatment of severe rheumatoid arthritis, may cause toxic reactions involving the skin, vasculature, blood cells, and kidneys.[8, 9] Infrequent reports of gold-induced neurologic toxicity include stroke, encephalopathy, cranial nerve palsies, and peripheral neuropathy.[10]

Gold-induced peripheral neuropathy has been associated with cumulative doses ranging from 30 to 2,600 mg. Gold sodium thiomalate is the most common preparation associated with neuropathy, although the other less frequently used salts are also implicated in nerve toxicity.[10] Affected patients complain of distal dysesthesias, numbness, weakness, and muscle cramps. Clinical examination shows distal sensory loss and weakness and diminished distal reflexes. Atrophy may be present in severely affected patients.[9] Myokymia has been identified in several patients with gold-induced neuropathy and may serve as a distinctive feature of this disorder.[9, 10]

EMG and NCS results may be normal, but may show prolonged distal latencies and mildly slow conduction velocities of sensory and motor nerves, in addition to denervation in distal muscles.[9, 10] Sural nerve biopsy may show axonal degeneration and segmental demyelination. The presence of elevated cerebrospinal fluid protein in some patients suggests radicular involvement.[1] Though early drug withdrawal in symptomatic patients usually results in favorable outcome, improvement may take weeks to months, and permanent sequelae may occur in severely affected patients.[9]

Antimicrobial Drugs

Chloramphenicol (Chloromycetin)

Although chloramphenicol was used frequently in the past, the development of safer antimicrobial drugs has led to the recommendations that this drug be used only for severe infections that are refractory to other antibiotics. Chloramphenicol may cause severe and sometimes fatal hematologic toxicity. Reports of neurologic toxicity include optic neuropathy and peripheral neuropathy. The peripheral neuropathy occurs in less than 30% of patients treated and may precede, follow, or begin simultaneously with optic neuropathy.[11–14]

Chloramphenicol is believed to cause a sensory neuropathy with sparing of motor fibers. Affected patients complain of severe paresthesias and their examinations show a stocking distribution of sensory loss to light touch and proprioception. The mechanism of nerve injury is unknown, although some researchers have proposed that chloramphenicol may interfere with vitamin B_{12} activity.[13]

The prognosis for recovery from chloramphenicol neuropathy is excellent on discontinuation of therapy. Prevention of neurotoxicity may be improved by using periodic visual acuity screening and patient questionnaires regarding the presence of paresthesias or visual changes during the course of treatment. Although several clinicians advocate the use of B complex vitamins for the treatment of chloramphenicol-induced nerve dysfunction, the efficacy of this practice is not established.[11, 13, 14]

Chloroquine

Chloroquine is an antimalarial agent that has recently been used for the treatment of severe rheumatoid arthritis, systemic lupus erythematosus, and a variety of dermatologic conditions. Though well known for its role in inducing a myopathy, chloroquine may also cause a sensorimotor polyneuropathy with both axonal and demyelinating features.[15, 16] Electron microscopy of affected nerves show abnormal inclusions in Schwann's cells similar to those seen in cases of amiodarone-induced neuropathy.[15]

Symptoms of chloroquine-induced peripheral neuropathy, variable sensory loss, and proximal or distal weakness usually begin after several months of treatment and resolve over weeks to months after discontinuation of the drug.[15, 16]

Dapsone

Dapsone is used to treat leprosy and dermatologic conditions such as dermatitis herpetiformis and for malaria prophylaxis. Although hematologic and gastrointestinal disturbances constitute the major adverse effects of this drug, toxic motor neuropathy is also well documented.[17]

The incidence of this dose-dependent neuropathy is unknown, but is likely uncommon. Affected patients complain predominantly of weakness, although some report pain and sensory loss.[17, 18] Neurologic examinations in reported cases of dapsone-induced neuropathy show weakness and atrophy involving hands and feet. Distal areflexia is common.[19] EMG and NCS results in such individuals show selective abnormalities in motor nerves and denervation in distal limb muscles. These findings suggest that dapsone causes an axonal neuropathy involving motor fibers. Recovery from the neuropathy is good, but may take months to years.[20]

Risk factors for developing dapsone neurotoxicity may be slow acetylation of the drug by *N*-acetyltransferase. Pretreatment screening of patients for slow acetylation may be helpful in determining those patients at increased risk for the development of neurotoxicity.

Isoniazid

Isoniazid (INH, isonicotinic acid) is one of the standard drugs used for the treatment of tuberculosis and early tuberculin skin test conversion. Isoniazid induces an axonal sensory motor polyneuropathy that is preventable with concurrent pyridoxine (vitamin B_6) supplementation. The finding that vitamin B_6 prevents INH-induced peripheral neuropathy has helped many patients to continue aggressive therapy that may have otherwise been intolerable.[21] Ethambutol, another drug used in multiple drug antituberculous regimens, may also cause a sensory motor polyneuropathy.[22]

The incidence of INH-induced peripheral neuropathy, according to one large retrospective study, is approximately 0.15%, although this report did not document if these patients had received pyridoxine supplementation.[23] Several risk factors for the development of INH neuropathy have been identified and include long duration of therapy, higher than standard doses (more than 5 mg per kg per day), poor nutrition, pregnancy, thyroid dysfunction, alcohol abuse, liver dysfunction, and slow acetylation of INH by *N*-acetyltransferase.[21, 24, 25]

Symptomatic patients complain of numbness and paresthesias of the fingers and toes, which may progress to painful dysesthesias, myalgias, and weakness. Neurologic examination in affected individuals may show distal weakness and sensory loss, diminished or absent muscle stretch reflexes, and gait disturbance. These abnormalities may begin within weeks to months after beginning treatment. EMG and NCS results in reported cases of INH neuropathy show evidence of an axonal sensory motor polyneuropathy, with sensory fibers more severely affected than motor fibers.[26–28] Pathologic specimens show axonal degeneration of small- and medium-diameter myelinated and unmyelinated fibers. Recovery of myelinated fibers after pyridoxine therapy has been documented by electron microscopy.[29]

After INH withdrawal and pyridoxine supplementation, recovery is usually good, although it may be slow and incomplete.[21, 24–28] Standard recommendation for pyridoxine supplementation during INH therapy is 25–50 mg per day. Higher than recommended doses of pyridoxine may make the neuropathy worse.[28]

The mode in which INH causes nerve damage is not well delineated, although it likely interferes with the metabolism of pyridoxine, which is an essential cofactor in protein, carbohydrate, and fatty acid metabolism.[21, 25, 28] Pyridoxine is also involved in the synthesis of sphingomyelin. Some propose that INH may actually cause a deficiency of vitamin B_6, which may become more significant with high drug dosages (more than 5 mg per kg per day) or in patients with poor nutritional status.[30] The lack of consistently low blood levels of pyridoxine in affected individuals, however, suggests the mechanism of nerve injury from INH is more complicated than simple vitamin B_6 deficiency.[21]

Metronidazole

Metronidazole is a synthetic nitroimidazole derivative used to treat bacterial and protozoal infections. More recent applications have been in the treatment of *Helicobacter pylori*–induced gastritis and peptic ulcer disease. Common side effects of metronidazole include nausea, vomiting, and anorexia. Nervous system toxicity may include seizures and peripheral neuropathy.[31, 32]

The incidence of metronidazole-induced neuropathy is unknown, although up to 50% of patients treated may have evidence of peripheral nerve dysfunction. Most researchers, however, believe symptomatic neuropathy to be unusual and characterize it as an axonal, predominantly sensory, neuropathy involving all fiber types. The mode of nerve injury is unknown.

Patients with metronidazole neuropathy complain of burning paresthesias of the hands and feet, and clinical examination shows distal sensory loss and diminished muscle stretch reflexes. EMG and NCS results show predominantly sensory nerve potential abnormalities, although minor abnormalities of motor nerves have occasionally been reported.[33] Sural nerve biopsy in affected patients has shown axonal degeneration of myelinated and unmyelinated sensory fibers of all sizes.[34]

Prevention of this toxic neuropathy is by identifying patients at risk for developing neurotoxicity and discontinuing the drug at the first sign of suggestive symptoms. Known risk factors include long-term metronidazole treatment and total dose exceeding 50 g.[35–38] Prognosis for recovery is usually favorable, but is variable and may be slow.

Nitrofurantoin (Furadantin)

Nitrofurantoin is widely used for the treatment of urinary tract infections and is generally well tolerated by patients, although it may cause gastrointestinal distress and rarely, in susceptible individuals, hemolytic anemia. Sensory motor polyneuropathy and a fulminating polyradiculoneuronopathy have been infrequently associated with its use. Electrophysiologic studies are lacking, although biopsy and necropsy specimens have shown wallerian degeneration of peripheral nerves.[39, 40]

Renal failure has long been identified as a major risk factor in the development of this toxic neuropathy, but renal insufficiency, in the absence of an elevated creatinine level, is also a significant hazard. Elevated nitrofurantoin levels have been reported in some with toxic neuropathy and renal insufficiency.[39]

The incidence of nitrofurantoin-induced neuropathy is likely uncommon in the absence of renal insufficiency, although subclinical impairment of nerve function has been well documented in normal volunteers treated with standard doses for 2 weeks. Symptomatic patients complain of distal paresthesias and sensory loss. Weakness, which variably follows the sensory disturbance, may be profound and may clinically resemble the Guillain-Barré syndrome.[41] The mechanism of nerve injury caused by nitrofurantoin is unknown, although it may involve interference with folic acid activity.[42]

Prevention of nitrofurantoin-induced neuropathy is likely best accomplished by physician and patient education. Nitrofurantoin is contraindicated in patients with renal failure and should be avoided in patients with renal insufficiency. Patients with dehydration, poor oral intake, or illness that could predispose to mild intravascular volume losses should be treated with alternative therapy. Clinicians should advise patients that they should discontinue the drug and contact the physician if they develop numbness or tingling while being treated with nitrofurantoin.

Nucleoside and Pyrimidine Analogues (Zalcitabine, Didanosine, and Stavudine)

The nucleoside and pyrimidine analogues are among many new drugs used to treat human immunodeficiency virus (HIV) infection. During the initial drug trials, it became apparent that a dose-dependent, axonal, sensory motor polyneuropathy is one of their main dose-limiting side effects. These drug-induced neuropathies are dose dependent: Risk factors for the development of toxic neuropathy in association with these drugs include preexisting peripheral neuropathy, advanced stage of HIV infection, alcohol abuse, nutritional deficiency, and high-dose regimens.[43, 44]

The signs, symptoms, and electrophysiologic abnormalities of zalcitabine-, didanosine-, and stavudine-associated peripheral neuropathies are similar to those of HIV-associated distal sensory neuropathy.[45] Affected patients develop distal paresthesias and potential weakness that evolve after weeks to months of treatment. Unlike HIV-associated distal sensory neuropathy, which progresses over months, didanosine-, zalcitabine-, and stavudine-associated neuropathies typically progress over weeks. The rate of progression of symptoms may help differentiate HIV-associated neuropathy from drug toxicity.

Drug withdrawal eventually leads to recovery, although it may be incomplete, and the peripheral neuropathy may continue to progress for several weeks after cessation of the responsible toxin.[43, 46, 44]

Prevention of the nucleoside and pyrimidine analogue–induced neuropathies is likely best achieved by using low-dose regimens, expectant management of high-risk individuals, and decreasing the drug dose or discontinuing therapy at the onset of symptoms. Some patients with neurotoxicity may be able to tolerate restarting the same drug at lower doses after they become asymptomatic.[47] Additional reports of neurotoxicity will likely come forth as additional antiretroviral agents become available to the clinician.[48]

Podophyllum Resin (Podophyllotoxin)

Podophyllum resins are topical solutions used for the treatment of genital condyloma acuminata. Several podophyllum derivatives are used as antineoplastic agents and carry similar risks of neurotoxicity (e.g., vincristine, etoposide). Systemic toxicity may result in multiorgan failure in addition to central and peripheral nervous system dysfunction. Nervous system toxicity can occur after topical application of the resin and has been reported in cases of accidental ingestion.[49]

Podophyllum causes an axonal sensory motor polyneuropathy that is usually noted after the onset of severe central nervous system (CNS) depression. The neuropathy, in combination with the encephalopathy, may be severe enough to require mechanical ventilation.[50] The neuropathy may progress for several months after discontinuation of the drug, and improvement is usually slow (weeks to months).[51] Autonomic nervous system involvement may also occur.[51]

EMG and NCS results show abnormal motor and sensory nerve action potentials and evidence of denervation in muscles. Reports of elevated cerebrospinal fluid protein suggest that some patients have involvement of nerve roots.[52]

Toxicity follows excessive systemic absorption of podophyllum, which may occur after application of the podophyllum resin to healthy tissue and to areas that are ulcerated or bleeding. Prevention of toxicity is therefore best achieved by avoiding topical application of podophyllum in patients with extensive disease and limiting the drug to abnormal but nonfriable tissue. More extensive condylomatous disease should be treated by other methods. In the event of systemic intoxication, immediate treatment should include thorough irrigation of the topically treated areas to remove residual drug, gastric lavage (in cases of ingestion), and supportive medical treatment. Hemodialysis in severe intoxication may be beneficial.[53]

Sulfonamides

Sulfanilamide was first developed in the early twentieth century. The newer, nonmethylated sulfa derivatives, unlike their older relatives, are rarely neurotoxic. One large review of patients treated with either sulfisoxazole or sulfamethoxazole showed an adverse reaction rate of approximately 3%, none of which involved the nervous system.[54] Poor renal function and slow acetylation of sulfonamides may increase the patients' risk of developing adverse affects as a result of treatment.

The incidence of peripheral neuropathy associated with sulfamethoxazole and sulfisoxazole is rare.[55] Reports of peripheral neuropathy with earlier types of sulfa drugs, even though relatively common, are poorly documented, and electrophysiologic and pathologic confirmation is lacking in many reports.[56, 57]

Antineoplastic Drugs and Immunomodulators

*Cisplatin (*cis*-dichlorodiammine Platinum)*

Cisplatin is a heavy metal widely used as a chemotherapeutic agent alone or in combination regimens for the treatment of solid tumors, particularly of the head and neck regions, reproductive organs, and bladder. Despite its notoriety as a peripheral nerve toxin, the mechanism by which cisplatin causes neuronal damage is not clear. Most researchers believe that the drug interferes with normal axonal transport, which then leads to axonal injury and subsequent segmental demyelination.[58]

Because of its frequent use in combination with other potentially neurotoxic drugs, the true incidence of cisplatin-induced neuropathy is unknown, although it is a common complication of platinum therapy. The toxicity is dose dependent and generally begins at cumulative doses of more than 200–250 mg per m^2 of body surface area.

Patients initially complain of numbness and tingling in the feet and then the hands, and the sensory disturbance may progress to severe sensory ataxia and gait disturbance. Leg cramps, Lhermitte's sign, and lancinating pain are common patient complaints.[59] In some patients, sensory signs and symptoms may progress for several weeks following discontinuation of cisplatin. Progression of symptoms after cessation of treatment, however, should prompt investigation for the possibility of tumor recurrence or progression.

Neurologic examination in patients with platinum-induced neuropathy shows loss of distal reflexes and early loss of vibratory sense at the toes. Later signs of neuropathy may include diminished proprioception and poor discrimination of light touch and pin prick in the distal lower extremities. The upper extremities are involved later than the lower extremities, and weakness is rarely noted. Lumbosacral plexopathy and cranial nerve toxicity has been reported in patients treated with intra-arterial administration of cisplatin.[60, 61]

Electrophysiologic studies generally show low-amplitude sensory nerve potentials with prolonged distal latencies and slow conduction velocities. Needle examination of distal muscles may show evidence of denervation. EMG and NCS results may be normal early in the course of the neuropathy.

The main site of cisplatin neurotoxicity is the large-diameter sensory nerves at the level of the axon or dorsal root ganglion.[58] Motor neurons are spared. Pathologic specimens show primarily axonal degeneration, although segmental demyelination is frequently present.[62] Autonomic involvement has been reported.[63]

Recovery of peripheral nerve function is variable and is most favorable when cisplatin is withdrawn immediately after the onset of signs or symptoms of peripheral neuropathy. Despite the potential hazards of neurotoxicity, the benefits of continuing cisplatin therapy, in some patients, exceeds the associated risks.

Cytarabine (Cytosine Arabinoside)

Cytarabine (Ara-C) is a chemotherapeutic agent used to treat acute leukemias and non-Hodgkin's lymphomas. Myelosuppression, gastrointestinal disturbances, and prominent CNS dysfunction constitute the most common adverse affects associated with its use. Peripheral neuropathy, although uncommon, has been reported with high-dose regimens (more than 200 mg per m^2 body surface area per day).[64, 65] Reports of peripheral nerve dysfunction associated with Ara-C include pure sensory neuropathy, sensory motor peripheral neuropathy, rapidly progressive polyradiculoneuropathy, and brachial plexopathy.[65]

Patients with cytarabine-induced peripheral neuropathy complain of predominantly sensory disturbances in the distal limbs. The lower extremities are more involved than upper extremities. Weakness may also occur and may be severe. The symptoms may begin after a few days to 2 weeks after the initiation of treatment.[64, 66, 67]

Reports of electrophysiologic studies and sural nerve biopsies in suspected cases of Ara-C–induced peripheral neuropathy are scarce and show a sensory motor polyneuropathy with mixed axonal and demyelinating features.[67] Some studies indicate root level injury as well.[64]

Short-term follow-up of patients with Ara-C neuropathy suggests incomplete recovery.[65–68] Early recognition of the peripheral nerve dysfunction and immediate withdrawal of Ara-C may prevent significant residual nerve dysfunction. Patients with pre-existing peripheral neuropathy may be at increased risk of developing Ara-C–induced neurotoxicity.[69]

Interferon

Interferon is an immunomodulating agent used to treat leukemia and is under investigation to establish its efficacy in the treatment of other disorders. Although interferon possibly causes peripheral nerve toxicity, reports are sporadic and are not well documented.[70] NCSs are rare, but in a few patients, the results have been normal.[71] There is one report of brachial plexopathy occurring after interferon treatment, although idiopathic brachial plexitis cannot be excluded in this case.[72]

Interleukin 2

Interleukin 2, another immunomodulator, is used in the treatment of renal cell carcinoma, melanoma, and other malignancies. Rare cases of brachial plexopathy and carpal tunnel syndrome have been associated with its use.[73, 74] Some speculate that increased vascular permeability and resultant soft-tissue edema may lead to compression of the median nerve in the carpal tunnel. Complete resolution of interleukin 2–induced carpal tunnel syndrome and associated limb edema after the completion of treatment may support this theory. The symptoms of median nerve compression may be severe enough to necessitate temporary splinting and analgesics, but rarely surgery.[74, 75]

The mode of injury in interleukin 2–induced brachial plexopathy is unknown, although signs and symptoms reportedly resolve over several weeks after discontinuation of the treatment.[73]

Taxol (Paclitaxel)

Taxol is an alkaloid derivative from the Pacific Yew that is used to treat breast and ovarian cancers. Taxotere, a semisynthetic derivative of Taxol, is under investigation for the treatment of ovarian and breast cancer, melanoma, and lung cancers.[76] Both Taxol and Taxotere produce a dose-dependent axonal sensory neuropathy, with infrequent motor nerve and autonomic nervous system involvement.[77–79] Nerve injury occurs at the level of both the axon and dorsal root ganglion. The signs and symptoms of Taxol-induced neuropathy usually begin at cumulative doses of more than 200 mg per m^2 of body surface area. Symptoms consist of paresthesias and numbness that may begin in the fingers before the feet and may involve the face and trunk. Painful dysesthesias are common. Weakness may include distal and proximal muscles and occurs in those patients with severe neuropathy.[77, 80] Neurologic assessment of affected patients shows a stocking-and-glove distribution of sensory loss to pin prick, light touch, and vibration, in addition to diminished or absent reflexes. Electrophysiologic studies show low-amplitude sensory potentials with slow sensory nerve conduction velocities.[81] Low-amplitude motor nerve compound muscle action potentials and slow motor nerve conduction velocities may be seen in patients with severe neuropathy.[82]

The mechanism of nerve injury in Taxol-induced neuropathy is not known. Both Taxol and Taxotere promote the polymerization of microtubules, and nerve biopsies have shown microtubule aggregates in axons, Schwann's cells, and dorsal root ganglion cells.[82] It has been proposed that the excessive microtubule polymerization may interfere with cellular function and axonal transport. Reports of varying histologic abnormalities in affected patients, however, suggest that more than one mechanism may be responsible for nerve injury.[77]

Vincristine (Vincristine Sulfate, Oncovin)

Vincristine is a *Vinca* alkaloid commonly used in the treatment of a variety of malignancies, including lymphomas, leukemias, sarcomas, and multiple myeloma and is well known for its peripheral nerve toxicity. Other *Vinca* alkaloids used to treat malignancies include vinblastine and a semisynthetic derivative, vindesine. Like vincristine, these *Vinca* alkaloids may also be toxic to peripheral nerves.[83] The mechanism of peripheral nerve injury is possibly related to the prevention of microtubule polymerization and resultant interference with axonal transport.

Dose-dependent peripheral nerve toxicity, in the form of sensory, motor, and autonomic neuropathies, often limits the clinical use of vincristine and frequently requires either dose reduction or discontinuation of the drug. The majority of patients undergoing standard cancer protocols using vincristine in combination with other chemotherapeutic agents develop peripheral nerve toxicity. Symptomatic patients complain of numbness and tingling in the hands and feet and later complain of distal weakness that may lead to difficulty with fine motor control. Signs of autonomic dysfunction include constipation, ileus, and orthostatic hypotension.[84] Vincristine-induced cranial neuropathies have also been reported.[85, 86] Peripheral nerve dysfunction may progress for several weeks after therapy has been stopped, although progressive symptoms should prompt an investigation to exclude recurrent tumor. Most patients stabilize or improve following discontinuation of therapy; however, some may be left with permanent disability.

EMG and NCS results commonly show low-amplitude sensory potentials and mild slowing of nerve conduction velocities. Histologic studies show axonal degeneration of large and small diameter fibers. Areas of segmental demyelination are frequently present.[87]

In the future, neuroprotectants may play a role in preventing vincristine-induced neuropathy; however, the current clinical practice is to discontinue or reduce the dose of vincristine at first sign of peripheral nerve dysfunction.[88]

Cardiovascular Drugs

Although several cardiovascular agents have been implicated as peripheral nerve toxins, amiodarone is the most clearly documented. Amiodarone is a benzofurane derivative that is used in the treatment of refractory supraventricular and ventricular tachycardias. Common side effects of treatment include corneal deposits, thyroid dysfunction, gastrointestinal disturbance, and photosensitivity.

Peripheral neuropathy has been reported in up to 6% of patients treated for several months with amiodarone.[89] Symptomatic complaints include distal paresthesias, which may be associated with weakness. Examination findings in these patients are variable and may range from absent reflexes to severe sensory loss, weakness, and atrophy.[90–92] Tremor and ataxia, which are more common than neuropathy, may occur concurrently with peripheral nerve dysfunction.[93, 94]

Amiodarone induces predominantly an axonal sensory motor peripheral neuropathy affecting small and large myelinated fibers. Some reports have shown prominent demyelination as well.[95] Histologic examination shows a characteristic Schwann's cell abnormality with cytoplasmic inclusion bodies. These inclusion bodies are believed to be abnormal lysosomes.[95–97]

EMG and NCS results show abnormalities in motor and sensory nerves and denervation of distal limb muscles. Myopathic features may be present concurrently with neuropathic abnormalities, and the myopathic features may predominate.[90, 91] The mechanism of amiodarone neural toxicity is unknown.

The prognosis for recovery from amiodarone-induced peripheral neuropathy is variable. Prevention of this neuropathy is best achieved by choosing alternative treatments when possible, although potentially fatal complications from the underlying arrhythmia may ensue on withdrawal of the medication. No risk factors have been identified for the development of amiodarone neuropathy, but most affected patients have been treated for several months before symptom onset.[90, 91]

Other instances of cardiovascular drug–associated peripheral neuropathies are not clearly documented, but may be the result of idiosyncratic phenomena. Flecainide, for example, can reportedly cause an axonal sensory polyneuropathy.[98] Paresthesias, and in rare cases, nerve conduction abnormalities, have been associated with captopril and with beta-blocker therapy for hypertension, but there is little solid evidence to support the causative role of these drugs.[99–101] The underlying cardiovascular disease may, however, play some role in the development of peripheral neuropathy. One study, however, suggested that up to 25% of cardiac patients, independent of the antiarrhythmic used, develop peripheral neuropathies.[102] Most of these patients were asymptomatic and found to have abnormal electrophysiologic studies. This same study, however, showed that 18% of cardiac patients not on treatment with antiarrhythmic drugs also had evidence of peripheral nerve dysfunction.

Amitriptyline

Amitriptyline is a tricyclic antidepressant commonly used for the treatment of painful neurologic conditions, including peripheral neuropathies. Sporadic acute polyradiculoneuronopathy has been reported as a rare consequence of amitriptyline overdose and an even less common result of conventional doses.[103–105] Some of these reports are questionable, however, and better clinical documentation with electrophysiologic and pathologic support is needed in the future.

Antiepileptic Drugs

Clinicians have recognized peripheral nerve dysfunction in association with long-standing phenytoin therapy for several decades. The usual reports consist of asymptomatic patients with diminished or absent distal muscle stretch reflexes, distal sensory deficits, or electrophysiologic abnormalities compatible with an axonal sensory motor polyneuropathy.[106] Sural nerve biopsies in a few patients have shown evidence of axonal degeneration and segmental demyelination.[107]

Treatment with phenytoin for more than 5 years and phenytoin intoxication appear to be risk factors for the development of peripheral nerve dysfunction.[106] Improvement in the electrophysiologic and clinical examination abnormalities following discontinuation of phenytoin has been reported.[107]

Phenobarbital, carbamazepine, and primidone have also been implicated in causing peripheral nerve dysfunction. One study suggested that more than 50% of patients treated with one or more antiepileptic drugs had either symptoms of neuropathy or electrophysiologic abnormalities.[108]

Disulfiram (Antabuse)

Disulfiram is used for the treatment of alcoholism. Disulfiram may cause many adverse effects, including hepatotoxicity, dermatitis, and neurologic disorders. An axonal, sensory motor peripheral neuropathy is one of the most common neurologic adverse effects associated with this drug.[109] Affected patients complain of numbness, burning dysesthesias, and weakness. Neurologic examination in these patients shows absent distal muscle stretch reflexes, distal weakness, and a stocking-and-glove distribution of sensory loss. Electrophysiologic studies show motor and sensory nerve abnormalities with denervation in distal limb muscles.[110, 111] Sural nerve biopsy has shown axonal degeneration of small and large myelinated fibers, and decreased numbers of myelinated fibers.[110, 112]

The mechanism of disulfiram-induced neuropathy is speculative, but may be secondary to one of its metabolites, carbon disulfide, a known neurotoxin.[111, 112]

Etretinate

Etretinate is a retinoid used to treat severe psoriasis. It has rarely been associated with an axonal sensory peripheral neuropathy that is reversible after withdrawal of the drug. Electrophysiologic findings are supportive of a sensory neuropathy, and sural nerve biopsy results have shown axonal degeneration of small and large myelinated fibers.[113, 114]

Lithium (Lithium Carbonate)

Lithium is an alkali metal used for the treatment of manic depressive disorders. Peripheral neuropathy has been sporadically reported in association with lithium intoxication. This toxic neuropathy may be underdiagnosed, however, because of the prominent and severe CNS dysfunction that precedes or occurs at the same time as the peripheral nerve dysfunction.[115] Some reports of peripheral neuropathy are dubious due to the lack of definite supportive electrophysiologic or pathologic findings.

Electrophysiologic findings in suspected cases of lithium-induced neuropathy include loss of amplitude and slow conduction velocities in motor and sensory nerves, in addition to distal muscle denervation.[115–118] Nerve conduction abnormalities, according to one study, are altered after 1 week of conventional therapy in normal volunteers.[118] Sural nerve biopsies show axonal degeneration and loss of myelinated fibers.[117]

The signs and symptoms of lithium-induced neuropathy are not usually recognized until the acute CNS disorder has resolved. Patients may complain of numbness and paresthesias, and clinical examination shows hyporeflexia or areflexia and weakness that may range from mild to profound.[115–117, 119] Recovery usually begins after drug withdrawal, but is often incomplete.[117] The neuropathy may continue to progress after discontinuation of the drug.[115, 116]

Prevention of lithium-induced peripheral neuropathy may be improved by frequent monitoring of lithium levels, especially in those patients with renal dysfunction or preexisting neuropathy, and adjusting dosages in those with renal impairment. Although hemodialysis rapidly lowers the serum levels of lithium in cases of intoxication, tissue levels are not immediately affected. There is no evidence to suggest that use of hemodialysis prevents peripheral nerve injury, although it can quickly improve signs of CNS depression.[118]

Pyridoxine (Vitamin B_6)

Pyridoxine is a water-soluble vitamin that functions as a coenzyme in many essential metabolic reactions and plays an important role in maintaining lipid integrity. Although toxicity is usually the result of self-medication with vitamins, iatrogenic pyridoxine toxicity has also been reported and may be devastating.[120–122] Pyridoxine has been prescribed by physicians for the treatment of INH-induced neuropathy, false morel mushroom poisoning, pyridoxine-dependent epilepsy,[121] infantile spasms,[123] carpal tunnel syndrome,[124] peripheral neuropathy, premenstrual syndromes,[122] as well as many other disorders. Its efficacy in many instances is dubious and potentially dangerous.

Peripheral nerve toxicity has been reported with pyridoxine doses as low as 200 mg per day, although some suggest that chronic ingestion of 50 mg per day may also result in peripheral nerve damage.[121, 122] Affected patients present with paresthesias and numbness and may progress to sensory ataxia. Most reports of pyridoxine neuropathy suggest a pure sensory axonal neuropathy, although severe cases involve the dorsal root ganglion. The nerve injury is usually reversible, except in patients with dorsal root ganglion involvement in whom permanent sequelae are common.[120, 122] The mechanism of injury is not clear, although many researchers speculate a direct toxic effect on nerve axons and sensory ganglion cells by pyridoxine or one of its metabolites.

Public and physician education regarding the potential hazards of pyridoxine supplementation is crucial in the prevention of vitamin B_6–induced peripheral neuropathy.

Conclusion

Drug-induced neuropathies are common and may lead to severe neurologic sequelae. Physicians must maintain a high index of suspicion for iatrogenic sources of nerve injury and elicit detailed medication histories in patients with peripheral neuropathies. Early recognition of drug-induced neuropathy and immediate withdrawal of the etiologic agent may be critical to favorable neurologic outcome. Continuing treatment with a known neurotoxin may become an issue in patients with life-threatening illnesses and no alternative treatment. The potential use of neuroprotective agents, in conjunction with known neurotoxic drugs, is currently under investigation and may substantially improve the efficacy of current drug therapy without increasing the risk of nerve injury.

References

1. Azulay JP, Blin O, Valentin P, et al. Regression of allopurinol-induced peripheral neuropathy after drug withdrawal. Eur Neurol. 1993;33:193.
2. Worth CT, Hussein SMA. Peripheral neuropathy due to long term ingestion of allopurinol. BMJ 1985;291:1688.
3. Kuncl R, Duncan G, Watson D, et al. Colchicine myopathy and neuropathy. N Engl J Med 1987;316:1562.
4. Van Der Naalt J, Haaxma-Reiche H, VanDenBerg A, et al. Acute neuromyopathy after colchicine treatment. Ann Rheum Dis 1992;51:1267.
5. Jonsson J, Gelpi J, Light J, et al. Colchicine-induced myoneuropathy in a renal transplant patient. Transplantation 1992;53:1369.
6. Older S, Finbloom D, Pezeshkpour G. Colchicine myonueuropathy and renal dysfunction. Ann Rheum Dis 1992;51:1343.
7. Schiff D, Drislane F. Rapid onset colchicine myoneuropathy. Arthritis Rheum 1992;35:1535.
8. Hill C, Pile K, Henderson D, et al. Neurological side effects in two patients receiving gold injections for rheumatoid arthritis. Br J Rheumatol. 1995;34:989.
9. Katrak SM, Pollock M, O'Brien CP, et al. Clinical and morphologic features of gold neuropathy. Brain 1980;103:671.
10. Fam A, Gordon D, Sarkozi J, et al. Neurologic complications associated with gold therapy for rheumatoid arthritis. J Rheumatol 1984;11:700.
11. Charache S, Finkelstein D, Leitman P, et al. Peripheral and optic neuritis in a patient with hemoglobin SC disease during treatment of *Salmonella* osteomyelitis with chloramphenicol. Johns Hopkins Med J 1977;140:121.

12. Joy Capt RJT, Scalettar R, Sodec D. Optic and peripheral neuritis. JAMA 1960;173:1732.
13. Ramillo O, Kinane B, McCracken G. Chloramphenicol neurotoxicity. Pediatr Infect Dis J 1988;7:359.
14. Wallenstein L, Snyder J. Neurotoxic reaction to chloromycetin. Ann Intern Med 1952;36:1526.
15. Estes M, Ewing-Wilson D, Chou S. Chloroquine neuromyotoxicity. Clinical and pathologic perspective. Am J Med 1987;82:447.
16. Tegner R, Tomé FMS, Godeau P. Morphological study of peripheral nerve changes induced by chloroquine treatment. Acta Neuropathol 1988;75:253.
17. Epstein F, Bohm M. Dapsone-induced peripheral neuropathy. Arch Dermatol 1976;112:1761.
18. Waldinger T, Siegle R, Weber W, et al. Dapsone-induced peripheral neuropathy. Case report and review. Arch Dermatol 1984;120:356.
19. Koller W, Gehlmann L, Malkinson F, et al. Dapsone-induced peripheral neuropathy. Arch Neurol 1977; 34:644.
20. Gutmann L, Martin J, Welton W. Dapsone motor neuropathy—an axonal disease. Neurology 1976;26:514.
21. Biehl JP, Vilter R. Effect of isoniazid on vitamin B6 metabolism. Its possible significance in producing isoniazid neuritis. Proc Soc Exp Biol Med 1954;185:389.
22. Tugwell P, James SL. Peripheral neuropathy with ethambutol. Postgrad Med J 1972;48:667.
23. Ormerod LP, Horsfield N. Frequency and type of reactions to antituberculous drugs: observations in routine treatment. Tuber Lung Disease 1996;77:37.
24. Tomkin G. Isoniazid as a cause of neuropathy and sideroblastic anemia. Practitioner 1973;211:773.
25. Snider DE. Pyridoxine supplementation during isoniazid therapy. Tubercle 1980;61:191.
26. Kalinowski SZ, Lloyd TW, Moyes EN. Complications in the chemotherapy of tuberculosis. Am Rev Respir Dis 1961;83(Suppl):359.
27. Aita J, Calame T. Peripheral neuropathy secondary to isoniazid-induced pyridoxine deficiency. A case report and review of the literature. Maryland State Med J 1972;21:68.
28. Nisar M, Watkin SW, Bucknall R, et al. Exacerbation of isoniazid induced peripheral neuropathy by pyridoxine. Thorax 1990;45:419.
29. Ochoa J. Isoniazid neuropathy in man: quantitative electron microscope study. Brain 1970;93:831.
30. Pellock J, Howell J, Kendig E, et al. Pyridoxine deficiency in children treated with isoniazid. Chest 1985;87:659.
31. Frytak S, Moertel C, Childs D. Neurologic toxicity associated with high dose metronidazole therapy. Ann Intern Med 1988;88:361.
32. Learned-Coughlin S. Peripheral neuropathy induced by metronidazole. Ann Pharmacother 1994;28:536.
33. Duffy L, Daum F, Fisher S, et al. Peripheral neuropathy in Crown's disease patients treated with metronidazole. Gastroenterology 1985;88:681.
34. Bradley WG, Karlsson I, Rassol L. Metronidazole neuropathy. BMJ 1977;2:610.
35. Schipper H, Beale F, Bush R, et al. Letter to the editor. N Engl J Med 1976;295:901.
36. Coxon A, Pallis CA. Metronidazole neuropathy. J Neurol Neurosurg Psychiatry 1976;39:403.
37. Rose GP, Dewar AJ, Stratford I. A biochemical neurotoxicity study relating the neurotoxic potential of metronidazole and nitrofurantoin with misonidazole. Int J Radiat Oncol Biol Phys 1982;8:781.
38. Snavely S, Hodges G. The neurotoxicity of antibacterial agents. Ann Intern Med 1984;101:92.
39. Loughridge LW, Belf MB. Peripheral neuropathy due to nitrofurantoin. Lancet 1962;2:1133.
40. Ellis FG. Acute polyneuritis after nitrofurantoin therapy. Lancet 1962;2:1136.
41. Holmberg L, Boman G, Bottinger L, et al. Adverse reactions to nitrofurantoin. Analysis of 921 results. Am J Med 1980;69:733.
42. Toole JF, Gergen J, Hayes D, et al. Neural effects of nitrofurantoin. Arch Neurol 1968;18:680.
43. Fichtenbaum C, Clifford D, Powderly W. Risk factors for dideoxynucleoside-induced toxic neuropathy in patients with the human immunodeficiency virus infection. J Acquir Immune Defic Syndr Hum Retrovirol 1995;10:169.
44. Simpson D, Tagliati M. Nucleoside analogue-associated peripheral neuropathy in human immunodeficiency virus infection. J Acquir Immune Defic Syndr Hum Retrovirol 1995;9:153.
45. Simpson D, Wolfe D. Neuromuscular complications of HIV infection and its treatment. AIDS 1991;5:917.
46. Berger AR, Arezzo JC, Schaumburg HH, et al. 2',3'-Dideoxycytidine (ddC) toxic neuropathy. A study of 52 patients. Neurology 1993;43:358.
47. Kieburtz K, Seidlin M, Lambert J, et al. Extended follow-up of peripheral neuropathy in patients with AIDS and AIDS-related complex treated with dideoxyinosine. J Acquir Immune Defic Syndr Hum Retrovirol 1992;5:60.
48. Cupler E, Dalakas M. Exacerbation of peripheral neuropathy by lamivudine. Lancet 1995;345:460.
49. Campbell AN. Accidental poisoning with podophyllin. Lancet 1980;1:206.
50. Chamberlain MJ, Reynolds AL, Yeoman W. Toxic effect of podophyllin application in pregnancy. BMJ 1972;3:391.
51. Filley CM, Graff-Radford N, Lacy J, et al. Neurologic manifestations of podophyllin toxicity. Neurology 1982;32:308.
52. Clark ANG, Parsonage M. A case of podophyllin poisoning with involvement of the nervous system. BMJ 1957;2:1155.
53. Slater G, Rumack B, Peterson R. Podophyllin poisoning. Systemic toxicity following cutaneous application. Obstet Gynecol 1978;52:94.
54. Koch-Weser J, Sidel V, Dexter M, et al. Adverse reactions to sulfisoxazole, sulfamethoxazole, and nitrofu-

rantoin. Manifestations and specific reaction rates during 2118 courses of therapy. Arch Intern Med 1971;128:399.
55. Craven W, Donofrio P. Sensory and autonomic polyneuropathy associated with trimethoprim sulfamethoxazole. Ann Neurol 1992;32:281.
56. Little SC. Nervous and mental effects of the sulfonamides. JAMA 1942;119:467.
57. Ornsteen AM, Furst W. Peripheral neuritis due to sulfanilamide. JAMA 1938;111:2103.
58. Boogerd W, Huinink W, Dalesio O, et al. Cisplatin induced neuropathy: central, peripheral and autonomic nerve involvement. J Neuro-Oncol 1990;9:255.
59. Siegal T, Haim N. Cisplatin-induced peripheral neuropathy. Frequent off-therapy deterioration, demyelinating syndromes and muscle cramps. Cancer 1990;66:1117.
60. Castellanos A, Glass JP, Yung A. Regional nerve injury after intra-arterial chemotherapy. Neurology. 187;37:834.
61. Frustaci S, Barzan L, Comoretto R, et al. Local neurotoxicity after intra-arterial cisplatin in head and neck cancer. Cancer Treat Rep 1987;71:257.
62. Thompson S, Davis L, Kornfeld M, et al. Cisplatin neuropathy. Clinical, electrophysiologic, morphologic and toxilogic studies. Cancer 1984;54:1269.
63. Rosenfeld C, Broder LE. Cisplatin-induced autonomic neuropathy. Cancer Treat Rep 1984;68:659.
64. Nevill TJ, Bernstead TJ, McCormick CW, et al. Horner's syndrome and demyelinating peripheral neuropathy caused by high dose cytosine arabinoside. Am J Hematol 1989;39:314.
65. Baker WJ, Royer G, Weiss R. Cytarabine and neurologic toxicity. J Clin Oncol 1991;9:679.
66. Powell B, Capizzi R, Lyerly E, et al. Peripheral neuropathy after high dose cytosine arabinoside, daunorubicin, and asparaginase consolidation for acute nonlymphocytic leukemia. J Clin Oncol 1986;4:95.
67. Borgeat A, DeMuralt B, Cooper MR. Peripheral neuropathy associated with high dose Ara-C therapy. Cancer 1986;58:852.
68. Russell JA, Powles RW. Neuropathy due to cytosine arabinoside. BMJ 1974;4:652.
69. Ventura G, Keating M, Castellanos A, et al. Reversible bilateral rectus muscle palsy associated with high dose cytosine arabinoside and mitoxantrone therapy. Cancer 1986;58:1633.
70. Smedley H, Katrok M, Sikora K, et al. Neurological effects of recombinant human interferon. BMJ 1983;286:262.
71. Dierckx RA, Michotte A, Schmedding E, et al. Unilateral seizures in a patient with hairy cell leukemia treated with interferon. Clin Neurol Neurosurg 1985;87:209.
72. Bernsen P, Chung R, Vingerhoets H, et al. Bilateral neuralgic amyotrophy induced by interferon treatment. Arch Neurol 1988;45:449.
73. Loh F, Herskovitz S, Berger A, et al. Brachial plexopathy associated with interleukin-2 therapy. Neurology 1992;42:462.
74. Puduvalli V, Sella A, Austin S, et al. Carpal tunnel syndrome associated with interleukin-2 therapy. Cancer 1996;77:1189.
75. Heys SD, Mills K, Eremin O. Bilateral carpal tunnel syndrome associated with interleukin-2 therapy. Postgrad Med J 1992;68:587.
76. Hilkens PHE, Verweij J, Stoter G, et al. Peripheral neurotoxicity induced by docetaxel. Neurology 1996;46:104.
77. Freilich R, Belmaceda C, Seidman A, et al. Motor neuropathy due to docetaxel and paclitaxel. Neurology 1996;47:115.
78. Gelmon K. The taxoids: paclitaxel and docetaxel. Lancet 1994;344:1267.
79. Hidalgo M, Benito J, Colomer R, et al. Recall reaction of a severe local peripheral neuropathy after paclitaxel extravasation. J Natl Cancer Inst 1996;88:1320.
80. Apfel S. Docetaxel neuropathy. Neurology 1996;46:2.
81. Sahenk Z, Barohn R, New P, et al. Taxol neuropathy. Electrodiagnostic and sural nerve biopsy findings. Arch Neurol 1994;51:726.
82. Lipton RB, Apfel SC, Dutcher J, et al. Taxol produces a predominantly sensory neuropathy. Neurology 1989; 39:368.
83. Obrist R, Paravicini U, Hartmann D, et al. Vindesine. A clinical trial with special reference to neurological side effects. Cancer Chemother Pharmacol 1979;2:233.
84. Carmichael S, Eagleton L, Ayres C, et al. Orthostatic hypotension during vincristine therapy. Arch Intern Med 1970;126:290.
85. Albert D, Wong V, Henderson E. Ocular complications of vincristine therapy. Arch Ophthal 1967;78:709.
86. Mahajan S, Ideda Y, Myers T, et al. Acute acoustic nerve palsy associated with vincristine therapy. Cancer 1981;47:2404.
87. McLeod JG, Penry R. Vincristine neuropathy: an electrophysiological and histological study. J Neurol Neurosurg Psychiatry 1969;32:297.
88. Van Kooten B, Van Diemen H, Groenhout K, et al. A pilot study on the influence of a corticotropin (4-9) analogue on vinca alkaloid-induced neuropathy. Arch Neurol 1992;49:1027.
89. Charness M, Morady F, Scheinman M. Frequent neurologic toxicity associated with amiodarone therapy. Neurology 1984;34:669.
90. Fraser AG, McQueen I, Watts A, et al. Peripheral neuropathy during long-term high-dose amiodarone therapy. J Neurol Neurosurg Psychiatry 1985;48:576.
91. Anderson NE, Lynch N, O'Brien KP. Disabling complications of amiodarone. Aust NZ J Med 1985;15:300.
92. Martinez-Arizala A, Sobol S, McCarty G, et al. Amiodarone neuropathy. Neurology 1983;33:643.
93. Coulter DM. Survey of neurological problems with amiodarone in the New Zealand Intensive Medicines Monitoring Programme. N Z Med J 1990;103:98.
94. Fraser AG, Mcqueen I. Adverse reactions during treat-

ment with amiodarone hydrochloride. BMJ 1983; 287:612.
95. Jacobs J, Costa-Jussa FR. The pathology of amiodarone neurotoxicity II. Peripheral neuropathy in man. Brain 1985;108:753.
96. Meier C, Kauer B, Müller U, Ludin HP. Neuromyopathy during chronic amiodarone treatment. A case report. J Neurology 1979;220:231.
97. Lemaire JF, Autret A, Biziere K, et al. Amiodarone neuropathy: further arguments for human drug-induced neurolipidosis. Eur Neurol 1982;21:65.
98. Palace J, Shah R, Clough C. Flecainide induced peripheral neuropathy. BMJ 1992;305:810.
99. Emara MK, Saadah AM. The carpal tunnel syndrome in hypertensive patients treated with beta-blockers. Postgrad Med J 1988;64:191.
100. Lipponi G, Lucantoni C, Antonicelli R, et al. Clinical and electromyographic evidence of carpal tunnel syndrome in a hypertensive patient with chronic beta-blocker treatment. Ital J Neurol Sci 1992;13:157.
101. Samanta A, Burden AC. Peripheral neuropathy due to captopril. BMJ 1985;291:1172.
102. Beghi E, Monticelli M, Bono A, et al. Antiarrhythmic drugs and polyneuropathy. J Neurol Neurosurg Psychiatry 1994;57:340.
103. Isaacs AD. Peripheral neuropathy after amitriptyline. BMJ 1963;1:1739.
104. LeWitt PA, Forno LS. Peripheral neuropathy following amitriptyline overdose. Muscle Nerve 1985;8:723.
105. Leys D, Pasquier F, Lamblin M, et al. Acute polyradiculoneuropathy after amitriptyline overdose. BMJ 1987;294:608.
106. So E, Penrey JK. Adverse effects of phenytoin on peripheral nerves and neuromuscular junction: a review. Epilepsia 1981;22:467.
107. Ramirez JA, Mendell J, Warmolts J, et al. Phenytoin neuropathy: structural changes in the sural nerve. Ann Neurol 1986;19:162.
108. Bono A, Beghi E, Bogliun G, et al. Antiepileptic drugs and peripheral nerve function: a multicenter screening investigation of 141 patients with chronic treatment. Epilepsia 1993;34:323.
109. Poulsen E, Andersen JR, Andersen M. Disulfuram therapy—adverse drug reactions and interactions. Acta Psychiatr Scand 1992;368(Suppl):59.
110. Gardner-Thorpe C, Benjamin S. Peripheral neuropathy after disulfuram administration. J Neurol Neurosurg Psychiatr 1971;34:253.
111. Moddel G, Bilbao J, Payne D, et al. Disulfuram neuropathy. Arch Neurol 1978;35:658.
112. Ansbacher L, Bosch P, Cancilla P. Disulfuram neuropathy: a neurofilamentous distal axonopathy. Neurology 1982;32:424.
113. Danon MJ, Carpenter S, Weiss V, et al. Sensory neuropathy associated with long term etretinate (ET) therapy. Neurology 1986;36(Suppl 1):321.
114. Hammer C, Carter C, Hanifin J. Peripheral neuropathy during etretinate therapy for psoriasis. J Am Acad Dermatol 1993;28:272.
115. Vanhooren G, Dehaene I, Van Zandycke M, et al. Polyneuropathy in lithium intoxication. Muscle Nerve 1990;13:204.
116. Chang Y, Yip P, Chiu Y, et al. Severe generalized polyneuropathy in lithium intoxication. Eur Neurol 1988;28:39.
117. Pamphlett RS, Mackenzie RA. Severe peripheral neuropathy due to lithium intoxication. J Neurol Neurosurg Psychiatry 1982;45:656.
118. Sansone M, Ziegler D. Lithium toxicity: a review of neurologic complications. Clin Neuropharmacol 1985;8:242.
119. Uchigata M, Tanabe H, Hasue I, et al. Peripheral neuropathy due to lithium intoxication. Ann Neurol 1981;9:414.
120. Albin RC, Albers J, Greenberg H, et al. Acute sensory neuropathy—neuronopathy from pyridoxine overdose. Neurology 1987;37:1729.
121. McLachlan R, Brown W. Pyridoxine dependent epilepsy with iatrogenic sensory neuronopathy. Can J Sci 1995;22:50.
122. Parry G, Bredesen D. Sensory neuropathy with low dose pyridoxine. Neurology 1985;35:1466.
123. Pietz J, Benninger C, Schäfer H, et al. Treatment of infantile spasms with high dose vitamin B_6. Epilepsia 1993;34:757.
124. Jacobson MD, Plancher K, Kleinman W. Vitamin B_6 (pyridoxine) therapy for carpal tunnel syndrome. Hand Clin 1996;12:253.

Chapter 16

Iatrogenic Disorders of the Neuromuscular Junction

Robert M. Pascuzzi

Objectives

- To recognize the signs and symptoms of impaired neuromuscular transmission
- To become familiar with the three iatrogenic causes of autoimmune myasthenia gravis (MG) (bone marrow transplantation [BMT], penicillamine therapy, and interferon-alfa therapy)
- To review those drugs that can produce clinically significant weakness from impairment of neuromuscular transmission in normal patients
- To outline those drugs that can exacerbate weakness in patients with underlying disorders of neuromuscular transmission
- To emphasize the potential for hypermagnesemia and other metabolic disorders to adversely affect neuromuscular transmission
- To recognize that the use of iodinated radiographic contrast is associated with clinical decompensation in patients with underlying junctional disorders

The hallmark of dysfunction of the neuromuscular junction (NMJ) is fluctuating weakness. Iatrogenic causes of NMJ disease can be separated into the following categories: (1) iatrogenic autoimmune MG, (2) drugs or conditions that impair neuromuscular transmission, leading to clinical weakness in otherwise normal patients, and (3) drugs or conditions that produce significant clinical manifestations in those patients with an underlying defect of neuromuscular transmission. Patients with MG or Lambert-Eaton syndrome (the myasthenic syndrome) may have worsening of symptoms on exposure to a variety of medications.

Underlying disorders of neuromuscular transmission may affect presynaptic release of acetylcholine (ACh) or the postsynaptic muscle fiber membrane at the end-plate. Similarly, adverse drug effects can occur presynaptically or postsynaptically. In a patient with a reduced safety factor for neuromuscular transmission, exposure to a drug or clinical state that further reduces the efficiency of neuromuscular transmission can result in significant clinical weakness.

Neuromuscular Junction and Neuromuscular Transmission

Familiarity with the NMJ and normal neuromuscular transmission is required to understand the clinical, laboratory, and experimental observations regarding iatrogenic junctional disorders.[1] The basic components of the NMJ and essential events in neuromuscular transmission are summarized in Figure 16.1. A single motor nerve terminal has approximately 200,000 synaptic vesicles that contain ACh. One quantum of ACh is defined as the number of transmitter molecules contained in a single vesicle (approximately 6,000–10,000 ACh molecules). ACh is released from vesicles by exo-

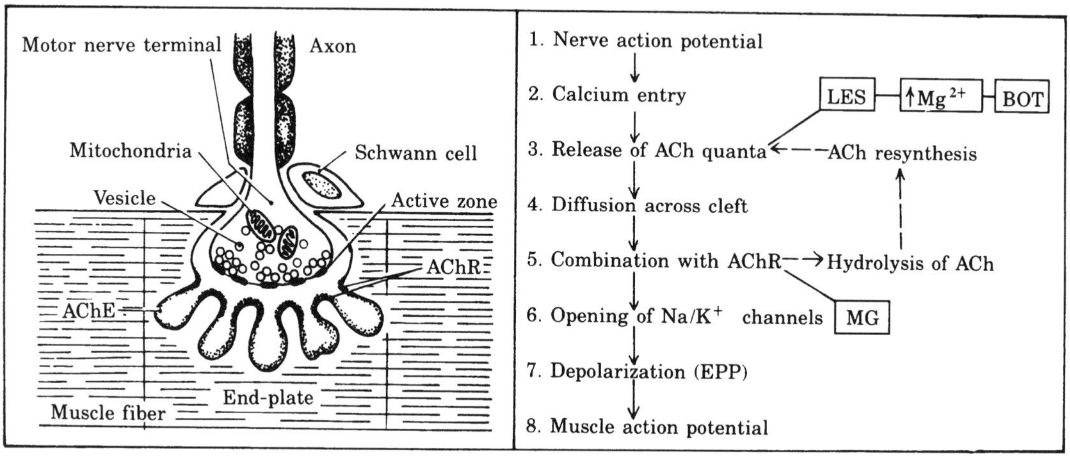

Figure 16.1. Schematic of the neuromuscular junction and the principal events of neuromuscular transmission. Presynaptic disorders affecting release of acetylcholine (ACh) include Lambert-Eaton syndrome (LES), hypermagnesemia (↑ Mg^{2+}), and botulinum toxin (BOT), whereas the main underlying postsynaptic disorder affecting ACh receptors is autoimmune myasthenia gravis (MG). Drugs adversely affecting neuromuscular transmission can act presynaptically, postsynaptically, and in some cases at both sites. (AChE = acetylcholinesterase; AChR = acetylcholine receptors; EPP = end-plate potential.)

cytosis, which occurs at specialized active zones or release sites at the nerve terminal. The active zones contain voltage-sensitive calcium channels. The postsynaptic end-plate contains acetylcholine receptors (AChR) located on the crests of junctional folds in the muscle fiber membrane. Acetylcholinesterase, which hydrolyses ACh, is located in the basement membrane. Most of the acetylcholinesterase is located in the valleys of the junctional folds. The receptors are concentrated on the crests of the junctional folds at a density of approximately 10^4 per μm^2. These AChRs are nicotinic receptors that bind nicotine but not muscarine. The nondepolarizing competitive antagonist curare inhibits the AChR, whereas atropine does not.

The binding of one or two ACh molecules to a specific region of the AChR produces a conformational change in the AChR, opening an ion channel and increasing sodium conductance. The ACh readily dissociates from the receptor, resulting in closure of the ion channel. After dissociation of ACh from AChR, acetylcholinesterase rapidly hydrolyses the neurotransmitter to choline and acetate. Choline is then taken up by the presynaptic nerve terminal for resynthesis into ACh by choline acetyltransferase.

Normally, when a single nerve action potential reaches the nerve terminal, 40–150 vesicles (or quanta) are simultaneously released. This release is mediated by the opening of voltage-sensitive calcium channels causing an influx of calcium at the nerve terminal. Calcium accumulation at the nerve terminal mediates the exocytosis of synaptic vesicles at the release sites or active zones of the presynaptic membrane. Cyclic adenosine monophosphate (AMP) also plays a role in the release of ACh. The postsynaptic depolarization of the muscle fiber membrane after a nerve-evoked release of a bolus of quanta is defined as the end-plate potential (EPP). A random small end-plate depolarization of approximately 1 mV is referred to as the *miniature end-plate potential* (MEPP) and is the result of single vesicles of ACh being released randomly from the nerve terminal. The *quantal content* refers to the number of vesicles or quanta released after a single nerve action potential invading the nerve terminal. Using intracellular microelectrode studies, the quantal content can be estimated by measuring the EPP amplitude and dividing that value by the MEPP amplitude. In general, presynaptic abnormalities of vesicle release (e.g., as from Lambert-Eaton syndrome, botulism, hypermagnesemia, and some drug effects) are char-

Table 16.1. Characteristics of Presynaptic and Postsynaptic Disorders as Shown by Microelectrode Studies of a Nerve-Muscle Preparation In Vitro

	Miniature End-Plate Potential Amplitude	Quantal Content	Miniature End-Plate Potential Frequency
Presynaptic disorder	Normal	Reduced	Normal or reduced
Postsynaptic disorder	Reduced	Normal	Normal

acterized by reduced quantal content (and normal MEPP amplitude), whereas postsynaptic disorders (e.g., MG and many drug effects) are associated with normal quantal content (and reduced MEPP amplitude) (Table 16.1).

The normal resting membrane potential is approximately –85 mV. Depolarization of 15–20 mV must occur in order to reach the threshold necessary to produce a self-propagating muscle fiber action potential. Therefore, if approximately 100 vesicles (or quanta) are released by a nerve action potential and if each vesicle of ACh produces approximately 1 mV depolarization, the resulting EPP would be approximately 100 mV (four to five times greater than that required to reach threshold for production of a self-propagating muscle fiber action potential). The excess depolarization of the EPP beyond that necessary to reach threshold is referred to as the *safety margin,* or *safety factor,* that allows neuromuscular transmission to occur, even if the nerve terminal becomes depleted of quanta. Once threshold is reached, a self-propagating muscle fiber action potential spreads away from the end-plate along the muscle fiber membrane and through the transverse tubule system at a rate of 3–5 m per second, eventually resulting in calcium release from the sarcoplasmic reticulum and activation of the muscle fiber contractile process. Any drug that impairs the presynaptic formation, storage, or release of ACh or postsynaptic receptor function can therefore potentially lead to clinical weakness.[2–5]

The NMJ disorders are characterized by fluctuating weakness. Often this includes extraocular, facial, and oropharyngeal muscles. Life-threatening respiratory failure and variable degrees of limb weakness may also occur. In some patients, individual muscle groups may be severely affected, whereas other muscle groups may be normal. Any patient with weakness of a lower motor neuron type or in which there are no upper motor neuron signs, particularly in the absence of sensory involvement, should be considered for NMJ disease. Patients with fluctuating weakness, especially those involving extraocular muscles or oropharyngeal muscles, should be thoroughly evaluated for NMJ dysfunction. Electrophysiologic studies in patients with NMJ disorders reveal a distinctive decremental response of the compound muscle action potential to slow rates of repetitive nerve stimulation. Figure 16.2 illustrates the basis for the typical decremental response (and explains, in part, the fluctuating character of junctional weakness). Evidence for milder NMJ dysfunction can be obtained by performing single-fiber electromyography, in which increased jitter can establish the presence of subclinical defects, whereas blocking of fiber potentials correlates with symptomatic weakness.

Myasthenia Gravis

The prototype NMJ disease is MG.[6] Familiarity with this disorder assists the clinician in recognizing others involving defective neuromuscular transmission. Furthermore, because MG is the most common of the junctional diseases, it represents the most common clinical setting in which the use of specific drugs may lead to clinical worsening. MG is an autoimmune disorder of neuromuscular transmission involving the production of autoantibodies directed against the nicotinic AChR. Receptor antibodies are detectable in the sera of 80–90% of patients with MG. The prevalence of MG is approximately 1 in 10,000–20,000. Women are affected approximately twice as often as men. Symptoms may begin at virtually any age, with a peak in women in the second and third decades and a peak in men in the fifth and sixth decades. Associated autoimmune diseases such as rheumatoid arthritis, systemic lupus erythematosus, and pernicious anemia are present in approximately 5% of patients. Thyroid disease occurs in approximately 10%, often

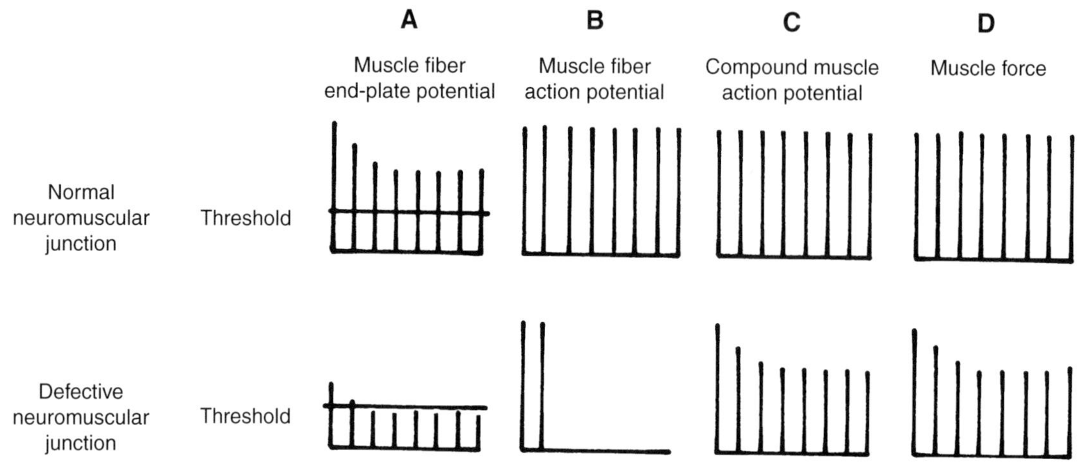

Figure 16.2. Schematic of the dynamics of neuromuscular transmission. Lines represent response to repetitive nerve stimulation at two per second in the normal neuromuscular junction (top row) and in the defective junction (bottom row), in which there is either a presynaptic or postsynaptic defect. (A) The gradual decline in the amplitude of the postsynaptic end-plate potential (EPP) is shown. (B) Each EPP exceeds the threshold necessary to produce a self-propagating muscle fiber action potential (AP) in the normal neuromuscular junction. In the defective neuromuscular junction, some of the EPPs do not reach threshold, and no AP is generated (transmission is blocked). (C) The compound muscle AP is the sum of all muscle fiber APs in one muscle group. In the defective junction, the compound muscle AP is reduced because of the progressive decline in the number of muscle fiber APs produced by each successive nerve stimulation. (D) There is a progressive decline in muscle strength with repetitive stimulation. Similarly, exercise in a patient with junctional disease produces progressive weakness or fluctuating symptoms.

in association with antithyroid antibodies. Approximately 10–15% of MG patients have thymoma, which is usually a benign tumor, and lymphoid hyperplasia with proliferation of germinal centers is present in 50–70% of patients.

The distinguishing feature of MG is fluctuating or fatigable weakness. Ocular symptoms are common; 25% of patients present with diplopia and 25% with ptosis. By 1 month into the course of illness, 80% of patients have some degree of ocular weakness. Presenting symptoms are bulbar in 10%, lower extremity in 10%, and generalized weakness in 10%. Respiratory failure is the presenting symptom in 1% of cases. Patients complain of symptoms from focal muscle dysfunction such as diplopia, ptosis, dysarthria, dysphagia, inability to work with arms raised over the head, or disturbance of gait. In contrast, patients with MG tend not to complain of generalized weakness, generalized fatigue, sleepiness, or muscle pain. In the classic case, fluctuating weakness is worse with exercise and improved with rest, and symptoms tend to increase as the day goes on. Many different factors can precipitate or aggravate weakness including physical stress, emotional stress, infection, or exposure to medications that impair neuromuscular transmission. Establishing an improvement in response to cholinesterase inhibitors (CEIs) is useful in making the diagnosis and also in management.

Similarly, other disorders of neuromuscular transmission, including Lambert-Eaton syndrome, botulism, organophosphate poisoning, hypermagnesemia, and snake envenomation, are characterized by fluctuating weakness. NMJ disorders should be suspected in any patient with unexplained weakness, especially those having a fluctuating course or cranial muscle involvement. Acute onset of weakness should prompt an assiduous review of the patient's medication history due to the large number of drugs that can potentially induce clinical weakness.

The spectrum of iatrogenic NMJ disorders is reviewed in the subsequent sections: iatrogenic autoimmune MG, metabolic disorders of neuromuscular transmission, botulinum toxin, drugs used in anesthesia, and drugs likely to cause weakness in patients with an underlying NMJ disease.

Iatrogenic Autoimmune Myasthenia Gravis

The three iatrogenic causes of autoimmune MG are D-penicillamine, interferon-alfa, and BMT.

D-Penicillamine

D-Penicillamine is used to treat Wilson's disease, rheumatoid arthritis, other chronic autoimmune diseases, and cystinuria. Use of D-penicillamine has been associated with a variety of immune-mediated complications, including polymyositis, systemic lupus erythematosus, nephritis due to immune complex deposition, scleroderma, and pemphigus. Since the initial reports of penicillamine-related autoimmune MG by Bucknall et al. and Czlonkowska in 1975, more than 100 such cases have been documented in the literature.[7, 8] The symptoms in penicillamine-induced MG are usually mild and may be limited to extraocular muscles, including isolated ptosis.[9] Patients develop AChR antibodies, classic electromyographic abnormalities, and the typical improvement with the use of CEIs. Nerve-muscle preparation studies from intercostal muscle biopsies have shown reduced MEPP amplitude typical for acquired MG. Other than taking penicillamine, the patients are indistinguishable from those with idiopathic autoimmune MG.[10–16] The diagnosis can be easily missed, especially in patients presenting with respiratory failure.[17] Myasthenia is reported to occur in 1–7% of all patients taking penicillamine.[18, 19] One group found MG in 5 of 71 consecutive patients with penicillamine-treated rheumatoid arthritis within a 2-year period.[19] The frequency of MG from penicillamine therapy may be less for patients with Wilson's disease than for those with rheumatoid arthritis, suggesting an underlying susceptibility to an immune-mediated process. Onset of MG symptoms typically occurs 2–12 months after the initiation of penicillamine.[20] In general, MG is less severe than idiopathic MG, although some patients require mechanical ventilation. Discontinuation of penicillamine leads to complete resolution of MG symptoms in 2–6 months in the majority of patients. By 1 year, MG symptoms have completely resolved in approximately 70% of patients, the titer of AChR antibodies improves, and the electrophysiologic abnormalities improve or resolve.[20, 21] The fact that some patients remain symptomatic long after stopping penicillamine suggests that in some cases, especially those with rheumatoid arthritis or other underlying autoimmune disease, MG may have been present subclinically before treatment with penicillamine and simply exacerbated by exposure to the drug. The management of MG involves discontinuation of penicillamine and the use of conventional treatments available for the treatment of autoimmune MG.[6]

The mechanism for penicillamine-induced MG is unclear.[22] Studies of penicillamine reaction with purified AChR from *Torpedo californica* show covalent attachment to two receptor subunits, alpha and gamma, presumed to result from reduction and formation of mixed disulfides.[12] Penicillamine modifies the equilibrium of ACh-binding properties of both purified receptor and receptor-rich membrane fragments.[12] Penicillamine given to normal rats in doses equivalent to human therapy results in no acute neuromuscular abnormalities.[23] Prolonged administration to guinea pigs in high doses results in a mild degree of neuromuscular block.[24] Therefore, there is little evidence to suggest that the drug has a direct effect on neuromuscular transmission. The latency to onset of symptoms and the presence of AChR antibodies indicate that the drug induces the autoimmune attack. Reduced sulfoxidation capacity observed in eight of nine patients with penicillamine-induced MG suggests that poor sulfoxidation may predispose the patient to developing MG.[25] Other drugs with similarities to penicillamine also used in the treatment of rheumatoid arthritis include tiopronin and pyrithioxin. An occasional association with MG has been reported with both drugs.[26, 27]

Interferon-alfa

Patients treated with interferon-alfa develop a variety of autoantibodies and autoimmune diseases. The initial reports of interferon-induced MG occurred in 1995, when a 66-year-old man was reported as having developed seropositive generalized MG approximately 6 months after starting interferon-alfa therapy for leukemia.[28] Subsequently, MG has developed in other patients during interferon alfa-2b treatment for malignancy.[29, 30] Patients treated for chronic active hepatitis C with interferon-alfa have also developed autoimmune MG, with onset 6–9 months after starting treatment. In one case, MG symptoms persisted for at least 7 months after stopping the drug.[31, 32] Fulminant myasthenic crisis may occur after interferon-alfa therapy.[33]

Regarding the mechanism of interferon-induced MG, the expression of interferon gamma at motor end-plates of transgenic mice results in generalized weakness, abnormal NMJ function, and improvement with CEIs. Immunoprecipitation analysis indicates that a previously unidentified 87-kD target antigen is recognized by sera from those transgenic mice and also from human MG patients. Such studies suggest that the expression of interferon gamma at motor end-plates in these transgenic mice provokes an autoimmune humoral response similar to that which occurs in human MG.[34]

Bone Marrow Transplantation

The third iatrogenic cause for autoimmune MG is BMT first reported in 1983 in association with thymoma and anti–skeletal muscle antibodies.[35, 36] Myasthenia occurs as one manifestation of the graft-versus-host disease.[37, 38] Acute graft-versus-host disease immediately after BMT is generally not associated with neurologic manifestations. In contrast, chronic graft-versus-host disease is associated with several neurologic problems, including polymyositis and MG.[39] Some patients develop both of these neuromuscular disorders, rendering the diagnosis difficult. MG seems more likely to occur in patients treated with BMT for aplastic anemia, some of whom have shown AChR antibodies before transplant. In BMT-associated MG, the clinical features are classic for autoimmune MG: AChR antibodies are present, and symptoms respond to CEIs and improve with immunosuppressive therapy.[40, 41] The onset of MG tends to be delayed from several months to as long as 10 years after BMT.[39, 42, 43] Myasthenia is a relatively uncommon neurologic complication of BMT. In one series of six children with neuromuscular complications of allogenic BMT, only one had MG, whereas four had myositis, and one had chronic inflammatory demyelinating polyneuropathy.[44] Patients respond to CEIs and immunosuppressive therapy typical for autoimmune MG.

Metabolic Impairment of Neuromuscular Transmission

Magnesium and Hypermagnesemia

Hypermagnesemia is an uncommon clinical situation associated with the use of magnesium-containing drugs.[45] Magnesium (Mg^{2+}) is contained in some antacids and laxatives. Magnesium sulfate ($MgSO_4$) is used in the treatment of preeclampsia and eclampsia, for hemodynamic control during anesthesia and the early postoperative period,[46] and in patients depleted of Mg^{2+} (such as in chronic alcoholism). Normal serum magnesium runs 1.5–2.5 mEq per liter (2–3 mg/dl), which is stabilized through exchange with tissue stores in bone, liver, muscle, and brain; also, serum Mg^{2+} concentration is maintained via renal excretion. Patients with renal failure are predisposed to developing hypermagnesemia and should avoid magnesium-containing antacids and laxatives for this reason.[47, 48] Elevated serum magnesium levels due to oral use of magnesium-containing compounds is very uncommon as long as the patient has normal renal function.[49, 50] Hypermagnesemia is occasionally seen with the use of enemas, but usually in patients with an underlying gastrointestinal tract disorder.[49, 51] In the treatment of preeclampsia, hypermagnesemia occurs commonly due to the administration of high doses of parenteral $MgSO_4$, at times resulting in serious side effects in the mother or the newborn.[52–54] The clinical features of hypermagnesemia correlate fairly well with the serum magnesium levels.[49, 55, 56] In treating preeclampsia, the neuromuscular transmission effects are monitored and used as a limiting factor in dosage. With serum levels above 5 mEq per liter, the muscle stretch reflexes become reduced, whereas levels of 9–10 mEq per liter are associated with absent reflexes and clinically significant weakness. In treating preeclampsia, muscle stretch reflexes are tested serially, and magnesium administration is stopped if the reflexes disappear.[53] Serum levels between 3.5 and 7 mEq per liter are usually associated with no significant adverse effects in preeclamptic women, but clinical weakness is common with levels greater than 10 mEq per liter, and death from respiratory failure can occur.[52, 53] Serum levels above 14 mEq per liter can induce acute cardiac arrhythmia, including heart block and arrest. Additional symptoms from autonomic nervous system involvement include dry mouth, dilated pupils, urinary retention, hypotension, and flushing skin thought to be from presynaptic blockade at autonomic ganglia.[57] Although patients can develop severe weakness, mental status is usually not directly affected.[56] Extraocular muscles tend to be spared. Reduced level of consciousness may occur indirectly as a result of hypoxia, hypercarbia, or hypotension.

Magnesium interferes with neuromuscular transmission by inhibiting release of ACh.[58] Magnesium competitively blocks calcium entry at the motor nerve terminal. There may also be a more mild postsynaptic affect. Clinically, hypermagnesemia resembles Lambert-Eaton syndrome more so than autoimmune MG.[59] In addition, magnesium can potentiate the action of neuromuscular blocking agents, which has been noted in women who had cesarean section after treatment with Mg^{2+} for preeclampsia.[60, 61] Patients with underlying junctional disorders are more sensitive to Mg^{2+}-induced weakness. Patients with MG[62–64] and Lambert-Eaton syndrome[65, 66] have been reported to have exacerbated symptoms in the setting of Mg^{2+} use, in spite of normal or only mildly elevated serum levels. Typically, increased MG symptoms occur with parenteral magnesium administration, but on occasion are seen with oral use.[66] Therefore, parenteral Mg^{2+} administration should be avoided and oral Mg^{2+} preparations used with caution in patients with known junctional disease (MG, Lambert Eaton syndrome, botulism, etc.).

The effects of standard parenteral doses of $MgSO_4$ on neuromuscular transmission of preeclampsia or preterm labor patients are significant, although largely subclinical. Train-of-four (TOF) recordings obtained from the thenar muscles before and 30 minutes after $MgSO_4$ infusion show an increase in tension of the contractile response in the control or baseline recordings, but the postinfusion TOF results show no increase, but rather a "fade" of the response.[67] These data suggest that in this patient population clinically relevant infusions of $MgSO_4$ produced significant changes in neuromuscular transmission, as manifested by loss of the treppe phenomenon and diminished TOF response.[67]

Effects of 60 mg per kg of $MgSO_4$ on residual neuromuscular block after administration of vecuronium are also significant.[46] Patients given Mg^{2+} immediately on recovery from vecuronium block or 1 hour later demonstrate rapid and profound recurarization, as measured by electromyography and TOF studies.

Treatment of the hypermagnesemic patient depends on the severity of clinical symptoms. Discontinuation of magnesium is the first step; if the patient is significantly weak, administration of intravenous calcium gluconate, 1 g over 3 minutes, can produce rapid, although temporary improvement (so long as the patient has normal renal function typical for a patient being treated for preeclampsia). If hypermagnesemia is more severe or if there are life-threatening side effects such as cardiac arrhythmia or renal failure, hemodialysis is indicated.[68] If patients have MG or Lambert-Eaton syndrome, they will respond poorly to calcium. Such patients may respond better to CEIs.[63]

Other Electrolyte Disorders

Weakness from hypokalemia is believed to result from decreased excitability of muscle cell membranes.[69] Hypokalemia is implicated as a potential factor in worsening MG symptoms, especially in the setting of corticosteroid therapy, but the relationship has received only limited study.[70] Diuretics may aggravate MG weakness, possibly by depleting potassium.[71] In spite of the crucial role of intracellular calcium concentration in ACh release, few data exist on the effects of hypocalcemia on neuromuscular transmission. Although hypocalcemia is well known to result in peripheral nerve hyperexcitability, tetany, and convulsive seizures, there is no clear establishment of a clinically significant effect on neuromuscular transmission.[45] Clinical decompensation of MG patients during plasma exchange, ostensibly from citrate used in the intravenous replacement fluids, is suggested to be mediated by citrate-induced hypocalcemia.[72]

Botulinum Toxin

As botulinum toxin A has been increasingly used to treat focal dystonia and spasticity, it has become apparent that there is potential for symptomatic complications from excess toxin. Botulinum toxin blocks ACh release at the presynaptic motor nerve terminal (and causes dysautonomia by blocking muscarinic autonomic cholinergic function as well). The intracellular target of botulinum toxin appears to be a protein of the ACh vesicle membrane. The toxin is a zinc-dependent protease that cleaves protein components of the neuroexocytosis apparatus.[73–75] Not only is its effect local at the site of injection into muscle, but there is also some degree of distant effect.[76] Dysphagia is a frequent side effect of botulinum injection for spasmodic dysphonia, typically lasting for approximately 2 weeks.[77] On occasion the dysphagia is severe, especially when patients report some degree of pretreatment dysphagia.[77] Prospective study of complications of botulinum toxin injections for cervical dystonia showed that before treatment 11% of patients had symptoms of dysphagia, whereas 22% had radiologic evidence for abnormal peristalsis.[78] After injections of botulinum toxin, new symptoms of dysphagia developed in an additional 33% of patients (those with pretreatment dysphagia were unchanged), and 50% developed new peristaltic abnormalities by radiographic study.[78] Single-fiber electromyography of the forearm muscle performed after treatment of cervical dystonia and hemifacial spasm shows an abnormal increase in mean jitter (suggesting impaired neuromuscular transmission), and 6 weeks after treatment there is increased fiber density indicating reinnervation.[79] In addition, mild abnormalities of cardiovascular reflexes suggest distant effects on autonomic function.[79] Previously undetected Lambert-Eaton syndrome has been unmasked in a patient after local botulinum toxin injection.[80] Clearly, botulinum toxin is relatively contraindicated in patients with a known defect of neuromuscular transmission. In addition, the clinician should be alert to the development of excessive weakness in the region of local injection, or even remote sites, particularly with higher doses of botulinum toxin.

Drugs Used in Anesthesiology

General Anesthetics

Patients with underlying junctional disease such as MG are well known for the propensity toward prolonged weakness after anesthesia for surgical procedures. The cause for such potential difficulty is likely to be multifactorial. General anesthetics may potentiate neuromuscular blocking drugs in myasthenic patients.[81] In addition, the inhalational anesthetics may have a direct effect on neuromuscular transmission. The routine administration of the inhalant anesthetic methoxyflurane is reported to unmask mild MG.[82] With repeated exposure the patient developed fatigue, weakness, and ptosis for several hours, which improved after CEI administration. In experimental studies some inhalational anesthetics appear to alter postjunctional sensitivity to ACh, affect ionic conductance, and induce shortening of ACh-activated channel open time.[83]

Local Anesthetics

In a normal person, local anesthetic use is unlikely to cause significant neuromuscular weakness. Intravenous lidocaine, procaine, and other local anesthetic agents can potentiate the effect of neuromuscular blocking drugs. There appear to be both presynaptic and postsynaptic effects. Interference with propagation of the nerve action potential at the nerve terminal and reduced ACh release may account for the presynaptic effects.[84] Local anesthetics also lead to reduced sensitivity of the postjunctional membrane to ACh.[85] Harvey observed procaine to induce acute myasthenic crisis in 1939, but subsequent studies provide evidence to the contrary.[86, 87]

Neuromuscular Blocking Drugs

Depolarizing and nondepolarizing neuromuscular blockers affect the muscle membrane potential. Neuromuscular blocking drugs may be modified by the degree of neuromuscular block, the associated disease state, acid-base status of the patient, and associated electrolyte imbalance. In patients with MG and Lambert-Eaton syndrome, relatively small amounts of nondepolarizing agents can produce profound and prolonged NMJ blockade. Prolonged paralysis from neuromuscular blockers may occur on occasion in patients without NMJ disease. Factors that may influence the duration of neuromuscular blockade include dosage and duration of therapy, concurrent drug use (including muscle relaxants, magnesium, and cimetidine), severity of underlying disease, electrolyte abnormalities, and renal insufficiency (which may lead to high drug concentrations).[88] Use of muscle relaxants for 1 week in a child resulted in a 6-week course of recovery.[89] Similarly, long-term weakness from vecuronium use is reported to occur in adults.[90, 91] Paralysis lasted 8 weeks after use of the neuromuscular blocker atracurium besilate.[92] Patients with metabolic acidosis, high serum magnesium levels, renal failure, and high blood levels of 3-desacetyl-vecuronium appear more likely to experience prolonged paralysis.[93] Prolonged neuromuscular blockade can be severe enough to produce neurogenic muscle atrophy.[94] Corticosteroids may even potentiate the effects of muscle relaxants.[95] Prolonged weakness in intensive care patients can result from a multitude of causes, some leading to peripheral neuropathy, myopathy, as well as junctional disturbance as previously mentioned. In many patients, there are multiple concomitant factors leading to paralysis.[96, 97]

Depolarizing agents including succinylcholine should be used with caution in patients with known NMJ disease. The inhibition of hydrolysis by CEIs results in prolonged duration of action. Patients with MG are less sensitive to this drug than the nondepolarizing agents. Occasionally, patients with MG have their disease unmasked by the use of these drugs. Pharmacologic effects of neuromuscular blockers are influenced by antibiotics, general anesthetics, local anesthetics, and antiarrhythmics, which may complicate clinical weakness. Newer neuromuscular blocking agents with shorter durations of action may still aggravate MG and Lambert-Eaton syndrome weakness. Occasional reports of reduced plasma cholinesterase levels by plasma exchange or by genetic abnormalities have been associated with reports of prolonged apnea and muscle weakness in patients receiving depolarizing neuromuscular blocking drugs.

Agents that Impair Neuromuscular Transmission and May Increase Weakness in Patients with Underlying Junctional Disorders

Antibiotics

In 1941 Robinson and Molitor showed that tyrothricin (gramicidin) could produce respiratory failure in animals.[98] In 1956 Pridgen reported respiratory arrest as a result of intraperitoneal neomycin in humans.[99] He noted four patients without prior neuromuscular symptoms who developed apnea from intraperitoneal neomycin sulfate, two of whom died. Subsequently, numerous case reports of neuromuscular weakness from antibiotic administration thought to be a result of impaired neuromuscular transmission have been reported in normal patients, those concurrently receiving neuromuscular blocking drugs, those with MG, those with other disorders that might alter pharmacokinetics, and patients with exposure to other drugs having an adverse effect on neuromuscular transmission.[100–105]

The aminoglycoside antibiotics are well established to impair neuromuscular transmission and produce clinically significant weakness, regardless of the method of administration.[103] Weakness appears to be dose dependent and reflected by serum levels. CEIs, infusion of calcium, and aminopyridines can partially reverse the weakness produced by aminoglycosides.[106–108] Microelectrode studies on nerve muscle preparations suggest that the effect is presynaptic, postsynaptic, or both and may depend on the specific aminoglycoside. Tobramycin appears to have predominantly presynaptic effects similar to hypermagnesemia with impairment of ACh release.[109–111] In contrast, netilmicin acts postsynaptically by blocking the binding of ACh to receptors, as is caused by curare.[109–111] Of the studies of amikacin, gentamicin, kanamycin, neomycin, netilmicin, streptomycin, and tobramycin, neomycin appears to be the most potent in interfering with neuromuscular transmission, whereas tobramycin would appear to be the least toxic in this regard.[109, 112–117]

Gentamicin, neomycin, streptomycin, tobramycin, and kanamycin have been reported to produce clinically significant muscle weakness on occasion in non-MG patients.[4] Patients with infantile botulism and MG can also have increased weakness on exposure to these antibiotics.[118–120]

Other antibiotics, including tetracyclines, sulfonamides, penicillins, amino acid antibiotics, and fluoroquinolones, have either been associated with anecdotal reports of increased weakness in myasthenic patients or implicated from in vitro studies to adversely affect neuromuscular transmission. Acute worsening of MG has been reported after administration of ciprofloxacin, a fluroroquinolone.[121] Exacerbation of MG has been reported with use of perfloxacin and also norfloxacin.[122, 123] Clindamycin and lincomycin are monobasic amino acid antibiotics that differ from aminoglycosides.[124, 125] The neuromuscular blockade produced by these drugs is not readily reversed with CEIs. These drugs have presynaptic and postsynaptic effects by microelectrode studies, with reduced MEPP frequency, reduced evoked transmitter release, and reduced sensitivity of the postjunctional AChR.[126, 127] Junctional effects of lincomycin can be reversed with increased calcium concentration or with use of aminopyridines.[128] However, CEIs may aggravate the effect. Clindamycin may also directly block muscle contractility.[127] Vancomycin may potentiate the neuromuscular blockade of succinylcholine.[129]

Colistin, colistimethate, and polymyxin B are reported to produce weakness, especially in patients with renal insufficiency and when used in combination with other neuromuscular blocking drugs or antibiotics.[130–135] Their mechanism of action includes reduced ACh release and, to some degree, postsynaptic blockade of the receptor.[136–138] Acute respiratory failure in MG may occur after a single intramuscular injection of colistimethate.[139] Colistin has been reported to cause acute weakness in patients with underlying MG.[140]

Although tetracycline has not been associated with weakness or abnormal in vitro abnormalities, several analogues of tetracycline including rolitetracycline and oxytetracycline are reported to exacerbate MG weakness. The mechanism for this effect is not known. Some studies show no deleterious effect of tetracycline.[109, 141]

Ampicillin is rarely reported to increase weakness of MG patients and increase the percent of decremental response on repetitive stimulation in rabbits with experimental MG.[142] Ampicillin also can lead to single-fiber electromyographic abnormalities.[143] In vitro studies on nerve-muscle preparations have not shown clear-cut abnormalities to indicate if the effect is presynaptic or postsynaptic.[142]

Myasthenic patients occasionally report increased weakness with erythromycin, and physiologic studies in normal humans suggest it has a presynaptic effect.[3, 144] Severe exacerbation of MG has been reported beginning 1 hour after taking 500 mg of azithromycin (Zithromax), a newer azalide antibiotic of the macrolide group. The patient required mechanical ventilation for 6 days. The same patient had previously had a similar exacerbation after taking another macrolide, erythromycin. Therefore, these antibiotics should also be used with caution in patients with MG.[145]

Clearly, the issue of antibiotic effects on neuromuscular transmission is complex and poses a vexing dilemma for the clinician. Nearly every antibiotic ever studied has demonstrated some deleterious effect or has been the subject of a clinical report suggesting exacerbation of MG. If a patient requires antibiotic treatment for an infection, the appropriate drugs should be used. When managing patients with junctional disease it behooves the clinician to remain alert to the potential for clinically significant adverse effects, especially if the patient becomes weaker with antibiotic use.

Cardiovascular Drugs

Quinidine and Quinine

Quinidine and its stereoisomer quinine can aggravate weakness in MG.[146] A number of reports suggest that quinidine can unmask previously undiagnosed or asymptomatic MG.[147–149] The drug acts presynaptically to impair the formation or release of ACh. In large doses, it may also have a postsynaptic effect with a curare-like action. A number of references in the literature suggest that quinine can also aggravate myasthenic weakness. Quinidine has been observed to potentiate weakness induced by nondepolarizing and depolarizing neuromuscular blocking drugs.[150, 151] Quinine has been used as a diagnostic test for MG in the past. Harvey and Whitehill in 1937 reported the differential effects of quinine and neostigmine in the diagnostic evaluation of MG.[152] Similarly, Eaton in 1943 pointed out the diagnostic usefulness of trials of neostigmine and alternatively, quinine.[153]

Sieb et al. studied the effects of quinoline derivatives quinine, quinidine, and chloroquine on neuromuscular transmission using conventional microelectrode and patch-clamp techniques.[154] All three derivatives reduce quantal content of the EPP by 37–45% and decrease the amplitude and decay time constant of the MEPP and miniature end-plate current. At progressively larger concentrations, the MEPP becomes undetectable. The effect on MEPP is not reversed by neostigmine. Single-channel patch-clamp analysis of quinine effects reveal a long-lived open-channel and a closed-channel block of AChR. Test results for competitive inhibition or desensitization of the AChR by quinine in these concentrations are negative. Quinoline drugs adversely affect both presynaptic and postsynaptic aspects of neuromuscular transmission at concentrations close to those used in clinical practice. Therefore, they should not be used, or used only with extreme caution, in disorders with a reduced safety margin of neuromuscular transmission.[154] I have cared for patients whose MG decompensated in the setting of quinine, 325 mg every evening, for the treatment of leg cramps. In both cases, the patients developed markedly increased weakness within hours to days of starting the medication. Anecdotal reports suggest that consumption of tonic water containing small amounts of quinine can result in exacerbation of myasthenic symptoms.

Beta-Blockers

Beta-adrenergic blocking drugs, including propranolol, oxprenolol, timolol, and practolol, have been observed on occasion to be associated with increasing weakncss in MG patients.[155–159] Although beta-blockers are unlikely to produce frank muscle weakness in normal patients, they are notorious for inducing subjective fatigue. Furthermore, occasional patients describe transient diplopia in the setting of beta-blocker use, which raises the question of an NMJ mechanism in such patients.[160] In vitro microelectrode studies of nerve-muscle preparations reveal that atenolol, labetalol, metoprolol, nadolol, propranolol, and timolol all produced dose-dependent reduction in neuromuscular transmission in rat skeletal muscle.[161, 162] Both presynaptic and postsynaptic effects have been observed. Reduced MEPP amplitude can be caused by any of the beta-blockers, suggesting a postsynaptic site of action. Presynaptic abnormalities include reduced MEPP frequency, and with metoprolol and propranolol, there is reduced quantal content. Propranolol seems to most markedly impair neuromuscular transmission, with atenolol having the least effect.[161, 162] The specific mechanism for the beta-blocker junctional effect is unclear.

In 10 patients with mild to moderate MG who received intravenous propranolol, 0.1 mg per kg at 1 mg per minute, there was no detectable effect on the decrement to repetitive nerve stimulation or on clinical tests, leading the investigators to conclude "there is no rapid deterioration of neuromuscular transmission in patients with moderately severe MG after injections with therapeutic doses of propranolol."[163] Such findings are consistent with my own observations in practice: The use of beta-blockers in MG patients is unlikely to cause significant worsening of their symptoms.

Calcium Channel Blockers

A variety of observations indicate that calcium channel blockers may adversely affect neuromuscular transmission. Presynaptic reduction in ACh release and also postsynaptic curare-like effects have been observed in experimental settings.[164–166] Calcium channel blockers can potentiate the effect of neuromuscular blocking drugs.[167, 168] Verapamil has been associated with increased weakness and respiratory failure with intravenous use in a patient with Duchenne's dystrophy.[169] A patient with Lambert-Eaton syndrome had exacerbated symptoms after receiving verapamil.[170] Verapamil is implicated as the cause of respiratory failure in a patient with MG.[3] Jonkers' group prospectively studied the effects of intravenous administration of verapamil on the decremental response to repetitive nerve stimulation and clinical function in 10 patients with mild to moderate MG.[163] Verapamil at doses of 0.1 mg per kg given at 1 mg per minute showed no adverse effects on neuromuscular transmission.

Protti et al. studied the effect of calcium channel blockers on transmitter release at normal human NMJ, observing that P-type calcium channel blockers blocked nerve-evoked muscle action potentials and inhibited evoked synaptic transmission.[171] But transmitter release was not affected either by nitrendipine, an L-type channel blocker, or omega-conotoxin GVIA, an N-type channel blocker. Those observations suggest that P-type channels mediate transmitter release at the motor nerve terminals.

Procainamide can lead to acute worsening of MG. Although the drug can induce autoimmune phenomena, the immediate onset of weakness and neuromuscular blockade would suggest a direct effect on neuromuscular transmission, as opposed to an indirect autoimmune process.[172, 173] Procainamide appears to act presynaptically in reducing formation of ACh or inhibiting its release, and there is some evidence to implicate postsynaptic factors as well. Bretylium may induce muscle weakness as well as potentiate the effect of neuromuscular blockers.[174]

Trimethaphan is a ganglionic blocking agent used occasionally for treating extreme hypertensive emergency and other acute vascular emergencies. It has been associated with acute neuromuscular weakness including respiratory failure, and there is speculation that it has a curare-like action at the NMJ. In addition, the drug can potentiate neuromuscular blockade in patients receiving nondepolarizing and depolarizing neuromuscular blocking drugs.[175–178]

Antiepileptic Drugs

Phenytoin has demonstrated presynaptic and postsynaptic effects on neuromuscular transmission in vitro.[179, 180] Occasional patients with MG have presented with increased weakness after treatment with phenytoin, mephenytoin, and trimethadione.[180–183] In some of these cases, the weakness has resolved after discontinuation of the anticonvulsant. In vitro studies of nerve-muscle preparations have shown that phenytoin reduces quantal release of ACh from the motor nerve terminal; also, it produces a simultaneous increase in spontaneous release of neurotransmitter (and therefore increases the MEPP frequency). Possible explanations for this effect include a reduction in the size of the nerve action potential at the motor nerve terminal, or perhaps a reduction in calcium influx into the motor nerve terminal. Postsynaptic effects have also been observed with phenytoin including reduction in the MEPP amplitude (thought to be related to desensitization of the end-plate).[184] Osserman and Genkins observed that barbiturates can aggravate MG weakness.[185] In vitro studies suggest that barbiturates and ethosuximide produce postsynaptic neuromuscular blockade, whereas carbamazepine has an effect on presynaptic junctional function.[186, 187] Trimethadione can induce a variety of autoimmune complications including systemic lupus and nephrotic syndrome.[188] Weakness with trimethadione use has been associated with autoantibodies against skeletal muscle, nuclear antigens, and thymus and has gradually resolved after removal of the drug.[182, 183]

Further study of antiepileptic drugs is needed before sweeping guidelines can be made regarding their use in patients with junctional disease. In my judgment, the overall risk of using anticonvulsants in MG patients is small.

Analgesics

Narcotic analgesics do not directly interfere with neuromuscular transmission in myasthenia.[189, 190] There may be an indirect effect on the myasthenic patient, however. Slaughter in 1950 demonstrated that CEIs (neostigmine) may potentiate the effects of morphine, codeine, hydromorphone, and opium alkaloids.[191] Grob reported sudden death abruptly after administration of morphine sulfate.[192] Due to the tendency of narcotic analgesics to produce respiratory depression, they should be used with caution in patients who have respiratory insufficiency from MG or other neuromuscular diseases.

Hormonal Medications

Corticosteroids

Approximately 50% of patients with MG receiving treatment with high-dose corticosteroids have an early exacerbation; in approximately 10% this exacerbation is severe, requiring mechanical ventilation or a feeding tube.[193] The mechanism for this exacerbation is unclear. Using a lower starting dose of corticosteroids, with a gradual increase over time, may reduce the risk of early exacerbation.[194] In experimental neuromuscular preparations, there appears to be some direct effect on neuromuscular transmission, including depolarization of nerve terminals, reduced ACh release, altered MEPPs, alteration of choline transport, and intracellular potassium depletion, some of which may be clinically significant mechanisms of action.[195–198]

Alternatively, the effect may be immune-mediated. Abramsky et al. found increased lymphocyte transformation in vitro in patients with prednisone-induced aggravation of weakness.[199] Nonreactive lymphocytes may be destroyed by corticosteroids, leading to enhanced proliferation of sensitized lymphocytes.[199–201]

Estrogen

Although poorly understood, it is commonly believed among neuromuscular clinicians that MG may fluctuate with the menstrual cycle and pregnancy, suggesting an influence of estrogen or progesterone on neuromuscular transmission, the immune system, or some other aspect of MG. On occasion estrogen therapy has been associated with increasing weakness in MG including parenteral use after 3–5 days.[202, 203] An isolated case occurred in a woman taking birth control pills.[204] Another patient experienced the onset of MG approximately 4 months following implant of levonorgestrel (Norplant).[205] Symptoms progressed over the next 9 months, and AChR antibodies were present. Within 1 week of removal of the implant, her symptoms markedly improved.[205]

Thyroid Imbalance

Hyperthyroidism and hypothyroidism can be associated with increasing myasthenic weakness.[206, 207] The mechanism is unclear. Any patient with underlying MG who develops progressive weakness should be screened for abnormal thyroid function unless there is an obvious alternative explanation.

Ophthalmologic Medications

Timolol, the beta-adrenergic blocking eye drop, has been reported to be associated with increased myasthenic weakness.[157, 159] Similar observations have been made with betaxolol hydrochloride.[208] Echothiophate is a long-acting cholinesterase inhibitor used in the treatment of open-angle glaucoma and has been reported to be associated with muscle weakness and fatigue. It has been temporally related to the use of the medication, resolving when the medication is stopped.[209] The mechanism of weakness is not clear, but might relate to long-acting cholinesterase inhibitor–induced cholinergic weakness.

Psychiatric Drugs

Phenothiazines

Chlorpromazine was reported to produce increased muscle weakness in a schizophrenic patient with MG by McQuillen et al. in 1963.[210] In vitro studies have demonstrated a postsynaptic effect with reduced MEPP and EPP amplitudes without change in quantal content or MEPP frequency.[211] Still other studies have implicated a presynaptic site. Chlorpromazine and promazine can antagonize applied ACh and may prolong effects of succinylcholine. Occasional reports note that in patients receiving chlorpromazine or phenelzine, subsequent administration of depolarizing neuromuscular blocking drugs results in prolonged neuromuscular blockade.

Lithium

Subjective weakness is a common side effect of lithium carbonate. Exacerbation or unmasking of MG is reported.[212] Lithium can prolong the effect of neuromuscular blockers.[213, 214] The mechanism for the lithium-induced junctional effect may result from its accumulation inside the presynaptic motor nerve terminal and becoming a competitive cation for calcium, thus reducing ACh synthesis and voltage-gated quantal release of ACh.[215] Other studies suggest that there is a reduced number of ACh receptors in denervated muscle preparations, raising the question that lithium may selectively increase the rate of breakdown of receptors without changing the rate of synthesis. The onset of weakness in a patient with MG can occur within days of starting lithium.

Amitriptyline, amphetamines, droperidol, haloperidol, imipramine, paraldehyde, and trichloroethanol have been found to impair neuromuscular transmission in experimental settings.[2, 3]

Chloroquine

Chloroquine is widely used for treatment of malaria, but on occasion is used in the treatment of autoimmune connective tissue disorders, including rheumatoid arthritis, discoid lupus, and even porphyria cutanea tarda. It has a variety of potential neurologic complications, including peripheral neuropathy and myopathy, as well as an effect on neuromuscular transmission. The mechanism of the chloroquine effect on neuromuscular transmission is controversial and may be multifactorial. Chloroquine appears to have a direct effect at the presynaptic level with reduced quantal content, as well as having a postsynaptic effect with reduced MEPP amplitude.[154] Clinical support for the direct effect stems from observation of weakness developing within the first week after beginning chloroquine therapy, with absent AChR antibodies, and rapidly resolving symptoms on drug withdrawal.[216] Chloroquine has been reported to directly reduce muscle membrane excitability. In addition, there is some belief that the drug may induce an autoimmune disorder similar to that triggered by D-penicillamine.[217, 218] Several patients with autoimmune diseases (rheumatoid arthritis and systemic lupus erythematosus) developed clinical, physiologic, and pharmacologic evidence for MG after prolonged use of chloroquine. These patients had AChR antibodies that eventually disappeared, as did the other abnormalities after discontinuation of the drug. In a review of 12 patients in whom chloroquine exacerbated or unmasked MG, approximately half were associated with long-term, high-dose therapy, whereas the remainder occurred in the setting of brief low-dose treatment for prevention of malaria.[219]

Iodinated Radiographic Contrast

Several studies have suggested that intravenous iodinated contrast can trigger or precipitate acute myasthenic worsening.[220–223] The initial reports of three patients in 1985 noted myasthenic crisis after administration of intravenous iodinated contrast.[220, 221] These patients had abrupt apnea and several days of severe myasthenic weakness. The occurrence is controversial and not uniformly observed.[224] Frank et al. reported on a similar experience with a patient, but found the overall risk of a severe reaction in MG patients to be only approximately 2–3% of all MG iodinated contrast exposures. One patient with Lambert-Eaton syndrome developed acute transient respiratory insufficiency after intravenous contrast infusion, speculated to be on the basis of acute hypocalcemia from calcium binding of the contrast agent and resulting presynaptic blockade with reduced ACh release.[222] Although iodinated contrast may have a direct effect on neuromuscular transmission, an indirect mechanism is also possible, as part of a more nonspecific allergic-type contrast reaction. On the other hand, because patients with an acute intravenous contrast reaction typically receive medications such as diphenhydramine, which have significant anticholinergic side effects, perhaps some of the increased weakness could result from drugs used to treat the acute contrast reaction.[225] In my own experience, acute myasthenic deterioration has occurred in several patients receiving iodinated contrast during computed tomographic scanning of the chest (looking for thymoma). For that reason, we routinely perform noncontrasted chest computed tomographic scanning (or magnetic resonance scanning) when screening MG patients for thymoma.

Miscellaneous Drugs

D-L-Carnitine (but not L-carnitine) has been associated with increased weakness in MG patients undergoing dialysis.[226] The mechanism is not known but may relate to the effect caused by hemicholinium or a postsynaptic block by the accumulation of acylcarnitine esters.[227] Emetine, used as an amoebicide and also the active ingredient of ipecac, has been observed to produce acute neuromuscular weakness as a side effect.[228, 229]

The following medications have also been the subject of reports suggesting a potential for aggravating MG weakness: intravenous sodium lactate, tetanus antitoxin, and trihexyphenidyl (Artane).[5, 230, 231] Cocaine use may cause acute exacerbation of MG.[232]

Laboratory studies of the following drugs have demonstrated an abnormal effect on neuromuscular transmission: Amantadine reduces postjunctional sensitivity to ACh by interacting with the AChR ion channel of the AChR.[233] Diphenhydramine can potentiate the neuromuscular block of barbiturates and neuromuscular blocking agents and reduce the amount of neurotransmitter released from the motor nerve terminal.[225] The H_2-receptor blocker roxatidine impairs neuromuscular transmission in rat sciatic nerve-gastrocnemius muscle preparation.[234]

Conclusion

Some may view the great wealth of information on iatrogenic NMJ disease as a tangled morass of anecdotal clinical reports and a cacophony of in vitro laboratory observations. If used thoughtfully, however, such knowledge can assist the clinician in diagnosing the patient with iatrogenic MG, defining a reversible cause for weakness in others, and reversing, if not preventing, progressive decline in the patient with an underlying NMJ disorder. Once again, the clinical neurologist remains the central figure in the diagnosis and management of a complex and potentially life-threatening clinical illness.

References

1. Pascuzzi RM. Introduction to the neuromuscular junction and neuromuscular transmission. Semin Neurol 1990;10:1.
2. Argov Z, Mastaglia FL. Disorders of neuromuscular transmission caused by drugs. N Engl J Med 1979; 30:409.
3. Howard JR. Adverse drug effects on neuromuscular transmission. Semin Neurol 1990;10:89.
4. Kaeser HE. Drug induced myasthenic syndrome. Acta Neurol Scand 1984;70(S100):39.
5. Engel WK, Festoff BW, Patten BM, et al. Myasthenia gravis. Ann Intern Med 1974;8:225.
6. Finley JC, Pascuzzi RM. The rational therapy of myasthenia gravis. Semin Neurol 1990;10:70.
7. Bucknall RC, Dixon A St J, Glick EN, et al. Myasthenia gravis associated with penicillamine treatment for rheumatoid arthritis. BMJ 1975;1:600.
8. Czlonkowska A. Myasthenia syndrome during penicillamine treatment. BMJ 1975;2:726.
9. Reynauld JP, Lee YS, Kornfeld P, Fries JF. Unilateral ptosis as an initial manifestation of D-penicillamine induced myasthenia gravis. J Rheumatol 1993;20:1592.
10. Masters CL, Dawkins RL, Zilko PJ, et al. Penicillamine-associated myasthenia gravis, antiacetylcholine receptor and antistriational antibodies. Am J Med 1977;63:689.
11. Russell AS, Lindstrom JM. Penicillamine-induced myasthenia gravis associated with antibodies to acetylcholine receptor. Neurology 1978;28:847.
12. Bever CT Jr, Chang HW, Penn AS, et al. Penicillamine-induced myasthenia gravis: effects of penicillamine on acetylcholine receptor. Neurology 1982;32:1077.
13. Vincent A, Newsom-Davis J, Martin V. Anti-acetylcholine receptor antibodies in D-penicillamine-associated myasthenia gravis [letter]. Lancet 1978;1:1254.
14. Vincent A, Newsom-Davis J. Acetylcholine receptor antibody characteristics in myasthenia gravis II. Patients with penicillamine-induced myasthenia or idiopathic myasthenia of recent onset. Clin Exp Immunol 1982;49:266.
15. Albers JW, Hodach RJ, Kimmel DW, Treacy WL. Penicillamine-associated myasthenia gravis. Neurology 1980;30:1246.
16. Fawcett PR, McLachlan SM, Nicholson LV, et al. D-Penicillamine-associated myasthenia gravis: immunological and electrophysiological studies. Muscle Nerve 1982;5:328.
17. Adleman HM, Winters PR, Mahan CS, Wallach PM. D-Penicillamine-induced myasthenia gravis: diagnosis obscured by coexisting chronic obstructive pulmonary disease. J Med Sci 1995;309:191.
18. Cooperative Systematic Studies of Rheumatic Disease Group. Toxicity of longterm low dose D-penicillamine therapy in rheumatoid arthritis. J Rheumatol 1987;14:67.
19. Andonopoulos AP, Terzis E, Tsibri E, et al. D-Penicillamine induced myasthenia gravis in rheumatoid arthritis: an unpredictable common occurrence? Clin Rheumatol 1994;13:586.
20. Drosos AA, Christou L, Galanopoulou V, et al. D-Penicillamine induced myasthenia gravis: clinical, serological and genetic findings. Clin Exp Rheumatol 1993;1:387.
21. Bruggemann W, Herath H, Ferbert A. Follow-up and immunologic findings in drug-induced myasthenia. Med Klin 1996;91:268.
22. Kuncl RW, Pestronk A, Drachman DB, Rechthand E. The pathophysiology of penicillamine-induced myasthenia gravis. Ann Neurol 1986;20:740.
23. Aldrich MS, Kim YI, Sanders DB. Effects of D-penicillamine on neuromuscular transmission in rats. Muscle Nerve 1979;2:180.
24. Burres SA, Richman DP, Crayton JW, Arnason BGW. Penicillamine-induced myasthenic responses in the guinea pig. Muscle Nerve 1979;2:186.
25. Seideman P, Ayesh R. Reduced sulphoxidation capacity in D-penicillamine induced myasthenia gravis. Clin Rheumatol 1994;13:435.
26. Menkes CJ, Job-Deslandre C, Bauer-Vinassac D, et al. Myasthénie induite par la tiopronine au cours du traitement de la polyarthrite rhumatoïde. Presse Med 1988;17:1156.
27. Kirjner M, LeBourges J, Camus JP. Myasthénie induite par la pyrithioxine au cours du traitement d'une polyarthrite rhumatoide. La Nouvelle Presse Medicale 1980;9:3098.
28. Perez A, Perella M, Pastor E, et al. Myasthenia gravis induced by alpha-interferon therapy. Am J Hematol 1995;49:365.
29. Batocchi AP, Evoli A, Servidei S, et al. Myasthenia gravis during interferon alpha therapy. Neurology 1995;45:382.
30. Lensch E, Faust J, Nix WA, Wandel E. Myasthenia gravis after interferon alpha treatment. Muscle Nerve 1996;19:927.
31. Piccolo G, Franciotta D, Versino M, et al. Myasthenia gravis in a patient with chronic active hepatitis C during interferon-alpha treatment [letter]. J Neurol Neurosurg Psychiatry 1996;60:348.
32. Mase G, Zorzon M, Biasutti E, et al. Development of myasthenia gravis during interferon-alpha treatment for anti-HCV positive chronic hepatitis. J Neurol Neurosurg Psychiatry 1996;60:348.

33. Konishi T. A case of myasthenia gravis which developed myasthenic crisis after interferon-alpha therapy for chronic hepatitis C. Rinsho Shinkeigaku 1996;36:980.
34. Gu D, Wogensen L, Calcutt N, et al. Myasthenia gravis-like syndrome induced by expression of interferon in the neuromuscular junction. J Exp Med 1995;181:547.
35. Smith CI, Aarli JA, Biberfeld, et al. Myasthenia gravis after bone marrow transplantation: evidence for a donor origin. N Engl J Med 1983;309:1565.
36. Smith CI, Aarli JA, Hammarstrom L, Persson MA. IgG subclass distribution of myasthenia gravis thymoma-associated antiskeletal muscle antibodies. Neurology 1984;34:1094.
37. Seely E, Drachman D, Smith BR, et al. Post bone marrow transplantation (BMT) myasthenia gravis: evidence for acetylcholine receptor abnormality [abstract]. Blood 1984;64(suppl 1):221a.
38. Bolger GB, Sullivan KM, Spence AM, et al. Myasthenia gravis after allogeneic bone marrow transplantation: relationship to chronic graft-versus-host disease. Neurology 1986;36:1087.
39. Nelson KR, McQuillen MP. Neurologic complications of graft-versus-host-disease. Neurol Clin 1988;6:389.
40. Smith CI, Norberg R, Moller G, et al. Autoantibody formation after bone marrow transplantation. Comparison between acetylcholine receptor antibodies and other autoantibodies and analysis of HLA and Gm markers. Eur Neurol 1989;29:128.
41. Hayashi M, Matsuda O, Ishida Y, Kida K. Change of immunological parameters in the clinical course of a myasthenia gravis patient with chronic graft-versus-host disease. Acta Paedriatr Jpn 1996;38:151.
42. Grau JM, Casademont J, Monforte R, et al. Myasthenia gravis after allogeneic bone marrow transplantation: report of a new case and pathogenetic considerations. Bone Marrow Transplant 1990;5:435.
43. Zaja F, Russo D, Silvestri F, et al. Myasthenia gravis after allogeneic bone marrow transplantation: a case report. Bone Marrow Transplant 1995;15:649.
44. Adams C, August CS, Maguire H, Sladky JT. Neuromuscular complications of bone marrow transplantation. Pediatr Neurol 1995;12:58.
45. Krendel DA. Hypermagnesemia and neuromuscular transmission. Semin Neurol 1990;10:42.
46. Fuchs-Buder T, Tassonyi E. Magnesium sulphate enhances residual neuromuscular block induced by vecuronium. Br J Anaesth 1996;76:565.
47. Randall RE, Cohen MD, Spray CC, Rossmeise EC. Hypermagnesemia in renal failure. Ann Intern Med 1964;61:73.
48. Castlebaum AR, Donofrio PD, Walker FO, Troost BT. Laxative abuse causing hypermagnesemia quadriparesis and neuromuscular junction defect. Neurology 1989;39:746.
49. Mordes JP, Wacker WEC. Excess magnesium. Pharmacol Rev 1978;29:273.
50. Lemcke B, Fuchs C. Magnesium load induced by ingestion of magnesium-containing antacids. Contrib Nephrol 1984;38:185.
51. Collins EN, Russell PW. Fatal magnesium poisoning. Cleve Clin Q 1949;16:162.
52. Flowers CJ. Magnesium in obstetrics. Am J Obstet Gynecol 1965;91:763.
53. Pritchard JA. The use of magnesium sulfate in preeclampsia/eclampsia. J Reprod Med 1979;23:107.
54. Lipsitz PJ. The clinical and biochemical effects of excess magnesium in the newborn. Pediatrics 1971;47:501.
55. Fishman RA. Neurological aspects of magnesium metabolism. Arch Neurol 1965;12:562.
56. Somjen G, Hilmy M, Stephen CR. Failure to anesthetize human subjects by intravenous administration of magnesium sulfate. J Pharmacol Exp Ther 1966;154:652.
57. Hutter OF, Kostial K. Effect of magnesium and calcium ions on the release of acetylcholine. J Physiol (Lond) 1954;124:234.
58. Del Castillo J, Engback L. The nature of the neuromuscular block produced by magnesium. J Physiol (Lond) 1954;124:370.
59. Swift TR. Weakness from magnesium containing cathartics. Muscle Nerve 1979;2:295.
60. De Silva AJC. Magnesium intoxication: an uncommon cause of prolonged curarization. Br J Anesth 1973;45:1228.
61. Ghoneim MM, Long JP. The interaction between magnesium and other neuromuscular blocking agents. Anesthesiology 1970;32:23.
62. Bashuk RG, Krendell DA. Myasthenia gravis presenting as weakness after magnesium administration. Muscle Nerve 1987;10:666.
63. Cohen BA, London RS, Goldstein PJ. Myasthenia gravis and preeclampsia. Obstet Gynecol 1976;48:35S.
64. George WK, Han CL. Calcium and magnesium administration in myasthenia gravis. Lancet 1962;2:561.
65. Gutmann L, Takamori M. Effect of magnesium on neuromuscular transmission in the Eaton-Lambert syndrome. Neurology 1973;23:977.
66. Streib EW. Adverse effects of magnesium salt cathartics in a patient with the myasthenic syndrome. Ann Neurol 1977;2:175.
67. Ross RM, Baker T. An effect of magnesium on neuromuscular function in parturients. J Clin Anesth 1996;8:202.
68. Alfrey AC, Terman DS, Brettschneider L, et al. Hypermagnesemia after renal homotransplantation. Ann Intern Med 1970;73:367.
69. Layzer RB. Mineral and Electrolyte Disorders. In RB Layzer (ed), Neuromuscular Manifestations of Systemic Disease. Philadelphia: FA Davis, 1985;47.
70. Critchley M, Herman KJ, Harrison M, Shields RA. Value of exchangable electrolyte measurement in the treatment of myasthenia gravis. J Neurol Neurosurg Psychiatry 1977;40:250.

71. Jenkins RB, Witorsch P, Smythe NPD. Aspects of treatment of crisis in myasthenia gravis. South Med J 1970;63:1127.
72. Wirguin I, Brenner T, Shinar E, Argov Z. Citrate-induced impairment of neuromuscular transmission in human and experimental autoimmune myasthenia gravis. Ann Neurol 1990;27:328.
73. Linial M. Bacterial neurotoxins—a thousand years later. Isr J Med Sci 1995;10:591.
74. Montecucco C, Schiavo G, Tugnoli V, de Grandis D. Botulinum neurotoxins: mechanism of action and therapeutic applications. Mol Med Today 1996;10:418.
75. Perie S, Lacau St-Guily J. Mode of action and effects of botulinum neurotoxin A. Ann Otolaryngol Chir Cervicofac 1996;113:73.
76. Olney RK, Aminoff MJ, Gelb DJ, Lowentein DH. Neuromuscular effects distant from the site of botulinum neurotoxin injection. Neurology 1988;38:1780.
77. Holzer SE, Ludlow CL The swallowing side effects of botulinum toxin type A injection in spasmodic dysphonia. Laryngoscope 1996;106:86.
78. Comella CL, Tanner CM, DeFoor-Hill L, Smith C. Dysphagia after botulinum toxin injections for spasmodic torticollis: clinical and radiographic findings. Neurology 1992;42:1307.
79. Girlanda T, Vita G, Nicolosi C, et al. Botulinum toxin therapy: distant effects on neuromuscular transmission and autonomic nervous system. J Neurol Neurosurg Psychiatry 1992;55:844.
80. Erbguth F, Claus D, Engelhardt A, et al. Systemic effects of local botulinum toxin injections unmasks the subclinical Lambert Eaton myasthenic syndrome. J Neurol Neurosurg Psychiatry 1993;56:1235.
81. Baraka A, Afifi A, Muallem M, et al. Neuromuscular effects of halothane suxamethion and tubocurarine in a myasthenic undergoing thymectomy. J Anesthesiol 1971;43:91.
82. Elder BF, Beal H, Dewald W, Sobb S. Exacerbation of subclinical myasthenia by occupational exposure to an anesthetic. Anesth Analg 1971;50:383.
83. Gage PW, Hamill OP. Effects of several inhalation anesthetics on the kinetics of postsynaptic conductance in mouse diaphragm. Br J Pharmacol 1976;57:263.
84. Matthews EK, Quilliam JP. Effects of central depressant drugs upon acetycholine release. Br J Pharmacol 1964;22:415.
85. Hirst GDS, Wood DR. On the neuromuscular paralysis produced by procaine. Br J Pharmacol 1971;41:94.
86. Harvey AM. The actions of procaine on neuromuscular transmission. Bull Johns Hopkins Hosp 1939;65:223.
87. Katz RL, Gissen AJ. Effects of intravenous and intraarterial procaine and lidocaine on neuromuscular transmission in man. Acta Anesthesiol Scand Suppl 1969;36:103.
88. Watling SM, Dasta JF. Prolonged paralysis in intensive care unit patients after the use of neuromuscular blocking agents: a review of the literature. Crit Care Med 1994;22:884.
89. Benzing G, Iannaccone ST, Bove KE, et al. Prolonged myasthenic syndrome after one week of muscle relaxants. Pediatr Neurol 1990;6:190.
90. Lagassa RS, Katz RI, Peterson M, et al. Prolonged neuromuscular blockade following vecuronium infusion. J Clin Anesth 1990;2:269.
91. Vanderheyden BA, Reynolds HN, Gerold KB, et al. Prolonged paralysis after long-term infusion. Crit Care Med 1992;20:304.
92. Branney SW, Haenel JB, Moore FA, et al. Prolonged paralysis with atracurium infusion: a case report. Crit Care Med 1994;22:1699.
93. Segredo V, Caldwell JE, Matthay MA, et al. Persistent paralysis after long-term administration of vecuronium. N Engl J Med 1992;327:524.
94. Gooch JL, Suchyta, MR, Baslbierz JM, et al. Prolonged paralysis after treatment with neuromuscular junction blocking agents. Crit Care Med 1991;19:1125.
95. Benzing G, Bove KE. Sedating drugs and neuromuscular blockade during mechanical ventilation. JAMA 1992;267:1775.
96. Hund EF. Neuromuscular complications in the ICU: the spectrum of critical illness-related conditions causing muscular weakness and weaning failure. J Neurol Sci 1996;136:10.
97. Maher J, Rutledge F, Remtulla H, Parkes A, et al. Neuromuscular disorders associated with failure to wean from the ventilator. Intensive Care Med 1995;21:737.
98. Robinson J, Molitor H. Some toxicological and pharmacological properties of gramicidin. J Pharmacol Exp Ther 1941;73:75.
99. Pridgen JE. Respiratory arrest thought to be due to intraperitoneal neomycin. Surgery 1956;40:571.
100. Benz HG, Lunn JN, Foldes FF. "Recurarisation" by intraperitoneal antibiotics. BMJ 1961;2:241.
101. Bodley PO, Brett JE. Postoperative respiratory inadequacy and the part played by antibiotics. Anesthesia 1962;17:438.
102. McQuillen MP, Canter HE, O'Rourke JR. Myasthenic syndrome associated with antibiotics. Arch Neurol 1968;18:402.
103. Pittinger CB, Eryasa Y, Adamson R. Antibiotic induced paralysis. Anesth Analg 1970;49:487.
104. Albiero L, Bamonte F, Ongini E, Parravicini L. Comparison of intramuscular effects in acute toxicity of some aminoglycoside antibiotics. Arch Int Pharmacodyn Ther 1978;233:343.
105. Burkett L, Bikhaze GB, Thomas KC, et al. Mutual potentiation of the neuromuscular effects of antibiotics and relaxants. Anesth Analg 1979;58:107.
106. Singh YN, Harvey AL, Marshall IG. Antibiotic induced paralysis of the mouse phrenic nerve hemidiaphragm preparation and reversibility by calcium and by neostigmine. Anesthesiology 1978;48:418.
107. Singh YN, Marshall IG, Harvey AL. Reversal of antibiotic induced muscle paralysis of 3-4-diaminopyridine. J Pharm Pharmacol 1978;32:249.

108. Maeno T, Enomoto K. Reversal of streptomycin induced blockade of neuromuscular transmission by 4-aminopyridine. Proc Jpn Acad 1980;56:486.
109. Capute AJ, Kim YI, Sanders DB. Neuromuscular blocking effects of therapeutic concentrations of various antibiotics on normal rat skeletal muscle. A quantitative comparison. J Pharmacol Exp Ther 1981;217:369.
110. Dretchen KL, Gergis SD, Sokoll MD, et al. Effect of various antibiotics on neuromuscular transmission. Eur J Pharmacol 1972;18:201.
111. Waterman PM, Smith RB. Tobramycin-curare interaction. Anesth Analg 1977;56:587.
112. Singh YN, Marshall IG, Harvey AL. Some effects of the aminoglycoside antibiotic amikacin on neuromuscular and autonomic transmission. Br J Anesthesiol 1978;50:109.
113. Torda T. The nature of gentamycin induced neuromuscular block. Br J Anesthesiol 1980;52:325.
114. Paradelis AG, Triantaphyllidis C, Giala MM. Neuromuscular activity of aminoglycoside antibiotics. Meth Find Exp Clin Pharmacol 1980;2:45.
115. Elmqvist D, Josefsson JO. The nature of the neuromuscular block produced by neomycin. Acta Physiol Scand 1962;54:105.
116. Dretchen KL, Sokoll MD, Gergis SD, et al. Relative effects of streptomycin on motor nerve terminal endplate. Eur J Pharmacol 1973;22:10.
117. de Rosayro M, Healy TEJ. Tobramycin and neuromuscular transmission in the rat isolated phrenic nerve diaphragm preparation. Br J Anesthesiol 1978;50:251.
118. L'Hommediau C, Stough R, Brown L, et al. Potentiation of neuromuscular weakness in infant botulism by aminoglycosides. J Pediatr 1979;95:1065.
119. Santos JI, Swenson P, Glasgow LA. Potentiation of clostridium botulinum toxin by aminoglycoside antibiotics. Clinical and laboratory observations. Pediatrics 1981;68:50.
120. Hokkanen E, Toibakka E. Streptomycin induced neuromuscular fatigue in myasthenia gravis. Ann Clin Res 1969;1:220.
121. Moore B, Safani M, Keesey J. Possible exacerbation of myasthenia gravis by ciprofloxacin. Lancet 1988;1:882.
122. Vial T, Chauplannaz G, Brunel P, et al. Exacerbation of myasthenia gravis by perfloxacin. Rev Neurol 1995; 251:286.
123. Rauser EH, Ariano RE, Anderson BA. Exacerbation of myasthenia gravis by norfloxacin. Ann Pharmacother 1990;24:207.
124. Samuelson RJ, Giesecke AH, Kallus FT, Stanley VF. Lincomycin-curare interaction. Anesth Analg 1975; 54:103.
125. Fogdall RP, Miller RD. Prolongation of a pancuroneum induced neuromuscular blockade by clindamycin. Anesthesiology 1974;41:407.
126. Rubbo JT, Gergis SD, Sokoll MD. Comparative neuromuscular effects of lincomycin and clindamycin. Anesth Analg 1977;56:329.
127. Wright JM, Collier B. Characterization of the neuromuscular block produced by clindamycin and lincomycin. Can J Physiol Pharmacol 1976;54:937.
128. Booij LHD, Miller RD, Crul JF. Neostigmine and 4-aminopyridine antagonism of lincomycin pancuroneum neuromuscular blockade in man. Anesth Analg 1978;57:316.
129. Albrecht RF, Lanier WL. Potentiation of succinylcholine-induced phase II block by vancomycin. Anesth Anal 1993;77:1300.
130. Parisi AF, Kaplan MH. Apnea during treatment with sodium colistimethate. JAMA 1965;194:298.
131. Gold GN, Richardson AP. An unusual case of neuromuscular blockade seen with therapeutic blood levels of colistin methanesulfonate. Am J Med 1966;41:316.
132. Pohlmann G. Respiratory arrest associated with intravenous administration of polymyxin B sulfate. JAMA 1966;196:81.
133. Lindesmith LA, Baines RD, Bigelow DB, Petty TL. Reversible respiratory paralysis associated with polymyxin therapy. Ann Intern Med 1968;68:38.
134. Pittinger C, Adamson R. Antibiotic blockade of neuromuscular function. Annu Rev Pharmacol 972;12:109.
135. McQuillen MP, Engbaek L. Mechanism of colistin induced neuromuscular depression. Arch Neurol 1975;32:235.
136. Wright JM, Collier B. The site of the neuromuscular block produced by polymyxin B and rolitetracycline. Can J Physiol Pharmacol 1976;54:926.
137. Durant NN, Lambert JJ. The action of polymyxin B at the frog neuromuscular junction. Br J Pharmacol 1981;72:41.
138. Viswanath DV, Jenkens HJ. Neuromuscular block of the polymyxin group of antibiotics. J Pharmacol Sci 1978;67:1275.
139. Decker DA, Fincham RW. Respiratory arrest in myasthenia gravis with colistimethate therapy. Arch Neurol 1971;25:141.
140. Herishanu Y. The effect of streptomycin and colistin on myasthenic patients. Conf Neurol 1969;31:370.
141. Hokkanen E. The aggregating effect of some antibiotics on the neuromuscular blockade in myasthenia gravis. Acta Neurol Scand 1964;40:346.
142. Argov Z, Brenner T, Abramsky O. Ampicillin may aggravate clinical and experimental myasthenia gravis. Arch Neurol 1986;43:255.
143. Girlanda P, Venuto C, Mangiapane R. Effect of ampicillin on neuromuscular transmission in healthy men. A single fiber electromyographic study. Eur Neurol 1989;29:36.
144. Herishanu Y, Taustein I. The electromyographic changes induced by antibiotics. Preliminary study. Conf Neurol 1971;33:41.
145. Cadisch R, Streit E, Hartmann K. Exacerbation of pseudoparalytic myasthenia gravis following azithromycin (Zithromax). Schweiz Med Wochenschr 1996;126:388.
146. Weisman SJ. Masked myasthenia gravis. JAMA 1949;141:917.

147. Stoffer SS, Chandler JH. Quinidine-induced exacerbation of myasthenia gravis in patients with Grave's disease. Arch Intern Med 1980;140:283.
148. Shy ME, Lange DJ, Howard JF, et al. Quinidine exacerbating myasthenia gravis: a case report and intracellular recordings. Ann Neurol 1985;18:120.
149. Miller RD, Way WL, Ketzumg BG. The neuromuscular effects of quinidine. Proc Soc Exp Biol Med 1968;129:215.
150. Grogono AW. Anesthesia for atrial fibrillation effect of quinidine on muscular relaxation. Lancet 1963;2:1039.
151. Way WL, Katzung BG, Larson CP. Recurarization with quinidine. JAMA 1967;200:153.
152. Harvey AM, Whitehill MR. Quinine as an adjuvant to prostigmine in the diagnosis of myasthenia gravis: a preliminary report. Bull Johns Hopkins Hosp 1937;61:216.
153. Eaton LM. Diagnostic tests for myasthenia gravis with prostigmine and quinine. Proceedings at the Staff Meetings of the Mayo Clinic 1943;18:230.
154. Sieb JP, Milone M, Engel AG. Effects of the quinoline derivatives quinine, quinidine and chloroquine on neuromuscular transmission. Brain Res 1996;712:179.
155. Herishanu Y, Rosenberg P. Beta blockers and myasthenia gravis. Ann Intern Med 1975;83:834.
156. Hughes RO, Zacharias FJ. Myasthenic syndrome during treatment with practolol. BMJ 1976;1:460.
157. Coppeto JR. Timolol associated myasthenia gravis. Am J Ophthalmol 1984;98:244.
158. Shaivitz SA. Timolol in myasthenia gravis. JAMA 1979;242:1611.
159. Verkijk A. Worsening of myasthenia gravis with timolol maleate eyedrops. Ann Neurol 1985;17:211.
160. Weber JCP. Beta adreno receptor antagonist and diplopia. Lancet 1982;2:826.
161. Harry JD, Linden RJ, Snow HM. The effects of three beta adreno receptor blocking drugs on isolated preparations of skeletal and cardiac muscle. Br J Pharmacol 1975;52:275.
162. Howard JF, Johnson BR, Quint SR. The effects of beta adrenergic antagonists on neuromuscular transmission in rat skeletal muscle. Society of Neuroscience Abstracts 1987;13:147.
163. Jonkers I, Swerup C, Pirskanen R, et al. Acute effects of intravenous injection of beta-adrenoreceptor and calcium channel antagonists and agonists in myasthenia gravis. Muscle Nerve 1996;19:959.
164. Van der Kloot W, Kita H. The effects of verapamil on muscle action potentials in the frog and crayfish and on neuromuscular transmission in the crayfish. Comp Biochem Physiol 1975;50:121.
165. Ribera AD, Nastuk WL. The actions of verapamil at the neuromuscular junction. Comp Biochem Physiol 1989;93:137.
166. Adams RJ, Rivner MH, Salazar J, Swift TR. Effects of oral calcium antagonists on neuromuscular transmission. Neurology 1984;34 (Suppl 1):132.
167. Bikhazi GB, Leung I, Foldes FF. Interaction of neuromuscular blocking agents with calcium channel blockers. Anesthesiology 1982;57:268.
168. Bikhazi GB, Leung I, Foldes FF. Calcium channel blockers increase potentency of blocking agents in vivo. Anesthesiology 1983;59:269.
169. Zalman F, Perloff JK, Durant NN, Campion DS. Acute respiratory failure following intravenous verapamil in Duchenne's muscular dystrophy. Am Heart J 1983;105:510.
170. Krendell DA, Hopkins LC. Adverse effect of verapamil in a patient with the Lambert Eaton syndrome. Muscle Nerve 1986;9:519.
171. Protti DA, Reisin R, Mackinley TA, Uchitel OD. Calcium channel blockers and transmitter release at the normal human neuromuscular junction. Neurology 1996;46:1391.
172. Drachman DA, Skom JH. Procainamide—a hazard in myasthenia gravis. Arch Neurol 1965;13:316.
173. Kornfeld P, Horowich SH, Genkins G, Papatestas AE. Myasthenia gravis unmasked by antiarrhythmic agents. Mt Sinai J Med 1976;43:10.
174. Campbell EDR, Montuschi E. Muscle weakness caused by bretylium tosylate. Lancet 1960;2:789.
175. Dale RC, Schroeder ET. Respiratory paralysis during treatment of hypertension with trimethaphan camsylate. Arch Intern Med 1976;136:816.
176. Wilson SL, Miller RN, Wright C, Hasse D. Prolonged neuromuscular blockade associated with trimethaphan. Case report. Anesth Analg 1976;55:353.
177. Nakamura K, Koide M, Imanaga TL. Prolonged neuromuscular blockade following trimethaphan infusion. Anesthesia 1980;35:1202.
178. Poulton TJ, James FM, Lockridge O. Prolonged apnea following trimethaphan in succinylcholine. Anesthesiology 1979;50:54.
179. Yarri Y, Pincus JH, Argov Z. Depression of synpatic transmission by diphenylhydantoin. Ann Neurol 1977;1:334.
180. Norris FH, Colella J, McFarlin D. Effect of diphenylhydantoin on neuromuscular synapse. Neurology 1964;14:869.
181. Brumlik J, Jacobs RS. Myasthenia gravis associated with diphenylhydantoin therapy for epilepsy. Can J Neurol Sci 1974;1:127.
182. Peterson HDC. Association of trimethadione therapy in myasthenia gravis. N Engl J Med 1966;274:506.
183. Booker HE, Chun RWM, Sanguino M. Myasthenia gravis syndrome associated with trimethadione. JAMA 1970;21:2262.
184. Yarri Y, Pincus JH, Argov Z. Phenytoin and transmitter release at the neuromuscular junction of the frog. Brain Res 1979;160:479.
185. Osserman KE, Genkins G. Studies in myasthenia gravis: review of a 20 year experience in over 1200 patients. Mt Sinai J Med 1971;38:497.
186. Thesleff S. The effect of anesthetic agents in skeletal muscle membrane. Acta Physiol Scand 1956;37:335.
187. Alderdice MT, Trommer BA. Differential effects of the

anticonvulsants phenobarbital, ethosuxamide and carbamazepine on neuromuscular transmission. J Pharmacol Exp Ther 1980;215:92.
188. Talamo RC, Crawford JD. Trimethadione nephrosis treated with cortisone and nitrogen mustard. N Engl J Med 1963;269:15.
189. Kim YI, Howard JF, Sanders DB. Depressant effects of morphine and meperidine on neuromuscular transmission in rat and human myasthenic muscles. Society of Neuroscience Abstracts 1979;5:482.
190. Sanders DB, Kim YI, Howard JF, et al. Intercostal muscle biopsy studies in myasthenia gravis: clinical correlations and the direct effects of drugs in myasthenic serum. Ann N Y Acad Sci 1981;377:544.
191. Slaughter D. Neostigmine and opiate analgesia. Arch Int Pharmacodyn 1950;83:143.
192. Grob D. Myasthenia gravis: current status of pathogenesis, clinical manifestations and management. J Chron Dis 1958;8:536.
193. Pascuzzi RM, Coslett HB, Johns TR. Long-term corticosteroid treatment of myasthenia gravis: report of 116 patients. Ann Neurol 1984;15:291.
194. Seybold ME, Drachman DB. Gradual increasing doses of prednisone in myasthenia gravis: reducing the hazards of treatment. N Engl J Med 1974;290:81.
195. Wilson RW, Ward MD, Johns TR. Corticosteroids—a direct effect at the neuromuscular junction. Neurology 1974;24:1091.
196. Hoffmann WW. Antimyasthenic action of corticosteroids. Arch Neurol 1977;34:356.
197. Dengler R, Rudel R, Warelas J, Birnberger KL. Corticosteroids and neuromuscular transmission. Pflugers Arch 1979;380:145.
198. Kim YI, Goldner MM, Sanders DB. Short term effects of prednisolone on neuromuscular transmission in normal rats and those with experimental autoimmune myasthenia gravis. J Neurol Sci 1979;41:223.
199. Abramsky O, Aharonov A, Teitelbaum B, Fuchs S. Myasthenia gravis and acetylcholine receptors. Arch Neurol 1975;32:684.
200. Cohen IR, Stavey L, Feldman M. Glucorticoids and cellular immunity in vitro. J Exp Med 1971;132:1055.
201. Stavey L, Cohen IR, Feldman M. Stimulation of rat lymphocyte proliferation by hydrocortisone during the induction of cell mediated immunity in vitro. Transplantation 1974;2:173.
202. Vacca JB, Knight WA. Estrogen therapy in myasthenia gravis. Mississippi Medicine 1957;54:337.
203. Frenkel M, Ehrlich EN. The influence of progesterone upon myasthenia gravis. Ann Intern Med 1964;60:971.
204. Bikerstaff ER. Neurological Complications of Oral Contraceptives. London: Oxford University Press, 1975.
205. Brittain J, Lange LS. Myasthenia gravis and levonorgestrel implant. Lancet 1995;346:1556.
206. Maclean B, Wilson JAC. See-saw relationship between hyperthyroidism and myasthenia gravis. Lancet 1954;1:950.
207. Thorner MW. Relation of myasthenia gravis to hyperthyroidism. Arch Intern Med 1939;64:330.
208. Alexander WD. Systemic effects with eye drops. BMJ 1981;282:1359.
209. Gesztes T. Prolonged apnea after suxamethonium injection associated with eye drops containing anticholinesterase agent. A case report. Br J Anesth 1966;38:408.
210. McQuillen MP, Gross M, Johns RJ. Chlorpromazine-induced weakness in myasthenia gravis. Arch Neurol 1963;8:286.
211. Argov Z, Yaari Y. The action of chlorpromazine at an isolated cholinergic synapse. Brain Res 1979;164:227.
212. Neil JF, Himmelhoch JM, Licata SM. Emergence of myasthenia gravis during treatment with lithium carbonate. Arch Gen Psychiatry 1976;33:1090.
213. Borden H, Clark MT, Katz H. The use of pancuronium bromide in patients receiving lithium carbonate. Can Anesth Soc J 1974;21:79.
214. Hill GE, Wong KC, Hodges MR. Potentiation of succinylcholine neuromuscular blockade by lithium carbonate. Anesthesiology 1976;44:439.
215. Vizi ES, Illes P, Ronai A, et al. The effect of lithium on acetylcholine release and synthesis. Neuropharmacology 1972;11:521.
216. Robberecht W, Bodnarik J, Bourgeois P, et al. Myasthenic syndrome caused by a direct effect of chloroquine on neuromuscular transmission. Arch Neurol 1989;46:464.
217. De Bleecker J, De Reuck J, Quatacker J, et al. Persistent chloroquine-induced myasthenia. Acta Clin Belg 1991;46:401.
218. Sghirlanzoni A, Mantsgazza R, Mora M, et al. Chloroquine myopathy and myasthenia-like syndrome. Muscle Nerve 1988;11:114.
219. Speak G. Malaria and myasthenics. Pharmaceutical Journal 1993;251:302.
220. Canal N, Franceschi M. Myasthenic crisis precipitated by iothalamic acid. Lancet 1983;1:1288.
221. Chagnac Y, Hadani M, Goldhammer Y. Myasthenic crisis after intravenous administration of iodinated contrast agent. Neurology 1985;35:1219.
222. Vanden Bergh P, Kelly JJ, Carter B, Munsat TL. Intravascular contrast media and neuromuscular junction disorders. Arch Neurol 1986;19:206.
223. Eliashiv S, Wirguin I, Brenner T, Argov Z. Aggravation of human and experimental myasthenia gravis by contrast media. Neurology 1990;49:1623.
224. Frank JH, Cooper GW, Black WC, Phillips LH. Iodinated contrast agents in myasthenia gravis. Neurology 1987;37:1400.
225. Abdel-Aziz A, Bakry N. The action and interaction of diphenhydramine (Benadryl) hydrochloride at the neuromuscular junction. Eur J Pharmacol 1973;22:169.
226. Bazzato G, Coli U, Landini S, et al. Myasthenia-like syndrome after D,L- but not L-carnitine. Lancet 1981;1:209.

227. DeGrandis D, Mezzina C, Fiaschi A, et al. Myasthenia due to carnitine treatment. J Neurol Sci 1980;46:365.
228. Brown PW. Results and dangers in the treatment of amebiasis. JAMA 1935;105:1319.
229. Ng KF. Blockade of adrenergic and cholinergic transmissions by emetine. Br J Pharmacol Chemother 1966;28:228.
230. Ionescu-Drinea M, Vioculescu V, Serbanescu G, Nicolau C. Association of myasthenic and neuritic symptoms following administration of antitetanic serum. Rev Roum Neurol 1973;10:239.
231. Ueno S, Takahashi M, Kajiyama K, et al. Parkinson's disease and myasthenia gravis: adverse effect of trihexiphenidyl on neuromuscular transmission. Neurology 1987;37:832.
232. Daras M, Samkoff LM, Koppel BS. Exacerbation of myasthenia gravis associated with cocaine use. Neurology 1996;46:271.
233. Tsai MC, Mansour NA, Eldefrawi AT, et al. Mechanism of action of amantadine on neuromuscular transmission. Mol Pharmacol 1978;14:787.
234. Bossa R, Chiericozzi M, Galatulas I, et al. The effects of roxatidine on neuromuscular transmission. In Vivo 1995;9:113.

Chapter 17
Drug-Induced Myopathies

Charles E. Schultz and John C. Kincaid

Objectives

- To recognize iatrogenic myopathies as an important but uncommon neurologic complication
- To become familiar with medications that have been associated with the development of myopathy
- To appreciate the incidence of drug-induced myopathies
- To recognize the clinical presentations of medication-induced myopathies
- To become familiar with the laboratory, electrophysiologic, and histopathologic results in these conditions
- To understand the course of the myopathy after adjusting the dosage of the medication or discontinuing it

General Considerations

Before exploring drug-induced myopathies, some basic terms need to be defined. *Myopathy* is a general term for any abnormal condition or disease of muscular tissue. *Myositis* is disease produced by inflammatory reactions against the muscle tissue. *Muscular dystrophy* is disease resulting from a biochemical defect within the muscle cell's metabolism. Diseases of the muscle must be differentiated from those of the neuromuscular junction, peripheral nerve, anterior horn cell, and central nervous system (CNS).

The most important step in the assessment of individuals with possible muscle disease is a careful history of the patient's symptoms, disease progression, family history, and medication list. The physical examination then provides important supportive information. A patient with myopathy often complains of difficulty arising from a low chair or a commode. The patient may have difficulty climbing stairs. Arm involvement is signaled by difficulty holding heavy objects or trouble using the arms above the shoulder level as when combing the hair. There are often complaints of enhanced muscular fatigue with repetitive or sustained activity, but weakness is present at the initiation of muscle use in myopathy. Pain in the muscles can be another symptom of muscle disease. The pain can be diffuse or localized in only some muscles. It can be present at rest and worsen with use, appear only with use, or persist after use. Cramps may be a symptom also.

The physical examination findings suggestive of a myopathy include symmetric distribution of primarily proximal weakness; preserved, atrophic, or rarely enlarged muscle bulk; and diminished muscle stretch reflexes congruent with muscle strength.[1] The findings making a myopathy less likely include asymmetric or distal weakness, fasciculations, tremor, sensory deficits, significant fatigue in the absence of initial weakness, and early absence of reflexes.

Laboratory findings suggestive of a myopathy include elevation of serum creatine kinase (CK) or aldolase level and in some cases myoglobinuria. CK is an enzyme that catalyzes the reversible transfer of high-energy phosphate between creatine and phosphocreatine, serving as a reservoir of high-energy phosphate in skeletal muscle. This enzyme is found in high concentrations in the heart and skeletal muscles and in much smaller concentrations in brain tissue. Because CK exists in relatively few organs, this test can be used as a specific index of injury to muscles. Aldolase is a glycolytic enzyme that is important in the intermediary glycolytic breakdown of glucose. This enzyme is also a helpful marker of skeletal muscle cell necrosis or increased membrane permeability. Myoglobin is a protein concentrated in muscles, serving as an oxygen reservoir. It is released into the serum when muscle damage takes place and can be detected in the urine. Traditionally, the presence in the urine was recognized only when amounts were high enough to cause red or brown coloration. Modern chemical assays detect its presence at levels below that.

Electromyographic findings of short-duration, low-amplitude, and at times polyphasic voluntary motor unit potentials with increased recruitment, normal nerve conductions, and normal repetitive motor nerve stimulation are suggestive of myopathy. The muscle's resting electrical activity may be normal or abnormal depending on the specific etiology.

The muscle biopsy can show a variety of findings, including an abnormality in the histochemical distinction between type I and type II muscle fibers, the normal size relationship between these fiber types, sarcoplasmic vacuole formation, mitochondria hypertrophy or clumping, muscle fiber necrosis, regeneration, central migration of nuclei, and infiltration of inflammatory cells.[1]

Several medications have been associated with the occurrence of muscle dysfunction. The actual incidence of these types of myopathy is incompletely known; however, they probably are more common than realized. Myalgia, muscle cramping, or asymptomatic elevation of CK level may indicate muscle dysfunction that is unappreciated in the absence of overt weakness. Medications may produce muscle disease by a direct effect on the muscle's biochemistry; by altering some essential aspect of systemic chemistry; by provoking an immunologic response against muscle; or by provoking a local toxic, necrotic, fibrotic reaction when injected directly into a muscle.

This chapter is concerned with therapeutic drugs and their ability to cause myopathy. We describe the clinical presentation, laboratory, electrophysiologic, and histopathologic findings and treatment options for these known medication-induced myopathies. There are a number of ways these conditions can be classified. In most real-world situations the clinician is faced with a clinical problem such as weakness or myalgia and a list of medications. We have therefore organized the discussion by generic drug name in alphabetic order. Focal myopathy due to local reaction from intramuscular injection of medication is discussed at the end of the chapter. Medications available and currently used in North America are the constituents of the list.

Albuterol (Salbutamol, Proventil, Ventolin)

Albuterol is the generic name widely used in the United States, whereas the World Health Organization recommends *salbutamol* as the name of the drug.[2] Albuterol stimulates beta-adrenergic receptors and is widely used for the treatment of asthma. There have been rare case reports of patients experiencing muscle spasms along with increased serum CK levels while taking this medication.[3] One study found elevated CK levels in 13 out of 93 patients with chronic obstructive pulmonary disease treated with either oral or inhaled albuterol.[4] Frank weakness has not been described. The muscle spasms and elevated CK levels resolved completely within 2 weeks when the albuterol dose was reduced or withdrawn.

Amiodarone (Cordarone)

Amiodarone, an antiarrhythmic drug, has rarely been linked to the development of a myopathy that occurs with the more commonly known peripheral neuropathy.[5] The clinical presentation includes marked weakness of proximal as well as distal muscle groups, although the latter may be neuropathic in origin.[6] The proximal weakness may come on months to years after the medication has been started. Ancillary test results show a moderate increase in CK levels.[7] Muscle biopsy results show a vacuolar myopathy. Vacuoles seen on light microscopy are present in type I and type II muscle fibers. On electron microscopy they correspond to autophagic vacuoles of varied size. These changes disappear on discontinuation of the drug. Gradual recovery of strength over a period of weeks or months after withdrawal of the drug is the reported outcome.

Amphotericin B (Fungizone)

A myopathy associated with amphotericin B treatment has been reported.[7, 8] The mechanism appears to be hypokalemia induced by the medication's effect on renal function. Clinical findings include severe muscle pain, swelling, weakness, and areflexia.[9] The weakness can be severe. Serum potassium concentrations of 3.0–3.5 mEq per liter may be associated with mild muscle weakness, myalgia, and easy fatigability.[10] Serum potassium levels of 2.5–3.0 mEq per liter are associated with the development of clinically significant muscle weakness, particularly of the proximal limb muscles.[8] When levels decrease below 2.0 mEq per liter, structural muscle damage, resulting at times in rhabdomyolysis, markedly elevated CK levels, and myoglobinuria, may occur.[11] The cranial musculature is spared in this myopathy.[8] Muscle histology shows segmental necrosis, degeneration, and vacuoles. Recovery is typically complete within a week after adequate potassium replacement, but recovery from rhabdomyolysis may take longer.

Chloroquine (Aralen) and Hydroxychloroquine (Plaquenil)

Chloroquine and hydroxychloroquine are antimalarial drugs also used in rheumatologic disease treatment. Both are known to cause a myopathy or peripheral neuropathy.[12] This may occur over periods of treatment ranging from a few weeks to several years and with varied drug doses.[13] Patients usually develop proximal muscle weakness and a moderate increase in CK level. Needle electromyography shows fibrillations and myopathic motor unit potentials. Histologically, a vacuolar degeneration of muscle fibers with particular involvement of type I muscle fibers is seen.[10] The myopathy is reversible with discontinuation of the drug, but improvement may take many months.[1, 7]

In patients with hydroxychloroquine exposure, the clinical presentation and muscle biopsy changes are similar to those of chloroquine but are less severe.[14] The milder degree of toxicity seen with hydroxychloroquine may be due to its faster metabolism and lower tissue drug levels.

Cimetidine (Tagamet)

Isolated case reports suggest that cimetidine, a histamine-receptor antagonist, can be a rare cause of a myopathy that occurs together with interstitial nephritis.[15–17] The clinical manifestation is proximal weakness developing over months.[18] The serum CK level is markedly elevated. The renal involvement is signaled by abnormal creatinine values and confirmed by biopsy. Muscle biopsy shows fragmentation of muscle fibers, areas of regeneration, and lymphocytic infiltrates.[10] Immunologic studies of B and T cells suggest activation of the cell-mediated immune system in the pathogenesis of both myopathy and nephritis.[18] Drug hypersensitivity is the presumed pathogenesis. Medication withdrawal and corticosteroid therapy resulted in improvement of the condition over approximately 6 weeks. Medication withdrawal alone is likely not sufficient to resolve the myopathy or nephritis.

Clofibrate (Atromid-S)

Clofibrate is a branched-chain fatty acid ester used therapeutically as a hypolipidemic agent.[19] Its use has been associated with the development of a myopathy in humans, as well as experimental animals.[13, 20] The myopathy can develop acutely shortly after beginning the medication or appear after months of therapy.[13] An increase in the dosage may precipitate the onset.

Clinically, it is manifested by muscle pain, tenderness, and proximal weakness.[21] Serum CK levels are usually markedly elevated when myopathy is manifest, but may be elevated in otherwise asymptomatic patients receiving the drug. The needle electromyographic examination may demonstrate normal motor unit action potentials in mildly affected individuals or show myopathic type abnormalities when obvious weakness is present.[22] Rest and spontaneous activity are normal. Muscle biopsies have shown scattered muscle fiber necrosis.[7] The myopathy may be more likely in patients with renal impairment.[21] Withdrawal of the drug has led to a gradual recovery over days to months.[7] The elevated enzyme levels may decrease before strength improves.

Several chemical relatives of clofibrate, referred to as fibric acids, include gemfibrozil, bezafibrate, and fenfibrate.[23] These have proven to be a less common cause of myopathy compared with clofibrate itself.[7]

Colchicine (ColBENEMID)

Colchicine is used for the treatment of gout, familial Mediterranean fever, primary biliary cirrhosis, and proliferative vitreoretinopathy.[23] Both myopathy and neuropathy are described and are more frequent in gout patients between 50 and 70 years of age who have mild chronic renal insufficiency.[7] Colchicine-associated myopathy may have a more rapid onset with concomitant use of drugs such as calcium channel blockers and cimetidine, which inhibit the cytochrome P450 system.[24] These patients typically present with distal sensory involvement, areflexia, and subacute painless proximal muscle weakness.[25] They typically are unable to lift objects above their shoulders or rise from a chair. Serum CK levels are usually elevated 10- to 20-fold. Nerve conduction study results commonly show a prolongation of the distal motor and sensory latencies in both the upper and lower limbs.[26, 27] Needle electromyography shows fibrillations and myopathic motor unit potentials. The muscle biopsy shows a vacuolar myopathy with accumulation of lysosomes and autophagic vacuoles, without necrosis.[28] The vacuoles react strongly with acid phosphatase. The mechanism of toxicity most likely involves a disruption of a microtubule-dependent cytoskeletal network that interacts with lysosomal enzymes. Resolution of the muscle weakness, neuropathy, and elevated serum CK level usually occurs within 4–6 weeks after discontinuation of colchicine.[10]

Corticosteroids

Corticosteroid myopathy is probably the most common drug-induced myopathy encountered in clinical practice. Two distinct types of corticosteroid-induced myopathy have been described: acute and chronic corticosteroid myopathy.[29]

The acute variety is infrequently encountered and is usually seen with high-dose systemic corticosteroid treatment such as gram quantities of methylprednisolone (Solu-Medrol) or 40–80 mg doses of dexamethasone given over several days.[30] Patients often present with a generalized proximal and distal muscle weakness, including the respiratory muscles, approximately 1 week after high doses of corticosteroids have been started.[7] There appears to be a direct correlation between the occurrence of an acute corticosteroid myopathy and the total dose and type of corticosteroids administered.[31] Also, the combination of corticosteroids and a nondepolarizing neuromuscular blocking agent such as pancuronium could increase the risk of developing the acute myopathy.[32] In most cases, the serum CK levels were high and at times accompanied by myoglobinuria.[29] The muscle biopsies show focal and diffuse necrosis and atrophy of all fiber types, without a predilection for type IIb fibers.[33] Once the corticosteroids are stopped, recovery is slow and extends over 6 months or longer.[29]

The chronic corticosteroid myopathy is the more familiar type of corticosteroid-induced myopathy.[29] The fluorinated corticosteroids (triamcinolone > betamethasone > dexamethasone) appear to produce weakness and myopathy more often than nonfluorinated corticosteroids (hydrocortisone > prednisone).[34, 35] One of the major physical complaints encountered with this myopathy is a progressive inability to arise from low chairs, climb stairs, and eventually elevate the arms over the head.[22] Some patients may have wasting of the thighs and upper arm muscles accompanying the weakness. There tends to be a relative sparing of the face, hand, and sphincter muscles. Muscle pain is usually mild at worse.

The serum CK levels are usually normal in chronic corticosteroid myopathy; elevated levels may suggest some other type of myopathy.[36] Creatine and 3-methylhistidine excretion in the urine is increased. The needle electromyographic study is usually normal, but may show small motor unit action potentials.[22] Positive sharp waves and fibrillation potentials are not seen. The muscle biopsy shows selective atrophy of type IIb, fast-twitch glycolytic muscle fibers.[37]

The etiology of chronic corticosteroid-induced myopathy is not entirely clear.[10] The mechanism of the myopathy is thought to be related to the basic cellular action of corticosteroids in inhibiting mRNA synthesis, as a result of which the translation and synthesis of muscle specific proteins is impaired.[38]

Chronic corticosteroid myopathy is usually reversible over months if the drug can be withdrawn or the dose reduced or a less myotoxic drug substituted.[10] A confusing situation can arise in some patients when the medication is tapered. A week or so after dosage lowering, the patient may complain of a diffuse aching and stiffness in the muscles and associated soft tissue. These symptoms are due to corticosteroid withdrawal and will improve over several weeks, only to recur again when the dose is lowered again. Studies now show that disuse of muscles due to physical inactivity may render them more susceptible to the effects of corticosteroids and that corticosteroid-induced muscle atrophy and weakness can be at least partially prevented or reversed by a regular exercise program. The level of creatine excretion may be helpful in monitoring recovery.[10]

Cyclosporine (Sandimmune, Sandimmune Neoral)

Cyclosporine is used to treat organ transplant patients and those with autoimmune disorders such as rheumatic diseases, multiple sclerosis, chronic inflammatory demyelinating polyneuropathy, and myasthenia gravis.[23] The reported cases suggest a cyclosporine-induced myopathy with or without a rhabdomyolysis.[7] In a postmarketing study, the incidence of myopathy was 0.17% in 3,017 patients followed over 1 year.[39] Symptoms were generalized severe muscle pain and weakness. Symptoms typically develop months after starting the drug and are 30 times more likely with concomitant colchicine or lovastatin use.[40] Serum CK levels are typically 10–20 times normal, and electromyography shows myopathic changes.[41] The muscle biopsy typically shows type II fiber atrophy, segmental necrosis, and ragged red fibers, with biochemical studies suggesting mitochondrial dysfunction. The myopathy tends to be dose dependent and subsides with a reduction in the dose or discontinuation of the drug.[42–44]

Didanosine (2',3'-dideoxyinosine, Videx)

Didanosine is a purine nucleoside analogue active against human immunodeficiency virus 1 (HIV-1) and HIV-2 infections including zidovudine-resistant isolates.[23] During phase I clinical trials, arthralgia or myopathy was reported in up to 4% of adult patients. Muscle atrophy (8%), myalgia (9%), and decreased strength (6%) were reported in pediatric patients during phase I trials. The serum CK levels were elevated in most cases. These symptoms were reversible with discontinuation of the drug.

D-Penicillamine (Cuprimine, Depen)

Convincing evidence suggests D-penicillamine can cause autoimmune adverse reactions such as pemphigus, nephritis, neuromuscular disorders, Sjögren's syndrome, and systemic lupus erythematosus.[45] Polymyositis or dermatomyositis has been reported in long-term treatment averaging approximately 16 months with D-penicillamine doses at 50–1,200 mg daily.[46] The most common clinical manifestations indicating myopathy are pain, tenderness, stiffness, and cramps, usually of the proximal muscle groups.[47] The serum CK levels are usually markedly elevated, up to 50 times higher than normal. The needle electromyography shows a myopathic type pattern. The muscle biopsy frequently shows perivascular mononuclear cell infiltration, suggesting cell-mediated immunity in the pathogenesis of this adverse effect.[10] The polymyositis appears to be an idiosyncratic reaction to D-penicillamine that does not have a relation to dose or duration of treatment.[48] Discontinuation of the drug usually results in improvement within 6 months.[49] Some cases may require the addition of corticosteroids to achieve recovery.

Emetine

Emetine is the principal alkaloid of ipecac, obtained from the dried root of *Cephaelis ipecacuanha*, and has been used for the treatment of amoebiasis since 1912.[7] This drug has also been abused by patients with anorexia nervosa to promote vomiting.[50] The adverse effects of prolonged treatment with emetine include cardiotoxicity, muscle weakness, muscle pain, tenderness, and stiffness of the proximal limb muscles.[51] Weakness of the neck flexors as well as proximal limb muscles may be found. Patients may have difficulty ambulating and demonstrate a Gower's sign.[22] The serum CK levels were elevated in some patients up to 14 times normal but were normal in other patients.[10] The needle electromyographic examination may show myopathic abnormalities in the proximal muscles.[22] The muscle biopsy typically shows type II fiber atrophy with muscle necrosis.[10] The mechanism of the myopathy is believed to be due to inhibition of protein synthesis and mitochondrial respiration by emetine and disruption of the cell membrane by high concentrations of the drug.[52] A gradual recovery over several months typically occurs after withdrawal of the drug.

Enalapril (Vasotec)

There is one reported case of myopathy resulting from enalapril, an angiotensin-converting enzyme inhibitor.[53] The patient developed a severe myalgia and proximal muscle weakness but had a normal CK level and electromyography result. Improvement occurred within 3 days after discontinuation of the drug.

Epsilon-Aminocaproic Acid (Amicar)

Epsilon-aminocaproic acid (EACA) is an antifibrinolytic agent used to treat patients with subarachnoid hemorrhage and hereditary angioneurotic edema.[13] A myopathy has been described in patients on long-term (4–6 weeks) treatment.[54] The occurrence myopathy does not appear to be correlated with treatment duration or dosage.[13] Patients develop significant muscle pain in the calves or about the shoulder and pelvic girdle regions that is accompanied by weakness in the proximal muscles.[22] The serum CK level is usually markedly elevated. Myoglobinuria and acute renal failure may occur.[13] The needle electromyographic examination shows a reduction in the amplitude and duration of the motor unit action potentials, along with profuse fibrillation potentials and positive sharp waves in the clinically affected muscles.[55] The muscle typically shows fiber necrosis with selective involvement of type I fibers.[10] The mechanism of EACA-induced myopathy is unknown, but EACA is an analogue of lysine and may substitute for it in the cellular membranes. Most patients experience a complete resolution of symptoms within a few weeks of cessation of EACA therapy, whereas severe cases may require several months for gradual recovery.[55]

Etretinate (Tegison)

Etretinate is an aromatic retinoid used for the treatment of pustular and erythrodermic psoriasis.[23] A significant portion of patients taking this drug report skeletal pain and muscle cramps. Frank myopathy is rare. Three reported patients developed an acute painful proximal muscle weakness with preserved tendon reflexes.[56] The CK level was slightly increased in two of the patients. The muscle biopsies showed necrotic fibers with accumulation of glycogen. In all cases, withdrawal of the drug led to a complete recovery within 2 weeks.

Gemfibrozil (Lopid)

See "Clofibrate (Antromid-S)" for discussion of this group of drugs.

Halothane (Fluothane), Isoflurane (Forane), Enflurane (Ethrane), and Succinylcholine Chloride (Anectine)

Halothane, isoflurane, and enflurane are inhalational anesthetic agents. Succinylcholine is a depolarizing neuromuscular blocking agent. These drugs are known to provoke malignant hyperthermia in susceptible individuals.[23] This inherited condition is characterized by vigorous muscle contraction and abrupt increase in body temperature provoked by exposure to these agents used in anesthesia.[10] Episodes of unexplained tachycardia, masseter spasm, and inability to intubate the patient are early warning signs of an impending malignant hyperthermia reaction.[57] Systemic features of impending crisis include sweating, cyanosis, hypotension, tachypnea, and a marked increase in body temperature (1–2°C increase every 5 minutes). Severe metabolic and respiratory acidosis soon develop. The laboratory abnormalities during the crisis include a striking increase of CK activity in the serum, hypercarbia, and hyperkalemia. Extensive muscle destruction can occur and result in myoglobinuria and renal failure.

Several myopathic diseases are also known to predispose patients to malignant hyperthermia attacks. These include multicore disease, central core disease, myotonia congenita, Schwartz-Jampel syndrome, and Duchenne's muscular dystrophy.[8]

The diagnosis of malignant hyperthermia can be made when an attack such as this occurs. Relatives should be considered to be at risk when a consistently elevated serum CK level is detected.[7] Elevation of CK level is not a completely satisfactory method for detecting this potentially fatal disease though, because it may not be present pre-exposure in some individuals.[57] The most sensitive diagnostic test for identifying the tendency for malignant hyperthermia is the halothane-caffeine contracture test. This test involves the bathing of skeletal muscle biopsy specimens (usually vastus lateralis) in a solution containing 1–3% halothane and caffeine or, alternatively, either drug alone. A positive test result shows an enhanced degree of contracture when exposed to these agents.

The incidence of this disorder is 1 in 20,000 anesthetized adults.[10] The basic defect is an autosomal dominantly inherited dysregulation of intracellular calcium, with the defective gene being located on the long arm of chromosome 19q12-13.2.[58] The calcium release channel of the sarcoplasmic reticulum, also known as the ryanodine receptor, is also coded in this region, and polymorphic DNA markers for the ryanodine receptor gene have been shown to cosegregate with malignant hyperthermia susceptibility trait.

During an acute attack, the cytosolic calcium concentration increases dramatically, which gives rise to a massive vigorous muscle contraction.[8] This is the cause of the hyperthermia, and the other features follow clinically from this process. As soon as an acute crisis is recognized, all anesthetic agents should be discontinued, and the patient should receive intravenous dantrolene therapy.[57] When malignant hyperthermia is diagnosed early and treated promptly, the mortality should be near zero. However, approximately two-thirds of untreated acute crises have a fatal outcome. Also, the discovery of a malignant hyperthermia attack requires that all relatives be informed of the possibility of latent malignant hyperthermia in other family members.

Hydroxychloroquine (PLAQUENIL)

See "Chloroquine (Aralen) and Hydroxychloroquine (Plaquenil)" for a discussion of this group of drugs.

Interferon (Intron A)

Interferon is used in the treatment of hairy cell leukemia, malignant melanoma, and hepatitis. Myalgia is a frequent side effect. Frank weakness is uncommon. One patient developed myopathy after being given interferon alpha-2b for hepatitis C infection.[59] After 19 weeks of treatment, the patient developed proximal muscle pain and weakness with an increase in serum CK levels. No muscle biopsy was performed. The patient returned to baseline after discontinuation of the interferon therapy.

Labetalol (Normodyne, Trandate)

Labetalol is a competitive antagonist at both alpha$_1$- and beta-adrenergic receptors and is used in the management of hypertension and treatment of pheochromocytoma.[23] Two children with renal disease and hypertension who were treated with labetalol developed a severe generalized myopathy.[60] These patients had proximal muscle weakness and markedly elevated CK levels. The muscle biopsy was consistent with a diagnosis of necrotic myopathy. Both patients achieved normal muscle strength within 2 months after discontinuing the drug, although one had persistent CK level elevation that normalized over the next year.

Levodopa (Larodopa, Dopar)

Levodopa, a metabolic precursor of dopamine, has been responsible for one reported case of myopathy in a patient treated for Parkinson's disease for 4 years.[61] The patient presented with proximal and distal muscle weakness and pain, eosinophilia, and elevated levels of CK and antinuclear antibodies. Muscle biopsy showed perivascular inflammation and type II muscle fiber atrophy. Nerve conductions showed a peripheral neuropathy pattern. After discontinuation of levodopa, the CK values returned to normal, the antinuclear antibody disappeared, and the eosinophilia subsided. The proximal muscle weakness gradually disappeared over 2–3 weeks; however, the severe distal muscle weakness persisted. The myopathy was thought to be part of a hypersensitivity vasculitis syndrome.

Leuprolide Acetate (Lupron)

Leuprolide acetate is a synthetic nonapeptide analogue of gonadotropin-releasing hormone and is used for treating endometriosis and palliative therapy of metastatic prostate cancer.[23] One reported case of myopathy appearing within 10 days of the first injection of the medication has been reported.[62] Muscle biopsy showed a myositis pattern. The serum CK level was elevated. The drug was withdrawn and corticosteroids were given because of the inflammatory pattern of the biopsy. Remission of the weakness and CK elevation occurred within 2 months. Withdrawing the corticosteroids did not produce relapse.

Lovastatin (Mevacor), Pravastatin (Pravachol), and Simvastatin (Zocor)

Lovastatin, pravastatin, and simvastatin are potent inhibitors of 3-hydroxy-3-methylglutaryl coenzyme A (HMG-CoA) reductase and reduce the blood concentration of low-density lipoproteins.[63] Lovastatin is associated with a myopathy that presents clinically with muscle pain, muscle cramps, proximal muscle weakness, and myotonia.[10] Approximately 0.2% of patients treated with lovastatin alone for 48 weeks develop these type of symptoms.[64] The serum CK level is elevated in excess of 2,000 U per liter.[7] The needle electromyographic examination demonstrates normal motor unit action potentials in mildly affected individuals or clear reductions in motor unit action potential duration and amplitude when significant weakness is present.[22] Fibrillation potentials and positive sharp waves are not prominent in this disorder. The muscle biopsy typically shows fiber necrosis, mononuclear cell infiltration with myophagocytosis, and regeneration.[7] Improvement generally occurs within 30 days after discontinuation of the drug.

The concomitant use of cyclosporine, erythromycin, nicotinic acid, or gemfibrozil with lovastatin may potentate the toxicity of lovastatin.[40, 65–67] Individuals with severe hepatobiliary dysfunction and renal insufficiency are at an increased risk of developing a toxic myopathy when taking lovastatin.[7]

Other HMG-CoA reductase inhibitors include pravastatin and simvastatin.[23] Pravastatin and simvastatin have been reported to cause a myopathy similar to that of lovastatin, with pravastatin being responsible for a reported case of dermatomyositis.[68–70] It is unclear whether patients experiencing myopathy from one of these medications can be switched to another without recurrence of the myopathy.

Nicotinic Acid (Niacin)

Nicotinic acid is a treatment for hyperlipoproteinemia. The term *niacin* was introduced to avoid confusion between the vitamin and the alkaloid nicotine.[23] Only in doses of more than 1 g per day has this drug been reported to cause a myopathy.[71] These patients develop proximal muscle weakness and pain with preserved tendon reflexes.[72] Three reported cases all had elevated serum CK levels and myalgia in the legs while on high doses of nicotinic acid.[71] Muscle biopsy was not performed on these patients. The symptoms resolved rapidly after discontinuing the nicotinic acid, and all patients had a complete recovery by 1 month.

Pancuronium (Pavulon), Vecuronium (Norcuron), Pipecuronium (Arduan), and Atracurium (Tracrium)

There have been numerous reports of drug-induced myopathy associated with pancuronium, vecuronium, pipecuronium, and atracurium, which are aminosteroid–based nondepolarizing neuromuscular blocking drugs.[73] The myopathy is often acute, presenting with a generalized prolonged paralysis of proximal and distal muscles, including the respiratory muscles. The incidence of this drug-induced myopathy is increased with concomitant use of high-dose corticosteroids.[74, 75] The serum CK level is typically elevated, and the electrophysiologic studies often confirm a myopathic process.[73] The muscle biopsy often shows atrophy and disorganization of myofibrils, including loss of myosin filaments. Once the neuromuscular blocking drug is discontinued, recovery may take longer than 6 months, and in some cases, may be incomplete.

Phenytoin (Diphenylhydantoin, Dilantin)

A myopathy has been reported as a hypersensitivity reaction to phenytoin. It appeared within the first 2 months of beginning treatment in five reported cases.[76] These patients' symptoms were fever, rash, lymphadenopathy, eosinophilia, proximal muscle weakness, and pain. Additionally, one of these patients had prominent bulbar involvement. The CK level was elevated without myoglobinuria. In one case, the muscle biopsy demonstrated necrosis and regeneration of muscle fibers without evidence of inflammation.[77] Patients typically return to baseline over 1–2 months with discontinuation of the phenytoin.[71] Depending on the severity of this hypersensitivity reaction, corticosteroids may be required to achieve resolution.[78]

Procainamide (Procanbid)

An analogue of the local anesthetic procaine, procainamide is used as an antiarrhythmic agent acting as a sodium channel blocker.[23] Procainamide therapy has been associated in one case with an interstitial form of myositis, usually as part of a lupus-like vasculitis.[79] This patient presented with proximal muscle pain and weakness. The CK level was normal. Muscle biopsy showed evidence of inflammation, regeneration, and necrosis. Drug withdrawal and azathioprine therapy resulted in complete recovery of the myopathy within months in one patient.[79] The author states that his patient was in such discomfort that his myopathy needed to be treated. Corticosteroids were his drug of choice; however, this patient had a previous history of a gastrectomy for peptic ulcer disease and would have been unable to tolerate the corticosteroids. His second choice for therapy was azathioprine.

Quinacrine (Mepacrine Hydrochloride, Atabrine)

Quinacrine was used extensively as an antimalarial agent during World War II and is currently used for the treatment of giardiasis.[7] Quinacrine-induced myopathy may include proximal muscle pain and weakness, sensorimotor neuropathy, and a cardiomyopathy. The CK level is usually mildly elevated. Muscle biopsy may show small groups of necrotic fibers with accompanying fibroblastic proliferation and slight lymphocytic infiltration. Gradual recovery is the rule over a period of weeks or months after withdrawal of the drug.

Tretinoin (Retin-A)

Tretinoin, a topical preparation used for the treatment of acne, is also used as a standard therapy for remission induction of acute promyelocytic leukemia.[10] When used to treat leukemia, one patient reportedly developed a myopathy.[80] The patient presented with acute localized leg pain. The CK level was two times normal. Muscle biopsy showed focal necrosis of the muscle fibers and infiltration of the endomysium and the perimysium with inflammatory cells. Complete recovery of the myopathy occurred in 6 weeks after withdrawal of the drug.

Vincristine (Oncovin, Vincasar PFS)

Vincristine is a *Vinca* alkaloid used for the treatment of lymphomas, leukemia, and some solid tumors.[81] Its most important toxic effect and one limiting its use as a therapeutic agent is a peripheral neuropathy. A severe direct myopathic effect of vincristine occurs much less frequently. A typical clinical presentation may include a mixed sensorimotor polyneuropathy, proximal muscle pain, proximal muscle weakness, and muscle wasting. Adults tend to be more sensitive to the toxic effects of vincristine than children. The CK level is often mildly elevated.[7] Nerve conduction studies often show an increase in distal sensory and motor latencies, with complete conduction block in several nerves.[81] The needle electromyography results show positive sharp waves and fibrillation potentials in the distally located muscles of the upper and lower extremities.[22] Motor unit action potentials in the proximal muscles have not been commented on in detail. The muscle biopsy may show areas of segmental necrosis and phagocytosis under the light microscope.[81] Under the electron microscope, fibers with myofibrillary disruption show accumulation of occasional fibrillary subsarcolemmal masses. The time until return of normal function and disappearance of paresthesias depends on the severity of symptoms at discontinuation of the drug. In cases of severe vincristine neuropathy and myopathy, resolution of symptoms may take months and may remain incomplete.

Zidovudine (Azidothymidine)

Zidovudine is a dideoxynucleoside analogue of thymidine used for the treatment of patients with HIV infection.[23] Its antiviral mechanism of action is to inhibit the RNA-dependent DNA polymerase (reverse transcriptase). Zidovudine has been shown to benefit patients with HIV myositis.[1]

Zidovudine is reported to produce a dose-related myopathy clinically and electrophysiologically similar to the myopathy caused by the HIV infection itself.[82, 83] The clinical features of a zidovudine-induced myopathy include progressive proximal muscle weakness with exercise-exacerbated myalgias in the thighs and calves.[83] Patients have typically been on zidovudine at full dose for 9 months before developing symptoms. The CK level is usually normal or moderately elevated.[84] The electromyography results may show fibrillations and positive waves in the proximal muscles, along with occasional complex repetitive discharges.[82, 83] The muscle biopsy of zidovudine-induced myopathy shows a distinctive pathologic alteration resembling ragged red fibers.[1] This evidence favors mitochondrial dysfunction. The muscle biopsy of HIV-induced myopathy usually shows only evidence of inflammation without evidence of ragged-red fibers.

Muscular weakness in some patients with acquired immunodeficiency syndrome has improved with reducing the zidovudine dosage or stopping the drug completely.[85] In a few cases, zidovudine has been reintroduced at lower dosages without a return of weakness.

Intramuscular Injection Myopathy

Localized areas of muscle damage due to needle insertion are produced by intramuscular injections of certain drugs. In the acute form, a relatively small number of patients develop local pain, swelling, hemorrhage, and sometimes abscess formation.[7] The incidence of this type of complications is approximately 0.4% per hospitalized patient per intramuscular injection.[86] Almost any drug may produce injection site complications; however, cephalothin, tetracycline, paraldehyde, colistimethate, and digoxin are the most likely to cause local effects. Intramuscular injections of lidocaine, phenytoin, diazepam, and digoxin can cause muscle necrosis at the injection site and an elevation in CK levels.

The chronic form of focal myopathy is provoked by frequent repeated intramuscular injections.[7] These disorders are characterized by fibrous contractures of muscle, often associated with induration and fibrosis of the overlying connective tissue and skin. The drugs most frequently involved include penicillin, streptomycin, chloromycetin, meperidine, pethidine, and pentazocine. The degree to which muscle is replaced by connective tissue is variable and depends on the frequency of the intramuscular injections and the duration over which the drug is administrated.

Conclusion

Many different medications may be responsible for causing a myopathy. The clinical presentation is the defining feature and typically includes myalgia and weakness. However, distal muscles may be involved in selected cases. The laboratory evaluation usually shows an elevated serum CK level; however, in some drug-induced myopathies, such as chronic corticosteroid myopathy, this may not hold true. The needle electromyographic examination may help support the clinical findings by showing short-duration, low-voltage, and at times, polyphasic motor unit potentials with increased recruitment at low efforts in the proximal muscles. A muscle biopsy may be helpful in selected cases, although it is not indicated in most circumstances. The importance in recognizing that a neurologic condition is drug induced is that discontinuation of the offending agent results in resolution of symptoms in most cases.

References

1. Griggs RC, Mendell JR, Miller RG. Evaluation and Treatment of Myopathies. Philadelphia: FA Davis, 1995;371.
2. McEvoy GK, Litvak K, Welsh OH, et al. Drug Information. Maryland: American Hospital Formulary Service, 1996;861.
3. Lisi DM. Muscle spasms and creatine phosphokinase elevation following salbutamol administration. Eur Respir J 1989;2:98.
4. Dyson AJ, Mackay AD. Two oral beta-adenergic stimulant drugs, pirbuterol and salbuterol, in reversible airway obstruction. Br J Dis Chest 1980;74:70.
5. Meier C, Kauer B, Muller U, Ludin HP. Neuromyopathy during chronic amiodarone treatment. A case report. J Neurol 1979;220:231.
6. Roth RF, Itabashi H, Louie J, et al. Amiodarone toxicity: myopathy and neuropathy. Am Heart J 1990;119: 1223.
7. Engel AG, Franzini-Armstrong C. Myology. New York: McGraw-Hill, 1994;1697.
8. Aminoff MJ. Neurology and General Medicine. New York: Churchill Livingstone, 1995;326, 934.
9. Drutz DJ, Fan JH, Tai TY. Hypokalemic rhabdomyolysis and myoglobinuria following amphotericin B therapy. JAMA 1970;211:824.
10. Jain KK. Drug-Induced Neurologic Disorders. Seattle: Hogrege and Huber, 1996;245.
11. Knochel JP. Neuromuscular manifestations of electrolyte disorders. Am J Med 1982;72:521.
12. Whisnant JP, Espinosa RE, Kierland RR, Lambert EH. Chloroquine neuromyopathy. Mayo Clin Proc 1963; 38:501.
13. Mastaglia FL. Adverse Effects of Drugs on Muscle. Drugs 1982;24:304.
14. Estes ML, Ewing-Wilson D, Chou SM, et al. Chloroquine neuromyotoxicity: clinical and pathologic perspective. Am J Med 1987;82:447.
15. Kimberly RP, Weinberg H, Rudd E. Great reduction in renal function associated with cimetidine. Arthritis Rheum 1980;23:614.
16. McGowan WR, Vermillion SE. Acute interstitial nephritis related to cimetidine therapy. Gastroenterology 1980;746.
17. Hake DH. Interstitial nephritis and cimetidine. Ann Intern Med 1981;94:416.
18. Watson AJ, Dalbow MH, Stachura I, et al. Immunologic studies in cimetidine-induced nephropathy and polymyositis. N Engl J Med 1983;308:142.
19. Cada DJ, Covington TR, Hussar DA, et al. Drug Facts and Comparisons. St. Louis: Wolters Kluwer, 1996;993.
20. Teravainen IW, Larsen A, Hillbom M. Clofibrate-induced myopathy in the rat. Acta Neuropathol 1977; 39:135.
21. Langer T, Levy RI. Acute muscular syndrome associated with administration of clofibrate. N Engl J Med 1968;279:856.
22. Dumitru D. Electrodiagnostic Medicine. Philadelphia: Hanley & Belfus, 1995;1106.
23. Gilman AG. Goodman and Gilman's The Pharmacologic Basis of Therapeutics. New York: McGraw-Hill, 1996;1.
24. Shiff D, Drislane FW. Rapid-onset colchicine myoneuropathy. Arthritis Rheum 1992;35:1535.
25. Kuncl RW, Duncan G, Watson D, et al. Colchicine myopathy and neuropathy. N Engl J Med 1987;316:1562.
26. Kontos HA. Myopathy associated with chronic colchicine toxicity. N Engl J Med 1962;266:38.
27. Kuncl RW, Cornblath DR, Avila O, Duncan G. Electrodiagnosis of human colchicine myoneuropathy. Muscle Nerve 1989;12:360.
28. Himmelmann F, Schroder JM. Colchicine myopathy in a case of familial Mediterranean fever: immunohistochemical and ultrastructual study of accumulated tubulin-immunoreactive material. Acta Neuropathol 1992; 83:440.
29. Dekhuijzen PN, Decramer M. Steroid-induced myopathy and its significance to respiratory disease. A known disease rediscovered. Eur Respir J 1992;5:997.
30. Williams TJ, O'Hehir RE, Czarny D, et al. Acute myopathy in severe acute asthma treated with intravenously administered corticosteroids. Am Rev Respir Dis 1988;137:460.
31. Shee CD. Risk factors for hydrocortisone myopathy in acute severe asthma. Respir Med 1990;84:229.
32. Op de Coul AAW, Lambregts PC, Koeman J, et al. Neuromuscular complications in patients given Pavulon (pancuronium bromide) during artificial ventilation. Clin Neurol Neurosurg 1985;87:17.
33. Van Marle W, Woods KL. Acute hydrocortisone myopathy. BMJ 1980;281:271.
34. Golding DN, Murray SM, Pearce GW, Thompson M. Corticosteroid myopathy. Ann Phys Med 1961;5:171.
35. Askari A, Vignos PJ, Moskowitz RW. Steroid myopathy in connective tissue disease. Am J Med 1976; 61:485.
36. Koehler PJ. Use of corticosteroids in neuro-oncology. Anti-Cancer Drugs 1995;6:19.
37. Rouleau G, Karpati G, Carpenter S, et al. Glucocorticoid excess induces preferential depletion of myosin in denervated skeletal muscle fibers. Muscle Nerve 1987;10:428.
38. Karpati G. Denervation and disuse atrophy of skeletal muscles: involvement of endogenous glucocorticoid hormones? Trends Neurosci 1984;7:61.

39. Arellano F, Krupp P. Muscular disorders associated with cyclosporin. Lancet 1991;337:915.
40. Norman D, Illingworth DR, Munson J, et al. Myolysis and acute renal failure in heart transplant recipient receiving lovastatin. N Engl J Med 1988;318:46.
41. Fernandez-Sola J, Campistol J, Casademont J, et al. Reversible cyclosporin myopathy. Lancet 1990;335:362.
42. Noppen M, Velkeniers B, Dierckx R, et al. Cyclosporine and myopathy. Ann Intern Med 1987;107:945.
43. Goy JJ, Stauffer JC, Deruaz JP, et al. Myopathy as a possible side-effect of cyclosporin. Lancet 1989; 1:1446.
44. Grezard O, Lebranchu Y, Birmele B, et al. Cyclosporin-induced muscular toxicity. Lancet 1990;335:177.
45. Carroll GJ, Will RK, Peter JB, et al. Penicillamine induced polymyositis and dermatomyositis. J Rheumatol 1987;14:995.
46. Zuckner J. Drug-related myopathies. Rheum Dis Clin North Am 1994;20:1017.
47. Aldrich TK, Prezant DJ. Adverse effects of drugs on the respiratory muscles. Clin Chest Med 1990;11:177.
48. Aydintug AO, Cervera R, D'Cruz D, et al. Polymyositis complicating D-penicillamine treatment. Postgrad Med J 1991;67:1018.
49. Halla JT, Fallahi S, Koopman WJ. Penicillamine-induced myositis: observations and unique features in two patients and review of the literature. Am J Med 1984;77:719.
50. Mateer JE, Farrell BJ, Chou SS, Gutmann L. Reversible ipecac myopathy. Arch Neurol 1985;42:188.
51. Klatskin G, Friedman H. Emetine toxicity in man: studies on the nature of early toxic manifestations, their relationship to the dose level, and their significance in determining safe dosage. Ann Intern Med 1948;28:892.
52. Duane DD, Engel AG. Emetine myopathy. Neurology 1970;20:733.
53. Leloet X, Moore N, Deshayes P. Pseudopolymyalgia rheumatica during treatment with enalapril. BMJ 1989;298:325.
54. Britt CW, Light RR, Peters BH, et al. Rhabdomyolysis during treatment with epsilon-aminocaproic acid. Arch Neurol 1980;37:187.
55. Lane RJM, McLelland NH, Martin AM, Mastaglia FL. Epsilon aminocaproic acid (EACA) myopathy. Postgrad Med J 1979;55:282.
56. Hodak E, David M, Gadoth N, Sandbank M. Etretinate-induced skeletal muscle damage. Br J Dermatol 1987;116:623.
57. Barash PG, Cullen BF, Stoelting RK. Handbook of Clinical Anesthesia. Philadelphia: Lippincott, 1991;14.
58. MacLennan DH, Duff C, Zorzato F, et al. Ryanodine receptor gene is a candidate for predisposition to malignant hyperthermia. Nature 1990;343:559.
59. Arai H, Tanaka M, Ohta K, et al. Symptomatic myopathy associated with interferon therapy for chronic hepatitis C. Lancet 1995;345:582.
60. Willis JK, Tilton AH, Harkin JC, Boineau FG. Possible myopathy due to labetalol. Pediatr Neurol 1990;6:275.
61. Wolf S, Goldberg LS, Verity MA. Neuromyopathy and periarteriolitis in a patient receiving levodopa. Arch Intern Med 1976;136:1055.
62. Crayton H, Bohlmann T, Sufit R, et al. Drug-induced polymyositis secondary to leuprolide acetate (Lupron) therapy for prostatic carcinoma. Clin Exp Rheumatol 1991;9:525.
63. Dujovne CA, Chremos AN, Pool JL, et al. Expanded Clinical Evaluation of Lovastatin (EXCEL) study results: IV. Additional perspectives on the tolerability of lovastatin. Am J Med 1991;91:1B-25S.
64. Tobert JA. Rhabdomyolysis in patients receiving lovastatin after cardiac transplantation. N Engl J Med 1988;318:47.
65. Ayanian JZ, Fuchs CS, Stone RM. Lovastatin and rhabdomyolysis. Ann Intern Med 1988;109:682.
66. Reaven P, Witztum JL. Lovastatin, nicotinic acid, and rhabdomyolysis. Ann Intern Med 1988;109:597.
67. Pierce LR, Wysowski DK, Gross TP. Myopathy and rhabdomyolysis associated with lovastatin-gemfibrozil combination therapy. JAMA 1990;264:71.
68. Deslypere JP, Vermeulen A. Rhabdomyolysis and simvastatin. Ann Intern Med 1991;114:342.
69. Berland Y, Coponat V, Durand C, et al. Rhabdomyolysis with simvastatin use. Nephron 1991;57:365.
70. Schalke BB, Schmidt B, Toyka K, et al. Pravastatin associated inflammatory myopathy. N Engl J Med 1992;327:649.
71. Litin SC, Anderson CF. Nicotinic acid-associated myopathy: a report of three cases. Am J Med 1989; 86:481.
72. Samuels MA, Feske S, Mesulam MM, et al. Office Practice of Neurology. New York: Churchill Livingstone, 1996;594.
73. Elliot JM, Bion JF. The use of neuromuscular blocking drugs in intensive care practice. Acta Anaesthesiol Scand 1995;39:70.
74. Danon MJ, Carpenter S. Myopathy with thick filament (myosin) loss following prolonged paralysis with vercuronium during steroid treatment. Muscle Nerve 1991;14:1131.
75. Griffin D, Fairman N, Coursin D, et al. Acute myopathy during treatment of status asthmaticus with corticosteroids and steroidal muscle relaxants. Chest 1992; 102:510.
76. Barclay CL, McLean M, Hagan N, et al. Severe phenytoin hypersensitivity with myopathy. Neurology 1992;42:2303.
77. Harney J, Glasberg M. Myopathy and hypersensitivity to phenytoin. Neurology 1983;33:790.
78. Haruda F. Phenytoin hypersensitivity: 38 cases. Neurology 1979;29:1480.
79. Fontiveros ES, Cumming WJ, Hudgson P. Procainamide-induced myositis. J Neurol Sci 1980;45:143.

80. Miranda N, Oliveria P, Frade MJ, et al. Myositis with tretinoin. Lancet 1994;344:1006.
81. Bradley WG, Lassman LP, Pearce GW, Walton JN. The neuromyopathy of vincristine in man: clinical, electrophysiological and pathological studies. J Neurol Sci 1970;10:107.
82. Simpson DM, Bender AN. Human immunodeficiency virus-associated myopathy: analysis of 11 patients. Ann Neurol 1988;24:79.
83. Chalmers AC, Greco CM, Miller RG. Prognosis in AZT myopathy. Neurology 1991;41:1181.
84. Mhiri C, Baudrimont M, Bonne G, et al. Zidovudine myopathy: a distinctive disorder associated with mitochondrial dysfunction. Ann Neurol 1991;29:606.
85. Simpson DM, Citak K, Godfrey E, et al. HIV or Zidovudine? Neurology 1994;44:360.
86. Greenblatt DJ, Allen MD. Intramuscular injection-site complications. JAMA 1978;240:542.

Chapter 18

Neurologic Complications of Anticoagulant and Antiplatelet Drugs

Linda S. Williams and José Biller

Objectives

- To appreciate the risk of intracranial hemorrhage (ICH) associated with heparin and coumarin compounds
- To learn the individual clinical risk factors that may increase the risk of anticoagulant-related ICH
- To appreciate the spinal cord, peripheral nerve, and ocular complications of anticoagulant and antiplatelet medications
- To learn common idiosyncratic and allergic effects of anticoagulant and antiplatelet medications
- To appreciate potential fetal effects of maternal use of anticoagulants and antiplatelet medications
- To increase familiarity with the risk-benefit analysis technique as applied to anticoagulant or antiplatelet medications

Anticoagulant and antiplatelet medications are among the most common drugs prescribed today. Although the potential benefit of these medications in reducing the risk and subsequent complications of arterial or venous thrombosis is great, the risk of hemorrhagic complications with many of these medications is not inconsequential. Although the majority of anticoagulant-related hemorrhages are minor, anticoagulants can cause life-threatening and fatal bleeding. Because of these potentially devastating complications, physicians must be informed both about the benefits and risks of anticoagulant and antiplatelet treatments.

There are three critical steps in the effective use of anticoagulant and antiplatelet drugs: (1) recognize the population that may benefit from their use, (2) understand the magnitude of both the benefit of the drug and risk of hemorrhage associated with the medication, and (3) recognize particular clinical factors that may increase or decrease the risk of hemorrhage in a particular patient. This chapter focuses on the neurologic risks of anticoagulant and antiplatelet medications, the foremost of which is ICH. Unless otherwise noted, ICH refers to either intra-axial or extra-axial intracranial bleeding. Other neurologic complications of anticoagulant and antiplatelet medications, including bleeding affecting the spinal cord, idiosyncratic allergic responses affecting the nervous system, and fetal central nervous system (CNS) effects, are also reviewed. Ototoxic complications of aspirin therapy are reviewed in Chapter 14.

Anticoagulants

Unfractionated Heparin

Unfractionated heparin is the most commonly used parenteral anticoagulant in the United States. Heparin is a heterogeneous sulfated mucopolysaccharide that is endogenously produced in mast cells. Commercial preparations of heparin consist of polysaccharides of variable molecular weight (usually 7,000–40,000 kD). Anticoagulant properties of heparin differ somewhat based on the tissue from which it was extracted; more protamine is required to neutralize a unit of heparin extracted from beef lung than a unit of heparin extracted from porcine mucosa.[1]

Heparin acts as an anticoagulant by binding with antithrombin-III and accelerating antithrombin-III neutralization of activated clotting factors. In small amounts, the heparin–antithrombin-III complex inactivates factor Xa; in larger amounts, the complex inactivates thrombin, thus preventing the conversion of fibrinogen to fibrin.[1] The anticoagulant effect of heparin occurs almost immediately after intravenous injection and lasts for approximately 6 hours after infusion is discontinued. Heparin activity is commonly measured by the degree of prolongation of the activated partial thromboplastin time.

Heparin is used to treat patients with acute arterial or venous thrombosis, such as acute myocardial infarction, pulmonary embolus, or deep venous thrombosis. It is also commonly used to maintain extracorporeal membrane circulation during cardiac surgery. Subcutaneous administration of heparin is used for prevention of deep venous thrombosis in immobilized patients and in pregnant women with venous thrombosis or hypercoagulable disorders.

Heparin in Acute Ischemic Stroke

The recently completed International Stroke Trial compared two doses of subcutaneous heparin (10,000 or 25,000 U daily) with or without 300 mg of aspirin in nearly 20,000 patients with recent (less than 48 hours) ischemic stroke.[2] Although ICH was uncommon, preliminary reports indicate that heparin-treated patients were significantly more likely to have ICH compared with patients not treated with heparin (1.2% versus 0.4%). Approximately half of the nonheparin group received aspirin. Further analysis of this large trial should provide more information about the long-term risks and benefits of subcutaneous heparin in patients with ischemic stroke.

Intravenous heparin has been more commonly used than subcutaneous heparin in acute stroke. The occurrence of ICH or hemorrhagic transformation of ischemic infarction in small series of patients treated with intravenous heparin is estimated to be between 0% and 6%.[3–7] Interpretation of these studies is difficult given the long or undefined time between symptom onset and exposure to heparin and the lack of standardized follow-up neuroimaging. Excessive prolongation of the activated partial thromboplastin time and large embolic infarcts may increase the risk of hemorrhage in patients with acute stroke.[8–10]

It is unclear whether heparin plays a role in transforming a bland infarct to a hemorrhagic infarct, although this transformation is usually not associated with neurologic worsening.[11, 12] Several studies indicate that the risk of transforming an ischemic to a hemorrhagic infarct is no greater in patients with early anticoagulation.[3, 13–16] One very small series suggests that patients with hemorrhagic infarct and a high risk of recurrent embolism can be anticoagulated with no significant risk of neurologic deterioration.[17]

Although heparin may not be associated with transformation of a bland infarct to a hemorrhagic infarct, it is likely that anticoagulation is associated with the development of intrainfarct hematoma.[5, 6, 8, 10, 11, 18–20] Intrainfarct hematoma is often associated with neurologic worsening and may be more associated with infarct size rather than intensity of anticoagulation.[11, 12, 18, 20, 21]

Heparin appears to be significantly safer in nonstroke patients. Intravenous heparin for other conditions such as acute myocardial infarction and deep venous thrombosis carries a risk of ICH of less than 1%.[22, 23]

Heparin and Neonatal Intraventricular Hemorrhage

Intravenous heparin is used to maintain patency and prolong longevity of venous catheters. The exposure of neonates to heparin via this route has been associated with an increased risk of germinal matrix hemorrhage.[24, 25] Because potential confounding variables in these case-control and cohort studies cannot be controlled for, the true presence and magnitude of the risk of heparin in premature infants cannot be assessed.

Heparin-Induced Thrombocytopenia

There are two types of heparin-induced thrombocytopenia. Type I usually occurs within the first 4 days after initiation of therapy and is clinically benign. Type II heparin-induced thrombocytopenia usually starts within 4–14 days after initiation of therapy and may be associated with new arterial or venous thrombotic events.[26–28] A complex of heparin and platelet factor 4 is the target antigen in this potentially immune-mediated allergic reaction.[29] This complex then triggers platelet activation and subsequent release of platelet-derived procoagulants.[30, 31] The decrease in platelet count usually begins within days of starting heparin. Arterial thrombosis, the so-called white clot syndrome, or venous thrombosis can occur.[32–34] In a series of 127 patients with heparin-induced thrombocytopenia, five patients developed thrombotic stroke; the most common complication in this series was deep venous thrombosis.[34] In a series from the Mayo Clinic, one-third of postendarterectomy carotid occlusions occurred in patients with heparin-induced thrombocytopenia.[35] Thrombocytopenia with venous thrombosis and ICH has also been reported with pentosan, a low-molecular-weight (LMW) heparin.[36, 37]

Low-Molecular-Weight Heparins

LMW heparins are produced by the depolymerization of heparin. They can be given subcutaneously and have a longer half-life than heparin. LMW heparins have been used extensively in patients with deep venous thrombosis and for prophylaxis of deep venous thrombosis without an increase in hemorrhagic complications as compared with conventional heparin.[38–42] Although perhaps safer than heparin, LMW heparins have been associated with systemic and, rarely, CNS bleeding complications.[43]

LMW heparins may be effective for treatment of acute stroke and do not appear to increase the risk of ICH.[44] In a randomized controlled study, two doses of subcutaneous nadroparin (4,100 antifactor Xa units daily or twice daily for 10 days) or placebo were tested in 312 patients within 48 hours of acute ischemic stroke. A dose-dependent effect of nadroparin was observed; patients treated with the medication were less likely to die or become dependent within 6 months after stroke. Symptomatic hemorrhagic transformation of the stroke occurred in only one patient in the placebo group. Asymptomatic hemorrhagic transformation occurred in 5% of the high-dose, 7% of the low-dose, and 9% of the placebo group (differences not significant). Because a follow-up computed tomography (CT) scan of the head was obtained in only 245 of the 312 patients, the precise risk of nadroparin-induced hemorrhagic transformation of ischemic infarction is not known.

Low-Molecular-Weight Heparinoids

LMW heparinoids are mixtures of sulfated glycosaminoglycans with low molecular weight. Because various components of heparin are combined to make the LMW heparinoids, a more selective mechanism of action can be obtained. Like LMW heparins, LMW heparinoids can be given subcutaneously. Danaparoid is a heparinoid that has been used for the treatment of venous thromboembolism. In a study of 188 patients with confirmed deep venous thrombosis or pulmonary embolism, high-dose danaparoid (intravenous loading dose of 2,000 U followed by 2,000 U subcutaneously twice daily) was shown to be safer and more effective than unfractionated heparin for preventing recurrence or extension of venous thromboembolism.[45]

Danaparoid has also been used in patients with acute stroke. Phase I and II trials of this medication in patients with acute ischemic stroke demonstrated no significant increase in risk of ICH.[46] The Phase III study (Trial of ORG 10172 for Acute Stroke Treatment) tested intravenous danaparoid against placebo in almost 1,300 patients with acute ischemic stroke. Analysis of this recently completed study should provide more information about the efficacy and safety of danaparoid in stroke patients.

Ancrod

Ancrod is a defibrinogenating medication made from the purification of Malayan pit viper venom.[47] In addition to lowering serum viscosity and fibrinogen levels by destabilizing the cross-linking of fibrin monomers, ancrod may also have weak thrombolytic activity.[48] Ancrod has been used in Canada and Europe for the treatment of peripheral vascular disease, for the treatment of deep vein thrombosis, and for prophylaxis of thromboembolism.[49–53] Ancrod is available in the United States on a compassionate-use basis for patients with heparin allergy or heparin-induced thrombocytopenia. Phase II trials of ancrod in patients with ischemic stroke have not shown an increase in ICH in ancrod-treated patients.[54, 55] A Phase III trial of ancrod in patients with acute ischemic stroke is ongoing.

Warfarin and Other Coumarin Compounds

The mechanism of action of all coumarin compounds (warfarin, dicumarol, phenprocoumon) is to block post-translational modification of factors II, VII, IX, and X by impairing vitamin K–dependent reactions. Dicumarol is erratically absorbed from the gut and is infrequently used.[1] Phenprocoumon (Marcumar, Falithrom) is more commonly used in Europe. Warfarin sodium is the most commonly used oral anticoagulant in North America.

The anticoagulant activity of warfarin takes effect within 3–5 days after oral administration. For this reason, patients with acute venous or arterial thrombus are often concomitantly given intravenous heparin until warfarin activity is therapeutic. Warfarin activity is commonly monitored using the International Normalized Ratio, which is a function of the observed prothrombin time ratio (PTR) and of the International Sensitivity Index (ISI) of the thromboplastin reagent used [$(PTR)^{ISI}$].

Warfarin is used chronically for primary and secondary stroke prevention in patients with atrial fibrillation (AF) and prosthetic heart valves, and it is used on a short-term basis for some patients with venous or arterial thrombosis. Despite proven efficacy in reducing thromboembolic complications in many of these disorders, chronic administration of coumarin compounds does increase the risk of hemorrhagic complications.[56–62]

The incidence of ICH in community-based studies of nonanticoagulated patients with CT or autopsy confirmation in more than 75% of cases ranges from 9 to 16 per 100,000 per year.[63–67] Chronic anticoagulation with coumarin compounds appears to increase this risk sevenfold to 12-fold.[68–70] The incidence of ICH is likely underestimated in pre-CT population studies.[71]

Patients with AF, who are at a higher risk of thromboembolism and thus stand to benefit more from anticoagulation, appear also to have a higher risk of ICH with warfarin treatment (Table 18.1). Information from several randomized clinical trials has estimated the risk of ICH in anticoagulated patients with AF to be from 0% to 1.8% per patient-year treated.[56–61] The Stroke Prevention in Atrial Fibrillation study indicated that this risk may be most elevated in patients older than age 75, but these patients are also at increased risk of thromboembolic stroke.[72]

Cohort studies of outpatients taking coumarin derivatives show that the risk of ICH in these more heterogeneous populations is slightly less than patients with AF (Table 18.2).[73–75] The risk of ICH per patient-year of treatment in these studies ranges from a low of 0.02% in a group of U.S. anticoagulation clinics to 0.6% in a similar setting in the Netherlands.[73, 75]

Because of this small but real risk of ICH in patients on warfarin, it is important to identify patients who may be at a higher risk of ICH based on other clinical factors (Table 18.3). Specific risk factors for ICH in patients taking warfarin include hypertension,[72, 76, 77] intensity of anticoagulation (AC),[72, 78] history of stroke or thromboembolism,[72, 78] increasing age,[72, 78] recent alcohol consumption,[76] and diabetes.[77] Because increasing age and intensity of AC have been identified as potential risk factors for hemorrhage in anticoagulated patients, it is essential to recognize that warfarin dose requirements decrease with age; one study estimated a 21% decline in warfarin dose over a 15-year period.[79]

Effects of Warfarin on the Fetus

Warfarin is teratogenic when given to pregnant women. Unlike heparin, warfarin readily crosses the placenta and so has potential teratogenic effects. Exposure to warfarin in the first trimester can cause bone abnormalities[80]; second- and third-trimester exposure has been associated with mental retardation, microcephaly, and optic atrophy[81]; congenital hydrocephalus and the Dandy-Walker malformation[82]; and congenital schizencephaly.[83] Maternal warfarin use has also rarely been associated with fetal ICH.[84–86]

Table 18.1. Risk of Intracranial Hemorrhage in Warfarin-Treated Atrial Fibrillation Patients

Study	Population	Treatment (Daily Dose)	Target/Mean INR or PTR	No. of Patients	Patient-Years of Follow-up	No. of Intracranial Hemorrhages	% Intracranial Hemorrhages per Patient-Year
SPAF I[57]	AF[a]	Warfarin	PTR 1.3–1.8/PTR 1.45	210	260	2	0.8
		ASA, 325 mg		552	720	2	0.3
		Placebo		568	731	2	0.3
SPAF II[58]	AF, age ≤75	Warfarin	INR 2.0–4.5/2.7	358	—[g]	6	0.6
		ASA, 325 mg		357	—	2	0.2
	AF, age >75	Warfarin		197	—	7	1.8
		ASA, 325 mg	INR 2.0–4.5/2.6	188	—	3	0.8
SPAF III[60]	AF + at least one thromboembolic risk factor[b]	Low-intensity, fixed-dose warfarin + ASA, 325 mg	INR 1.2–1.5/1.3	521	558	5	0.9
		Adjusted-dose warfarin	INR 2–3/2.4	523	581	3	0.5
Pooled data[59, f]	AF	Warfarin	PTR 1.2–1.5, INR 2–4.2[c]	1,225	1,889	10	0.5
		Placebo		1,236	1,802	2	0.1
		ASA, 75–325 mg		888	1,132	—[d]	—
		Placebo		904	1,133	—	—
EAFT[61]	AF and TIA or minor stroke	Warfarin	INR 2.5–4.0	225	507	0	0
		ASA, 300 mg		404	838	2	0.2
		Placebo		378	715	1	0.1
VA[56]	AF, males	Warfarin	PTR 1.2–1.5[e]	260	468	1	0.2
		Placebo		265	450.5	0	—

ASA = aspirin; EAFT = European Atrial Fibrillation Trial; INR = International Normalized Ratio; PTR = prothrombin time ratio; SPAF = Stroke Prevention in Atrial Fibrillation Study; VA = Veterans Affairs Stroke Prevention in Nonrheumatic Atrial Fibrillation Study; AF = atrial fibrillation; TIA = transient ischemic attack.

[a]Patients older than age 75 not eligible for warfarin for most of study period.

[b]Thromboembolic risk factors: congestive heart failure or left ventricular fractional shortening of ≤25%, previous thromboembolism, systolic blood pressure of >160 mm Hg at study enrollment, or female age >75 years.

[c]See individual trials for target and mean PTRs/INRs.

[d]Intracranial hemorrhages occurring on ASA or placebo were not reported in this publication.

[e]PTR reported as "in range" in 56% of the measurements, "below range" in 29%, and "above range" in 15%.

[f]Data from Atrial Fibrillation, Aspirin, Anticoagulation Study (AFASAK); Boston Area Anticoagulation Trial for Atrial Fibrillation Study (BAATAF); Canadian Atrial Fibrillation Anticoagulation Study; SPAF; and VA.

[g]Patient-years of follow-up not reported.

Table 18.2. Risk of Intracranial Hemorrhage in Patients on Warfarin in Cohort Studies

Study	Population	Treatment	Target/Actual AC	No. of Patients	No. of Patient-Years of Follow-up	No. of Intracranial Hemorrhages	% Intracranial Hemorrhages per Patient-Year
Palareti et al.[74]	Outpatients in Italian AC clinics	64% on warfarin	INR ≤2.8 in 71%; INR >2.8 in 29%	2,745	2,011	4	0.2
		36% on acenocoumarin	68% of measures within target, 26% above, and 6% below				
van der Meer et al.[73]	Outpatients in the Netherlands AC clinics: 1988	87% on phenprocoumon	77% of measures in target range in both 1988 and 1991[a]	6,814	6,085	38[b]	0.62
	1991			6,512	5,784	35[c]	0.61
Fihn et al.[75]	Outpatients in U.S. AC clinics	Warfarin	Low-intensity (PTR 1.3–1.5)/ mean PTR = 1.47[d]; high-intensity (PTR 1.5–1.8)/ mean PTR = 1.643	2,376[e]	3,702	7[f]	0.02

AC = anticoagulation; INR = International Normalized Ratio; PTR = prothrombin time ratio.

[a]Specific target ranges were not reported. In 1988 there were fewer bleeding complications with increasing target range; in 1991 no effect of target range on bleeding complications was found.

[b]Eight patients did not have computed tomography or autopsy.

[c]Five patients did not have computed tomography or autopsy.

[d]Number of patients receiving low- and high-intensity AC not given.

[e]Four hundred seventy-one patients were retrospectively included.

[f]The number of intracranial hemorrhages is estimated; 20% of 37 life-threatening or fatal hemorrhages were intracranial hemorrhages.

Table 18.3. Risk Factors for Intracranial Hemorrhage in Patients on Anticoagulation

Study	Population	No. of Patients	Risk Factors	OR (95% CI), *P* value
Hylek and Singer[78]	Consecutive cases of ICH	121 cases; 363 controls	PTR (per unit)	4.5 (2.6–8.0), P <.001
			Cerebrovascular disease	2.3 (1.4–3.7), P <.001
			Prosthetic valve	2.1 (1.2–3.8), P = .01
			Age (per decade)	1.4 (1.2–1.7), P <.001
SPAF[72]	Patients with AF on warfarin	1,100	History of thromboembolism	6.3, P = .003
			Systolic BP ≥160	4.4, P = .02
			Age >75 years	3.7, P = .05
			Diastolic BP ≥90	3.6, P = .04
Juvela et al.[76]	Consecutive cases of ICH[a]	156 cases; 332 controls	Hypertension[b]	6.6 (3.9–11.3), P <.001
			Alcohol in last 24 hrs	
			1–40 g	0.33 (0.16–0.72), P <.01
			41–120 g	4.34 (2.2–9.4), P <.001
			>120 g	11.35 (3.0–42.8), P <.001
			Alcohol in last week	
			1–150 g	2.0 (1.14–3.49), P <.05
			151–300 g	4.3 (1.6–11.7), P <.01
			>300 g	6.5 (2.4–17.7), P <.001
Dawson et al.[77]	Consecutive series of patients with chronic lower limb ischemia on warfarin	376 cases[c]	Diabetes mellitus	5.4, P <.01
			Systolic BP ≥160	4.8, P <.01

AF = atrial fibrillation; SPAF = Stroke Prevention in Atrial Fibrillation Study; BP = blood pressure (mm Hg); ICH = any intracranial hemorrhage; PTR = prothrombin time ratio.
[a]Age range of this population was 16–60 years.
[b]Systolic BP of ≥170 mm Hg or diastolic BP of ≥95 mm Hg.
[c]Two of the 18 cases of ICH did not have computed tomography or autopsy.

Spinal, Peripheral Nervous System, Ocular, and Rare Complications of Anticoagulants

Just as anticoagulants increase the risk of ICH, heparin and coumarin compounds also increase the risk of bleeding at other sites. The most common extracranial nervous system structures affected by bleeding are the spinal cord, peripheral nerves, and the eye.

The spinal cord may be compromised by intramedullary hemorrhage or by epidural hemorrhage and secondary compression.[87–92] Epidural hemorrhage may occur after lumbar puncture in anticoagulated patients.[93, 94] Spinal epidural hemorrhage has also been reported in patients taking aspirin,[95, 96] but the widespread use of aspirin and the rarity of spinal epidural hematoma make the association of the two purely speculative. Spinal subarachnoid hemorrhage may occur spontaneously,[91] after chiropractic manipulation,[97] or after lumbar puncture[98] in anticoagulated patients. The cauda equina syndrome can occur in anticoagulated patients as a primary syndrome or as a result of intratumor hemorrhage.[99, 100]

Intratumor hemorrhage is a potential complication of antiplatelet or anticoagulant treatment in patients with intracranial tumors.[101, 102] Despite this potential risk, patients with primary glial tumors have been anticoagulated with warfarin without bleeding complications.[103, 104] ICH resulting from a meningioma in a patient taking aspirin has been reported.[105] Cerebral siderosis, a rare disorder usually linked to repeated subarachnoid hemorrhage, has been reported in a patient anticoagulated with warfarin.[106]

Heparin and warfarin have frequently been associated with retroperitoneal or iliopsoas hemorrhage and subsequent femoral, obturator, or lumbar plexus neuropathy.[107–113] Brachial plexus compression can also occur spontaneously or after intravascular procedures in anticoagulated patients.[114, 115] The median nerve in the carpal tunnel is another potential site of peripheral nerve compression secondary to anticoagulant-related hemorrhage.[116, 117]

Hemorrhage into various tissues of the eye is another possible neurologic complication of anticoagulation. Although not common, ocular hyphaema, subretinal hemorrhage, intraocular hemorrhage, and subconjunctival hemorrhage have all been reported in anticoagulated patients.[118–122]

Methods of Reversing Anticoagulation

Patients with excessive anticoagulation who are receiving intravenous heparin but who do not have evidence of hemorrhage or who have minor hemorrhage can be treated by discontinuing the heparin infusion. The duration of action of intravenous heparin is dose dependent; the half-life of 200 and 400 U per kg doses is 96 and 152 minutes, respectively.[1] The half-life of heparin given subcutaneously is less predictable, but generally longer than when administered intravenously.

Anticoagulated patients with active bleeding may require rapid reversal of anticoagulation. Fresh frozen plasma is indicated for treatment of heparin overdose accompanied by hemorrhage. Protamine sulfate, given by slow intravenous injection, can also be used to neutralize the effects of heparin. Approximately 1 mg of protamine sulfate antagonizes 100 U of USP heparin[1]; the dose of protamine is calculated based on the amount of heparin given in the preceding 3–4 hours. The effect of protamine lasts approximately 2 hours; thus, coagulation activity must be monitored frequently so repeat doses can be given if necessary.

Excessive anticoagulation and hemorrhage caused by warfarin is also treated with transfusion of 20 ml per kg of fresh frozen plasma to replete the vitamin K–dependent clotting factors. Adults usually require 2–3 U of fresh frozen plasma.[1] If serious bleeding is not present, warfarin may be discontinued temporarily and reinstituted once the International Normalized Ratio reaches a desirable level. For serious hemorrhages in warfarin-treated patients, 10 mg of phytonadione (vitamin K_1) subcutaneously is required to provide prolonged reversal of anticoagulation; response usually develops within 4–24 hours after administration. For minor hemorrhages, or if a patient will need continued oral anticoagulation, doses of phytonadione should not exceed 0.5–1.0 mg.[1]

Antiplatelet Medications

Aspirin

Aspirin is the most commonly used antiplatelet medication. It irreversibly inhibits platelet cyclooxygenase, thereby blocking the formation of thromboxane A_2 and subsequent platelet aggregation. The inhibition of platelet aggregation also results in decreased release of adenosine diphosphate (ADP) from platelets, which normally serves to induce further platelet clumping.

Aspirin has been proven effective for the primary prevention of myocardial infarction (MI) and for the secondary prevention of stroke, MI, and vascular death.[123–126] In patients with cardiovascular disease, antiplatelet therapy produces a 25% relative risk reduction in MI, stroke, or death; a 32% relative risk reduction in nonfatal MI; a 27% relative risk reduction in nonfatal stroke; and a 15% relative risk reduction in cardiovascular death.[125] Aspirin has also been proven effective in reducing the short-term risk of MI, stroke, or death in patients with evolving MI and the short-term risk of recurrent stroke in patients with acute ischemic stroke.[2, 127]

The risk of ICH in patients taking aspirin for primary prevention of vascular events may be slightly elevated, although no trial of aspirin has demonstrated a statistically significant risk (Table 18.4). The U.S. Physicians' Health Study compared 325 mg of aspirin every other day to placebo in 22,074 male physicians.[123] There were 23 patients with hemorrhagic stroke in the aspirin group compared with 12 in the placebo group (odds ratio of 2.14, 95% confidence interval of 0.96–4.77, $P = .06$). A similar study in British physicians using 500 mg of aspirin daily reported a 1.6% per year risk of "probable hemorrhagic stroke" in aspirin-treated patients.[124] This rate of ICH was slightly although not significantly less than in placebo patients (2.1% per year). Other large studies of aspirin in doses

Table 18.4. Risk of Intracranial Hemorrhage in Patients in Aspirin Trials

Study	Population	Treatment (Daily Dose)	No. of Patients	No. of Patient-Years of Follow-up	No. of Intracranial Hemorrhages	% Intracranial Hemorrhages per Patient-Year
USPHS[123]	U.S. male physicians	ASA, 162.5 mg	11,037	54,650	23	0.04
		Placebo	11,034	54,636	12	0.02 ($P = .06$)
Peto et al.[124]	British male physicians	ASA, 500 mg	3,429	18,820	—[a]	1.6[a]
		Placebo	1,710	9,470	—[a]	2.1[a]
UK-TIA[133]	Patients with recent TIA or minor ischemic stroke	ASA, 1,200 mg	815	—[b]	13[c]	—
		ASA, 300 mg	806	—	—	—
		Control	814	—	3	—
Swedish Cooperative Study[134]	Patients with ischemic stroke	ASA, 1,500 mg	253	—[b]	3	—
		Placebo	252	—	2	—
Dutch TIA[136]	Patients with TIA or minor ischemic stroke[d]	ASA, 30 mg	1,555	—[b]	13	—[b]
		ASA, 283 mg	1,576	—	15	—
SALT[132]	Patients ages 50–79 years with TIA, minor ischemic stroke, or retinal artery occlusion	ASA, 75 mg	676	—[b]	10	—
		Control	684	—	3	—
Bousser et al.[135]	Patients with TIA or ischemic stroke	ASA, 1,000 mg	198	—[b]	1	—[b]
		ASA, 1,000 mg + dipyridamole, 225 mg	202	—	2	—
		Placebo	204	—	2	—

USPHS = U.S. Physicians Health Study; ASA = aspirin; SALT = Swedish Aspirin Low-dose Trial; TIA = transient ischemic attack.
[a]Numbers of ICH not reported; results given as "probable hemorrhagic stroke" rate per 10,000 patient-years.
[b]Patient-years of follow-up not reported.
[c]Intracranial hemorrhages in combined aspirin treatment groups; intracranial hemorrhages by aspirin treatment group not reported.
[d]Approximately 40% of patients had head computed tomography at study entry.

from 75 to 500 mg daily have also shown a slight but not statistically significant preponderance of hemorrhagic strokes in patients on aspirin.[128–131] The large number of patients treated in these studies is reassuring; if the risk of ICH is elevated by chronic use of aspirin, the magnitude of this risk is extremely small.

The risk of aspirin-related ICH in patients with recent stroke also appears small (see Table 18.4). Studies comparing aspirin to other antiplatelet agents for the prevention of stroke, MI, or vascular death in patients with recent ischemic stroke have shown a risk of ICH of less than 1% in aspirin-treated patients.[132–136] The Swedish Aspirin Low-Dose Trial compared 75 mg aspirin with placebo in patients with recent transient ischemic attack, minor ischemic stroke, or retinal artery occlusion.[132] Although there was no significant difference in total ICH between aspirin and placebo groups, fatal hemorrhagic stroke was significantly more common in aspirin-treated patients (5 versus 0, $P = .03$). No other trial of aspirin reported similar findings. The European Stroke Prevention Study compared 975 mg of aspirin and 225 mg of dipyridamole daily with placebo for the prevention of recurrent stroke or death.[137] This trial did not report the number of ICH in the 2,500 patients treated; any bleeding was significantly more likely in the aspirin-dipyridamole group but fatal stroke was more common in the placebo group. Although many of these studies did not report patient-years of follow-up, the consistently small number of ICH in both treatment and placebo groups suggests that aspirin does not significantly increase the risk of ICH in patients with recent stroke. Maternal use of aspirin has rarely been associated with fetal ICH.[138, 139]

Ticlopidine

Ticlopidine is an antiplatelet drug that acts by inhibiting the ADP pathway for platelet activation. The most serious side effects with ticlopidine are neutropenia and agranulocytosis, although transient thrombotic thrombocytopenia and thrombotic thrombocytopenic purpura with ICH have rarely occurred.[140, 141]

Ticlopidine does not appear to significantly increase the risk of ICH when compared with either placebo or aspirin. The Canadian American Ticlopidine Study tested ticlopidine, 250 mg twice daily, against placebo in 1,072 patients with recent thromboembolic stroke.[142] The composite outcome of stroke, MI, or vascular death occurred significantly less often in ticlopidine-treated patients. Two patients in the treatment group had ICH, and two patients in the placebo group had subarachnoid hemorrhage. The Ticlopidine Aspirin Stroke Study compared ticlopidine, 250 mg twice daily, with aspirin, 650 mg twice daily, in 3,069 patients with recent transient or mild persistent focal cerebral or retinal ischemia.[143] Ticlopidine was shown to be slightly more effective than aspirin for the prevention of subsequent fatal or nonfatal stroke and for the composite outcome of nonfatal stroke or death. No ICH was reported in either treatment group; aspirin was significantly more likely to cause gastrointestinal hemorrhage (1.4% versus 0.5%).

Clopidogrel

Clopidogrel is the most recent antiplatelet medication to show efficacy in a large randomized, controlled trial.[144] Clopidogrel is a novel thienopyridine that acts by irreversibly inhibiting the binding of ADP to platelets, thus decreasing ADP-dependent activation of the major fibrinogen receptor on the platelet surface. Clopidogrel, 75 mg daily, was compared with aspirin, 325 mg daily, in 19,185 patients with either recent atherothrombotic stroke, recent MI, or symptomatic peripheral arterial disease. The occurrence of ICH was slightly more frequent in patients taking aspirin (0.49% versus 0.35%), but this difference was not statistically significant.

Risk-Benefit Analysis

To effectively use anticoagulant and antiplatelet medications, the magnitude of both the benefit and the risk of the treatment must be known. The patient for whom the therapy is being considered should be similar to the population in which the drug was studied so that the estimated benefits and risks of the drug will be applicable to the patient. One way of weighing these factors is to construct a risk-benefit table.

First, the risk of developing the outcome of interest must be determined from either randomized

Table 18.5. Risk-Benefit Analysis for a 65-Year-Old Man with Atrial Fibrillation

Risk of Stroke Untreated (%/yr)	Risk of Stroke with Warfarin (%/yr)	Absolute Stroke Risk Reduction (%/yr)	Risk of Major Hemorrhage with Warfarin (%/yr)	(%/yr)	(%/yr)
			1.3*	2	5
			Net Benefit-Risk		
4.5*	1.4*	3.1	1.8	1.1	(1.9)
3	1	2	0.7	0	(3)

Note: Numbers in parentheses indicate negative benefit.
*Estimate of these risks taken from Atrial Fibrillation Investigators. Risk factors for stroke and efficacy of antithrombotic therapy in atrial fibrillation. Analysis of pooled data from five randomized controlled trials. Arch Intern Med 1994;154:1449; other estimates are theoretical.

controlled trials or population-based studies. The relative and absolute risk reductions in the outcome of interest are obtained from the randomized controlled trials. The risk of the adverse event of interest is also obtained from the randomized controlled trials' results. Special attention should be paid to the inclusion and exclusion criteria of the trial to ensure that the patient for whom the medication is intended does not differ significantly from the study population. Identification of any clinical factors that affect the benefit or the risk of the medication should be sought from the published results. To calculate the risk–benefit ratio, the absolute risk reduction in the outcome is compared with the risk of the adverse event of interest.

This process is illustrated by a common clinical situation. Consider the risk-benefit analysis for treating a 65-year-old man with new-onset AF and asymptomatic cardiac disease (Table 18.5). Assumptions about risk of stroke, relative and absolute risk reductions due to treatment, and risk of hemorrhage are taken from pooled data from five anticoagulation in AF trials.[59] The yearly risk of stroke without warfarin is estimated to be 4.5%. The estimated treatment benefit is a relative risk reduction of 68% (absolute stroke risk decreased 3.1%, from 4.5% to 1.4%). The yearly risk of major hemorrhage on warfarin is estimated at 1.3%. The net benefit-risk is calculated by subtracting the major hemorrhage risk from the absolute risk reduction, and is thus 1.8 (3.1 – 1.3), indicating a positive benefit for treating this patient.

A similar conclusion about the risk-benefit of warfarin in this example may be reached by comparing the number needed to treat to prevent one outcome to the number needed to treat to cause one adverse event. The reciprocal of the absolute risk reduction gives the number needed to treat to prevent an outcome; in this case, 32 patients (1/0.031) must be treated with warfarin to prevent one stroke. The reciprocal of the major hemorrhage risk gives the number needed to treat to cause one major hemorrhage; in this case 77 (1/0.013). Because the benefit of preventing one stroke is achieved by treating fewer patients than the number necessary to cause one major hemorrhage, warfarin can be assumed to be beneficial.

As the risk of bleeding increases (represented by the theoretical increase to 2% or 5% per year) or as the baseline risk of stroke decreases (represented by the theoretical 3% per year), the potential benefit from treatment is reduced or even reversed. These theoretical calculations illustrate the importance of recognizing risk factors that influence either the risk of the outcome or the risk of an adverse event; small changes in either estimate can quickly shift the net risk–benefit equation.

Conclusion

Anticoagulant and antiplatelet medications are commonly used for both treatment of acute arterial and venous thrombosis and for prophylaxis of thrombosis. Although these medications are effective for treating and preventing serious and even life-threatening conditions, the risk of hemorrhage secondary to the disruption of coagulation must always be considered. Neurologic complications of anticoagulants and antiplatelet agents are usually related to intraparenchymal or ICH, spinal cord hemorrhage, bleeding causing peripheral nerve compression, or ocular hemorrhage. All physicians prescribing anticoagulants must know how to rapidly reverse anticoagulation if serious bleeding does occur. In addition to the risk of bleeding, physicians prescribing anticoagulants and platelet antiaggregants should be aware of other allergic and idiosyncratic reactions patients may experience when taking these medications. For individual patients, the risk-benefit ratio of a given medication can be estimated.

References

1. AMA Drug Evaluations (6th ed). Chicago: American Medical Association, 1986;603.
2. The International Stroke Trial Collaborative Group. The International Stroke Trial. Preliminary results part II: effects of heparin [abstract]. Stroke 1997;28:231.
3. Cerebral Embolism Study Group. Immediate anticoagulation of embolic stroke: a randomized trial. Stroke 1983;14:668.
4. Duke RJ, Bloch RF, Turpie AGG, et al. Intravenous heparin for the prevention of stroke progression in acute partial stable stroke: a randomized controlled trial. Ann Intern Med 1986;105:825.
5. Ramirez-Lassepas M, Quinones MR. Heparin therapy for stroke: hemorrhagic complications and risk factors for intracerebral hemorrhage. Neurology 1984;34:114.
6. Bogousslavsky J, Regli F. Anticoagulant-induced intracerebral bleeding in brain ischemia. Evaluation in 200 patients with TIAs, emboli from the heart, and progressing stroke. Acta Neurol Scand 1985;71:464.
7. Camerlingo M, Casto L, Censori B, et al. Immediate anticoagulation with heparin for first-ever ischemic stroke in the carotid artery territories observed within 5 hours of onset. Arch Neurol 1994;51:462.
8. Babikian VL, Kase CS, Pessin MS, et al. Intracerebral hemorrhage in stroke patients anticoagulated with heparin. Stroke 1989;20:1500.
9. Fisher CM, Adams RD. Observations on brain embolism with special reference to the mechanism of hemorrhagic infarction. J Neuropathol Exp Neurol 1951;10:92.
10. Cerebral Embolism Study Group. Immediate anticoagulation of embolic stroke: brain hemorrhage and management options. Stroke 1984;15:779.
11. Moulin T, Crépin-Leblond T, Chopard J-L, Bogousslavsky J. Hemorrhagic infarcts. Eur Neurol 1993;34:64.
12. Hart RG, Easton JD. Hemorrhagic infarcts. Stroke 1986;17:586.
13. Furlan AJ, Cavalier SJ, Hobbs RE, et al. Hemorrhage and anticoagulation after nonseptic embolic brain infarction. Neurology 1982;32:280.
14. Koller RL, Kovacs AG. Recurrent embolic cerebral infarction and anticoagulation. Neurology 1982;32:283.
15. Lodder J, Van der Lugt PJM. Evaluation of the risk of immediate anticoagulation treatment in patients with embolic stroke of cardiac origin. Stroke 1983;14:42.
16. Rothrock JF, Dittrich HC, McAllen S, et al. Acute anticoagulation following cardioembolic stroke. Stroke 1989;20:730.
17. Pessin MS, Estol CJ, Lafranchise F, Caplan LR. Safety of anticoagulation after hemorrhagic infarction. Neurology 1993;43:1298.
18. Cerebral Embolism Study Group. Cardioembolic stroke, early anticoagulation and brain hemorrhage. Arch Intern Med 1987;147:636.
19. Bogousslavsky J, Regli F, Uske A, Maeder P. Early spontaneous hematoma in cerebral infarct: is primary cerebral hemorrhage overdiagnosed? Neurology 1991;41:837.
20. Beghi E, Goliun G, Cavaletti G, et al. Hemorrhagic infarction: risk factors, clinical and tomographic features and outcome. A case-control study. Acta Neurol Scand 1989;80:226.
21. Ott BR, Samani A, Kleefield J, Funkenstein HH. The clinical spectrum of hemorrhagic infarction. Stroke 1986;17:630.
22. Drapkin A, Merskey C. Anticoagulant therapy after acute myocardial infarction: relation of therapeutic benefit to patient's age, sex, and severity of infarction. JAMA 1972;222:541.
23. Handley AJ, Emerson PA, Fleming PR. Heparin in the prevention of deep vein thrombosis after myocardial infarction. BMJ 1972;2:436.
24. Malloy MH, Cutter GR. The association of heparin exposure with intraventricular hemorrhage among very low birth weight infants. J Perinatol 1995;15:185.
25. Lesko SM, Mitchell AA, Epstein MF, et al. Heparin use as a risk factor for intraventricular hemorrhage in low-birth-weight infants. N Engl J Med 1986;314:1156.
26. Warkentin TE, Levine MN, Hirsh J, et al. Heparin-induced thrombocytopenia in patients treated with low-molecular-weight heparin or unfractionated heparin. N Engl J Med 1995;332:1330.
27. Chong BH. Heparin-induced thrombocytopenia. Br J Haematol 1995;89:431.
28. AbuRahma AF, Boland JP, Witsberger T. Diagnostic and therapeutic strategies of white clot syndrome. Am J Surg 1991;162:175.
29. Greinacher A, Pötzch B, Amiral J, et al. Heparin-associated thrombocytopenia: isolation of the antibody and

characterization of a multimolecular PF4-heparin complex as the major antigen. Thromb Haemost 1994; 71:247.

30. Chong BH, Pitney WR, Castaldi PA. Heparin-induced thrombocytopenia: association of thrombotic complications with heparin-dependent IgG antibody that induces thromboxane synthesis and platelet aggregation. Lancet 1982;2:1246.
31. Warkentin TE, Hayward CPM, Boshkov LK, et al. Sera from patients with heparin-induced thrombocytopenia generate platelet-derived microparticles with procoagulant activity: an explanation for the thrombotic complications of heparin-induced thrombocytopenia. Blood 1994;84:3691.
32. Towne JB, Bernhard VM, Hussey C, Garancis JC. White clot syndrome. Peripheral vascular complications of heparin therapy. Arch Surg 1979;114:372.
33. Benhamou AC, Gruel Y, Barsotti J, et al. The white clot syndrome or heparin associated thrombocytopenia and thrombosis (WCS or HATT): (26 cases). Int Angiol 1985;4:303.
34. Warkentin TE, Kelton JG. A 14-year study of heparin-induced thrombocytopenia. Am J Med 1996;101:502.
35. Atkinson JL, Sundt TM Jr, Kazmier FJ, et al. Heparin-induced thrombocytopenia and thrombosis in ischemic stroke. Mayo Clin Proc 1988;63:353.
36. Tardy-Poncet B, Tardy B, Brelac F, et al. Pentosan polysulfate-induced thrombocytopenia and thrombosis. Am J Hematol 1994;45:252.
37. Rosenthal E, Tiger F, Benoit P, et al. Thrombopenia and fatal intracerebral hemorrhage caused by pentosan polysulfate [letter]. Presse Med 1988;17:126.
38. Bergqvist D, Benoni G, Bjorgell O, et al. Low-molecular-weight heparin (enoxaparin) as prophylaxis against venous thromboembolism after total hip replacement. N Engl J Med 1996;335:696.
39. Geerts WH, Jay RM, Code KI, et al. A comparison of low-dose heparin with low-molecular-weight heparin as prophylaxis against venous thromboembolism after major trauma. N Engl J Med 1996;335:701.
40. Anderson DR, O'Brien BJ, Levine MN, et al. Efficacy and cost of low-molecular-weight heparin compared with standard heparin for the prevention of deep vein thrombosis after total hip arthroplasty. Ann Intern Med 1993;119:1105.
41. Levine M, Gent M, Hirsh J, et al. A comparison of low-molecular-weight heparin administered primarily at home with unfractionated heparin administered in the hospital for proximal deep-vein thrombosis. N Engl J Med 1996;334:677.
42. Koopman MMW, Prandoni P, Piovella F, et al. Treatment of venous thrombosis with intravenous unfractionated heparin administered in the hospital as compared with subcutaneous low-molecular-weight heparin administered at home. N Engl J Med 1996; 334:682.
43. Sternlo JE, Hybbinette CH. Spinal subdural bleeding after attempted epidural and subsequent spinal anaesthesia in a patient on thromboprophylaxis with low molecular weight heparin. Acta Anaesthesiol Scand 1995;39:557.
44. Kay R, Wong KS, Yo YL, et al. Low-molecular-weight heparin for the treatment of acute ischemic stroke. N Engl J Med 1995;333:1588.
45. de Valk HW, Banga JD, Wester JWJ, et al. Comparing subcutaneous danaparoid with intravenous unfractionated heparin for the treatment of venous thromboembolism. A randomized controlled trial. Ann Intern Med 1995;123:1.
46. Biller J, Massey EW, Marler JR, et al. A dose escalation study of ORG 10172 (low molecular weight heparinoid) in stroke. Neurology 1989;39:262.
47. Reid H, Chan K, Thean P. Prolonged coagulation defect (defibrination syndrome) in Malayan viper bite. Lancet 1963;1:621.
48. Pollak VE, Glas-Greenwalt P, Olinger CP, et al. Ancrod causes rapid thrombolysis in patients with acute stroke. Am J Med Sci 1990;299:319.
49. Tonnensen K, Sager P, Gormsen J. Treatment of severe foot ischemia by defibrination with ancrod: a randomized blind study. Scand J Clin Lab Invest 1978;38:431.
50. Sharp A, Warren B, Paxton A, Allington MJ. Anticoagulant therapy with a purified fraction of Malayan pit viper venom. Lancet 1968;1:493.
51. Davies JA, Merrick MV, Sharp AA, Holt JM. Controlled trial of ancrod and heparin in the treatment of deep vein thrombosis of the lower limb. Lancet 1972;1:113.
52. Barrie WW, Wood EH, Crumlish P, et al. Low-dosage ancrod for prevention of thrombotic complications after surgery for fractured neck of femur. BMJ 1974:4:130.
53. Lowe G, Marrice J, Fulton A, et al. Subcutaneous ancrod after operation for fractured hip: a dose-ranging and feasibility study. Thromb Haemostasis 1978;40: 134.
54. Olinger CP, Brott TG, Barsan WG, et al. Use of ancrod in acute or progressing ischemic cerebral infarction. Ann Emerg Med 1988;17:1208.
55. The Ancrod Stroke Study Investigators. Ancrod for the treatment of acute ischemic brain infarction. Stroke 1994;25:1755.
56. Ezekowitz MD, Bridgers SL, James KE, et al. Warfarin in the prevention of stroke associated with nonrheumatic atrial fibrillation. N Engl J Med 1992;327: 1406.
57. Stroke Prevention in Atrial Fibrillation Investigators. Stroke Prevention in Atrial Fibrillation study. Final results. Circulation 1991;84:57.
58. Stroke Prevention in Atrial Fibrillation Investigators. Warfarin versus aspirin for prevention of thromboembolism in atrial fibrillation: Stroke Prevention in Atrial Fibrillation II Study. Lancet 1994;343:687.
59. Atrial Fibrillation Investigators. Risk factors for stroke and efficacy of antithrombotic therapy in atrial fibrilla-

tion. Analysis of pooled data from five randomized controlled trials. Arch Intern Med 1994;154:1449.

60. Stroke Prevention in Atrial Fibrillation Investigators. Adjusted-dose warfarin versus low-intensity, fixed-dose warfarin plus aspirin for high-risk patients with atrial fibrillation: Stroke Prevention in Atrial Fibrillation III randomised clinical trial. Lancet 1996;348:633.
61. EAFT (European Atrial Fibrillation Trial) Study Group. Secondary prevention in non-rheumatic atrial fibrillation after transient ischaemic attack or minor stroke. Lancet 1993;342:1255.
62. Coulshed DS, Fitzpatrick MA, Lee CH. Drug treatment associated with heart valve replacement. Drugs 1995; 49:897.
63. Broderick JP, Phillips SJ, Whisnant JP, et al. Incidence rates of stroke in the eighties: the end of the decline in stroke? Stroke 1989;20:577.
64. Ashok PP, Radhakrishnan K, Sridharan R, et al. Incidence and pattern of cerebrovascular diseases in Benghazi, Libya. J Neurol Neurosurg Psychiatry 1986; 49:519.
65. Bamford J, Sandercock P, Dennis M, et al. A prospective study of acute cerebrovascular disease in the community: the Oxfordshire Community Stroke Project—1981–86. 2. Incidence, case fatality rates and overall outcome at one year of cerebral infarction, primary and subarachnoid hemorrhage. J Neurol Neurosurg Psychiatry 1990;53:16.
66. Giroud M, Gras P, Chadan N, et al. Cerebral haemorrhage in a French prospective population study. J Neurol Neurosurg Psychiatry 1991;54:595.
67. Thrift AG, Donnan GA, McNeil JJ. Epidemiology of intracerebral hemorrhage. Epidemiol Rev 1995;17:361.
68. Franke CL, de Jonge J, van Swieten JC, et al. Intracerebral hematomas during anticoagulant treatment. Stroke 1990;21:726.
69. Wintzen AR, de Jonge H, Loeliger EA, Bots GTAM. The risk of intracerebral hemorrhage during oral anticoagulant treatment: a population study. Ann Neurol 1984;16:553.
70. Fogelholm R, Eskola K, Kiminkinen T, Kunnamo I. Anticoagulant treatment as a risk factor for primary intracerebral haemorrhage. J Neurol Neurosurg Psychiatry 1992;55:1121.
71. Drury I, Whisnant JP, Garraway WM. Primary intracerebral hemorrhage: impact of CT on incidence. Neurology 1984;34:653.
72. Stroke Prevention in Atrial Fibrillation Investigators. Bleeding during antithrombotic therapy in patients with atrial fibrillation. Arch Intern Med 1996;156:409.
73. van der Meer FJM, Rosendaal FR, Vandenbroucke JP, Briët E. Assessment of a bleeding risk index in two cohorts of patients treated with oral anticoagulants. Thromb Haemostasis 1996;76:12.
74. Palareti G, Leali N, Coccheri S, et al. Bleeding complications of oral anticoagulant treatment: an inception-cohort, prospective collaborative study (ISCOAT). Lancet 1996;348:423.
75. Fihn SD, Callahan CM, Marin DC, et al. The risk for and severity of bleeding complications in elderly patients treated with warfarin. Ann Intern Med 1996; 124:970.
76. Juvela S, Hillbom M, Palomäki H. Risk factors for spontaneous intracerebral hemorrhage. Stroke 1995;26: 1558.
77. Dawson I, van Bockel JH, Ferrari MD, et al. Ischemic and hemorrhagic stroke in patients on oral anticoagulants after reconstruction for chronic lower limb ischemia. Stroke 1993;24:1655.
78. Hylek EM, Singer DE. Risk factors for intracranial hemorrhage in outpatients taking warfarin. Ann Intern Med 1994;120:897.
79. Wynne HA, Kamali F, Edwards C, et al. Effect of ageing upon warfarin dose requirements: a longitudinal study. Age Ageing 1996;25:429.
80. Holzgreve W, Carey JC, Hall BD. Warfarin-induced fetal abnormalities. Lancet 1976;2:914.
81. Golbus MS. Teratology for the obstetrician: current status. Obstet Gynecol 1980;55:269.
82. Kaplan LC, Anderson GG, Ring BA. Congenital hydrocephalus and Dandy-Walker malformation associated with warfarin use during pregnancy. Birth Defects: Original Article Series 1982:18(3 Pt A):79.
83. Pati S, Helmbrecht GD. Congenital schizencephaly associated with in utero warfarin exposure. Reproductive Toxicology 1994;8:115.
84. Moore KL. The Developing Human (3rd ed). Philadelphia: Saunders, 1982;56.
85. Raivio KO, Ikonen E, Saarikoski S. Fetal risks due to warfarin therapy during pregnancy. Acta Paediatrica Scand 1977;66:735.
86. Ville Y, Jenkins E, Shearer MJ, et al. Fetal intraventricular haemorrhage and maternal warfarin [letter]. Lancet 1993;34:1211.
87. Zeidman SM, Olivi A. Cervical intramedullary hemorrhage as a result of anticoagulant therapy. J Spinal Disord 1993;6:456.
88. Murphy MA, Nye DH. Thoracic intramedullary haematoma as a complication of warfarin: case report and literature review. Aust N Z J Surg 1991;61:789.
89. Constantini S, Ashkenazi E, Shoshan Y, et al. Thoracic hematomyelia secondary to coumadin anticoagulant therapy: a case report. Eur Neurol 1992;32:109.
90. Rodriguez y Baena R, Gaetani P, Tancioni F, Tartara F. Spinal epidural hematoma during anticoagulant therapy. A case report and review of the literature. J Neurosurg Sci 1995;39:87.
91. Bersen RA, Hoogenraad TU. A spinal haematoma occurring in the subarachnoid as well as in the subdural space in a patient treated with anticoagulants. Clin Neurol Neurosurg 1992;94:35.
92. Groen RJ, Ponssen H. The spontaneous spinal epidural

hematoma. A study of the etiology. J Neurol Sci 1990; 98:121.
93. Messer HD, Forshan VR, Brust JC, Hughes JE. Transient paraplegia from hematoma after lumbar puncture. A consequence of anticoagulant therapy. JAMA 1976; 235:529.
94. Sadjadpour K. Hazards of anticoagulation therapy shortly after lumbar puncture [letter]. JAMA 1977; 237:1692.
95. Heye N. Is there a link between acute spinal epidural hematoma and aspirin? Spine 1995;20:1931.
96. Franscini L, Ballmer PE, Sturzenegger M, et al. Evaluation of back pain secondary to spinal epidural hematoma associated with aspirin intake and a partial platelet glycoprotein Ia/IIa deficiency. Arch Intern Med 1994;154:2768.
97. Dabbert O, Freeman DG, Weis AJ. Spinal meningeal hematoma, warfarin therapy, and chiropractic adjustment. JAMA 1970;214:2058.
98. Owens EL, Kasten GW, Hessel EA II. Spinal subarachnoid hematoma after lumbar puncture and heparinization: a case report, review of the literature, and discussion of anesthetic implications. Anesth Analges 1986;65:1201.
99. Willems J, Anne A, Herregods P, et al. A cauda equina syndrome in a patient treated with oral anticoagulants. Paraplegia 1994;32:277.
100. Malbrain ML, Kamper AM, Lambrecht GL, et al. Filum terminale ependymoma revealed by acute cauda equina compression syndrome following intratumoral and spinal subarachnoid hemorrhage in a patient on oral anticoagulants. Acta Neurol Belg 1994;94:35.
101. Wolfe MW. Intracranial hemorrhage during systemic anticoagulation in patients with cerebral metastasis [letter]. Arch Intern Med 1988;148:1878.
102. Chee CP, Bailey IC, Refsum SE. Spontaneous massive haemorrhage into acoustic neuroma during anticoagulation therapy. Br J Neurosurg 1987;1:489.
103. Altschuler I, Moosa H, Selker RG, et al. The risk and efficacy of anticoagulant therapy in the treatment of thromboembolic complications in patients with primary malignant brain tumors. Neurosurgery 1990;27:74.
104. Choucair AK, Silver P, Levin VA. Risk of intracranial hemorrhage in glioma patients receiving anticoagulant therapy for venous thromboembolism. J Neurosurg 1987;66:357.
105. Spektor S, Ashkenazi E, Israel Z. Intracranial haemorrhage from a meningioma in a patient receiving aspirin prophylaxis: a case report. Acta Neurochir 1995; 134:51.
106. deSouza NM, Cox TC, Hoare RD, Clarke CR. Cerebral siderosis: a complication of anticoagulant therapy? Am J Neuroradiol 1993;14:774.
107. Niakan E, Carbone JE, Adams M, Schroeder FM. Anticoagulants, iliopsoas hematoma and femoral nerve compression. Am Fam Physician 1991;44:2100.
108. Jamjoom ZA, al-Bakry A, al-Momen A, et al. Bilateral femoral nerve compression by iliacus hematomas complicating anticoagulant therapy. Surgery Today 1993;23:535.
109. Peuchal X, Liote F, Kuntz D. Bilateral femoral neuropathy caused by iliacus hematomas during anticoagulation after cardiac catheterization. Am Heart J 1992; 123:262.
110. Zarranz JJ, Simon R, Salisachs P. Acute anticoagulant-induced compressive lumbar plexus neuropathy. A clinico-pathological study. Eur Neurol 1981;20:469.
111. Wallach HW, Oren ME. Sciatic nerve compression during anticoagulation therapy. Computerized tomography aids in diagnosis. Arch Neurol 1979;36:448.
112. Emery S, Ochoa J. Lumbar plexus neuropathy resulting from retroperitoneal hemorrhage. Muscle Nerve 1978;1:330.
113. Chiu WS. The syndrome of retroperioneal hemorrhage and lumbar plexus neuropathy during anticoagulant therapy. South Med J 1976;69:595.
114. Frangides C, Kounis NG. Anticoagulant-induced shoulder hematoma producing brachial plexus neuropathy—case reports. J Angiology 1992;43:701.
115. Luce EA, Futrell JW, Wilgis EF, Hoopes JE. Compression neuropathy following brachial arterial puncture in anticoagulated patients. J Trauma 1976;16:717.
116. Bonantz E, Seabol KE. Acute carpal tunnel syndrome in a patient taking Coumadin: case report. J Trauma 1993;35:143.
117. Copeland J, Wells HG Jr, Puckett CL. Acute carpal tunnel syndrome in a patient taking Coumadin. J Trauma 1989;29:131.
118. Mathis A, Camuzet F. [Anticoagulants and the eye]. [French] Année Thérapeutique et Clinique en Ophtalmologie 1982;33:299.
119. Holden R. Spontaneous hyphaema as a result of systemic anticoagulation in previously abnormal eyes. Postgrad Med J 1991;67:1008.
120. Brown GC, Tasman WS, Shields JA. Massive subretinal hemorrhage and anticoagulant therapy. Can J Ophthalmol 1982;17:227.
121. Simel PJ. Anticoagulation, intraocular bleeding and pupillary paralysis following Choyce intraocular lens implantation. Journal of the American Intra-ocular Implant Society 1978;4:117.
122. Browne TR, Wray SH. Subconjuctival hemorrhage as a complication of ophthalmodynamometry in an anticoagulated patient. Am J Ophthalmol 1973;76:981.
123. Steering Committee of the Physicians' Health Study Research Group. Final report on the aspirin component of the ongoing Physicians' Health Study. N Engl J Med 1989;321:129.
124. Peto R, Gray R, Collins R, et al. Randomised trial of prophylactic daily aspirin in British male doctors. BMJ 1988;296:313.
125. Antiplatelet Trialists' Collaboration. Collaborative review of randomized trials of antiplatelet therapy-I:

prevention of death, myocardial infarction, and stroke by prolonged antiplatelet therapy in various categories of patients. BMJ 1994;308:81.
126. Antiplatelet Trialists' Collaboration. Secondary prevention of vascular disease by prolonged antiplatelet treatment. BMJ 1988;296:320.
127. ISIS-2 (Second International Study of Infarct Surival) Collaborative Group. Randomised trial of intravenous steptokinase, oral aspirin, both, or neither among 17,187 cases of suspected acute myocardial infarction: ISIS-2. Lancet 1988;2:349.
128. Juul-Möller S, Edvardsson N, Jahnmatz B, et al. Double-blind trial of aspirin in primary prevention of myocardial infarction in patients with stable chronic angina pectoris. The Swedish Angina Pectoris Aspirin Trial (SAPAT) Group. Lancet 1992;340:1421.
129. ISIS-3 (Third International Study of Infarct Survival) Collaborative Group. ISIS-3: a randomised comparison of streptokinase vs tissue plasminogen activator vs anistreplase and of aspirin plus heparin vs aspirin alone among 41,299 cases of suspected acute myocardial infarction. Lancet 1992;339:753.
130. Hirsh J, Dalen JE, Fuster V, et al. Aspirin and other platelet-active drugs. The relationship between dose, effectiveness and side effects. Chest 1992;102S:327S.
131. Krupski WC, Weiss DG, Rapp JH, et al. and the VA Cooperative Asymptomatic Carotid Artery Stenosis Study Group. Adverse effects of aspirin in the treatment of asymptomatic carotid artery stenosis. J Vasc Surg 1992;16:588.
132. The SALT Collaborative Group. Swedish Aspirin Low-Dose Trial (SALT) of 75 mg aspirin as secondary prophylaxis after cerebrovascular ischaemic events. Lancet 1991;338:1345.
133. UK-TIA Study Group. United Kingdom Transient Ischaemic Attack (UK-TIA) aspirin trial: interim results. BMJ 1988;296:316.
134. Swedish Cooperative Study. High-dose acetylsalicylic acid after cerebral infarction. Stroke 1987;18:325.
135. Bousser MG, Eschwege E, Haguenau M, et al. "AICLA" controlled trial of aspirin and dipyridamole in the secondary prevention of athero-thrombotic cerebral ischemia. Stroke 1983;14:5.
136. The Dutch TIA Trial Study Group. A comparison of two doses of aspirin (30 mg vs. 283 mg a day) in patients after a transient ischemic attack or minor ischemic stroke. N Engl J Med 1991;325:1261.
137. European Stroke Prevention Study Group. European Stroke Prevention Study (ESPS): principal end points. Lancet 1987;2:1351.
138. Karlowicz MG, White LE. Severe intracranial hemorrhage in a term neonate associated with maternal acetylsalicylic acid ingestion. Clin Pediatr 1993;32:740.
139. Rumack CM, Guggenheim MA, Rumack BH, et al. Neonatal intracranial hemorrhage and maternal use of aspirin. Obstet Gynecol 1981;58(5 Suppl):52S.
140. Page Y, Tardy B, Zeni F, et al. Thrombotic thrombocytopenic purpura related to ticlopidine. Lancet 1991;337:1219.
141. Capra R, Marciano N, Fieni F, et al. Cerebral hemorrhage and thrombotic thrombocytopenic purpura during ticlopidine treatment: case report. Acta Neurol Belg 1992;92:83.
142. Gent M, Easton JD, Hachinski VC, et al. The Canadian-American ticlopidine study (CATS) in thromboembolic stroke. Lancet 1989;1:1215.
143. Hass WK, Easton JD, Adams HP, et al. A randomized trial comparing ticlopidine hydrochloride with aspirin for the prevention of stroke in high-risk patients. N Engl J Med 1989;321:501.
144. CAPRIE Steering Committee. A randomised, blinded, trial of clopidogrel versus aspirin in patients at risk of ischaemic events (CAPRIE). Lancet 1996;348:1329.

Chapter 19

Neurologic Complications of Thrombolytic Therapy

Michael A. Sloan

Objectives

- To define the types of neurologic complications that occur after thrombolytic therapy in diverse clinical settings
- To understand the frequency, types, risk factors, causes, management, and outcome of intracranial and spinal hemorrhage occurring after thrombolytic therapy for acute myocardial infarction
- To understand the frequency, risk factors, and management of ischemic stroke occurring after thrombolytic therapy for acute myocardial infarction and other disorders
- To understand the frequency, risk factors, and other associations of brain hemorrhage occurring after thrombolytic therapy for acute ischemic infarction
- To appreciate the rationale for and hemorrhagic complications of thrombolytic therapy for intracerebral and subarachnoid hemorrhage (SAH)
- To describe the peripheral neuromuscular complications of thrombolytic therapy

Neurologic disorders are feared complications of thrombolytic therapy. The most serious adverse event, intracranial hemorrhage (ICH), was first identified in early studies of therapeutic thrombolysis for presumed acute ischemic stroke patients.[1–6] These investigations were limited, however, by lack of availability of computed tomography (CT) scans to exclude patients with hematomas and clear cerebrospinal fluid (CSF), significant hypertension before or during neurologic worsening, use of combined anticoagulant and thrombolytic therapy, and frequent presence of a systemic fibrinolytic state.[1, 2, 5–9] Despite these limitations, such experiences delayed investigation of therapeutic thrombolysis into the 1980s and 1990s. Extensive recent clinical work has shown that thrombolytic therapy may be effective for selected patients with acute myocardial infarction (AMI),[10–98] deep vein thrombosis,[7, 99–109] pulmonary embolism,[110–125] peripheral arterial occlusive disease,[7, 126] and hyperacute ischemic cerebral infarction (ACI).[127–215] However, in these and other publications, a variety of central and peripheral neurologic complications have been reported, including stroke (ICH[216–245] and ischemic cerebral infarction[246–260]), spinal epidural hemorrhage,[261–266] Guillain-Barré syndrome,[267–269] neuropathies,[270–273] and myopathies.[272] This chapter analyzes the different types of neurologic complications, with emphasis on risk factors, clinical features, diagnosis, and management, where information is available.

A variety of central nervous system (CNS) complications have been described after thrombolytic therapy for each thromboembolic disorder. These include ICH, parenchymatous intracerebral hemorrhage (PIH), subdural hematoma (SDH), epidural hematoma (EPH), SAH, intraventricular hemorrhage (IVH), ischemic cerebral infarction (CI), and ischemic cerebral infarction with hemorrhagic transformation (HI). The average frequency of ICH after therapeutic thrombolysis in available large studies is 0.47% for AMI[10–12, 15, 18, 19, 21, 23–34, 90–92, 235] (Table 19.1), 0.21% for deep venous thrombosis,[7, 99–109] and 0.98% for pulmonary embolism.[110–125] Each of these complications has been best studied in the setting of AMI. It is therefore essential to define the specific characteristics of these disorders in order to identify risk factors and underlying causes to facilitate optimal patient care.

PIH refers to primary bleeding within brain parenchyma. These lesions are generally thought to be nonterritorial, compact, or confluent blood collections that have, on CT scan, a homogeneous density and sharp edge, often with a surrounding mass effect occurring after several days.[31, 33, 84, 85, 235] In two AMI studies, PIH was classified on the basis of focal neurologic deficits associated with focal collections of blood within brain parenchyma seen on CT scan with neither a normal brain image at the time of onset of neurologic symptoms nor evidence of preceding CI.[31, 33, 235] In patients with ACI, PIH refers to a blood collection in a region remote from the presumed CI site.

Extraparenchymal hemorrhage may also occur. First, SDH may be diagnosed if a high- or mixed-density fluid collection is seen in the subdural space.[31, 33, 235] There may be sulcal effacement and mass effect on CT scan. Second, EPH may be diagnosed if a high-density fluid collection is seen in the cranial or spinal epidural space.[261–266] SAH may be diagnosed if a high-density fluid collection is seen in the subarachnoid space. IVH may be diagnosed if a high-density fluid collection is seen in the ventricular system. Both SAH and IVH may be primary or secondary to PIH extension.

Ischemic CI is defined as a focal neurologic deficit that lasts longer than 24 hours, with or without a corresponding lesion on neuroimaging studies.[31, 235] Cardioembolic, lacunar, and border zone infarctions have been described.[32]

Hemorrhagic transformation or conversion of CI (HI) refers to secondary bleeding believed to occur either with early reperfusion into a damaged vascular bed with impaired autoregulation or because of development of collateral circulation into the same vascular bed. HIs are strictly territorial, and CT scans show mixed areas of hypodensity and hyperdensity, with an indistinct edge and no significant mass effect at an early stage.[84] HI may be diagnosed by the appearance of blood with the presumed CI location if (1) blood densities were not present on the initial CT image, or (2) blood densities on the first CT scan are surrounded by a region of radiolucency consistent with ischemic CI.[32] The extent of HI may range from petechial change (variable hypodensity or hyperdensity) to confluent hematoma, thus mimicking primary PIH.[32] Thus, it may be extremely difficult to distinguish confluent HI from PIH on a CT scan.[32, 33] In some of these cases, there may also be signs of early CI, such as hemispheric sulcal effacement, that may facilitate lesion classification.

Stroke Complicating Thrombolysis for Acute Myocardial Infarction

General Aspects

The occurrence of stroke has long been known to be a serious but infrequent complication of AMI. In the prethrombolytic era, stroke was reported to complicate the course of AMI in 1.7–3.2% of patients,[274–277] with a mortality of 54–61%.[70, 71] A typical stroke occurred during the first week after AMI, although as many as 33% occurred within 24 hours of AMI onset. The occurrence of stroke correlated with anterior or apical infarction,[274, 275] large infarct size,[274] atrial arrhythmias,[275] cardiac pump failure or Killip Class IV,[275] and history of previous stroke.[275] Most, if not all, strokes were attributed to cerebral embolism. Anticoagulant therapy for AMI was complicated by CNS hemorrhage in 0.05–0.14% of treated patients.[278, 279]

In the thrombolytic era, a number of changes in the characteristics of stroke have occurred. First, the reported occurrence rate of stroke complicating AMI in placebo-controlled,[10–20] comparative,[10–12, 15, 18, 19, 21, 23–34, 90, 92, 235] (see Table 19.1), and many smaller trials[35–49, 51–59, 240] has decreased. This has been observed in trials using streptokinase (SK),[10–15, 21–25, 90, 92, 235] anisoylated plasminogen-SK activator complex (APSAC),[16, 17, 25] recombinant tissue plasminogen activator (rt-PA),[18–23, 25–29, 31–34, 91, 235] recombinant single

Table 19.1. Cerebrovascular Complications in Large Comparative Coronary Thrombolysis Trials

Study	Reference	Stroke Incidence		Stroke Subtypes No. (%)			
		No.	%	ICH	CI	NS	SDH
Streptokinase							
GISSI-1	10–12	49/5,860	0.8	8 (16)	9 (19)	32 (65)	—
ISIS-2	15	61/8,592	0.7	7 (11)	—	54 (89)	—
GISSI-2	21, 23	54/6,199	0.9	15 (28)	24 (44)	15 (28)	—
ISG	22, 23	44/4197	1.0	15 (34)	22 (50)	7 (16)	—
Netherlands[a]	24	24/2,469	1.0	24 (100)	—	—	—
ISIS-3[b]	25	141/13,607	1.0	25 (18)	66 (47)	50 (35)	—
EMERAS	90	34/2,234	1.5	18 (53)	16 (47)	—	—
GUSTO-I +sch[c]	235	117/9,841	1.2	41 (35)	62 (53)	10 (9)	7 (6)
GUSTO-I +ivh[c]	235	144/10,410	1.4	57 (40)	73 (51)	12 (8)	9 (6)
INJECT + ivh	92	30/3,066	1.00	11 (37)	9 (30)	10 (33)	—
Subtotal[d]		698/66,715		227 (33)	281 (40)	190 (27)	16 (2)
Percent of all patients[e]			1.05	0.34	0.42	0.29	0.02
Recombinant tissue plasminogen activator (rt-PA)							
ASSET	18, 19	28/2,516	1.1	7 (25)	11 (39)	10 (36)	—
TAMI[f]	26–28	13/1,696	0.8	11 (85)	—	—	6 (4)
Burroughs-Wellcome	29	9/1,900	0.5	9 (100)	—	—	—
TIMI-2	31–33						
150 mg		23/908	2.5	12 (52)	9 (39)	—	2 (9)
100 mg		33/3,016	1.1	11 (33)	20 (61)	—	2 (6)
GISSI-2	21, 22	70/6,182	1.1	19 (28)	28 (40)	23 (32)	—
ISG	22, 23	68/4,190	1.6	25 (37)	26 (38)	17 (25)	—
ISIS-3[b]	25	188/13,569	1.4	76 (40)	55 (29)	57 (31)	—
MITI[g]	34	22/1,413	1.6	15 (68)	7 (32)	—	—
GUSTO-I[h]	235	161/10,396	1.5	72 (45)	79 (49)	9 (6)	8 (5)
LATE	91	65/2,836	2.3	30 (46)	35 (54)	—	—
Subtotal[d]		680/48,622		287 (42)	270 (40)	116 (17)	18 (3)
Percent of all patients[e]			1.40	0.59	0.56	0.24	0.04
Anisoylated plasminogen streptokinase activator complex							
ISIS-3[b]	25	172/13,599		54 (31)	45 (26)	73 (43)	—
Percent of all patients[e]			1.26	0.40	0.33	0.53	—

Table 19.1. *continued.*

Study	Reference	Stroke Incidence No.	Stroke Incidence %	Stroke Subtypes No. (%) ICH	CI	NS	SDH
Accelerated rt-PA and reduced streptokinase							
GUSTO-I[i]	235	170/10,374		84 (49)	67 (39)	12 (7)	16 (9)
Percent of all patients[e]			1.64	0.81	0.65	0.12	0.15
Recombinant single chain urokinase plasminogen activator (r-scuPA)							
	30	15/1,698		8 (53)	7 (47)	—	—
Percent of all patients[e]			0.88	0.47	0.41	—	—
Reteplase							
INJECT[j]	92	77/3,084		23 (62)	10 (27)	4 (11)	—
Percent of all patients[e]			1.2	0.77	0.33	0.13	—
Total[d]		1,772/143,712		677 (38)	680 (38)	395 (22)	50 (3)
Percent of all treated patients			1.23	0.47	0.47	0.27	0.03

GISSI-1 = Gruppo Italiano per lo studio della streptochinasi nell'Infarto Miocardico; ISIS-2 = Second International Study of Infarct Survival; GISSI-2 = Gruppo Italiano per lo studio della Sopravvivenza nell'Infarto Miocardico; ISG = International Study Group; Netherlands = Netherlands Cooperative Registry, Thoraxcenter, University Hospital of Erasmus University; ISIS-3 = Third International Study of Infarct Survival; ASSET = Anglo-Scandinavian Study of Early Thrombolysis; TIMI-2 = Thrombolysis in Myocardial Infarction, Phase II; TAMI = Thrombolysis and Angioplasty in Myocardial Infarction, 1–3; MITI = Myocardial Infarction Triage and Intervention Project; GUSTO-I = Global Utilization of Streptokinase and rt-PA for Occluded Coronary Arteries; EMERAS = Estudio Multicéntrico Estreptoquinasa Repúblicas de América del Sur; LATE = Late Assessment of Thrombolytic Efficacy; INJECT = International Joint Efficacy Comparison of Thrombolytics; No. = number of patients with specific stroke subtypes in each study; ICH = definite intracerebral hemorrhage; CI = definite ischemic cerebral infarction; NS = stroke subtype unspecified or "probable" ischemic infarction or "probable" intracranial hemorrhage; SDH = subdural hematoma; sch = subcutaneous heparin; ivh = intravenous heparin.

[a]For the Netherlands Study, 1,791 of 2,469 (72.5%) patients were treated with streptokinase. In this study, no attempt was made to distinguish parenchymatous ICH from hemorrhagic transformation of ischemic cerebral infarction.

[b]In ISIS-3, duteplase rt-PA was used. Only definite stroke subtype diagnoses were categorized as ICH or CI, whereas probable diagnoses were assigned to the NS category. In addition, "definite" ICH included patients with parenchymatous intracerebral hemorrhage, subarachnoid hemorrhage, and hemorrhagic infarction.

[c]In GUSTO-I, the streptokinase groups were defined by concomitant use of subcutaneous or intravenous heparin. The ICH group contains intracerebral hemorrhage and intracerebral hemorrhage plus subdural hematoma. The SDH group contains patients with subdural hematoma and subdural hematoma plus intracerebral hemorrhage.

[d]In the subtotal and total lines, the numbers in parentheses refer to the percentage of strokes in each group.

[e]Numbers refer to the reported occurrence rate of each stroke subtype in the entire population treated with each thrombolytic agent or thrombolytic agent combination in the cited studies.

[f]In the TAMI studies, six of 13 (46.2%) stroke patients had been treated with rt-PA, four of 13 (30.8%) stroke patients had been treated with streptokinase, and one of 13 (7.7%) stroke patients had been treated with rt-PA and urokinase. Because the number of individuals treated with each thrombolytic regimen in this study (N = 1,696) was not stated, all intracranial hemorrhages were assigned to the rt-PA group to facilitate analysis.

[g]In the MITI Project, 1,137 of 1,413 (80.5%) patients received rt-PA. Hemorrhagic stroke was defined by the appearance of blood on the computed tomography (CT) scan, and no attempt was made to distinguish between parenchymatous intracerebral hemorrhage and hemorrhagic infarction. Ischemic infarction was defined as a stroke with the CT scan either not being performed or failing to show blood. Because the number of individuals suffering stroke after use of specific thrombolytic agents was not stated, all strokes were assigned to the rt-PA group to facilitate analysis.

[h]In the GUSTO-I trial, "accelerated" rt-PA was given (100 mg over 90 mins) with intravenous heparin. See text for definitions of ICH, SDH, and CI.

[i]In the GUSTO-I trial, "accelerated" rt-PA (1.0 mg per kg, <90 mg, over 60 mins), "reduced" streptokinase (1.0 million U over 60 mins), and intravenous heparin were given.

[j]In the INJECT trial, two cases in the reteplase group were assessed by investigators as hemorrhagic, but no CT scan or autopsy data were available.

Table 19.2. Overall Stroke-Related Mortality in Previous Large Coronary Thrombolysis Trials

Study	Reference	Agent	No. of Patients (%)[a]	Mortality: Treatment Group No. (%)	Mortality: Control Group No. (%)
GISSI	10–12	SK	11,712 (23)	23/54 (43)	24/45 (53)
ISIS-2[b]	15	SK	17,187 (34)	36/86 (42)	44/112 (39)
EMERAS	90	SK	4,534 (9)	20/34 (59)	10/25 (40)
ASSET	18, 19	rt-PA	5,011 (10)	11/51 (22)	6/34 (18)
TIMI-2[c]	31–33	rt-PA	3,924 (8)	21/56 (38)	—
MITI[d]	34	rt-PA	1,413 (3)	14/22 (64)	27/94 (29)
LATE	91	rt-PA	5,711 (11)	30/65 (46)	14/34 (41)
AIMS	16, 17	APSAC	1,258 (2)	4/8 (50)	3/4 (75)
Total			50,750 (100)	159/376 (42)	128/348 (37)

SK = streptokinase; rt-PA = recombinant tissue plasminogen activator; APSAC = anisoylated plasminogen-streptokinase activator complex; ASA = acetylsalicylic acid; ICH; intracerebral hemorrhage; SDH = subdural hematoma; CI = ischemic cerebral infarction.
[a]Plain numbers are numbers of patients, while numbers in parentheses are percentages of total patients where stroke-related mortality can be evaluated.
[b]Includes SK and SK plus ASA groups.
[c]Includes ICH, SDH, and CI cases.
[d]Includes ICH and CI cases.

chain urokinase plasminogen activator (r-scuPA),[30] reteplase,[92] and various combination or front-loaded thrombolytic therapy regimens.[85] The incidence of stroke in treated groups is 0.5–2.5% (mean, 1.13%) and in control groups it is 0–1.0% (mean, 0.81%).[10–30] This apparent reduction in overall stroke risk may be due to improved treatment of general and high-risk AMI patients or exclusion of patients at high risk of stroke.[12, 18, 24–27,31] Second, the distribution of stroke subtypes has shifted to include PIH, SDH, SAH, ICH, EPH, and HI (see Table 19.1). The wide variation in stroke rates, specifically for hemorrhagic stroke subtypes, could have been due to chance, different effects of the various thrombolytic agents, or different intensity of the evaluation and reporting of stroke complications.[11, 12, 15, 16, 18, 31–33, 235] For example, more recent comparative trials have low rates of stroke, unspecified type.[31, 32, 92, 235] Third, the occurrence, location, and timing of PIH may have implications for patient selection, both for AMI and ACI patients (vide infra).

In placebo-controlled studies[10–20] using SK,[10–15] rt-PA,[18–20] and APSAC,[16, 17] overall stroke-related mortality is similar between treatment and control groups (Table 19.2). Several large trials have reported that ICH has a higher stroke-related mortality than ischemic stroke. Data from GISSI-2[21–23] and ISIS-3[25] suggest a slight but significant improvement in combined stroke survival at day 35 (0.7% versus 0.5%, with $2P < .05$), and a slight but significant improvement in ICH survival at day 35, either alone (0.3% versus 0.2%, with $2P < .00001$) or combined (0.2% versus 0.1%, with $2P < .00001$) with rt-PA therapy. For the concomitant antithrombotic therapies, use of aspirin plus subcutaneous heparin versus aspirin alone was associated with a slight but significant increase in ICH occurrence and a slight but significant increase in ICH survival, either alone (0.2% versus 0.1%, with $2P < .05$) or combined (0.2% versus 0.1%, with $2P < .01$).[21–23, 25] In GUSTO-I, 41% of all stroke patients died, with no significant differences in fatality rates between the four thrombolytic/antithrombotic regimens.[235] However, there were strong differences in mortality by stroke subtype. The 60% ICH mortality in GUSTO-I confirms the experience in other large coronary thrombolysis trials.[26–28, 31, 33] However, the higher ICH mortality in GUSTO-I compared with the Burroughs-Wellcome duteplase rt-PA trial (44%) and TIMI-2 trial (52%) might be explained by the more aggressive combined thrombolytic/antithrombotic regimens used in that study.[29, 31, 33] The 17% mortality for CI in GUSTO-I compares favorably with the 21% in TIMI-2, 35% in GISSI-2, and 57% in MITI.[21, 23, 31, 32, 34] The 32.4% mortality among patients with HI in GUSTO-I[235] is higher than the 12.5% in TIMI-2,[32] suggesting that the HIs may have been more severe, the affected patients had more serious cardiac disease, or some other reason. There was a 72.1% mortality in the stroke of unknown cause group in GUSTO-I, somewhat higher than the 54.8% mortality for strokes of unknown cause in GISSI-2.[21, 23, 235] These findings suggest that many strokes of unknown cause may be unrecognized ICHs or are strokes that affect patients who have more serious cardiovascular disease and thus are more likely to die, or there is some other reason.

In ISIS-2, there was no difference in occurrence of disabling stroke between treatment and control groups, although partial recovery with minor residual was more frequent in ischemic stroke (41%) than hemorrhagic stroke (22%).[15] In TIMI-2, there was no significant difference in occurrence of partial recovery with major residual between CI (21%) and ICH (17%).[31] In MITI, 7 of 11 (67%) ICH and 19 of 56 (34%) CI were discharged to a nursing home, suggesting an increased disability rate in ICH survivors.[34] In GUSTO-I, the proportions of patients with varying degrees of residual neurologic disability did not significantly differ by treatment assignment. Approximately two-thirds of ICH survivors were moderately to severely disabled, and one-half of HI survivors were severely disabled whereas 38% of CI survivors had minimal or no disability. In the GUSTO-I North American Quality of Life substudy, patients with severe or moderate disability had significantly diminished time trade-off values (0.71 ± 0.31 or 0.81 ± 0.34) compared with patients with minor or no residual deficits (0.89 ± 0.15 or 0.92 ± 0.17) or other patients without stroke (0.87 ± 0.20). Moreover, the data indicate that the majority of patients who survive a stroke after thrombolysis for AMI do not rate their outcomes as "worse than death."[235]

Intracranial Hemorrhage

ICH has been reported to occur during[18, 31, 33, 48, 53, 54] and usually within 24 hours or less after infusion,[11, 12, 14, 15, 18, 24, 25, 31, 33, 235] irrespective of the dosage or aggressiveness of the thrombolytic or antithrombotic regimen. In two studies, 65–77% of ICHs occurred within 24 hours of study entry.[31, 33, 235] The overall average frequency of PIH is 0.47%, with 0.34% for SK, 0.59% for rt-PA, 0.40% for APSAC, 0.47% for r-scuPA, 0.77% for reteplase, and 0.81% for combined rt-PA and SK (see Table 19.1). As many as 77% of ICHs occur in lobar or subcortical lobar sites[31, 33, 235]; 15–33% are multiple ICHs,[29, 31, 33, 235, 243] and up to 15% may be combined PIH and SDH.[243] On brain images, PIH are confluent (80%), mottled (20%), and usually (76%) have blood fluid levels.[26, 243] These patterns of PIH location and imaging characteristics are more typical of coagulopathy-induced or other nonhypertensive causes of PIH.[85] Patients typically develop an acute change in the level of consciousness, coma, unifocal or multifocal neurologic symptoms and signs, nausea, vomiting, headache, and seizures.[27, 33] Acute hypertension may also be observed.[33] In many cases, onset is catastrophic and rapidly fatal.[14, 15, 18, 31, 33, 74, 75, 79] Patients with spinal EPH develop back pain, motor or sensory loss at or below the level of the hematoma, or urinary or fecal incontinence that may evolve over hours.[261–266] Thus, changes in neurologic function, particularly in the first 24 hours after treatment, should be highly suspicious of CNS hemorrhage.

Risk Factors

On the basis of available data, putative risk factors for ICH have been identified. These include age, gender, systolic hypertension, diastolic hypertension, excess pulse pressure, type and dosage of thrombolytic agent, anticoagulant therapy at study entry, prior neurologic disease, low body weight, dementia, head or face trauma, and use of concomitant medications. Table 19.3 shows the most well-established risk factors for ICH after coronary thrombolysis.

The mortality in elderly patients with AMI, even if treated with SK[45, 66, 232] or rt-PA,[25, 66, 280] increases dramatically from age of younger than 65 years to older than 75 years.[281, 282] In the GUSTO-I trial, 30-day mortality was 2.8% in patients younger than 65 years old, 9.1% in patients 65–74 years old, 19.1% in patients 75–84 years old, and 30.3% in patients older than 85 years old.[234] Because the elderly constitute an ever increasing proportion of the population at risk and only 30% of eligible patients receive thrombolytic therapy, investigators have sought to extend treatment to this age group.[283–289] A meta-analysis of five large trials suggested that thrombolytic therapy may significantly reduce mortality in the elderly (17.9%) when compared with control subjects (22.1%).[11, 12, 14, 16, 18, 284] A recent cost-effectiveness analysis suggested that SK therapy in elderly patients may be beneficial.[288] Data from the GUSTO-I trial suggest that the accelerated rt-PA regimen is associated with lower mortality in patients 85 years and younger.[234] In addition, data from the National Registry of Myocardial Infarction show that the proportion of elderly AMI patients receiving thrombolytic therapy has increased over time (ages 75–84 years: 16% from 1990–1991, 21.4% from 1993–1994; ages 85+ years: 5.3% from 1990–1991, 9.1% from 1993–1994).[290] However, elderly patients may be more likely to have bleeding complications.[66, 280, 291] Some investigators have expressed concern that elderly patients may have more defects in cerebrovascular integrity, particularly because older age is associated with silent vascular disease.[28, 53] In small studies, older age was variably associated with an increased risk of ICH in patients treated with rt-PA.[28, 55, 66] In three large trials, both SK and rt-PA were associated with an excess of strokes in older patients (>70 years: 2.7% rt-PA, 1.6% SK; <70 years: 0.9% rt-PA, 0.8% SK).[21–23] In TIMI-2 and GUSTO-I, older patients had a significantly increased frequency of PIH when age was treated as a continuous variable.[31, 235] In TIMI-3B, which used 0.8 mg per kg rt-PA (maximum, 80 mg; mean, 63 mg), there were four ICHs (0.55%): two of 30 (6.7%) in patients older than age 75 and two of 699 (0.2%) in patients 75 years and younger (P = .01).[240] In GUSTO-I, age was the most important factor independently associated with ICH risk.[235] Hemorrhagic strokes occurred in 0.3% of patients younger than 65 years, 1% of patients between 65 and 74 years, 1.6% of patients between 75 and 84 years, and 1.7% of patients older than age 85 years.[234] In the aggregate, although thrombolytic therapy for elderly AMI patients may be associated with more strokes, the overall reduction in mortality suggests that the benefits of careful thrombolysis may outweigh the risks.[85]

Table 19.3. Risk Factors for Intracranial Hemorrhage After Coronary Thrombolysis

Age
Low body weight
Prior neurologic or cerebrovascular disease
Dementia
Head or facial injury within 2 weeks of study entry
Anticoagulant therapy at study entry
Diastolic blood pressure
Type and dosage of thrombolytic regimen

Recent work has examined the relationship between a history of hypertension or acute hypertension and ICH occurrence after thrombolytic therapy. Gorelick and colleagues reported a patient with poorly controlled hypertension who had a fatal cerebellar PIH after intracoronary SK.[75] In ISIS-2, although persistent severe hypertension was a relative contraindication, the mortality with systolic blood pressure of more than 175 mm Hg was 5.7% in patients treated with SK versus 8.7% in controls.[15] O'Connor and colleagues found lower blood pressure in four patients with ICH than in nine patients with CI.[28] In a small retrospective study, Anderson and colleagues reported that transient systolic blood pressure of more than 150 mm Hg was associated with ICH.[66] Althouse and colleagues reported that two of nine (22%) patients with transient systolic blood pressure of more than 180 mm Hg before rt-PA treatment versus one of 147 (0.7%) patients without this level of blood pressure before rt-PA treatment had ICH.[64] In TIMI-2, PIH was more frequent among patients with chronic hypertension than among patients without chronic hypertension (0.9% versus 0.7%), although this difference was not statistically significant.[31] However, PIH occurred in two of 22 (9.1%) patients with systolic blood pressure of more than 180 mm Hg or diastolic blood pressure of more than 110 mm Hg before study entry compared with nine of 647 (1.4%) patients without elevated blood pressure. One patient, who initially had severe hypertension that was then controlled at the time of study entry, subsequently had recurrent severe hypertension despite treatment and suffered a PIH. In GISSI-2, diastolic blood pressure of more than 110 mm Hg was associated with ICH.[21, 23] In the 19 ICH cases identified in the Thrombolytic Predictive Instrument Project, Selker and colleagues reported that an "excess pulse pressure" (extent to which pulse pressure exceeded 40 mm Hg for systolic blood pressures of more than 120 mm Hg) was strongly associated with ICH.[226] For each 10-point pulse pressure excess, the relative risk for ICH was increased by 1.85 (P = .0002; 95% CI = 1.34–2.55) by itself and 1.76 (P = .001; 95% CI = 1.26–2.46) when adjusted for age. In GUSTO-I, multivariable analysis of 268 ICH cases showed that diastolic blood pressure, hypertension, an interaction between hypertension and lower age, and systolic blood pressure, but not excess pulse pressure, were each independently associated with ICH risk.[235] For diastolic hypertension, the ICH frequencies were 0.58% (70–79 mm Hg), 0.69% (80–89 mm Hg), 0.95% (90–99 mm Hg), and 0.76% (≥100 mm Hg). For systolic hypertension, the ICH frequencies were 0.45% (100–124 mm Hg), 0.72% (125–149 mm Hg), 0.93% (150–174 mm Hg), and 1.71% (≥175 mm Hg). For both systolic and diastolic blood pressures, the mortality was highest in patients with the lowest blood pressures, with no substantial change as systolic and diastolic blood pressures increased. There was no significant interaction between the effect of treatment assignment (rt-PA or SK) and blood pressure at study entry or rates of death within 30 days of randomization or death plus disabling stroke.[237] Although a significant incremental elevation in blood pressure may contribute to ICH occurrence in some cases, it is still possible that severe hypertension at the time of recognition of change in neurologic function may reflect a systemic response to an acute cerebrovascular insult and not be its cause.

Patients with body weight of less than 70 kg, particularly women, have higher rt-PA concentrations during the infusion and, with more fibrinogenolysis, may have a greater risk of bleeding complications.[24, 28, 53] In ISIS-2, body mass index was not associated with risk of hemorrhagic stroke, although data collection was limited.[23] In GUSTO-I, low body weight was the second most important factor independently associated with ICH risk.[235]

In coronary thrombolysis trials, potential study patients with history of acute ischemic cerebrovascular disease within 3 months of study entry have generally been excluded.[84, 281] In the TIMI-2 pilot and early clinical trial, patients with acute cerebrovascular disease within the 6 months before AMI presentation were excluded.[31] In the initial phase of the study, three of 30 (10%) patients with a history of stroke, intermittent cerebral ischemic attack, or other neurologic disease had PIH compared with eight of 639 (1.2%) without stroke histories. At this point, the protocol was changed to make patients with histories of stroke or intermittent cerebral ischemic attacks ineligible. Because the observed excess risk of PIH was based on the observation of only three patients who had PIH in the high-risk group, the estimated increased risk was imprecise (95% CI = 1.97–22.81). In the GUSTO-I trial, the frequency of ICH was 2.9% in patients with a history of transient ischemic attacks and 2.4% in patients with a history of stroke.[235] In a multivariable analysis, prior cerebrovascular disease was the third most important factor independently associated with ICH risk. In the GUSTO-I case control study, patients with a history of stroke had a moderate increase in ICH risk (OR = 2.8, 95% CI = 1.1–6.6).[241]

Other neuropathology may be associated with increased risk of ICH. In TIMI-2, three of five autopsied PIH patients had cortical neuritic plaques; two of three had plaque frequencies consistent with the diagnosis of Alzheimer's disease had the patients been demented.[33] In the GUSTO-I case control study, dementia was strongly associated with ICH occurrence (OR = 3.4, 95% CI = 1.2–10).[241] Therefore, it may be informative to briefly evaluate cognitive and neurologic function in older patients before giving thrombolytic therapy.

The type, dosage, and rate of delivery of the thrombolytic agent are associated with ICH risk (see Table 19.1). Plasminogen activators have different mechanisms of action with varying effects on the fibrinolytic system.[7–9, 292–295] SK binds to plasminogen, induces a conformational change, and forms plasminogen activator. Spontaneous deacylation of APSAC regenerates the active site of plasmin. Urokinase directly activates plasminogen.

These exogenous plasminogen activators can produce severe hypofibrinogenemia, with a resulting bleeding diathesis. On the other hand, rt-PA forms a complex with plasminogen and fibrin that allows for plasmin generation on the fibrin surface. rscu-PA may act via a fibrin-dependent neutralization of a competitive inhibitor.[8, 292, 295] Both rt-PA and rscu-PA are endowed with fibrin selectivity, but at clinically effective doses significant hypofibrinogenemia can still occur. In some studies using rt-PA, a dose-response relationship for induction of a systemic fibrinolytic state has been shown.[31, 53, 59, 296, 297] Plasmin may also cleave factor V and VIII, which are essential for thrombin generation. As a result, marked prolongation of the prothrombin time and activated partial thromboplastin time (aPTT) is common, particularly with SK and urokinase (UK).

Plasma fibrinogen degradation products are higher in patients treated with SK than in patients treated with rt-PA.[292, 298] In patients treated with rt-PA, there are modest direct correlations between rt-PA levels at 50 minutes and fibrinogen degradation products at 5 hours, and modest inverse correlations between rt-PA levels at 50 minutes and fibrinogen and plasminogen levels at 5 hours.[298] However, several other studies have shown poor correlation between residual plasma rt-PA level and residual fibrinogen level, as well as between the extent of the fibrinolytic state and bleeding complications.[44, 53, 292, 297–303] In 12 published cases, ICH occurred in association with severe hypofibrinogenemia.[29, 33, 39, 53, 54, 57, 75, 77] On occasion, marked elevation of fibrinogen degradation products have also been observed.[53, 54] In the majority of case reports, the aPTT has been markedly prolonged.[29, 44, 53, 54, 57, 74, 75, 77–79] In TIMI-2, limited data show that there were no important differences in fibrinogen, fibrinogen degradation products, rt-PA antigen, or plasminogen levels between patients with PIH, CI, or between these groups and the other patients without cerebrovascular complications who had plasma specimens analyzed.[31] Taken together, these data confirm the observations of others that there may be a poor correlation between the existence of systemic fibrinolytic state and ICH occurrence.

In ISIS-3, "definite or probable ICH" occurred in 0.24% of SK patients, 0.66% of duteplase rt-PA patients, and 0.55% of APSAC patients, respectively.[25] It has recently been stated that the 30-U dose of APSAC contains approximately 1.2 million U of SK, somewhat less than the 1.5 million U of SK used in clinical practice. Thus, the higher ICH frequency for APSAC is difficult to explain on the basis of dosage.[87] In TIMI-2, 12 of 908 (1.3%) patients treated with 150 mg of alteplase rt-PA and intravenous heparin and 11 of 3,016 (0.7%) patients treated with 100 mg of alteplase rt-PA and intravenous heparin developed PIH.[31] This apparent dose-response relationship was confounded by the effect of more restrictive entry criteria in the 100-mg rt-PA group, such as exclusion of patients with blood pressure of more than 180 mm Hg or history of acute cerebrovascular disease. In other large trials using 100 mg of alteplase rt-PA or 1.5 million U of SK with or without heparin, ICH occurred in 0.4–0.6% of patients.[10–12, 18, 19, 21–24, 26–29, 34, 40, 91, 235] Several studies employed various accelerated or "front-loaded" rt-PA regimens.[69–71, 73] In four studies, 3 of 721 (0.42%) patients had ICH.[69–71, 73] In eight small studies (total of 760 patients) using combination thrombolytic therapy (rt-PA plus UK or rt-PA plus SK), the reported ICH occurrence rate was 0.7% for rt-PA plus UK and 0.5% for rt-PA plus SK.[87] In GUSTO-I, ICH frequencies were 0.46% for SK plus subcutaneous heparin, 0.57% for SK plus intravenous heparin, 0.7% for accelerated rt-PA plus intravenous heparin, and 0.88% for accelerated rt-PA plus SK plus intravenous heparin.[235] In multivariable analysis, the combination regimen and accelerated rt-PA regimen were each associated with a significant increase in ICH occurrence.

Adjunctive anticoagulant and antiplatelet therapies may contribute to the occurrence of CNS bleeding. The role of anticoagulation in the production of ICH after thrombolytic therapy has been reviewed.[87, 231] One study found that patients taking oral anticoagulants before admission had an increased risk of ICH after thrombolytic therapy (OR = 5.7, 95% CI = 1.1–29.4).[24] Increased bleeding may in part relate to the use of intravenous or subcutaneous heparin. Heparin binds to antithrombin III, inducing a conformational change that accelerates inactivation of thrombin and factors Xa, IXa, and VIIIa. It may also impair platelet function, increase bleeding time, and increase capillary permeability. Heparin effects may also be influenced by hepatic function and bioavailability of the drug.[304, 305] In ISIS-2, there was a small excess of major bleeding requiring transfusion whether or not aspirin was used, but it was dependent on planned use of intravenous and subcutaneous heparin.[15] In several trials, the ICH occurrence rate was similar in patients who received 100 mg of alteplase rt-PA alone,[19, 21, 22, 31] 100 mg of alteplase rt-PA and intravenous heparin,[29, 31] and 100 mg of alteplase rt-PA and subcutaneous heparin,[21, 22, 25] although the latter is not likely to be therapeutic in the first 24 hours of use. In TIMI-2, the proportion of patients with or without PIH or CI who had at least one aPTT greater than 90 seconds was not different.[31] In GUSTO-I, aPTTs were significantly higher at 6 and 12 hours than at 24 hours after study entry.[235] Higher aPTTs and frequencies of major hemorrhage were found in patients who had lighter body weight, were an older age, were female, and did not smoke. In addition, ICH frequencies were similar or higher with higher aPTT compared with lower aPTTs at 12 hours after study entry.[238]

In GUSTO-2A, use of higher dose heparin (5,000-U bolus; 1,000 U per hour infusion for 72–120 hours in patients weighing less than 80 kg, 1,300 U per hour infusion for 72–120 hours in patients weighing 80 kg or more) was associated with an increased ICH frequency in patients treated with thrombolytics: 0.9% heparin plus rt-PA and 2.7% heparin plus SK.[228] In 26 ICH patients, the aPTT at 12 hours was significantly elevated compared with event-free patients (116 ± 46 seconds versus 87 ± 36 seconds, $P = .03$). In TIMI-9A, ICH occurred in 1.9% of patients treated with high-dose heparin (weight-adjusted regimen as in GUSTO-2A).[229] Patients who developed a major hemorrhage were significantly older and had significantly higher aPTTs at 12 hours after thrombolysis. In HIT-3, ICH occurred in 0% patients treated with heparin (15 IU per kg per hour for 48–72 hours).[230]

Hirudin, a direct antithrombin, has also been associated with ICH after thrombolytic therapy. Hirudin forms an essentially irreversible complex with thrombin by binding both at catalytic and substrate (fibrinogen) recognition sites (anion-binding exosite) of thrombin. It can also reduce activation and adhesion of platelets by inhibiting thrombin and displace factor Xa from endothelial cells.[306–310] In GUSTO-2A, use of recombinant desulfatohirudin (0.6 mg per kg bolus, 0.2 mg per kg per hour infusion for 72–120 hours) was associated with an increased ICH frequency: 1.7% rt-PA plus hirudin and 3.2% SK plus hirudin.[228] In TIMI-9A, use of recombinant desulfatohirudin (0.6 mg per kg bolus, 0.2 mg per kg per hour infusion for 96 hours) was associated with a 1.7% frequency of ICH.[229] In HIT-3, use of recombinant (Leu^1, Thr^2)63-desulfatohirudin (0.4 mg per kg bolus, 0.15 mg per kg per hour infusion for 48–72 hours) with rt-PA therapy was associated with a 2.7% frequency of ICH.[230] In GUSTO-2B, which used hirudin, 0.1 mg per kg bolus and 0.1 mg per kg per hour infusion for 72–120 hours, or heparin, 5,000 U bolus and 1,000 U per hour infusion for 72–120 hours, ICH occurred in 0.3% patients treated with hirudin and 0.2% patients treated with heparin.[239]

These latter results indicate that more potent or excessive antithrombin regimens substantially increase the risk of ICH in patients receiving thrombolytic therapy for AMI. In GUSTO-2A[228] and TIMI-9A,[229] major hemorrhage and ICH were associated with more prolonged aPTTs, suggesting the need to more closely monitor aPTTs in these patients. In TIMI-9A, data suggest that patients who received hirudin, are older, have reduced creatinine clearance, or have congestive heart failure may have reduced clearance of the drug and increased ICH risk.[229]

The role of concomitant aspirin therapy in these patients is controversial. The possible increased risk of ICH in U.S. physicians taking aspirin has prompted investigators to delay use of aspirin until 1 day after thrombolytic treatment.[311] In one small study, combined rt-PA and aspirin therapy prolonged the bleeding time, with maximal effect at 4 hours.[312] However, ICH did not occur in that study, and it is well known that ICH usually occurs more than 4 hours after initiation of thrombolytic therapy. In ISIS-3, a small but significant excess of strokes attributed to "definite or probable ICH" in patients treated with aspirin plus heparin (0.56%) versus heparin alone (0.40%) was observed.[25] The relevance of these findings is unclear.

It is possible that use of other medications in conjunction with thrombolytic therapy places patients at risk for ICH. A number of drugs, such as nonsteroidal anti-inflammatory agents, nitrates, and propranolol may affect platelet function and contribute to bleeding. Calcium channel antagonists have been shown to inhibit platelet aggregation and arachidonic acid metabolism.[313, 314] In TIMI-2, use of calcium channel antagonists at study entry was associated with an increased frequency of PIH (1.5%) compared with patients not taking these drugs (0.045%) and was not the result of any one agent's effect.[31] However, in the GUSTO-I case control study, calcium channel antagonist use was not associated with hemorrhagic stroke (OR = 1.3, 95% CI = 0.86–1.8), but was associated with any stroke (OR = 1.5, 95% CI = 1.1–2.0). Beta-blocker use was associated with hemorrhagic stroke (OR = 1.6, 95% CI = 1.1–2.4), but not with any stroke (OR = 1.2, 95% CI = 0.86–1.7). Nonsteroidal anti-inflammatory drug use was not associated with hemorrhagic stroke (OR = 1.6, 95% CI = 0.91–2.9) or any stroke (OR = 1.5, 95% CI = 0.97–2.5).[241]

Head injury before study entry has been associated with ICH occurrence after therapy. In TIMI-2, one patient who developed a symptomatic SDH had a history of head injury 8 years previously.[31, 50] Another patient had syncope and trivial head injury after an acute inferior wall MI and developed acute SDH during the infusion. In another study, one patient developed a cerebellar PIH after unrecognized syncope and head trauma.[20]

SDHs are a rare (0.03%) complication of thrombolytic therapy for AMI. Acute and chronic SDHs are believed to grow by direct rebleeding.[315, 316] Experimental and clinical studies suggest that the fibrinolytic system is activated in chronic SDH.[316–320] Once an SDH is formed, red blood cells accumulate in the hematoma at a daily rate of 5–10% of total volume. The outer wall of the SDH neomembrane surface contains plasminogen and plasminogen activator, whereas the SDH fluids have low plasminogen values; the latter presumably due to consumption. Fibrinogen degradation products are present in high concentrations and are incorporated into newly formed fibrin strands. Such clots are defective and cannot provide effective local hemostasis. Any minor trauma can produce rebleeding or plasmatic effusion. Moreover, these events can lead to a self-perpetuating growth cycle and clinical symptoms. Thrombolytic agents may enhance fibrinolytic activity within a SDH, promote bleeding, and produce symptoms. In the GUSTO-I case control study, head and face injury within 2 weeks of study entry was strongly associated with ICH occurrence (OR = 7.6, 95% CI = 2.9–20.0), particularly SDH.[241]

It has been suggested that sex may be associated with ICH risk after thrombolysis. In GISSI-2 and ISG, female sex was found to be predictive of ICH risk.[21–23, 227] In another study, male sex was associated with ICH risk.[220] In GUSTO-I, univariable analysis indicated that female sex was predictive of ICH, but this effect was lost in multivariable analysis.[235] The combination of age, weight, and blood pressure may contain the confounding information that would explain the lack of an independent relationship between female sex and ICH.

It has been suggested that brief (less than 10 minutes) cardiopulmonary resuscitation (CPR) should not be a contraindication to thrombolytic therapy. Califf and colleagues found no difference in transfusion requirements or in the incidence of hemothorax and hemopericardium in 62 patients receiving brief CPR when compared with 676 patients not requiring CPR.[321] Scholz and colleagues found that prolonged CPR (mean duration, 36 ± 32 minutes; range, 4–120 minutes) was not associated with an increased risk of bleeding complications.[322] However, prolonged CPR can cause global hypoxic-ischemic encephalopathy and border zone parenchymal and vascular tissue disruption, perhaps with an increased risk of ICH. In TIMI-2, six of 23 (26%) patients had life-threatening ventricular arrhythmias, either before (3), during (1), or after (2) rt-PA infusion and before onset of neurologic symptoms.[33] Ventricular fibrillation occurred before or during the rt-PA infusion in four of 23 (17.4%) patients with ICH and 181 of 3,901 (46.4%) patients without ICH. At present, data that address this point in larger clinical trials are not available.

Available data indicate that the risk of ICH after thrombolytic therapy for AMI can be predicted for individual patients.[224, 235, 241] In a multiple logistic regression analysis of data on ICH patients from a number of clinical trials, Simoons et al. suggested that four variables known at hospital admission appeared to be related to ICH occurrence: elderly age (older than 65 years), low body weight (less than 70 kg), hypertension on admission (systolic blood pressure of 170 mm Hg or more, diastolic blood pressure of 95 mm Hg or more, or both), and alteplase rt-PA regimen.[224] In patients receiving alteplase rt-PA, the odds ratios were 3.2 (95% CI = 1.8–5.6) for elderly age, 2.5 (95% CI = 1.4–4.4) for low body weight, and 2.0 (95% CI = 1.0–3.9) for hypertension on admission. Assuming an overall ICH risk of 0.75%, the risk estimate varied from 0.26% for a patient without ICH risk factors who

Table 19.4. Causes of Intracranial Hemorrhage After Thrombolytic Therapy for Acute Myocardial Infarction

Acute hypertension
Combined thrombolytic, anticoagulant, and antiplatelet therapy
Cerebrovascular pathology
Cerebral amyloid angiopathy
Arteriovenous malformation
Microaneurysm or other microvascular lesions
Berry aneurysm
Head injury before treatment
Brain tumors
Cocaine use
Endocarditis
Septicemia or meningoencephalitis
Vasculitis

received SK to 5.0% for an elderly hypertensive patient with low body weight treated with alteplase rt-PA. These risk estimates have been extended in the GUSTO-I trial, which showed the continuous nature of the ICH risk in relation to several baseline demographic characteristics.[235] For example, the median ICH risk for a 70-year-old patient with a history of stroke, weighing 65 kg, and an entry blood pressure of 170/95 might be 1% + 1% + 2.4% + 1% + 1% = 6.4%. The GUSTO-I multivariable model had a c-index of 0.53, suggesting that much predictive power resided in other variables, such as, perhaps, history of head and facial trauma within a few weeks and history of dementia.[241] Future studies should develop a more refined predictor of ICH risk and compare it with mortality reduction benefits of various thrombolytic therapies in order to match AMI patients with optimal thrombolytic and antithrombotic regimens.[236]

Hemorrhage and hemorrhagic stroke have been reported to occur between less than 24 hours and 4 weeks after thrombolytic treatment in patients receiving coronary artery bypass graft surgery and percutaneous transluminal coronary angioplasty.[31, 47, 58, 59, 323, 324] Abnormal bleeding after cardiopulmonary bypass is well known and is believed to be due to an acquired defect in formation of the platelet plug. Platelets are activated by passage through the oxygenation apparatus, causing secondary release and partial depletion of alpha granules. The severity of the defect relates to duration of cardiopulmonary bypass and use of platelet active drugs. This defect is, in general, rapidly reversible and can be prevented.[325, 326] In clinical settings, the profile of illness, presenting features, findings on brain images, and presence or absence of anticoagulant therapy have infrequently been reported. In addition, it may not be possible to distinguish between PIH and HI in these cases. In only one instance was the ICH site specified (posterior fossa).[47] In TIMI-2, there was no increase in PIH occurrence in patients who received immediate or delayed coronary angiography and percutaneous transluminal coronary angioplasty.[31]

Causes

A number of conditions and preexisting lesions may contribute to ICH occurrence after thrombolytic treatment in specific individuals. These factors are summarized in Table 19.4. Although autopsy investigations have been performed in a number of studies, specific results have infrequently been reported or have been unrevealing. Nonetheless, a number of cerebrovascular lesions have been described that may be the underlying cause of bleeding in patients treated with thrombolytic agents.

Cerebral amyloid angiopathy (CAA) is recognized as an important cause of ICH in elderly people.[327, 328] CAA is characterized by an acellular thickening in the walls of arterioles and small- to medium-sized arteries and veins. Both the media and adventitia are infiltrated by amyloid. Such changes are found in vessels in the superficial cerebral cortex, although they may be found in the brain stem and cerebellum.[328, 329] Ultrastructural studies of patients with multiple ICH or infarcts[329–331] associated with CAA have demonstrated segmental fibrinoid degeneration of small vessels,[331, 332] petechiae in cortical and subcortical locations,[331] and occasional microaneurysms.[331, 332] The microaneurysms have sometimes been present in the basal ganglia.[329] Many serum proteins are present in vessel walls affected by CAA, implying leakiness of the vessels.[332] Blood vessels infiltrated by CAA are believed to be brittle and unable to withstand trauma or blood pressure changes.[328]

Recent work has explored the role of molecular genetic analysis of patients with CAA-related ICH. In a recent autopsy study, Greenberg and colleagues found a significant and independent effect of apoE genotype and severity of CAA: One copy of apoε4 increased the odds ratio for moderate-to-severe CAA by 2.9-fold, whereas two copies of apoε4 increased the odds ratio 13.1-fold.[333] The frequency of the apoε4 allele was 0.40 in CAA-related ICH cases and 0.14 in control cases. This effect remained after controlling for the presence of Alzheimer's disease. In another study, Greenberg and colleagues showed that the frequency of the apoε4 allele was more common in patients with multiple lobar hemorrhages and patients who have first lobar hemorrhage at a younger age.[334] Graffagnino and colleagues recently reported a case of sporadic CAA-associated ICH with a mutation in exon 2 of cystatin C (a cysteine protease inhibitor), identical to the one associated with the Icelandic variety of hereditary cerebral hemorrhage with amyloidosis.[335] Alberts and colleagues recently reported cases of ICH associated with thrombolytic therapy in which a mutation in the endoglin gene was found.[336] In another study, Alberts and colleagues reported that the apoε4 genotype may be associated with higher ICH mortality and worse functional outcome.[337]

CAA-related ICH typically occurs in elderly patients who are frequently demented. Many cases have also been reported in the sixth and seventh decades.[329] The hemorrhages are single, multiple, or sequential. They are located in the lobar and subcortical lobar regions.

Limited pathologic data are available to explore the relationship between CAA and ICH after thrombolytic therapy for AMI. Ramsay and colleagues reported a 56-year-old man with an inferior wall AMI who developed fatal multiple left temporoparietal PIHs and a left SDH after receiving 1.5 million U SK.[78] Histologic section results were positive for amyloid. Kase and colleagues reported a 67-year-old hypertensive woman with an inferior wall AMI who developed three ICHs after receiving 100 mg of alteplase rt-PA.[57] Evacuation of one hematoma was performed and histologic sections revealed no evidence of CAA. Pendlebury and colleagues reported a 60-year-old woman with an inferior wall AMI who developed fatal right frontal and left temporal lobe PIHs after receiving 100 mg of alteplase rt-PA.[79] On microscopic examination, blood vessels in intact and hemorrhagic areas stained positive for CAA. Kirschenbaum and colleagues reported one case of CAA-associated ICH occurring after synergistic therapy with rt-PA and prourokinase.[61] Sloan and colleagues reported that three of five PIH patients in TIMI-2 who were autopsied had evidence of CAA (severe in two) by Congo Red stain and immunohistochemistry.[33] Wijdicks and Jack reported one case of PIH associated with severe CAA found at surgery.[81] Leblanc and colleagues found CAA in a surgical specimen of PIH after thrombolysis for AMI and noted that hemostasis was difficult to achieve.[82] The suspicion that CAA may be a potential cause of PIH in AMI patients treated with thrombolytic agents may be based on the lobar location, multiplicity, and the increasing frequency in older patients.[84–86]

Arteriovenous malformations (AVMs) are vascular anomalies composed of tangles of abnormally fragile arteries and veins that are prone to parenchymatous, subarachnoid, and intraventricular bleeding. Pathologic and magnetic resonance studies have demonstrated that the natural history of AVMs may be complicated by subclinical episodes of thrombosis or bleeding.[338] It is possible that blood clots formed either spontaneously or to limit the extent of bleeding episodes may be inadvertently lysed by thrombolytic agents. Two cases of PIH due to AVM rupture after thrombolytic therapy for AMI have been reported. Proner and colleagues described a patient who developed a right frontoparietal PIH 10 hours after initiation of therapy with 100 mg of alteplase rt-PA.[76] At surgery, an AVM with gross signs of recent bleeding was removed. In TIMI-2, one patient who received 100 mg of alteplase rt-PA developed a left temporoparietal PIH on day 2.[31, 33] CT showed a serpentine structure coursing medially and inferiorly from the hematoma, suggestive of an AVM.

Illicit drug users who suffer AMI as a result of their drug use may be at risk for ICH after thrombolytic therapy. Lovecchio and Nelson reported fatal ICH complicating thrombolytic therapy for a cocaine-induced AMI.[216] Sloan and colleagues described an intravenous drug user who developed massive anterior wall AMI due to *Staphylococcus aureus* prosthetic value endocarditis; intravenous thrombolysis was given, and the patient died of multiple PIHs.[225] Herzog and colleagues described a patient with mitral valve prolapse and streptococcal endocarditis who had a small occipital PIH 3 days after receiving 120 mg of rt-PA over 2 hours and percutaneous transluminal coronary angioplasty for AMI.[221] DiSalvo and colleagues reported fatal multifocal PIH, SAH, and IVH in a patient with unsuspected native valve infective endocarditis who received thrombolytic therapy for probable coronary artery embolism.[219] Autopsy demonstrated multiple supratentorial and infratentorial hematomas, IVH, and SAH; multiple microabscesses in both supratentorial and infratentorial compartments; and infiltration of numerous blood vessels by polymorphonuclear leukocytes consistent with vasculitis. Potential underlying lesions in these settings include septic arteritis, HI, or (less likely) rupture of a mycotic aneurysm. Reynard and colleagues describe a patient with simultaneous staphylococcal septicemia and meningoencephalitis and AMI with cardiogenic shock who developed a fatal ICH after thrombolytic therapy.[223]

ICH has also been observed after thrombolysis of an occluded coronary artery bypass graft and prosthetic valve thrombosis.[217, 218, 339] In the setting of prosthetic valve thrombosis, PIH and SDH were associated with transient neurologic deficits.[217, 339] Both primary and metastatic brain tumors may occasionally be complicated by intratumoral hemorrhage. Anecdotal experience suggests that the rate of ICH in brain tumors after thrombolytic therapy for AMI has been excessively high.[291] Srinivasan and colleagues reported a case of ICH occurring after thrombolysis in a patient with unsuspected vasculitis.[245]

Various other lesions have been described in patients with spontaneous PIH. These include Charcot-Bouchard microaneurysms,[340–345] miliary aneurysms with lipohyalinosis,[345] degeneration of medial smooth muscle cells with or without miliary aneurysms, fibrinoid necrosis with or without miliary aneurysms, fibrin globes ("bleeding globes"),[345] and pseudoaneurysms.[346] Microaneurysms may be found in any brain region, but often at the gray-white junction (30%) or in the pons (15%). Associated abnormalities may include fibrin presence at or near the lumenal surface; thrombus in the cavity; microscopic hemorrhages in the subcortical white matter, basal ganglia, and internal capsule; and, rarely, CAA. Because these lesions exist, particularly in elderly hypertensive patients, it is tempting to speculate that they may be responsible for the occurrence of some PIH cases that occur after thrombolytic therapy for AMI. For example, lesion location, multiplicity, fragility, and microscopic evidence of hemorrhage suggest that some instances of single or multiple PIH could be explained on this basis. At present, no direct evidence exists to prove that these lesions could be unmasked by thrombolytic therapy. Finally, SAH was reported to accompany 13% of ICH cases in the GUSTO-I trial.[243] Although a handful of other cases have been described, clinical details have been provided in only two cases.[25, 26, 42, 44, 45] The paucity of cases described in detail may reflect incomplete evaluation of ICH cases or lack of susceptibility of congenital aneurysms to rupture after thrombolytic therapy.

Spinal Hemorrhage

Thrombolytic therapy with rt-PA, SK, and UK in diverse settings has rarely been complicated by the occurrence of spinal hemorrhage, specifically EPH.[261–266] Mustafa and Gallino reported a 49-year-old man who received 1.5 million U of SK and intravenous heparin for anterior wall AMI and developed transient severe low back pain 16 hours later.[261] Two days later, he developed left leg numbness and weakness; CT showed a posterior epidural cystic lesion in the flaval ligament at L4. Heparin was discontinued. Myelopathy revealed complete block at L4–L5; lumbar laminectomy revealed an EPH. Dickman and colleagues described a 67-year-old man who presented with occlusion of the left femoral artery.[262] Lumbar epidural anesthesia was followed by surgical placement of an intra-arterial catheter through which UK was infused. Three hours later, the patient complained of back pain, and the epidural catheter was removed. However, back pain persisted and paraplegia developed. Myelography showed complete blockage due to a dorsal extradural mass from T12–L4. At emergency surgery, a large solidified hematoma beneath the ligamentum flavum was completely removed, with complete neurologic recovery within 3 days. Krolick and Cintron reported a 69-year-old man with recent minor head trauma who received 100 mg of rt-PA, intravenous heparin, and aspirin for inferior wall AMI who developed a complete C5 level neurologic defect 9 hours after initiation of treatment.[263] Myelography showed a high grade block at C6–C7; CT demonstrated an epidural lesion from C2 to C7. Emergency decompression demonstrated an EDH from C2 to C6, but there was no neurologic recovery. Onishchuk and Carlsson described a 69-year-old man who presented with a left superficial femoral artery occlusion.[264] In the operating room, placement of an epidural catheter at L3–L4 was traumatic; the catheter was removed and inserted at L2–L3. The patient received intravenous heparin and UK via the catheter. Postoperatively, the catheter was removed. On the first postoperative day, the patient had full movement of his legs. He developed a groin hematoma that resolved with bed rest. On the fourth postoperative day, he could not move his legs; MRI showed an EPH from T10 to L2. Emergency decompressive laminectomy was performed, but no neurologic recovery occurred over the next several weeks. Sawin and colleagues described two patients with spinal EPH complicating thrombolytic therapy for AMI.[265] The first was a 60-year-old woman who received 100 mg of rt-PA and intravenous heparin for anterolateral wall AMI. Eighteen hours later she developed severe midthoracic back pain. Over the next few hours, she developed complete flaccid paralysis and T12 level sensory loss. MRI revealed EPH over multiple levels with severe cord deformation. Emergency laminectomies of T8–T11 with irrigation and aspiration of ventral clot resulted in immediate neurologic improvement and complete recovery 6 months later. The second patient was a 68-year-old woman who received 100 mg of rt-PA and intravenous heparin for lateral wall AMI. Twenty hours later, she noted midscapular pain and transient leg weakness and urinary incontinence. Eight hours later, she had acute quadriparesis with urinary and fecal incontinence. MRI showed an epidural mass from C2 to L2. Multilevel cervicothoracic decompressive laminectomies were performed with resolution of upper and truncal motor and sensory function, persistent paraplegia, and modest improvement in lower extremity sensory function. Finally, Connolly and colleagues described a 69-year-old man who received 100 mg of rt-PA and intravenous heparin for anterolateral wall AMI.[266] Approximately 12.5 hours after initiation of treatment, he had acute neck pain and a normal head CT. At that point, the patient also had mild left-hand weakness. On day 10, he was diagnosed as having an incomplete left-sided Brown-Séquard syndrome. MRI showed a nonenhancing epidural mass posterior to the cord at C5 with marked thecal compression and intramedullary signal abnormality consistent with edema. He had 5/5 strength and was ambulatory. Follow-up MRI 1 week later showed complete resolution of the epidural mass and its associated cord compression.

Diagnosis and Management of Central Nervous System Hemorrhage Occurring After Thrombolytic Therapy for Acute Myocardial Infarction

Any change in neurologic function, particularly during the first 24 hours after treatment, should be regarded as strongly indicative of CNS hemorrhage until proven otherwise. Emergent CT and MRI scanning and application of the aforementioned definitions aid in identification of the type of CNS hemorrhage. Early involvement of neurologists, neurosurgeons, and hematologists optimizes treatment decisions.[84, 292]

It is reasonable to discontinue thrombolytic, anticoagulant, antiplatelet, or combined therapies as soon as symptoms and signs are recognized. Because CNS hemorrhage is a serious complication, it is useful to document the severity of the coagulopathy to the extent possible. For fibrinogen determinations, the sulfite precipitation test provides higher and more accurate levels than the Clauss chronometric method, although the Clauss method is believed to provide the best indication of functional fibrinogen levels. The presence of a lytic state is best documented by the reptilase time. Assays for coagulation factors V and VIII have not been routinely performed in coronary thrombolysis trials because they are repleted during cryoprecipitate and fresh frozen plasma therapy.[292] However, knowledge of coagulation factor levels at or near the time of symptom onset may be as important, from academic and clinical perspectives. The bleeding time has been shown to correlate with spontaneous bleeding after rt-PA therapy and should be measured.[312]

Once PIH, SAH, SDH, IVH, or EPH is documented, the patient should be given 10 U of cryoprecipitate, which will increase the fibrinogen level approximately 0.70 g per liter and the factor VIII level by approximately 30% in a 70-kg adult. Fresh frozen plasma may be used as a source of factors V and VIII and as a volume expander in carefully selected cases. In patients who are receiving heparin therapy, 1 mg of protamine for every 100 U of heparin given in the preceding 4 hours may be administered. If the bleeding time is abnormal, infusion of 6–8 U of platelets is indicated. In rare cases, antifibrinolytic agents, such as ε-aminocaproic acid (Amicar) may be necessary. It should be recognized that these replacement therapies may theoretically be complicated by coronary reocclusion.[292] Blood pressure should be managed judiciously with an appropriate balance between competing cardiologic and neurologic concerns.[84] For patients with ICH, the decision to use various measures to reduce increased intracranial pressure, such as corticosteroids, mannitol, hyperventilation, and ventriculostomy, may be based on the consensus of the management team. Angiography may be necessary when an aneurysm or AVM is suspected.

Neurosurgical evacuation of PIH, SDH, and cranial EPH has been reported either by craniotomy or stereotactic aspiration. In TIMI-2, 5 of 23 (21.7%) PIH patients had surgical evacuation of the hematoma and three died.[33] In GUSTO-I, 47 of 268 (17.5%) patients had neurosurgical intervention.[242] For all patients with ICH, surgical evacuation was associated with a higher likelihood of survival without disability (OR = 2.1, 95% CI = 0.95–4.7). The prognosis for patients with both PIH and SDH was very poor, regardless of treatment strategy. In the absence of a randomized clinical trial, physicians caring for patients with ICH occurring after thrombolysis should consider neurosurgical intervention in carefully selected cases. For patients with spinal EPH and significant neurologic deficits occurring after thrombolysis, early decompressive laminectomy should be performed to minimize long-term disability.

Prognosis of Intracranial Hemorrhage Occurring After Thrombolytic Therapy for Acute Myocardial Infarction

The mortality and morbidity of ICH occurring after thrombolysis for AMI have already been described. In the Thrombolysis and Angioplasty for Myocardial Infarction I–III protocols and the Duke Cardiovascular Databank, 13 of 1,696 patients had ICH, of whom eight of 13 (62%) died.[26–28] The CT findings associated with mortality included multiple intracranial bleeding sites, significant mass effect with midline shift, and large-volume PIH.[26] In TIMI-2, fatal PIHs tended to be larger than nonfatal PIHs.[33] In GUSTO-I, univariable analysis revealed that Glasgow Coma Scale score and age were significant clinical predictors of 30-day mortality and that median ICH volume from quantitative three-dimensional analysis (64 cubic centimeters [dead] versus 44 cubic centimeters [alive]), hydrocephalus, herniation, mass effect, intraventricular extension, and multiple ICH sites were significant neuroimaging predictors of 30-day mortality.[244] Multivariable analysis showed that Glasgow Coma Scale score, time from initiation of thrombolytic therapy to ICH onset, ICH volume, and age were independent predictors of 30-day mortality.[244a] Ongoing work will develop a nomogram to facilitate bedside clinical decision making.

Ischemic Cerebral Infarction

General Aspects

Some investigators have expressed concern that thrombolytic therapy for AMI may lyse mural thrombi and lead to cerebral and other systemic embolism.[246–249] The range of the reported frequencies of definite CI in large or comparative coronary thrombolysis trials are 0.15–0.75% for SK,[10–12, 21–23, 25, 90, 92, 235] 0.43–1.24% for rt-PA,[18, 19, 21–23, 25, 31–34, 91, 235] 0.33% for APSAC,[15] 0.65% for accelerated rt-PA plus SK,[235] 0.41% for r-scuPA,[30] 0.35% for UK, and 0.33% for reteplase.[92] Because the frequencies of stroke of unknown type are 0.29%, 0.24%, 0.53%, 0.12%, unknown, and 0.13%, respectively, the actual frequencies of definite CI complicating therapy for each thrombolytic agent may be somewhat higher (see Table 19.1). Based on the pharmacologic properties of the various agents, a causative role could be inferred if ischemic strokes occurred at a time consistent with their duration of action (less than 24 hours).[12] Clinical studies in the prethrombolytic[274–278] and thrombolytic eras[11, 12, 15–18, 27] and echocardiographic studies of patients not treated with thrombolytic agents[347–350] indicate that most ischemic infarcts occur in the first few weeks and months after AMI. Of 29 CI in TIMI-2, 9 (31%) occurred within the first 24 hours, 4

(14%) between 24 and 48 hours, 5 (17%) during the remainder of the first week, 9 (31%) during the second week, and 2 (7%) during the remainder of the first month after AMI.[32] Taken together, these data suggest that overall embolic stroke risk has not increased as a result of thrombolytic therapy. However, individual patients with dilated cardiomyopathy or chronic aneurysmal dilatation, particularly if left ventricular thrombus is present, may be at increased risk of cerebral embolization after thrombolytic therapy.[251, 347–350]

Risk Factors

In five studies, age (particularly older than 70 years) was strongly associated with CI.[12, 21, 22, 31, 250] In two studies, anterior infarct, poor Killip class, and nonwhite race were associated with CI.[12, 31] In GUSTO-I, the factors associated with CI in univariable analysis were history of stroke, previous coronary artery bypass surgery, diabetes mellitus, previous AMI, prior angina pectoris, history of hypertension, and older age (per 10 years).[250] Ongoing research will develop a multivariable predictor for CI occurrence after thrombolytic therapy for AMI.

Clinical Features

In TIMI-2, 23 of 29 (79%) CI involved the cerebral cortex; nine (31%) had multiple CI.[32] Compared with ICH, patients with CI present more commonly with focal neurologic deficits and less commonly with decreased level of consciousness; headache, vomiting, and coma are uncommon. These differences in presentation should be viewed with caution because the number of patients analyzed is small and CT scans are necessary to definitively distinguish between CI and ICH. Of 28 CIs thought to be cardioembolic in origin, 17 (61%) had strong evidence for at least one cardiac abnormality (mural clot, wall motion abnormality, aneurysm, or atrial fibrillation) known to be associated more specifically with embolism than AMI. Border zone infarction has rarely been documented following cardiovascular surgery[351]; one TIMI-2 patient had multiple border zone CIs after repair of an aortic dissection.[32] Twelve (41%) patients had CI temporally associated with invasive cardiovascular procedures (coronary artery bypass graft in five, aortic dissection repair in one, ventricular septal defect repair in one, cardiac catheterization in three, and percutaneous transluminal coronary angioplasty in two). However, the frequencies of CI that occurred after coronary angiography, percutaneous transluminal coronary angioplasty, and the invasive treatment strategy were not increased compared with other studies.[31]

Management

If the patient has an acute focal neurologic deficit and the initial CT scan result is normal, ischemic cerebral dysfunction may be presumed. Depending on the nature of the neurologic deficits, anticoagulant therapy with intravenous heparin may be appropriate while the diagnostic evaluation (repeat CT scanning, MRI, echocardiography, carotid duplex, transcranial Doppler, and so forth) is under way. In the patient with major neurologic deficits, it may be prudent to withhold anticoagulant therapy, repeat the CT scan in 3–5 days, and then begin anticoagulant therapy if HI is absent. If HI is present, anticoagulant therapy may be started 7–10 days later. However, anticoagulant therapy may be started sooner based on clinical considerations. The utility of cerebral angiography in this setting is unclear. However, for a carotid territory stroke, evidence of surgically important carotid disease (70% or more diameter reduction stenosis) should be sought. Long-term antithrombotic therapy or surgery for secondary stroke prevention may be planned by considering the site of AMI, cardiologic and neurologic status, documented vascular lesions, and other factors.[86, 87]

Other Settings

A number of clinical studies have evaluated the judicious use of SK, UK, and rt-PA to lyse prosthetic valve thrombosis. In 11 studies, four of 82 (5%) patients had transient neurologic deficits attributable to cerebral embolism.[216, 252–256, 352–357] Hirschl and colleagues described a 63-year-old woman who presented in cardiogenic shock and received 100 mg of rt-PA for thrombosis of a CarboMedics (CarboMedics, Austin, TX) mitral valve prosthesis.[256] During fibrinolytic therapy, multiple cerebral emboli occurred, and she was left with severe aphasia and right hemiplegia.

Pape and colleagues reported a 66-year-old woman with atrial fibrillation and congestive heart failure who received 50 mg of rt-PA for mobile thrombosis on a St. Jude (St. Jude Medical SC, St. Paul, MN) mitral valve prosthesis shown on transthoracic echocardiography.[255] Forty-five minutes into the infusion, she developed a massive left hemisphere stroke and died 48 hours later. Autopsy revealed a left middle cerebral artery embolus. Dzavik and colleagues reported one patient who had thrombosis of a mitral valve prosthesis detected by transesophageal echocardiography.[257] Twelve hours after initiation of thrombolytic therapy, a massive fatal stroke occurred. Roudaut and colleagues reported the occurrence of four fatal strokes (three with mitral valve prostheses) in 75 patients with prosthetic valve thrombosis (5%) treated with thrombolytic therapy.[258] Therefore, in some patients with left-sided valve prostheses, particularly if they are hemodynamically stable, thrombolytic therapy may not be the treatment of choice.[258] Finally, Dejaeger and colleagues reported a 58-year-old man with massive pulmonary embolus who received 1.75 million U of SK over 15 hours.[259] Twenty-two hours after the end of the SK infusion, the patient developed somnolence and right hemiplegia, associated with increasing fibrinogen levels. It was thought that the unusually early and marked increase in plasma fibrinogen levels may have been due to a rebound effect.

Intracranial Hemorrhage Occurring After Thrombolytic Therapy for Acute Ischemic Cerebral Infarction

General Aspects

In cases of thrombolytic therapy for ACI, one must be concerned about bleeding into both normal brain and ischemic brain. It is therefore necessary to first review concepts and existing data pertaining to CT findings in ACI and hemorrhagic transformation of ischemic infarcts. This provides the background for discussion of complications in older clinical studies of intravenous and intra-arterial thrombolysis, as well as the more recently published randomized clinical trials.[1–6, 127–215]

Six studies have shown that CT scans obtained within 2, 3, 5, 6, 12, and 14 hours of stroke onset may demonstrate evidence of ischemic cerebral injury.[190, 358–362] One study suggested that early demonstration of a lesion on CT scan may not correlate with patient outcome, as defined by the Glasgow Outcome Scale and the attending physician's assessment of the patient at hospital discharge.[359] Moulin and colleagues reported on early CT signs within 14 hours of onset of acute middle cerebral artery (MCA) territory infarction: hyperdense MCA sign, attenuation of the lenticular nucleus, loss of the insular ribbon, and hemispheric sulcal effacement.[362] Early CT was abnormal in 55 of 62 (88%) patients with CT performed within 6 hours of stroke onset. The CT signs were significantly associated with subsequent MCA infarction location and extension: attenuation of the lenticular nucleus and deep infarct, hemispheric sulcal effacement and superficial infarct, and loss of the insular ribbon and large infarct. Hyperdense MCA sign was never found in isolation and was always associated with the three other signs in extended MCA infarct. The presence of two or three signs (attenuation of the lenticular nucleus, loss of the insular ribbon, hemispheric sulcal effacement) was associated with extended MCA infarct ($P < .001$) and poor outcomes ($P < .001$). These results corroborate the findings of other investigators.[359] Limitations of this analysis include its retrospective nature and uncertain application to patients seen within 3 hours of stroke onset.

Hemorrhagic Infarction

It is well known that transformation of a "bland" CI to an HI or parenchymatous hemorrhage (confluent HI) may occur.[16, 362–397] Hemorrhagic infarction describes multifocal secondary bleeding into brain infarcts via diapedesis through damaged capillary and venular walls, forming petechiae of varying sizes. When large areas of petechiae merge to form confluent purpura or parenchymatous hematoma, an intracerebral hemorrhage detectable by CT scan may occur.[364] A number of investigators[2, 366, 383, 392] believe that HI can result from restoration of blood flow into a recently ischemic area that contains abnormal blood vessels lacking autoregulatory capacity,[392, 393, 395, 396] perhaps potentiated by hypertension.[393, 397] Restoration of blood flow may occur either by reopening the occluded vessel or by establishment of collateral circulation.[364, 381, 394] Experimental studies in rats, cats, and monkeys showed that when ischemia is followed by reperfusion, permeability changes in the blood-brain barrier occur at some time between 2 and 6 hours after the onset of ischemia.[398–402] Brain capillaries may expand and rupture in this setting, with the extent of disruption related to the duration and degree of ischemia.[402] Thus, mild (petechial) to moderate HIs are believed to result from diapedesis through ischemic endothelium, usually without vessel rupture. When vessel walls necrose, hemorrhage may be focal and severe. Four experimental studies using norepinephrine infusion, hypercarbia, or aortic obstruction[2, 403–405] and one clinical report of patients with permanently occluded MCAs[394] have shown that induction of significant acute hypertension may produce HI, presumably by accentuation of blood flow through leptomeningeal collaterals via retrograde flow into damaged cerebral vessels.[405]

In autopsy series, cardioembolic stroke appears to have a higher propensity for hemorrhagic transformation (57–76% prevalence)[364, 366, 378, 383, 385] than nonembolic studies (2–21% prevalence).[371–385, 406] The reported difference may reflect ascertainment bias because lethal infarcts are more often large with mass effect, brain herniation, or hemorrhagic transformation.[376, 378] However, HI has also been documented in small- to moderate-sized infarctions.[358, 391] Clinical CT studies of nonanticoagulated patients indicate that HI occurs in 5–43% of cases.[372–377, 394, 395] Autopsy[385] and clinical[363, 377, 379, 382] studies suggest that the majority of HIs occur within 3–4 days after stroke onset, but may occur within hours after onset[396] or as late as 10–14 days after onset.[377, 382] Parenchymatous hematomas (confluent HI) occur in 2.0–8.6% of cases.[373–375, 395, 396]

It is estimated that as many as 95% of HIs in nonanticoagulated patients are asymptomatic,[363, 372, 377, 379] whereas parenchymatous hematomas are generally associated with clinical worsening except for the smallest ones.[389] One experimental study suggests that anticoagulation does not increase the likelihood of HI, but may accentuate the degree of hemorrhage on CT.[407] Several studies report that the estimated incidence of clinical deterioration is 5–20%, with a mortality as high as 55%.[364, 370, 372, 373, 378–381, 396] The period of active bleeding is transient, and anticoagulation therapy administered after the appearance of HI on CT does not normally result in clinical or roentgenographic worsening.[370, 386] In fact, some patients may be improving at the time HI is detected.[408]

Intracranial Hemorrhage Occurring After Thrombolysis: Experimental and Clinical Studies

Recent reviews have summarized experimental studies of thrombolytic therapy for acute cerebral ischemia.[9, 83, 87, 409–413] The occurrence of HI is common in animals treated with rt-PA and placebo.[87] In three studies, administration of SK, particularly when delayed for 6–24 hours, may be associated with a greater frequency of hemorrhagic complications.[414–416] Confluent HI has been observed in animals treated at 60 minutes,[415] 3 hours,[417] 3.5 hours,[418] 6 hours,[415] 8 hours,[419] and 24 hours[414, 419] after vascular occlusion. In rare instances, a confluent HI may occur in placebo-treated animals.[418]

The rationale, data on safety and efficacy, and ongoing analyses of clinical studies of thrombolytic therapy in ACI have recently been reviewed.[87, 150, 386, 387, 412, 413] These clinical reports have been designed as either angiographically controlled or clinical outcome evaluations of intravenous or intra-arterial therapy with SK, UK, rt-PA, prourokinase, and ancrod. Patients with carotid, vertebrobasilar, or any territory stroke have been treated by a wide variety of protocols initiated at various times after symptom onset. ICHs have been reported in numerous studies from the pre-CT scan and CT scan eras (Table 19.5). The types of hemorrhage include HI, confluent HI, PIH, ICH of unspecified type, extension to the subarachnoid space or intraventricular system, or SDH. Hemorrhages have occurred in patients treated with SK, UK, alteplase rt-PA, duteplase rt-PA, and prourokinase administered by intravenous and intra-arterial routes. Of the 2,597 patients covered in Table 19.5, there were 171 (6.6%) HI, 70 (2.1%) confluent HI, 7 (0.3%) PIH, and 10 (0.4%) ICH of unspecified type. In carotid territory distribution studies, the proportions of HI, confluent HI, PIH, and ICH of unspecified type are 104 of 696 (14.9%; range, 0–100%), 47 of 696 (6.8%; range, 0–25%), five of 696 (0.7%; range, 0–20%), and six of 696 (0.9%;

Table 19.5. Central Nervous System Hemorrhage (Intracranial Hemorrhage) in Clinical Studies of Thrombolytic Therapy for Acute Ischemic Stroke

Author	Reference	Agent	Route	Time Window	Vascular Territory	No.	HI (%)	CHI (%)	PIH (%)	ICH-NS (%)
Intravenous studies										
Meyer	1, 2	SK	IV	<72 hrs	Carotid	37	1 (2.7)	3 (8.1)	—	—
Fletcher	5	u-PA	IV	<36 hrs	—	31	1 (3.2)	1 (3.2)	—	2 (6.5)
Abe	136, 137	u-PA	IV	<720 hrs	—	216	—	—	—	1 (0.5)
Atarashi	144	u-PA	IV	<120 hrs	—	191	2 (1)	—	—	—
Otomo	145	u-PA	IV	<120 hrs	—	176	2 (1.1)	—	—	—
Otomo	153	u-PA	IV	<120 hrs	—	184	3 (1.6)	—	—	—
Otomo	153	rt-PA	IV	<120 hrs	—	171	2 (1.2)	—	—	—
Terashi	159	rt-PA	IV	<72 hrs	—	171	8 (4.7)	—	—	—
Terashi	159	u-PA	IV	<72 hrs	—	171	8 (4.7)	—	—	—
Hennerici	161	rt-PA	IV	2–18 hrs	MCA/BA	12	—	—	1 (8.3)	—
Abe	162	rt-PA	IV	<72 hrs	—	14	3 (2.1)	—	—	—
Abe	162	u-PA	IV	<72 hrs	—	77	6 (4.1)	—	—	—
Mori	166	drt-PA	IV	<6 hrs	Carotid	19	8 (42.1)	—	—	2 (10.5)
von Kummer	167–169	rt-PA	IV	<6 hrs	ICA/MCA	32	9 (28.1)	3 (9.4)	1 (3.1)	—
Yamaguchi	170	rt-PA	IV	<6 hrs	—	58	12 (21)	—	—	—
Pilz	175	rt-PA	IV	<8 hrs	BA	17	1 (5.9)	3 (17.7)	—	—
Pilz	175	rt-PA	IV	<6 hrs	MCA	5	1 (20)	—	—	—
Hamann	180	u-PA + rscu-PA	IV	<6 hrs	MCA	3	1 (33.3)	—	—	—
Brott	183	rt-PA	IV	<1.5 hrs	ICA/MCA/ACA	74	3 (4.1)	2 (2.7)	1 (1.4)	—
Haley	184	rt-PA	IV	1.5–3.0 hrs	ICA/MCA	20	4 (20.0)	1 (5)	1 (5)	—
Sperling	186	rt-PA	IV	<6 hrs	—	12	1 (8.3)	—	—	—
Brucker	187	rt-PA +u-PA	IV/IA	<6 hrs	ICA/MCA = 19; BA = 9	28	8 (28.6)	2 (7.1)	—	—
Okada	190	rt-PA	IV	<6 hrs	ICA/MCA	10	4 (40)	1 (10)	—	—
del Zoppo	182	drt-PA	IV	<8 hrs	ICA/MCA	104	21 (20.2)	11 (10.6)	2 (1.9)	—
Trouillas	191	rt-PA	IV	<7 hrs	Carotid	43	1 (2.3)	3 (7.0)	—	—
Yamaguchi	192	drt-PA	IV	<7 hrs	Carotid	51	1 (2.0)	4 (7.8)	—	—
Jansen	198	rt-PA	IV	<6 hrs	Intracranial carotid	16	—	1 (6.7)	—	—
Overgaard	200	drt-PA	IV	<6 hrs	Cortical/MCA	23	2 (8.7)	—	—	—
Demchuk	202	rt-PA	IV	<5 hrs	?	16	—	2 (12.5)	—	—
Huemer	205	rt-PA	IV	<6 hrs	BA	16	—	1 (6.7)	1 (6.7)	—

Intra-arterial studies										
del Zoppo	149	SK/u-PA	IA	<8 hrs	Carotid	20	4 (20)	—	—	—
del Zoppo	150	rt-PA	IA	<1 hr	MCA	3	1 (33.1)	1 (33.3)	—	—
Hacke	151	SK/u-PA	IA	<24 hrs	VBA	43	1 (2.3)	3 (7.0)	—	—
Mori	152, 165	u-PA	IA	<12 hrs	ICA = 8; MCA = 31; BA = 5	44	4 (9.1)	6 (13.6)	—	—
Theron	154	SK/u-PA	IA	<1 hr	ICA/MCA	12	—	3 (25)	—	—
Buteux	155	rt-PA	IA	—	PCA	1	—	—	1 (100)	—
Brückman	156	drt-PA	IA	<6 hrs	MCA	1	—	1 (100)	—	—
Pfeiffer	173	SK/u-PA	IA	<8 hrs	VBA	20	3 (15)	1 (5)	—	—
Ikeda	160	u-PA	IA	<3 hrs	ICA/MCA	13	3 (23.1)	—	—	—
Matsumoto	171	u-PA	IA	<24 hrs	ICA/MCA	39	9 (23.1)	4 (10.3)	—	—
Matsumoto	171	u-PA	IA	<24 hrs	BA/PCA	11	1 (9.1)	—	—	—
Herderscheé	177	rt-PA	IA	< 6 hrs	BA	2	1 (50)	—	—	—
Jansen	198	tPA/UK	IA	<6 hrs	Intracranial carotid	16	6 (37.5)	3 (18.8)	—	—
Lanzieri	199	UK	IA	<6 hrs	MCA	8	—	—	—	—
Ueda	428	tPA/UK	IA	<7.5 hrs	Carotid	34	15 (14.7)	2 (5.8)	—	—
Tirschwell	201	UK	IA	?	15 carotid, 8 basilar	23	—	2 (8.7)	—	—
Zeumer	194	UK/rt-PA	IA	<8 hrs	VBA	28	—	2 (7.1)	—	—
Brandt	193	UK/rt-PA	IA	<48 hrs	VBA	51	3 (5.3)	3 (5.3)	—	—
LaMonte	195	UK	IA	<8 hrs	Carotid	11	—	—	—	—
Casto	207	UK	IA	<5 hrs	Carotid	5	1 (20)	—	—	—
Frey	203	rt-PA	IA	<6 hrs	Carotid	6	1 (16.7)	—	—	—
					BA	1	1 (100)			
Sasaki	206	drt-PA	IA	<6 hrs	ICA/MCA	53	12 (20)	1 (2.8)	—	—
Sasaki	206	drt-PA	IA	<6 hrs	BA	9	2 (22.2)	—	—	—
PROACT I	420	rproUK	IA	<6 hrs	MCA	26	—	—	—	4 (15.4)
Total						2,597	171 (6.6)	70 (2.1)	7 (0.3)	10 (0.4)

SK = streptokinase; u-PA = urokinase; rproUK = recombinant prourokinase; HI = hemorrhagic infection; rt-PA = alteplase recombinant tissue plasminogen activator; CHI = confluent hemorrhagic infection; drt-PA = duteplase recombinant tissue plasminogen activator; PIH = parenchymatous intracerebral hematoma; ICA = internal carotid artery; ICH = intracranial hemorrhage; MCA = middle cerebral artery; ICH-NS = intracranial hemorrhage of unspecified type; ACA = anterior cerebral artery; PCA = posterior cerebral artery; BA = basilar artery; VBA = vertebral and basilar arteries; UK = urokinase; rpronk = recombinant prourokinase; rscu-PA = recombinant single chain urokinase plasminogen activator.

Table 19.6. Thrombolytic Therapy for Acute Ischemic Stroke: Definitions for Intracranial Hemorrhage in Randomized Clinical Trials

Hemorrhage Type	ECASS	MAST-I
PIH	—	Intracerebral hemorrhage
Confluent HI, total infarct	—	Hemorrhagic infarction III
Confluent HI, >30% infarct	Parenchymal hematoma II	Hemorrhagic infarction II
Confluent HI, < 30% infarct	Parenchymal hematoma I	—
Petechial HI, large	Hemorrhagic infarction II	Hemorrhagic infarction I
Petechia HI, small, marginal	Hemorrhagic infarction I	Hemorrhagic infarction I

ECASS = European Cooperative Acute Stroke Study; MAST-I = Multicenter Acute Stroke Trial in Italy; PIH = parenchymal intracerebral hemorrhage in vascular territory of cerebral infarction; HI = hemorrhagic infarction.

range, 0–10.5%), respectively. In the Prolyse in Acute Cerebral Thromboembolism (PROACT I) trial, 26 patients were randomized to receive 6 mg of intra-arterial r-prourokinase.[420] The frequency of brain hemorrhage with neurologic deterioration in patients who received r-prourokinase was 15.7% versus 14.3% in patients who received placebo. The frequency of brain hemorrhage with deterioration was 22.3% r-prourokinase versus 20% placebo for high-dose heparin and 6.7% r-prourokinase versus 11.1% placebo for low-dose heparin.[420] In vertebrobasilar territory distribution studies, the proportions of HI, confluent HI, PIH, and ICH of unspecified type are 6 of 212 (2.8%; range, 0–50%), 14 of 212 (6.6%; range, 0–20%), one of 212 (0.5%), and 0%, respectively. In some studies, the exact nature of the hemorrhagic complication could only be inferred. In one study, confluent HI occurred in one patient in the placebo group.[185]

Intracranial Hemorrhage and Outcome: Randomized Trials

The main results of five randomized trials of thrombolytic therapy for ACI have been reported.[208–215] Brain hemorrhage has occurred in each trial. Definitions for the types of brain hemorrhage for the European Cooperative Acute Stroke Study (ECASS)[212] and Multicenter Acute Stroke Trial in Italy (MAST-I)[211] are shown in Table 19.6. Data on mortality and ICH in each trial are shown in Table 19.7.

The three SK trials—that is, MAST-E,[209, 215] MAST-I,[211] and ASK[210, 214]—were terminated prematurely due to unacceptably high rates of death and ICH. Early (10 days or less) mortality was 17.8% in ASK,[210, 214] 19% (SK), and 34% (SK plus ASA) ($P \leq .001$) in MAST-I,[211] and 34% ($P < .01$ versus placebo) in MAST-E,[209, 215] respectively. Symptomatic brain hemorrhage was 6% (SK, $P < .01$ versus placebo) and 10% (SK plus ASA, $P < .001$ versus placebo) in MAST-I,[211] 9.8% (0–3 hours) and 14.3% (3–4 hours) in ASK,[210, 214] and 21.2% ($P < .001$ versus placebo) in MAST-E.[209,215] In MAST-I, informed consent was not always obtained, and the onset time was not always established.[211]

The two rt-PA trials—that is, ECASS[212] and NINDS[213]—were completed with the NINDS trial being unequivocally positive in favor of rt-PA versus placebo. Thirty-day mortality was 17.9% (intention to treat) and 14.9% (target population) in ECASS and 12.9% in the NINDS trials. There were no significant differences in mortality between treatment or placebo groups in either trial at 30 or 90 days. Although some investigators have expressed concern that thrombolysis in ACI may be associated with life-threatening brain edema,[147, 421] herniation from space-occupying edema was not significantly more common in the rt-PA–treated group than in the placebo group in ECASS.[212] The frequency of ICH in ECASS was higher than in NINDS, irrespective of exclusion of patients with clinical or CT scan violations in ECASS. Symptomatic hemorrhage occurred in 19.8% (intention to treat, $P < .001$ versus placebo) and 19.4% (target population, $P < .001$ versus placebo) in ECASS and 6.4% ($P < .001$ versus placebo) in NINDS. The overall incidence of total (symptomatic and asymptomatic) ICH was not significantly different between the treatment groups. In both intention to treat and target population analyses for ECASS, HI

Table 19.7. Intracranial Hemorrhage After Thrombolytic Therapy: Randomized Clinical Trials in Acute Ischemic Stroke[a]

					Mortality		Intracranial Hemorrhage	
Trial	**Reference**	**Agent**	**Dose**	**Entry Time**	**Treatment**	**Control**	**Treatment**	**Control**
NINDS	213	rt-PA	0.9 mg/kg (maximum, 90 mg), 10% bolus, 60' infusion	3 hrs	30 days: 12.9%	15.8%	Sx: 6.4%	0.6%
					90 days: 17.4%	20.6%	Asx: 4.5%	2.9%
ECASS	212	rt-PA	1.1 mg/kg (maximum, 100 mg), 10% bolus, 60' infusion	6 hrs	30 days:		Sx:	
					ITT 17.9%	12.3%	19.8%[b]	6.5%
					TP 14.6%	11.7%	19.4%[b]	6.8%
					90 days:		Asx:	
					ITT 22.4%	15.8%	23%	30.3%
					TP 19.4%	14.8%	24.3%	29.9%
MAST-E	209, 215	SK	1.5 million U over 60 mins	6 hrs	10 days: 34%[c]	18.2%	Sx: 21.2%[b]	2.6%
					90 days: 44.9%[e]	34.4%	Asx: 45.3%	41.3%
MAST-I	211	SK	1.5 million U over 60 mins ± ASA, 300 mg	6 hrs	10 days:		Sx:	
					SK 19%	13%	6%[d]	
					SK + ASA 34%[a]		10%[b]	0.6%
					180 days:		Asx:	
					SK 28%	29%	18%	10%
					SK + ASA 44%[d]		20%	

Table 19.7. *continued*

					Mortality		Intracranial Hemorrhage	
Trial	**Reference**	**Agent**	**Dose**	**Entry Time**	**Treatment**	**Control**	**Treatment**	**Control**
ASK	210, 214	SK	1.5 million U over 60 mins	4 hours	7 days: 17.8%	 10.8%	0–3 hrs: Sx: 9.8%	 0%
					30 days 31%	 16.3%	Asx: 19.5%	 6.9%
					90 days: 36%	 21.5%	3–4 hours: Sx: 14.3%	 3.6%
							Asx: 18.8%	 15.3%

NINDS = National Institute of Neurological Disorders and Stroke; ECASS = European Cooperative Acute Stroke Study; MAST-E = Multicenter Acute Stroke Study—Europe; MAST-I = Multicenter Acute Stroke Study—Italy; ASK = Australian Streptokinase Study; rt-PA = recombinant tissue plasminogen activator; SK = streptokinase; ASA = aspirin; ITT = intention to treat; TP = target population; Sx = symptomatic hemorrhage; Asx = asymptomatic hemorrhage.

[a]Hemorrhagic infarctions were assigned to the asymptomatic hemorrhage group.

[b]P <.001.

[c]P = .002.

[d]P <.01.

[e]P <.05.

was significantly more frequent in the placebo-treated groups, whereas confluent HI and PIH were more frequent in the rt-PA–treated groups ($P < .001$ for both analyses). Treatment with rt-PA was associated with an increased risk of confluent HI and PIH (OR = 3.6, 95% CI = 2.6–6.1; $P = .0001$).[422] In ECASS, 19 (6.3%) rt-PA patients and seven (2.4%) placebo-treated patients died from ICH ($P = .02$). In the target population, there was no significant difference in the frequency of hemorrhage-related death (10 deaths, 4.2%, for rt-PA; 7 deaths, 2.7%, for placebo; $P = .37$), presumably due to exclusion of a high number of hemorrhages in patients with major protocol violations randomized to rt-PA. In the NINDS trial, symptomatic ICH during the first 36 hours occurred more commonly in the rt-PA–treated group ($P < .001$). The frequency of asymptomatic ICH was similar in the rt-PA–treated group (14 of 312, 4.5%) and placebo-treated groups (9 of 312, 2.9%). At 90 days, 17 of 28 (61%) patients with symptomatic ICH had died.

Risk Factors

A number of clinical characteristics may be important in the pathogenesis of ICH in this setting. In three small studies, there was no relationship between ICH and patient age.[182–184, 189] In ECASS, age (by decades) was associated with an increased risk of confluent HI and PIH (OR = 1.3, 95% CI = 1.0–1.7; $P = .0328$).[422] In two small studies there was a trend for patient weight to be inversely correlated with combined HI, confluent HI, and PIH; ICH patients weighed 65 ± 11.9 kg and non-ICH patients weighed 78 ± 17.5 kg.[183, 184, 189] Evidence of a relation between blood pressure at entry and ICH is conflicting. In three small studies, there was no relationship between ICH and history of hypertension.[182–184, 189] In one study, there was no relationship between blood pressure and ICH occurrence.[422] However, in two studies, diastolic blood pressure (104 ± 10 mm Hg versus 86 ± 14 mm Hg, $P < .01$) and mean blood pressure (127 ± 18 versus 108 ± 17, $P < .02$) were higher in patients with ICH compared with patients without ICH.[183, 184, 189] It is possible that the blood pressure management criteria may have contributed to the lower observed rate of symptomatic ICH in the NINDS trial.[213]

Evidence for a relation between the type and dose of thrombolytic agent and ICH occurrence is accumulating. The SK trials adopted the dosage from the coronary thrombolysis experience without a dose range finding study, so it is difficult to know if the dose used had an effect on ICH occurrence.[209–211, 214, 215] In two studies using alteplase rt-PA, an apparent dose-response relationship with combined HI, confluent HI, and PIH was observed (0.97 mg per kg with hemorrhage versus 0.74 mg per kg without hemorrhage), although it was not seen in terms of dose per square meter or actual dose administered.[183, 184, 189] In a study using duteplase rt-PA, no dose-response relationship was apparent between rt-PA dose and combined HI, confluent HI, and PIH.[182] The reasons for these discrepant results may include small numbers of patients, differences in thrombolytic activity between agents, differences in rt-PA dosages, and other factors. In randomized trials, there was a significantly higher ICH rate in ECASS (1.1 mg per kg)[212] than in NINDS (0.9 mg per kg).[213]

Limited data are available on the hematologic aspects of thrombolytic therapy for ACI. In one study, there was a dose-response relationship between rt-PA dose and changes in fibrinolytic parameters.[166] In another study, levels of fibrin degradation products and D-dimers were higher in the hemorrhagic transformation group than in the nonhemorrhagic group.[423] However, another study reported that changes in hemostasis were not different between patients who did and did not have hemorrhage.[151] In two studies, cerebellar PIH occurred in association with sustained severe hypofibrinogenemia.[183, 184] However, in another study, the 3 hours' post-treatment fibrinogen level was not related to the combined occurrence of confluent HI and PIH.[189] In several studies, concomitant heparin and a hemorheologic agent were administered.[149–151, 167–169, 180, 187] In three studies, there was no relationship between ICH and subsequent heparin use or prior aspirin use.[182–184, 424, 425] In one recent study of 30 consecutive patients treated with rt-PA (NINDS protocol) followed immediately by intravenous heparin, HI occurred in 16% of patients, and symptomatic ICH (confluent HI and PIH) occurred in 3%.[425] In one study, the three patients with confluent HI or PIH had PTTs of more than 120 seconds.[167–169] Whether combined thrombolytic and anticoagulant therapy for ACI is safe

Table 19.8. Risk Factors for Intracranial Hemorrhage After Thrombolytic Therapy for Acute Ischemic Stroke

Demographics
Age
Blood pressure
Thrombolytic agents
Type
Dose
Clinical factors
Time to treatment
Stroke severity
Early infarct on computed tomographic scan

and efficacious can be addressed only in a controlled clinical trial.

Many patients have moderate to severe deficits before treatment is given. Although one clinical study[152, 165] suggested that ICH may be more common in unconscious patients, two other studies[183, 184, 189] showed no relationship between ICH and initial summed NIH Stroke Scale score. In three studies, patients treated later, particularly more than 6 hours after symptom onset, were more likely to suffer ICH.[152, 165, 170, 182] In ECASS, severe stroke on admission (Scandinavian Stroke Scale score ≤14) was associated with an increased risk of HI (OR = 2.5, 95% CI = 1.6–4.0, P = .0001).[422] In the NINDS trial, an NIH Stroke Scale Score of more than 20 was strongly associated with symptomatic ICH (OR = 11).[426] Patients with HI,[149, 152, 155, 156, 165, 175, 180, 182, 187] confluent HI,[152, 158, 165, 173, 175, 182–184] and PIH[161, 183, 184] may be clinically stable[149, 152, 155, 156, 165, 182–184, 187] or deteriorate[151, 158, 161, 167–169, 171, 173, 175, 180, 182–184, 187] after the hemorrhagic complication. In many cases, patients with ICH die either as a result of the stroke severity, the ICH, or both.[151, 152, 160, 161, 165, 167–169, 171, 175, 180, 184]

Data on the radiologic aspects of ICH following thrombolytic therapy for ACI are also accumulating. Toni and colleagues reported in an observational study of 150 consecutive patients that baseline CT findings were significantly associated with HI: early hypodensity (OR = 56.76, 95% CI = 17.79–181), mass effect (OR = 6.07, 95% CI = 1.86–19.8), and hyperdense MCA sign (OR = 7.71, 95% CI = 3.25–18.22).[360] Early focal hypodensity was the only independent predictor of HI among baseline findings. On repeat CT scan, medium- and large-sized lesions and mass effect were associated with HI. Patients with HI and confluent HI did not differ in terms of frequency of early deterioration or poor outcome at 30 days. Moulin and colleagues found HI in 43% of patients with large infarct and was an intrainfarct hematoma in 47% of HI cases.[362] Intrainfarct hematoma was associated with a large infarct (78%) versus a limited infarct (22%), with a P of <.02. In the NINDS trial, the presence of early infarct signs on CT (16 patients) was associated with symptomatic hemorrhage (OR = 7.8, 95% CI = 2.2–27).[426] In ECASS, early ischemic change on CT scan was associated with HI (OR = 3.5, 95% CI = 2.3–5.3, P = .001).[422]

A method to predict the risk of symptomatic brain hemorrhage following thrombolytic therapy for ACI is needed. At this time, one may estimate the risk by extrapolating from the coronary thrombolysis trials and include the clinical and radiographic factors from the randomized cerebral thrombolysis experience (Table 19.8). Hommel and colleagues have calculated the relative risks and 95% CI for symptomatic brain hemorrhages in each trial: MAST-E = 8.14 (2.95–22.44); MAST-I = 6.17 (2.17–17.53); ECASS = 2.66 (1.14–6.24); and NINDS = 10 (2.36–42.43).[427] Future research should create a nomogram for predicting ICH risk based on baseline demographic, clinical, and radiographic variables. Standardized ways to define ICH, measure stroke severity, and interpret early CT scans would be valuable.

The previously mentioned findings are consistent with the observations that the risk of HI is higher when the residual cerebral blood flow is markedly reduced.[422, 428] In fact, both single-photon emission CT (SPECT)[428–431] and xenon-enhanced CT[432] have been shown to demonstrate areas of low or absent perfusion[428–432] and volume of vascular territory with severe flow compromise.[429, 432] In one study, frank absence of brain perfusion on SPECT was associated with the largest volume of infarction.[429] In addition, SPECT independently added to the predictive power of the Canadian Neurological Stroke Scale by distinguishing between focal decrease or absence of brain perfusion in patients studied within 72 hours of stroke onset. Hanson and colleagues showed that among 15 patients studied within 3 hours of stroke onset, a threshold value of the SPECT perfusion defect was found above which all patients suffered massive cerebral edema or HI.[430] Ueda and colleagues found that HI was significantly more likely to occur in patients with reduced regional cerebral blood flow before intra-arterial thrombolytic therapy with UK or rt-PA.[428] Kaufmann and colleagues reported that intra-arterial thrombolytic therapy was complicated in six patients who had large volumes of severe MCA territory ischemia on xenon-enhanced CT scan (i.e., 57 ± 25% of territory with flow less than 8 ml per 100 g per min versus 14 ± 15% in uncomplicated cases, $P = .01$).[432] These data suggest that pretreatment cerebral blood flow studies may help in selecting patients for thrombolytic therapy. The SPECT Safe Thrombolysis Study (SSTS) has been designed with this aim in mind.[433]

Thrombolytic Therapy for Intracerebral and Subarachnoid Hemorrhage

Parenchymatous Intracerebral Hemorrhage

Primary parenchymal hemorrhage leads to tissue destruction and mass effect with compression. Early removal of the mass might relieve compression of the microcirculation, reduce edema formation, reduce intracranial pressure, remove toxic and vasoactive blood by-products, and perhaps improve outcome.[434] Using stereotactic techniques, the hematoma coordinates are determined.[434–443] Through a burr hole, a catheter is placed in the hematoma. Aspiration of the liquid or solid part of the hematoma is attempted. Bleeding vessels are occluded or coagulated. If a significant amount of clot persists, a silicone catheter is inserted into the hematoma bed, and a thrombolytic agent (UK, rt-PA) may be infused at 6- to 8-hour intervals for up to several days. Similarly, thrombolytic agents may be infused via a ventricular catheter to facilitate removal of ventricular clot in selected cases. Serial CT scans are obtained to document response to therapy. Experimental studies in macaques,[435] rabbits,[436, 438] rats,[435] and dogs[444–446] and in vitro[439] using UK[435, 438, 444–446] and rt-PA4[439, 441] demonstrate that thrombolytic agents promote clot lysis,[432, 438] clot absorption,[441, 444] and clot aspiration.[441]

Stereotactic hematoma evacuation with the assistance of UK[434, 436, 437, 439, 440, 442, 443] or rt-PA[439, 441] has been carried out in preliminary open studies of patients with putaminal,[437, 439] basal ganglia,[439] subcortical lobar,[436] thalamic,[436] cerebellar,[436, 442] and intraventricular[447, 448] hematomas. In one study, there was no significant difference in mortality between craniotomy and stereotactic aspiration with UK in cases treated within the first 3 days or later after onset.[436] Good to very good outcomes have been reported in several studies,[437–440, 447] but some patients may have done well even without surgery.[439] In these preliminary studies, intracranial bleeding complications occurred in 0%[437, 442, 447] to 4%[437, 439, 440] of patients.

Aneurysmal Subarachnoid Hemorrhage

CT scan studies of patients with aneurysmal SAH have convincingly shown that thick subarachnoid clot can accurately predict the site and severity of vasospasm after SAH and resultant delayed ischemic neurologic deficits.[449, 450] Analysis of diverse experimental and clinical investigations indicates that early rather than later removal of subarachnoid clot offers the best chance to prevent vasospasm.[451, 452] Under normal circumstances, CSF lacks intrinsic fibrinolytic (rt-PA) activity.[453, 454] The rationale for intrathecal thrombolytic therapy after aneurysm clipping is to augment the limited fibrinolytic activity of the CSF, promote rapid clot lysis, and thereby promote clearance of entrapped erythrocytes before hemolysis and release of spasmogens near vessels in the subarachnoid space.[453, 454] Experimental studies with small numbers of pigs,[455, 456] cynolmogous monkeys,[454, 457–459] dogs,[460] and cats[461] using plasmin or various doses of rt-PA have resulted in near complete disappearance of subarachnoid clot,[457–459] significant reduction in the occurrence of angiographic vasospasm,[457–459] lower frequency of structural vessel wall changes,[455, 456, 460] and reduced CSF outflow resistance.[461] In addition, PIH, IVH, EPH, and SDH did not occur.[454–460]

Initial open clinical studies[462–466] using single[462–464] or multiple[465, 466] injections of various doses of rt-PA in patients classified as Hunt and Hess grade III or IV[466] or at high risk of developing vasospasm (Fisher grade III)[449–452] have been reported. Results indicate partial to total blood removal, demonstrated by serial postoperative CT scans over several days,[462–465] and reduced frequency of severe vasospasm demonstrated by angiography[462–464, 466] or transcranial Doppler[464] and hypodense areas on CT scan.[463] Thrombolytic therapy did not result in systemic fibrinolysis in three studies.[462, 465, 466] In three studies,[462, 463, 466] bleeding complications were frequent and included subgaleal bleeding,[463] oozing from the incision site, oozing from the ventriculostomy site,[466] and facial bruising.[463] In one study, one of five patients received 15 mg of rt-PA after clipping of a large right internal carotid artery aneurysm.[462] Postoperatively he did not awaken, and CT scan showed a large right-sided SDH, which was evacuated. The next day, however, residual right-sided SDH and a right-sided temporal PIH were removed. A second patient in that study had a thin, asymptomatic EPH that was partially aspirated the day after surgery. In another study, one of 10 patients developed a small EPH that required delayed burr hole drainage.[466] In another study, two of 30 patients developed ICH.[463] One had development of PIH after operation from which a good recovery was made with conservative therapy. The second patient required evacuation of an EPH from which a good recovery was made. Sasaki and colleagues conducted a multicenter trial of various doses of rt-PA given three times daily via a cisternal drain over 5 days after early aneurysm clipping.[467] One patient received surgery to remove a delayed-onset EPH. In addition, several cases of "increased SAH" were noted, presumably due to rt-PA treatment.

Findlay and colleagues recently reported the results of a multicenter, randomized, blinded, placebo-controlled trial to evaluate the role of intracisternal rt-PA to prevent vasospasm after SAH.[468] Although the overall incidence of angiographic vasospasm was similar between the groups (74.4% for placebo, 64.6% for rt-PA), there was a trend toward lesser severity of vasospasm ($P = .07$), lower mean flow velocities on transcranial Doppler, reduced delayed neurologic worsening, reduced use of hypervolemia and hypertensive treatment, lower 14-day mortality, and improved 3-month outcome rate. Intracranial bleeding occurred in nine of 48 (18.8%) rt-PA patients and seven of 43 (16.3%) placebo-treated patients. In each treatment group, two patients had severe life-threatening bleeds, and two patients had moderate bleeds. Neither of the severe bleeding complications in the rt-PA group was fatal.

Thrombolytic Therapy and Neuromuscular Complications

Both SK[469–471] and APSAC[472] have been associated with low back pain, at times severe, during treatment for AMI. Guillain-Barré syndrome has been reported to follow treatment with SK.[267–269] In the case of Kaiser and colleagues, oligoclonal bands in the CSF and serum were specific for SK, suggesting SK antibody complex mediated damage to the local blood-nerve barrier.[268] Seaberg and Generalovitch described a patient, who 3 hours after receiving intravenous SK for AMI after an unsuccessful right subclavian vein catheterization, was found to have a markedly elevated right hemidiaphragm on chest radiography.[270] Subsequent CT and fluoroscopy revealed paralysis of the right phrenic nerve by a hematoma. Segal and Adair reported an AMI patient who fell to the ground, striking his shoulder and arm immediately before rt-PA was administered and thereafter developed a triceps muscle compartment syndrome.[473] Burnside and colleagues described a patient in whom a volar forearm compartment syndrome developed 3 days after thrombolytic therapy for AMI associated with a disrupted forearm vein after unsuccessful catheterization.[474] After surgical decompression, the patient was left with a sensory deficit over the forearm. Blankenship reported the case of a patient treated with SK who developed inflammation of the infusion site.[475] This was followed by permanent ulnar and median neuropathy. Gillanders and colleagues reported a patient who developed spontaneous iliopsoas hemorrhage occurring after intravenous SK therapy.[272] Cadman reported a case of femoral neuropathy complicating femoral artery puncture and intra-arterial thrombolysis.[271] Piazza and colleagues described a patient who developed a femoral neuropathy associated with CT-detectable iliacus muscle hematoma after therapy with UK, heparin, and aspirin for AMI.[273] Treatment for this lesion may include discontinuation of anticoagulants and early surgical decompression.

Conclusion

Thrombolytic therapy may be complicated by diverse central and peripheral neurologic disorders. ICH is the most feared adverse event, in view of its high mortality. Evidence is accumulating to permit an accurate assessment of risks and benefits for specific patients, particularly in the AMI and ACI settings. This exercise allows the clinician to maximize the efficacy and safety of thrombolytic therapy. The frequency of cerebral embolism is low after thrombolysis, but high-risk subgroups may exist. In these instances, caution is warranted. Spinal and peripheral neurologic complications are rare.

References

1. Meyer JS, Gilroy J, Barnhart ME, et al. Anticoagulants plus streptokinase therapy in progressive stroke. JAMA 1963;189:373.
2. Meyer JS, Gilroy J, Barnhart ME, et al. Therapeutic Thrombolysis in Cerebral Thromboembolism: Randomized Evaluation of Intravenous Streptokinase. In CH Millikan, W Siekert, JP Whisnant (eds), Cerebral Vascular Diseases. New York: Grune & Stratton, 1964;200.
3. Hass WK, Clauss RM, Goldberg AF. Special problems associated with surgical and thrombolytic treatment of strokes. Arch Surg 1966;92:27.
4. Araki G, Minakami K, Mihara H. Therapeutic effects of urokinase in cerebral infarction. Rinsho to Kenkyu 1973;50:3317.
5. Fletcher AP, Alkjaersig N, Lewis M. A pilot study of urokinase therapy in cerebral infarction. Stroke 1976;7:135.
6. Hanaway J, Torack R, Fletcher AP, et al. Intracranial bleeding associated with urokinase therapy for acute ischemic hemispheral stroke. Stroke 1976;7:143.
7. del Zoppo GJ, Zeumer H, Harker LA. Thrombolytic therapy in stroke: possibilities and hazards. Stroke 1986;17:595.
8. Verstraete M, Collen D. Thrombolytic therapy in the 80s. Blood 1986;67:1529.
9. Sloan MA. Thrombolysis and stroke: past and future. Arch Neurol 1987;44:748.
10. Gruppo Italiano per lo Studio della Streptochinasi nell'Infarto Miocardico (GISSI). Effectiveness of intravenous thrombolytic treatment in acute myocardial infarction. Lancet 1986;1:397.
11. Rovelli F, Devita C, Feruglio GA, et al. GISSI trial: early results and late follow-up. J Am Coll Cardiol 1987;10(Suppl):33B.
12. Maggioni AP, Franzoni MG, Farnia ML, et al. Cerebrovascular events after myocardial infarction. BMJ 1991;302:1428.
13. The ISAM Study Group. A prospective trial of intravenous streptokinase in acute myocardial infarction (ISAM). N Engl J Med 1986;314:1465.
14. Schroder R, Neuhaus KL, Leizorovicz A, et al. A prospective placebo-controlled double-blind multicenter trial of intravenous streptokinase (ISAM): long-term mortality and morbidity in acute myocardial infarction. J Am Coll Cardiol 1987;9:197.
15. ISIS-2 (Second International Study of Infarct Survival). Randomized trial of intravenous streptokinase, oral aspirin, both or neither among 17,187 cases of suspected acute myocardial infarction: ISIS-2. Lancet 1988;2:349.
16. AIMS Trial Study Group. Effect of intravenous APSAC on mortality after acute myocardial infarction: preliminary report of a placebo-controlled clinical trial. Lancet 1988;1:545.
17. AIMS Trial Study Group. Long-term effect of intravenous anistreplase in acute myocardial infarction: final report of the AIMS study. Lancet 1990;335:427.
18. Wilcox RG, Olsson CG, Skene AM, et al. Trial of tissue plasminogen activator for mortality reduction in acute myocardial infarction: Anglo-Scandinavian Study of Early Thrombolysis (ASSET). Lancet 1988;2:525.
19. Wilcox RG, von der Lippe G, Olsson CG, et al. Effects of alteplase on acute myocardial infarction. 6-month results from the ASSET Study. Lancet 1990;335:1175.
20. Van de Werf F, Arnold AER for the European Cooperative Study Group. Intravenous tissue plasminogen activator and size of infarct, left ventricular function, and survival in acute myocardial infarction. BMJ 1988; 297:1371.
21. Gruppo Italiano per lo Studio della Sopravvivenza nell'Infarto Miocardico, GISSI-2. A factorial randomized trial of alteplase versus streptokinase and heparin versus no heparin among 12,490 patients with acute myocardial infarction. Lancet 1990;336:65.
22. International Study Group. In-hospital mortality and clinical course of 20,891 patients with suspected acute myocardial infarction randomized between alteplase and streptokinase with or without heparin. Lancet 1990;336:71.
23. Maggioni AP, Franzosi MG, Santoro E, et al. The Gruppo Italiano per lo Studio della Sopravvivenza nell'Infarto Miocardico II (GISSI-II), and the International Study Group. The risk of stroke in patients with acute myocardial infarction after thrombolytic and antithrombotic treatment. N Engl J Med 1992;327:1.
24. de Jaegere PP, Arnold AP, Balk AH, et al. Intracranial hemorrhage in association with thrombolytic therapy: incidence and clinical predictive factors. J Am Coll Cardiol 1992;20:289.
25. ISIS-3. A randomized comparison of streptokinase vs. tissue plasminogen activator vs. anistreplase and of aspirin plus heparin vs. aspirin alone among 41,299 cases of suspected acute myocardial infarction. ISIS-3 (Third International Study of Infarct Survival) Collaborative Group. Lancet 1992;339:753.
26. Uglietta JP, O'Connor CM, Boyko OB, et al. CT patterns of intracranial hemorrhage complicating thrombolytic therapy for acute myocardial infarction. Radiology 1991;181:555.

27. O'Connor CM, Aldrich H, Massey EW, et al. Intracranial hemorrhage after thrombolytic therapy for acute myocardial infarction: clinical characteristics and in hospital outcome. J Am Coll Cardiol 1990;15(Suppl):213A.
28. O'Connor CM, Califf RM, Massey EW, et al. Stroke and acute myocardial infarction in the thrombolytic era: clinical correlates and long-term prognosis. J Am Coll Cardiol 1990;16:533.
29. Kase CS, Pessin MS, Zivin JA, et al. Intracranial hemorrhage after coronary thrombolysis with tissue plasminogen activator. Am J Med 1992;92:384.
30. Vermeer F, Massberg I, Meyer J, et al. Saruplase, a new fibrin specific thrombolytic agent: efficacy and safety in the first 1000 patients. J Am Coll Cardiol 1991; 17(Suppl):152A.
31. Gore JM, Sloan M, Price TR, et al. Intracerebral hemorrhage, cerebral infarction, and subdural hematoma after acute myocardial infarction and thrombolytic therapy in the thrombolysis in myocardial infarction study. Thrombolysis in Myocardial Infarction, Phase II, Pilot and Clinical Trial. Circulation 1991;83:448.
32. Sloan MA, Price TR, Terrin ML, et al. Ischemic cerebral infarction after rt-PA and heparin therapy for acute myocardial infarction. The TIMI-II pilot and randomized trial combined experience. Stroke 1997;28:1107.
33. Sloan MA, Price TR, Petito CK, et al. for the TIMI Investigators. Clinical features and pathogenesis of intracerebral hemorrhage after rt-PA and heparin therapy for acute myocardial infarction: the TIMI II pilot and randomized clinical trial combined experience. Neurology 1995;45:649.
34. Longstreth WT, Litwin PE, Weaver WD for the MITI Project Group. Myocardial infarction, thrombolytic therapy, and stroke: a community-based study. Stroke 1993;24:587.
35. Amery A, Roeber G, Vermeulen HJ, et al. Single blind randomized multicenter trial comparing heparin and streptokinase treatment in recent myocardial infarction. Acta Med Scand 1969;505(Suppl):5.
36. European Working Party. Streptokinase in recent myocardial infarction: a controlled multicenter trial. BMJ 1971;3:325.
37. Bett JHN, Castaldi PA, Hale GS, et al. Australian multicenter trial of streptokinase in acute myocardial infarction. Lancet 1973;1:57.
38. Ness PM, Simon TL, Cole C, et al. A pilot study of streptokinase therapy in acute myocardial infarction: observations on complications in relation to trial design. Am Heart J 1974;88:705.
39. European Cooperative Study Group. Streptokinase in acute myocardial infarction. N Engl J Med 1979; 301:794.
40. Rutsch W, Schartl M, Mathey D, et al. Percutaneous transluminal coronary recanalization. Procedure, results, and acute complications. Am Heart J 1981;102:1178.
41. Weinstein J. Treatment of myocardial infarction with intracoronary streptokinase: efficacy and safety data from 209 United States cases in the Hoeschst-Roussel Registry. Am Heart J 1982;104:894.
42. Gans W, Gelt I, Shaw PK, et al. Intravenous streptokinase in evolving acute myocardial infarction. Am J Cardiol 1984;53:1209.
43. Urban PL, Cowley M, Goldberg S, et al. Intracoronary thrombolysis in acute myocardial infarction: clinical course following successful myocardial reperfusion. Am Heart J 1984;108:873.
44. Aldrich MS, Sherman SA, Greenberg HS. Cerebrovascular complications of streptokinase infusion. JAMA 1985;253:1777.
45. Lew AS, Hod H, Cercek B, et al. Mortality and morbidity rates of patients older and younger than 75 years with acute myocardial infarction treated with intravenous streptokinase. Am J Cardiol 1987;59:1.
46. PRIMI Study Group. Randomized double blind trial of recombinant prourokinase against streptokinase in acute myocardial infarction. Lancet 1989;i:863.
47. Topol EJ, Morris DC, Smalling RD, et al. A multicenter, randomized, placebo-controlled trial of a new form of intravenous recombinant tissue-type plasminogen activator (Activase) in acute myocardial infarction. J Am Coll Cardiol 1987;9:1205.
48. Topol EJ, Califf RM, George BS, et al. A randomized trial of immediate versus delayed elective angioplasty after intravenous tissue-plasminogen activator in acute myocardial infarction. N Engl J Med 1987;317:581.
49. de Bono DP. Thrombolysis with intravenous human recombinant tissue-type plasminogen activator in acute myocardial infarction: the European experience. J Am Coll Cardiol 1987;10(Suppl):75B.
50. Passamani E, Hodges M, Herman M, et al. The Thrombolysis in Myocardial Infarction (TIMI) Phase II Pilot Study: tissue plasminogen activator followed by percutaneous transluminal coronary angioplasty. J Am Coll Cardiol 1987;10(Suppl):51B.
51. National Heart Foundation of Australia Coronary Thrombolysis Group. Coronary thrombolysis and myocardial salvage by tissue plasminogen activator given up to four hours after onset of myocardial infarction. Lancet 1988;i:203.
52. Neuhaus K-L, Tebbe U, Gottwik M, et al. Intravenous recombinant tissue plasminogen activator (rt-PA) and urokinase in acute myocardial infarction. Results of the German Activator Urokinase Study (GAUS). J Am Coll Cardiol 1988;12:581.
53. Califf RM, Topol EJ, George BS, et al. Hemorrhagic complications associated with the use of intravenous tissue plasminogen activator in treatment of acute myocardial infarction. Am J Med 1988;85:353.
54. Carlson S, Aldrich MS, Greenberg HS, et al. Intracerebral hemorrhage complicating intravenous tissue plasminogen activator treatment. Arch Neurol 1988; 45:1070.
55. Althouse R, Maynard C, Olsufka M, et al. Risk factors for hemorrhagic and ischemic stroke in myocardial

infarct patients treated with tissue plasminogen activator. J Am Coll Cardiol 1989;13(Suppl):153A.
56. Tebbe U, Tanswell P, Seifried E, et al. Single bolus injection of recombinant tissue-type plasminogen activator in acute myocardial infarction. Am J Cardiol 1989;64:448.
57. Kase CS, O'Neal AN, Fisher M, et al. Intracranial hemorrhage after use of tissue plasminogen activator for coronary thrombolysis. Ann Intern Med 1990;112:17.
58. Hsia J, Hamilton WP, Kleiman N, et al. A comparison between heparin and low dose aspirin as adjunctive therapy with tissue plasminogen activator for acute myocardial infarction. N Engl J Med 1990;323:1433.
59. Smalling RW, Schumacher R, Morris D, et al. Improved infarct-related arterial patency after high dose, weight adjusted, rapid infusion of tissue-type plasminogen activator in myocardial infarction: results of a multicenter randomized trial of two dosage regimens. J Am Coll Cardiol 1990;15:915.
60. Eleff SM, Borel C, Bell WR, et al. Acute management of intracranial hemorrhage in patients receiving thrombolytic therapy. Case reports. Neurosurg 1990;26:876.
61. Kirschenbaum JM, Flaherty JT, Bahr RD, et al. Coronary thrombolysis with low dose synergistic combinations of prourokinase and recombinant tissue plasminogen activator. Circulation 1990;82(Suppl III):III-537.
62. The GUSTO Investigators. An international randomized trial comparing four thrombolytic strategies for acute myocardial infarction. N Engl J Med 1993;329:673.
63. Grines CL, Nissen SE, Booth DC, et al. A prospective, randomized trial comparing combination half dose t-PA with streptokinase to full dose t-PA in acute myocardial infarction. Preliminary report. J Am Coll Cardiol 1990;15:4A.
64. Althouse R, Maynard C, Cerqueira MD, et al. The Western Washington Myocardial Infarction Registry and Emergency Department tissue plasminogen activator treatment trial. J Am Coll Cardiol 1990;16:1298.
65. Bassand JP, Cassagnes J, Machecourt J, et al. A multicenter double-blind trial aimed at comparing the efficiency and safety of alteplase and anistreplase in acute myocardial infarction. Circulation 1990;82(Suppl III):III-665.
66. Anderson JL, Karagounis L, Allen A, et al. Older age and elevated blood pressure are risk factors for intracerebral hemorrhage after thrombolysis. J Am Coll Cardiol 1991;18:166.
67. O'Connor CM, Meese R, MacKrell J, et al. Reduced hemorrhagic complications following APSAC therapy in acute myocardial infarction by withholding heparin. J Am Coll Cardiol 1992;19:91A
68. Tranchesi B, Caramelli B, Gegara O, et al. Efficacy and safety of ridogrel versus aspirin in coronary thrombosis with alteplase for myocardial infarction. J Am Coll Cardiol 1992;19:92A.
69. Wall TC, Califf RM, George BS, et al. Accelerated plasminogen activator dose regimens for coronary thrombolysis. J Am Coll Cardiol 1992;19:482.
70. von Essen R, Neuhaus KL, Markreiter M, et al. Double bolus of r-PA in the dosage finding. Results of the GRECO-II-Study. J Am Coll Cardiol 1992;19:274A.
71. Neuhaus KL, von Essen R, Tebbe U, et al. Improved thrombolysis in acute myocardial infarction with front-loaded administration of alteplase: results of the rt-PA-APSAC Patency Study (TAPS). J Am Coll Cardiol 1992;19:885.
72. Cherng WF, Chiang CW, Kuo CT, et al. A comparison between intravenous streptokinase and tissue plasminogen activator with early intravenous heparin in acute myocardial infarction. Am Heart J 1992;123:841.
73. Carney RJ, Murphy GA, Brandt TR, et al. Randomized angiographic trial of recombinant tissue-type plasminogen activator (alteplase) in myocardial infarction. J Am Coll Cardiol 1992;20:17.
74. Weisberg LA. The fluid blood level in intracranial hematoma due to anticoagulant medication. J Neurol Neurosurg Psychiatry 1987;50:1076.
75. Gorelick PB, Parik M, McDonald L. Intracoronary streptokinase and fatal cerebellar hemorrhage. Ill Med J 1987;171:28.
76. Proner J, Rosenblum BR, Rothman A. Ruptured arteriovenous malformation complicating thrombolytic therapy with tissue plasminogen activator. Arch Neurol 1990;47:105.
77. Da Silva VF, Bormanis J. Intracerebral hemorrhage after combined anticoagulant-thrombolytic therapy for myocardial infarction: two case reports and a short review. Neurosurgery 1992;30:943.
78. Ramsay DA, Penswick JL, Robertson DM. Fatal streptokinase-induced intracerebral haemorrhage in cerebral amyloid angiopathy. Can J Neurol Sci 1990;17:336.
79. Pendlebury WW, Iole ED, Tracy RP, et al. Intracerebral hemorrhage related to cerebral amyloid angiopathy and t-PA treatment. Ann Neurol 1991;29:210.
80. Kase CS. Intracranial Hemorrhage After Coronary Thrombolysis with Tissue Plasminogen Activator. In W Hacke, GJ del Zoppo, M Hirschberg (eds), Thrombolytic Therapy in Acute Ischemic Stroke. Berlin: Springer-Verlag, 1991;75.
81. Wijdicks CFM, Jack CR. Intracerebral hemorrhage after fibrinolytic therapy for acute myocardial infarction. Stroke 1993;24:554.
82. Leblanc R, Haddad G, Robitaille Y. Cerebral hemorrhage from amyloid angiopathy after coronary thrombolysis. Neurosurgery 1992;31:586.
83. Sloan MA, del Zoppo GJ, Brott TG. Thrombolysis and Stroke. In DG Julian, W Kubler, RM Norris, et al. (eds), Thrombolysis in Cardiovascular Disease. New York: Marcel-Dekker, 1989;361.
84. Sloan MA, Price TR. Intracranial hemorrhage following thrombolytic therapy for acute myocardial infarction. Semin Neurol 1991;11:385.

85. Sloan MA, Gore JM. Ischemic stroke and intracranial hemorrhage following thrombolytic therapy for acute myocardial infarction. A risk-benefit analysis. Am J Cardiol 1992;69:21A.
86. Sloan MA. Stroke associated with thrombolytic therapy for acute myocardial infarction. Heart Dis Stroke 1992;1:287.
87. Sloan MA. Thrombolysis and Intracranial Hemorrhage. In E Feldmann (ed), Intracerebral Hemorrhage. Armonk, NY: Futura, 1994;99.
88. TIMI Research Group. Immediate versus delayed catheterization and angioplasty following thrombolytic therapy for acute myocardial infarction: TIMI IIA results. JAMA 1988;260:2849.
89. TIMI Study Group. Comparison of invasive and conservative strategies after treatment with intravenous tissue plasminogen activator in acute myocardial infarction: results of the Thrombolysis in Myocardial Infarction (TIMI) Phase II Trial. N Engl J Med 1989;320:618.
90. EMERAS (Estudio Multicéntrico Estreptoquinasa Repúblicas de América del Sur) Collaborative Group: randomized trial of late thrombolysis in patients with suspected acute myocardial infarction. Lancet 1993;342:767.
91. LATE Study Group. Late assessment of thrombolytic efficacy (LATE) study with alteplase 6–24 hours after onset of acute myocardial infarction. Lancet 1993;342:759.
92. International Joint Efficacy Comparison of Thrombolytics. Randomized double blind comparison of reteplase double-bolus administration with streptokinase in acute myocardial infarction. Trial to investigate equivalence. Lancet 1995;346:329.
93. Kaufmann HH, McAllister P, Taylor M, et al. Intracerebral hematoma related to thrombolysis for myocardial infarction. Neurosurgery 1993;33:898.
94. Levine MN, Goldhaber SZ, Gore JM, et al. Hemorrhagic complications of thrombolytic therapy in the treatment of myocardial infarction and venous thromboembolism. Chest 1995;108:291S.
95. Lauer JE, Meyer JJ, Mirro MJ. Hemorrhagic complications of thrombolytic therapy. Chest 1995;108:1520.
96. Conrad AR, Feffer SE, Rajan RT, et al. Intracranial hemorrhage complicating acute myocardial infarction in the era of thrombolytic therapy. South Med J 1997;90:5.
97. Fibrinolytic Therapy Trialists (FTT) Collaborative Group. Indications for fibrinolytic therapy in suspected acute myocardial infarction: collaborative overview of early mortality and major morbidity results from all randomised trials of more than 1000 patients. Lancet 1994;343:311.
98. Collins R, Peto R, Baigent C, Sleight P. Aspirin, heparin, and fibrinolytic therapy in suspected acute myocardial infarction. N Engl J Med 1997;336:847.
99. Robertson BR, Wilsson IM, Nylander G. Value of streptokinase and heparin in treatment of acute deep venous thrombosis; a coded investigation. Acta Chir Scand 1968;134:202.
100. Kakkar VV, Flonce C, Houle CT, et al. Treatment of deep vein thrombosis: a trial of heparin, streptokinase and arvin. BMJ 1979;1:806.
101. Tibbutt OA, Williams EW, Walker ME, et al. Controlled trial of ancrod and streptokinase in the treatment of deep vein thrombosis of lower limbs. Br J Haematol 1974;27:407.
102. Porter JM, Seamon AJ, Connon HH, et al. Comparison of heparin and streptokinase in the treatment of venous thrombosis. Am Surg 1974;41:511.
103. Elliott MS, Immelman EJ, Jeffery P, et al. A comparative randomized trial of heparin versus streptokinase in the treatment of acute proximal venous thrombosis: an interim report of a prospective trial. Br J Surg 1979;66:838.
104. Schulman S, Lockner D, Gronquist S, et al. A comparative randomized trial of low dose versus high dose streptokinase in deep vein thrombosis of the thigh. Thromb Haemost 1984;51:261.
105. Goldhaber SZ, Meyerovitz MF, Green D, et al. Randomized controlled trial of tissue plasminogen activator in proximal deep venous thrombosis. Am J Med 1990;98:235.
106. Turpie AG, Levine MN, Hirsh J, et al. Tissue plasminogen activator (rt-PA) vs heparin in deep vein thrombosis. Chest 1990;97(Suppl):172.
107. Bounameaux H, Banga JD, Bluhmki E, et al. Double-blind randomized comparison of systemic continuous infusion of 0.25 versus 0.5 mg/kg/24 h of alteplase over 3 to 7 days for treatment of deep venous thrombosis: results of the European Thrombolysis with rt-PA in Venous Thrombosis (ETTT) trial. Thromb Haemost 1992;67:306.
108. Goldhaber SZ, Polak JF, Feldstein MI, et al. Efficacy and safety of repeated boluses of urokinase in the treatment of deep vein thrombosis. Am J Cardiol 1994;73:75.
109. Moia M, Mannucci P, Pini M, et al. A pilot study of pro-urokinase in the treatment of deep vein thrombosis. Thromb Haemost 1994;72:430.
110. Urokinase Pulmonary Embolism Trial Study Group. Urokinase pulmonary embolism trial: phase I results. JAMA 1970;214:2163.
111. Ly B, Arnesen H, Erie H, et al. A controlled trial of streptokinase and heparin in the treatment of major pulmonary embolism. Acta Med Scand 1978;203:465.
112. Tibbutt DA, Davies JA, Anderson JA, et al. Comparisons by controlled clinical trial of streptokinase and heparin in treatment of life-threatening pulmonary embolism. BMJ 1974;1:343.
113. Urokinase Pulmonary Embolism Trial Study Group. Urokinase/streptokinase embolism trial: phase 2 trial results. JAMA 1974;229:1606.
114. Verstraete M, Miller GAN, Bounemeaux H, et al. Intravenous and intrapulmonary recombinant tissue-type

plasminogen activator in the treatment of acute massive pulmonary embolism. Circulation 1988;77:353.

115. Goldhaber SZ, Kessler CM, Heit J, et al. A randomized controlled trial of recombinant tissue plasminogen activator versus urokinase in the treatment of acute pulmonary embolism. Lancet 1988;2:293.

116. Goldhaber SZ, Kessler CM, Heit J, et al. Recombinant tissue-type plasminogen activator versus a novel dosing regimen of urokinase in acute pulmonary embolism: a randomized controlled trial. J Am Coll Cardiol 1992; 20:24.

117. A Collaborative Study by the PIOPED Investigators. Tissue plasminogen activator for the treatment of acute pulmonary embolism. Chest 1990;97:528.

118. Levine M, Hirsh J, Weitz J, et al. A randomized trial of single bolus dosage regimen of recombinant tissue plasminogen activator in patients with acute pulmonary embolism. Chest 1990;98:1473.

119. Marini C, DiRicco G, Rossi G, et al. Fibrinolytic effects of urokinase and heparin in acute pulmonary embolism: a randomized clinical trial. Respiration 1988;54:162.

120. The UKEP Study. Multicentre trial on two local regimens of urokinase in massive pulmonary embolism. Eur Heart J 1987;8:2.

121. Meyer G, Sors H, Charbonnier B, et al. Effects of intravenous urokinase versus alteplase on total pulmonary resistance in acute massive pulmonary embolism: a European multicenter double-blind trial. J Am Coll Cardiol 1992;19:239.

122. Dalla-Volta S, Palla A, Santolicandro A, et al. Alteplase combined with heparin versus heparin in the treatment of acute pulmonary embolism: Plasminogen Activator Italian Multicenter Study 2. J Am Coll Cardiol 1992; 20:520.

123. Goldhaber SZ, Haire WD, Feldstein ML, et al. Alteplase versus heparin in acute pulmonary embolism: randomized trial assessing right ventricular function and pulmonary perfusion. Lancet 1993;341:507.

124. Sors H, Pacouret G, Azarian R, et al. Hemodynamic effects of bolus vs 2 h infusion of alteplase in acute massive pulmonary embolism: a randomized controlled multicenter trial. Chest 1994;106:712.

125. Goldhaber SZ, Agnelli G, Levine MN, et al. Reduced dose bolus alteplase vs conventional alteplase infusion for pulmonary embolism thrombolysis: an international multicenter randomized trial. Chest 1994;106:718.

126. Berridge DC, Makin GS, Hopkinson BR. Local low dose intra-arterial thrombolytic therapy: the risk of stroke or major haemorrhage. Br J Surg 1989;76:1230.

127. Sussman BJ, Fitch TSP. Thrombolysis with fibrinolysin in cerebral arterial occlusion. JAMA 1958;167:1705.

128. Herndon RM, Meyer JS, Johnson JF, et al. Treatment of cardiovascular thrombosis with fibrinolysin. Am J Cardiol 1960;30:540.

129. Clarke RL, Clifton EE. The treatment of cerebrovascular thrombosis and embolism with fibrinolytic agents. Am J Cardiol 1960;30:546.

130. Meyer JS, Herndon RM, Gotch F. Therapeutic Thrombolysis. In CH Millikan, W Siekert, JP Whisnant (eds), Cerebral Vascular Disease: Third Princeton Conference. New York: Grune & Stratton, 1961;160.

131. Atkin N, Nitzberg S, Dorsey J. Lysis of intracerebral thromboembolism with fibrinolysin: report of a case. Angiology 1964;15:436.

132. Brooks J, Davis D, Devivo G. Blood hypercoagulability in acute cerebrovascular syndromes: its control with urokinase therapy. J Lab Clin Med 1970;76:879.

133. Larcan A, Laprevote-Heully MC, Lambert H, et al. Indications de thrombolytique au cours de accidents vasculaires cérébraux thrombosants traités pars ailleurs par OMB (ZATA). Therapie 1977;32:259.

134. Malinovsky NN, Kozlov VA. Embolism of the Cerebral Arteries. In Anticoagulant and Thrombolytic Therapy in Surgery. St. Louis: Mosby, 1979;239.

135. Labauge A, Bland J-M, Salvaing P, et al. Traitment fibrinolytique et anticoagulant dans 37 cas d'occlusions arterielles: cervicocerebrales d'origin thromboembolique. In Proceedings of the Fifth International Congress on Thromboembolism. Bologna, Italy, 1978. Pisa, Italy: Quaderni della Coagulazione, 1980;362.

136. Abe T, Kasawa M, Naito I, et al. Clinical evaluation for efficacy of tissue culture urokinase (TCUK) on cerebral thrombosis by means of multicenter double-blind study. Blood Vessels 1981;12:321.

137. Abe T, Sazawa M, Naito I, et al. Clinical effect of urokinase (60,000 U/d) on cerebral infarction: comparative study by means of multicenter double-blind test. Blood Vessels 1981;12:342.

138. Zeumer H, Hacke W, Kolmann HL, et al. Lokale fibrinolyse bei basilaris thrombose. Dtsch Med Wochenschr 1982;102:728.

139. Zeumer H, Hacke W, Ringelstein EB. Intra-arterial thrombolysis in vertebrobasilar thromboembolic disease. Am J Neuroradiol 1983;4:401.

140. Nenci GG, Gresele P, Taramelli M, et al. Thrombolytic therapy for thromboembolism of vertebrobasilar artery. Angiology 1983;34:561.

141. Miyakawa T. The cerebral vessels and thrombosis. Rinsho Ketseuki 1984;25:1018.

142. Zeumer H, Hundgen R, Ferbert A, et al. Local intraarterial fibrinolytic therapy in inaccessible internal carotid occlusion. Neuroradiology 1984;76:315.

143. Zeumer H. Vascular recanalization techniques in interventional neuroradiology. J Neurol 1985;231:287.

144. Atarashi J, Otomo E, Araki G, et al. Clinical utility of urokinase in the treatment of acute stage of cerebral thrombosis: multicenter double-blind study in comparison with placebo. Clin Eval 1985;13:659.

145. Otomo E, Araki G, Itch E, et al. Clinical efficacy of urokinase in the treatment of cerebral thrombosis: multicenter double-blind study in comparison with placebo. Clin Eval 1985;13:711.

146. Bruckman H, Ferbert A, del Zoppo GJ, et al. Acute vertebrobasilar thrombosis: angiologic-clinical compari-

son and therapeutic implications. Acta Radiol 1986; (Suppl 369):38.
147. Koudstaal PJ, Stibbe J, Vermeulen M. Fatal ischemic brain oedema after early thrombolysis with tissue plasminogen activator in acute stroke. BMJ 1988;297:1571.
148. Henze TH, Breer A, Tebbe U, et al. Lysis of basilar artery occlusion with tissue plasminogen activator. Lancet 1987;2:1391.
149. del Zoppo GJ, Ferbert A, Otis S, et al. Local intra-arterial fibrinolytic therapy in acute carotid territory stroke. Stroke 1988;19:307.
150. del Zoppo GJ. Thrombolysis: New Concepts in the Treatment of Stroke. In M Hennerici, G Sitzer, H-D Weger (eds), Carotid Artery Plaques. Basel: Karger, 1988;247.
151. Hacke W, Zeumer H, Ferbert A, et al. Intraarterial fibrinolytic therapy improves outcome in patients with acute vertebrobasilar occlusive disease. Stroke 1988;19:1216.
152. Mori E, Tabuchi M, Yoshida T, et al. Intracarotid urokinase with thromboembolic occlusion of the middle cerebral artery. Stroke 1988;19:802.
153. Otomo E, Tohgi H, Hirai T, et al. Clinical efficacy of AK-124 (tissue plasminogen activator) in the treatment of cerebral thrombosis: study by means of multicenter double-blind comparison with urokinase. Yakuri To Chiryo 1988;16:3775.
154. Theron J, Courtheoux P, Casasco A, et al. Local intra-arterial fibrinolysis in carotid territory. Am J Neuroradiol 1989;10:753.
155. Buteux G, Jubault V, Suisse A, et al. Local recombinant tissue plasminogen activator to clear cerebral artery thrombosis developing soon after surgery. Lancet 1988;1:1143.
156. Brückman H, Ferbert A. Putamenal haemorrhage after recanalization of an embolic MCA occlusion treated with tissue plasminogen activator. Neuroradiology 1989;31:95.
157. The Ancrod Stroke Study Investigators. Ancrod for the treatment of acute ischemic brain infarction. Stroke 1994;25:1755.
158. Zeumer H, Freitag H-J, Grzyska U, et al. Interventional neuroradiology: local intra-arterial fibrinolysis in acute vertebrobasilar occlusion. Technical developments and recent results. Neuroradiology 1989;31:336.
159. Terashi A, Kobayashi Y, Katayama Y, et al. Clinical effects and basic studies of thrombolytic therapy on cerebral thrombosis. Semin Thromb Hemost 1990; 16:236.
160. Ikeda S, Muraishi K. Intra-arterial urokinase infusion therapy for the superacute intracranial major artery occlusions. Stroke 1990;21(Suppl I):I-95.
161. Hennerici M, for the German t-PA-Stroke Study Group. Fibrinolysis of intracranial arteries. Stroke 1990;21(Suppl I):I-129.
162. Abe T, Tarashi A, Tohgi H, et al. Clinical efficacy of intravenous administration of SM-9527 (t-PA) in cerebral thrombosis. Clin Eval 1990;18:39.
163. Asplund K, Carlberg B. Thrombolysis in Stroke: Timing of Recanalization and its Clinical Consequences. In W Hacke, GJ del Zoppo, M Hirschberg (eds), Thrombolytic Therapy in Acute Ischemic Stroke. Berlin: Springer-Verlag, 1991;46.
164. Hacke W. Intraarterial Urokinase Plasminogen Activator and Streptokinase in Carotid and Vertebrobasilar Territory Stroke: Clinical Outcome. In W Hacke, GJ del Zoppo, M Hirschberg (eds), Thrombolytic Therapy in Acute Ischemic Stroke. Berlin: Springer-Verlag, 1991;131.
165. Mori E. Fibrinolytic Recanalization Therapy in Acute Cerebrovascular Thromboembolism. In W Hacke, GJ del Zoppo, M Hirschberg (eds), Thrombolytic Therapy in Acute Ischemic Stroke. Berlin: Springer-Verlag, 1991;137.
166. Mori E, Yoneda Y, Tabuchi M, et al. Intravenous recombinant tissue plasminogen activator in acute carotid artery territory stroke. Neurology 1992;42:976.
167. von Kummer R, Forsting M, Sartor K, et al. Intravenous Recombinant Tissue Plasminogen Activator in Acute Stroke. In W Hacke, GJ del Zoppo, M Hirschberg (eds), Thrombolytic Therapy in Acute Ischemic Stroke. Berlin: Springer-Verlag, 1991;161.
168. von Kummer R, Forsting M, Hutschenreuter M, et al. Angiography in acute stroke due to occlusions of intracerebral arteries before and after treatment with intravenous recombinant tissue plasminogen activator. Stroke 1990;21(Suppl I):I-94.
169. von Kummer R, Hacke W. Safety and efficacy of intravenous tissue plasminogen activator and heparin in acute middle cerebral artery stroke. Stroke 1992; 23:646.
170. Yamaguchi T, Hayakama T, Kikuchi H, et al. Thrombolytic Therapy in Embolic and Thrombotic Cerebral Infarction: A Cooperative Study. In W Hacke, GJ del Zoppo, M Hirschberg (eds), Thrombolytic Therapy in Acute Ischemic Stroke. Berlin: Springer-Verlag, 1991;168.
171. Matsumoto K, Satoh K. Topical Intra-Arterial Urokinase Infusion for Acute Stroke. In W Hacke, GJ del Zoppo, M Hirschberg (eds), Thrombolytic Therapy in Acute Ischemic Stroke. Berlin: Springer-Verlag, 1991;207.
172. Möbius E, Berg-Dammer E, Kühne D, et al. Local Thrombolytic Therapy in Acute Basilar Artery Occlusion: Experience with 18 Patients. In W Hacke, GJ del Zoppo, M Hirschberg (eds), Thrombolytic Therapy in Acute Ischemic Stroke. Berlin: Springer-Verlag, 1991;213.
173. Pfeiffer G, Thayssen G, Arlt A, et al. Vertebrobasilar Occlusion: Outcome With and Without Local Intra-Arterial Fibrinolysis. In W Hacke, GJ del Zoppo, M Hirschberg (eds), Thrombolytic Therapy in Acute Ischemic Stroke. Berlin: Springer-Verlag, 1991;216.
174. Biniek R, Ringelstein EB, Brückman H, et al. Recanalization of Acute Middle Cerebral Artery Occlusion Monitored by Transcranial Doppler Sonography. In W Hacke, GJ del Zoppo, M Hirschberg (eds), Throm-

bolytic Therapy in Acute Ischemic Stroke. Berlin: Springer-Verlag, 1991;221.

175. Pilz P, Ladurner G, Griebnitz E. Neuropathological Findings After Thrombolytic Therapy in Acute Ischemic Stroke. In W Hacke, GJ del Zoppo, M Hirschberg (eds), Thrombolytic Therapy in Acute Ischemic Stroke. Berlin: Springer-Verlag, 1991;224.

176. Siepmann G, Müller-Jensen M, Goossens-Merkt H, et al. Local Intra-Arterial Fibrinolysis in Acute Middle Cerebral Artery Occlusion. In W Hacke, GJ del Zoppo, M Hirschberg (eds), Thrombolytic Therapy in Acute Ischemic Stroke. Berlin: Springer-Verlag, 1991;240.

177. Herderscheé D, Limburg U, Hijdra A, et al. Recombinant tissue plasminogen activator in two patients with basilar artery occlusion. J Neurol Neurosurg Psychiatry 1991;54:71.

178. Herderscheé D, Limburg M, Hijdra A, et al. Treatment of Acute Ischemic Stroke with Recombinant Tissue Plasminogen Activator: Evaluation with Regional Cerebral Blood Flow Single Photon Emission Computed Tomography. In W Hacke, GJ del Zoppo, M Hirschberg (eds), Thrombolytic Therapy in Acute Ischemic Stroke. Berlin: Springer-Verlag, 1991;244.

179. Wildemann B, von Kummer R, Hutschenreuter M, et al. Basilar Artery Occlusion Associated with Protein C Deficiency: Successful Treatment Using Recombinant Tissue Plasminogen Activator Infusion. In W Hacke, GJ del Zoppo, M Hirschberg (eds), Thrombolytic Therapy in Acute Ischemic Stroke. Berlin: Springer-Verlag, 1991;255.

180. Hamann G, Haass A, Pindur G, et al. Prourokinase Therapy in Stroke. In W Hacke, GJ del Zoppo, M Hirschberg (eds), Thrombolytic Therapy in Acute Ischemic Stroke. Berlin: Springer-Verlag, 1991;262.

181. The rt-PA/Acute Stroke Study Group. An open safety/efficacy trial of rt-PA in acute thromboembolic stroke: final report. Stroke 1991;22:153.

182. del Zoppo G, Poeck K, Pessin MS, et al. Recombinant tissue plasminogen activator in acute thrombotic and embolic stroke. Ann Neurol 1992;32:78.

183. Brott TG, Haley EC, Levy DE, et al. Urgent therapy for stroke. Part I. Pilot study of tissue plasminogen activator administered within 90 minutes. Stroke 1992;23:632.

184. Haley EC, Levy DE, Brott TG, et al. Urgent therapy for stroke. Part II. Pilot study of tissue plasminogen activator administered 91–180 minutes from onset. Stroke 1992;23:641.

185. Haley EC, Brott TG, Sheppard GL, et al. for the TPA Bridging Study Group. Pilot randomized trial of tissue plasminogen activator in acute ischemic stroke. Stroke 1993;24:1000.

186. Sperling B, Overgaard K, Videbk C, et al. Evaluation of thrombolytic therapy in acute ischemic stroke with pre- and posttreatment rCBF measurements. Presented at the Second International Symposium on Thrombolytic Therapy for Acute Stroke, San Diego, May 1992.

187. Brucker B, Laich E, Bhm-Jurkovic H, et al. Relation of thrombolytic reperfusion and of collateral circulation to outcome in patients suffering cerebral main artery occlusion. Presented at the Second International Symposium on Thrombolytic Therapy for Acute Stroke, San Diego, May 1992.

188. Wardlaw JM, Warlow CP. Thrombolysis in acute ischemic stroke. Does it work? Stroke 1992;23:1826.

189. Levy DE, Brott TG, Haley EC Jr, et al. Factors related to intracranial hematoma formation in patients receiving tissue-type plasminogen activator for acute ischemic stroke. Stroke 1994;25:291.

190. Okada Y, Sadoshima S, Nakane H, et al. Early computed tomographic findings for thrombolytic therapy in patients with acute brain embolism. Stroke 1992;23:20.

191. Trouillas P, Nighoghossian N, Getenet J-C, et al. Open trial of intravenous tissue plasminogen activator in acute carotid territory stroke. Correlations of outcome with clinical and radiological data. Stroke 1996;27:882.

192. Yamaguchi T, Hayakawa T, Kikuchi H. Intravenous Tissue Plasminogen Activator in Acute Thromboembolic Stroke: A Placebo-Controlled, Double-Blind Trial. In G del Zoppo, E Mori, W Hacke (eds), Thrombolytic Therapy in Acute Ischemic Stroke II. New York: Springer-Verlag, 1993;59.

193. Brandt T, von Kummer R, Müller-Küppers M, et al. Thrombolytic therapy of acute basilar artery occlusion. Variables affecting recanalization and outcome. Stroke 1996;27:875.

194. Zeumer H, Freitag MJ, Zanella F, et al. Local intra-arterial fibrinolytic therapy in patients with stroke: urokinase versus recombinant tissue plasminogen activator (rt-PA). Neuroradiology 1993;35:159.

195. LaMonte MP, Hurst RW, Raps EC, et al. Selective intra-arterial thrombolysis for acute cerebral ischemia: a case control comparison. Neurology 1995;45(Suppl 4):A469.

196. Komiyama M, Nishijima Y, Nishio A, et al. Extravasation of contrast medium from the lenticulo-striate artery following local intracarotid fibrinolysis. Surg Neurol 1993;39:315.

197. Wolpert SM, Bruckmann H, Greenlee R, et al. and the rt-PA Acute Stroke Study Group. Neuroradiologic evaluation of patients with acute stroke treated with recombinant tissue plasminogen activator. Am J Neuroradiol 1993;14:3.

198. Jansen O, von Kummer R, Forsting M, et al. Thrombolytic therapy in acute occlusion of the intracranial internal carotid artery bifurcation. AJNR Am J Neuroradiol 1995;16:1977.

199. Lanzieri CF, Tarr RW, Landis D, et al. Cost-effectiveness of emergency intra-arterial intracerebral thrombolysis: a pilot study. AJNR Am J Neuroradiol 1995; 16:1987.

200. Overgaard K, Sperling B, Boysen G, et al. Thrombolytic therapy in acute ischemic stroke: a Danish pilot study. Stroke 1993;24:1439.

201. Tirschwell DL, Coplin WM, Longstreth WT, et al. Intraarterial urokinase for acute ischemic stroke: experience with 23 patients. Neurology 1997;48(Suppl): A271.
202. Demchuk A, Hoyte K, Newcommon N, et al. Open label rt-PA therapy for acute ischemic stroke: the Calgary experience. Neurology 1997;48(Suppl):A272.
203. Frey JL, Greene KA, Khayata MH, et al. Intrathrombus administration of tissue plasminogen activator in acute cerebrovascular occlusion. Angiology 1995;46:649.
204. Barr JD, Horowitz MB, Mathis JM, et al. Intraoperative urokinase infusion for embolic stroke during carotid endarterectomy. Neurosurgery 1995;36:606.
205. Huemer H, Niederwieser V, Ladurner G. Thrombolytic treatment for acute occlusion of the basilar artery. J Neurol Neurosurg Psychiatry 1995;58:227.
206. Sasaki O, Takeuchi S, Koike T, et al. Fibrinolytic therapy for acute embolic stroke: intravenous, intracarotid, and intra-arterial local approaches. Neurosurgery 1995;36:246.
207. Casto L, Moschini L, Camerlingo M, et al. Local intraarterial thrombolysis for acute stroke in the carotid artery territories. Acta Neurol Scand 1992;86:308.
208. Adams HP, Brott TG, Furlan AJ, et al. Guidelines for thrombolytic therapy for acute stroke: a supplement to the guidelines for the management of patients with acute ischemic stroke. Stroke 1996;27:1711.
209. Hommel M, Boissel JP, Cornu C, et al. for the MAST Study Group. Termination of trial of streptokinase in severe acute ischaemic stroke. Lancet 1994;345:57.
210. Donnan GA, Davis SM, Chambers BR, et al. Trials of streptokinase in severe acute ischaemic stroke. Lancet 1995;345:578.
211. Multicentre Acute Stroke Trial-Italy (MAST-I) Group. Randomised controlled trial of streptokinase, aspirin, and combination of both in treatment of acute ischaemic stroke. Lancet 1995;346:1509.
212. Hacke W, Kaste M, Fieschi C, et al. for the ECASS Study Group. Intravenous thrombolysis with recombinant tissue plasminogen activator for acute hemispheric stroke: the European Cooperative Acute Stroke Study (ECASS). JAMA 1995;274:1017.
213. The National Institute of Neurological Disorders and Stroke rt-PA Stroke Study Group. Tissue plasminogen activator for acute ischemic stroke. N Engl J Med 1995;333:1581.
214. Donnan GA, Davis SM, Chambers BM, et al. for the Australian Streptokinase (ASK) Trial Study Group. Streptokinase for acute ischemic stroke with relationship to time of administration. JAMA 1996;276:961.
215. The Multicenter Acute Stroke Study—Europe Study Group. Thrombolytic therapy with streptokinase in acute ischemic stroke. N Engl J Med 1996;335:145.
216. Lovecchio F, Nelson L. Intraventricular bleeding after the use of thrombolytics in a cocaine user. Am J Emerg Med 1996;14:663.
217. Lopez FG, Mata GV, Toral AR, et al. Thrombolytic treatment for massive thrombosis of prosthetic cardiac valves. Intensive Care Med 1993;19:145.
218. Taylor MA, Santoain EC, Aji J, et al. Intracerebral hemorrhage complicating urokinase infusion into an occluded aortocoronary bypass graft. Catheter Cardiovasc Diagn 1994;31:206.
219. DiSalvo TG, Tatter SB, O'Gara PT, et al. Fatal intracerebral hemorrhage following thrombolytic therapy of embolic myocardial infarction in unsuspected infective endocarditis. Clin Cardiol 1994;17:340.
220. More RS, Vincent R. Intracerebral hemorrhage after thrombolytic therapy for acute myocardial infarction. Postgrad Med J 1992;68:800.
221. Herzog C, Henry T, Zimmer S. Bacterial endocarditis presenting as acute myocardial infarction: a cautionary note for the era of reperfusion. Am J Med 1991;90:392.
222. Masuoka H, Kotani H, Yazu T, et al. An autopsy case of intracranial hemorrhage during tissue plasminogen activator infusion. Heart and Vessels 1993;8:163.
223. Reynard CA, Calain P, Pizzolato GP, et al. Severe acute myocardial infarction during a staphylococcal septicemia with meningoencephalitis. A possible contraindication to thrombolytic treatment. Intensive Care Med 1992;18:247.
224. Simoons ML, Maggioni AP, Knatterud G, et al. Individual risk assessment for intracranial hemorrhage during thrombolytic therapy. Lancet 1993;342:1523.
225. Sloan MA, Kittner SJ, Feeser BR, et al. Illicit drug use in young adults with intracerebral hemorrhage. The Baltimore-Washington Cooperative Young Stroke Study. Submitted to Neurology.
226. Selker HP, Beshansky JR, Schmid CH, et al. Presenting pulse pressure predicts thrombolytic therapy-related intracranial hemorrhage: Thrombolytic Predictive Instrument (TPI) Project results. Circulation 1994;90:1657.
227. White HD, Barbash GI, Modan M, et al. for the Investigators of the International Tissue Plasminogen Activator/Streptokinase Mortality Study. After correcting for worse baseline characteristics, women treated with thrombolytic therapy for acute myocardial infarction have the same mortality and morbidity as men except for a higher incidence of hemorrhagic stroke. Circulation 1993;88:2097.
228. The Global Use of Strategies to Open Occluded Coronary Arteries (GUSTO) IIa Investigators. Randomized trial of intravenous heparin versus recombinant hirudin for acute coronary syndromes. Circulation 1994;90:1631.
229. Antman EM. Hirudin in acute myocardial infarction: safety report from the Thrombolysis and Thrombin Inhibition in Myocardial Infarction (TIMI) 9A Trial. Circulation 1994;90:1624.
230. Neuhaus KL, von Essen R, Tebbe U, et al. Safety observations from the pilot phase of the randomized r-Hirudin for Improvement of Thrombolysis (HIT-III) study: a study of the Arbeitsegemeinschaft Leitender Kardiologischer Krankenhausartze (ALKK). Circulation 1994;90:1638.

231. Sobel BE. Intracranial bleeding, fibrinolysis and anticoagulation. Causal, connective and clinical implications. Circulation 1994;90:2147.
232. Maggioni AF, Maseri A, Fresco C, et al. on behalf of the Investigators of the Gruppo Italiano per lo studio della streptochinasi nell'Infarto Miocardico (The Gruppo Italiano per lo Studio della Sopravvivenza nell'Infarto Miocardico II-aissi-2). Age related increase in mortality among patients treated with first myocardial infarction treated with thrombolysis. N Engl J Med 1993;329:1442.
233. Lee KL, Woodlief LH, Topol EJ, et al. for the GUSTO-I Investigators. Predictors of 30 day mortality in the era of reperfusion for acute myocardial infarction. Results from an international trial of 41,021 patients. Circulation 1995;91:1659.
234. White HD, Barbash GI, Califf RM, et al. for the GUSTO-I Investigators. Age and outcome with contemporary thrombolytic therapy. Results from the GUSTO-I trial. Circulation 1996;94:1826.
235. Gore JM, Granger CB, Simoons ML, et al. for the GUSTO-I Investigators. Stroke after thrombolysis. Mortality and functional outcomes in the GUSTO-I trial. Circulation 1995;92:2811.
236. Hillegass WB, Jolis JG, Granger CB, et al. Intracranial hemorrhage risk and new thrombolytic therapies in acute myocardial infarction. Am J Cardiol 1994;73:444.
237. Aylward PE, Wilcox RG, Horgan JH, et al. for the GUSTO-I Investigators. Relation of increased arterial blood pressure to mortality and stroke in the context of contemporary thrombolytic therapy for acute myocardial infarction: a randomized trial. Ann Intern Med 1996;125:891.
238. Granger CB, Hirsh J, Califf RM, et al. for the GUSTO-I Investigators. Activated partial thromboplastin time and outcome after thrombolytic therapy for acute myocardial infarction. Results from the GUSTO-I trial. Circulation 1996;93:870.
239. The global use of strategies to open occluded coronary arteries (GUSTO) IIb Investigators. A comparison of recombinant hirudin with heparin for the treatment of acute coronary syndromes. N Engl J Med 1996; 335:775.
240. Bovill EG, Tracy RP, Knatterud GL, et al. Hemorrhagic events during therapy with recombinant tissue plasminogen activator, heparin and aspirin for unstable angina. (Thrombolysis in Myocardial Ischemia, Phase III B trial.) Am J Cardiol 1997;79:391.
241. Granger C, White H, Simoons M, et al. Risk factors for stroke following thrombolytic therapy: case control study from the GUSTO trial. J Am Coll Cardiol 1995;25(Suppl):232A.
242. Mahaffey KW, White HD, Granger CB, et al. for the GUSTO Investigators. Neurosurgical evacuation for intracranial hemorrhage associated with improved outcome in GUSTO. J Am Coll Cardiol 1995;25(Suppl): 232A.
243. Gebel J, Sila C, Sloan M, et al. Hemorrhagic stroke complicating coronary artery thrombolysis in the GUSTO trial. Stroke 1996;27:176.
244. Sloan MA, Sila CA, Mahaffey KW, et al. for the GUSTO-I Investigators. Clinical and radiographic factors associated with mortality following intracranial hemorrhage after thrombolysis for acute myocardial infarction. Stroke 1996;27:183.
244a. Mahaffey KW, Granger CB, Sloan, MA, et al. Mortality prediction model for patients with intracranial hemorrhage following thrombolysis. Presented at the XIX Congress of The European Society for Cardiology, Stockholm, Sweden, August 24–28, 1997.
245. Srinivasan G, Boschman C, Roth SI, et al. Unsuspected vasculitis and intracranial hemorrhage following thrombolysis. Clin Cardiol 1997;20:84.
246. Cranston RE, Olfson MA, Buchsbaum HW, et al. Plasminogen activator and cerebral infarction [letter]. Ann Intern Med 1988;108:766.
247. Stafford PJ, Strachan CJL, Vincent R, et al. Multiple microemboli after disintegration of clot during thrombolysis for acute myocardial infarction. BMJ 1989; 299:1310.
248. Bodenheimer MM, Sauer D, Shareif B, et al. Relation between myocardial infarct location and stroke. J Am Coll Cardiol 1994;24:61.
249. Bautista RED. Embolic stroke following thrombolytic therapy for myocardial infarction in a patient with preexisting ventricular thrombi. Stroke 1995;26:324.
250. Mahaffey KW, Granger CB, White HD, et al. for the GUSTO Investigators. Risk factors for ischemic stroke in patients with acute myocardial infarction treated with thrombolytic therapy. J Am Coll Cardiol 1996;27 (Suppl):81A.
251. Bellone P, Domenicucci S, Chiarella F, et al. Chronic aneurysmatic dilatation: a possible source of lethal embolization in patients with acute myocardial infarction undergoing thrombolysis. Int J Cardiol 1996;56:201.
252. Witchitz S, Veyrat C, Moisson P, et al. Fibrinolytic treatment of thrombus on prosthetic heart valves. Br Heart J 1980;44:545.
253. Ledain LD, Ohayon JP, Colle JP, et al. Acute thrombotic obstruction with disc valve prostheses: diagnostic considerations and fibrinolytic treatment. J Am Coll Cardiol 1986;7:743.
254. Silber H, Khan SS, Matloff JM, et al. The St. Jude valve, thrombolysis as the first line therapy for cardiac valve thrombosis. Circulation 1993;87:30.
255. Pape LA, Love DG, Gore JM. Massive thromboembolic stroke and death after thrombolytic therapy of St. Jude prosthetic mitral valve thrombosis: documentation by transthoracic Doppler echocardiography. Am Heart J 1994;128:406.
256. Hirschl MM, Gwechenberger M, Zehetgruber M, et al. Severe complications following thrombolytic therapy for acute thrombosis of a prosthetic mitral valve. Clin Invest 1994;72:466.

257. Dzavik V, Cohen G, Chan KL. Role of transesophogeal echocardiography in the diagnosis and management of prosthetic valve thrombosis. J Am Coll Cardiol 1991;18:1829.
258. Roudaut R, Labbe T, Lorient-Roudaut M, et al. Mechanical cardiac valve thrombosis. Is fibrinolysis justified? Circulation 1992;86(Suppl II):II-8.
259. Dejaeger PH, van de Werf F, Vermylen J, et al. Thromboembolic complications after streptokinase therapy of pulmonary emboli. Acta Cardiol 1988;43:61.
260. Yasaka M, Yamaguchi T, Yonehara T, et al. Recurrent embolization during intravenous administration of tissue plasminogen activator in acute cardioembolic stroke. Angiology 1994;45:481.
261. Mustafa MH, Gallino R. Spontaneous spinal epidural hematoma causing cord compression after streptokinase and heparin therapy for acute coronary occlusion. South Med J 1988;81:1202.
262. Dickman CA, Shedd SA, Spetzler RF, et al. Spinal epidural hematoma associated with epidural anesthesia. Complications of systemic heparinization in patients receiving peripheral vascular thrombolytic therapy. Anesthesiology 1990;72:947.
263. Krolick MA, Cintron GB. Spinal epidural hematoma causing cord compression after tissue plasminogen activator and heparin therapy. South Med J 1991;89:670.
264. Onishchuk JL, Carlsson C. Epidural hematoma associated with epidural anesthesia: complications of anticoagulant therapy. Anesthesiology 1992;77:1221.
265. Sawin PD, Traynelis VC, Follett KA. Spinal epidural hematoma following coronary thrombolysis with tissue plasminogen activator. J Neurosurg 1995;83:350.
266. Connolly ES, Winfree CJ, McCormick PC. Management of spinal epidural hematoma after tissue plasminogen activator. Spine 1996;21:1694.
267. Taylor BV, Mastaglia FL, Stell R. Guillain-Barré syndrome complicating treatment with streptokinase. Med J Aust 1995;162:214.
268. Kaiser R, Kaufmann R, Czygan M, et al. Guillain-Barré syndrome following streptokinase threapy. Clin Invest 1993;71:795.
269. Barnes D, Hughes RA. Guillain-Barré syndrome after treatment with streptokinase. BMJ 1992;304:1225.
270. Seaberg DC, Generalovitch T. Hemorrhagic compression of the phrenic nerve after streptokinase infusion. Am J Emerg Med 1989;7:185.
271. Cadman PJ. Case report: femoral nerve palsy complicating femoral artery puncture and intra-arterial thrombolysis. Clin Radiol 1995;50:345.
272. Gillanders IA, Nakielner R, Channer KS. Spontaneous iliopsoas hemorrhage: an unusual complication of streptokinase therapy. Postgrad Med J 1990;66:862.
273. Piazza I, Girardi A, Giurita G, et al. Femoral nerve palsy secondary to anticoagulant-induced iliacus hematoma. A case report. Int Angiol 1990;9:125.
274. Thompson PL, Robinson JS. Stroke after acute myocardial infarction: relation to infarct size. BMJ 1978;2:457.
275. Konrad MS, Coffey CE, Coffey MS, et al. Myocardial infarction and stroke. Neurology 1984;34:1403.
276. Drapkin A, Merskey C. Anticoagulant therapy after acute myocardial infarction: relation of therapeutic benefit to patient's age, sex, and severity of infarction. JAMA 1972;222:541.
277. Veterans Administration Cooperative Study. Anticoagulants in acute myocardial infarction: results of a cooperative clinical trial. JAMA 1973;225:724.
278. Report of the Working Party Medical Research Council. Assessment of short-term anticoagulant administration after cardiac infarction. BMJ 1969;1:335.
279. Hart RG. Prevention and Treatment of Cardioembolic Stroke. In AJ Furlan (ed), The Heart and Stroke. Berlin: Springer-Verlag, 1987;17.
280. Chaitman BR, Thompson B, Wittry MD, et al. The use of tissue plasminogen activator for acute myocardial infarction in the elderly: results for the Thrombolysis in Myocardial Infarction Phase I Open-Label Studies, and the Thrombolysis in Myocardial Infarction Phase II Pilot Study. J Am Coll Cardiol 1989;14:1159.
281. Cragg DR, Friedman HZ, Bonema JD, et al. Outcome of patients with acute myocardial infarction who are ineligible for thrombolytic therapy. Ann Intern Med 1991;115:173.
282. Weaver WD, Litwin PE, Martin JS, et al. Effect of age on use of thrombolytic therapy and mortality in acute myocardial infarction. J Am Coll Cardiol 1991;18:657.
283. Pfeiffer MA, Moyé LA, Braunwald E, et al. Selection bias in the use of thrombolytic therapy in acute myocardial infarction. JAMA 1991;266:528.
284. Grines CL, DeMaria AL. Optimal utilization of thrombolytic therapy for acute myocardial infarction: concepts and controversies. J Am Coll Cardiol 1990;16:223.
285. Muller DMW, Topol EJ. Selection of patients with acute myocardial infarction for thrombolytic therapy. Ann Intern Med 1990;113:949.
286. Kennedy JW. Expanding the use of thrombolytic therapy for acute myocardial infarction [editorial]. Ann Intern Med 1990;113:907.
287. Gurwitz JH, Goldberg RJ, Gore JM. Coronary thrombolysis for the elderly? JAMA 1991;263:1720.
288. Krumholz HM, Pasternak RC, Weinstein MC, et al. Cost effectiveness of thrombolytic therapy with streptokinase in elderly patients with suspected acute myocardial infarction. N Engl J Med 1992;327:7.
289. Hendra TJ, Marshall AJ. Increased prescription of thrombolytic treatment to elderly patients with suspected acute myocardial infarction associated with audit. BMJ 1992;304:423.
290. Gurwitz JH, Gore JM, Goldberg RJ, et al. for the participants in the National Registry of Myocardial Infarction: recent age related trends in the use of thrombolytic therapy in patients who have had acute myocardial infarction. Ann Intern Med 1996;124:283.
291. Califf RM, Fortin DF, Tenaglia AN, et al. Clinical risks of thrombolytic therapy. Am J Cardiol 1992;69:12A.

292. Sane DC, Califf RM, Topol EJ, et al. Bleeding during thrombolytic therapy for acute myocardial infarction: mechanisms and management. Ann Intern Med 1989;111:1010.
293. Hirsch DR, Goldhaber SZ. The bleeding time: its potential utility among patients receiving thrombolytic therapy. Am Heart J 1990;119:158.
294. Sherry S. Dissimilar systemic and local adverse effects of thrombolytic therapy. Am J Cardiol 1988;61:1344.
295. Marder VJ, Sherry S. Thrombolytic therapy: current status. N Engl J Med 1988;318:1512.
296. Bovill E, Stump D, Tracy R, et al. Dose response relationship of rt-PA infusion to induction of systemic fibrinogenolysis in the thrombolysis in myocardial infarction (TIMI) trial. Blood 1987;70:367a.
297. Bovill EG, Terrin ML, Stump DC, et al. Hemorrhagic events during therapy with recombinant tissue-type plasminogen activator, heparin, and aspirin for acute myocardial infarction. Results of the Thrombolysis in Myocardial Infarction (TIMI), Phase II Trial. Ann Intern Med 1991;115:256.
298. Rao A-K, Pratt C, Burke A, et al. Thrombolysis in myocardial infarction (TIMI) trial. Phase I. Hemorrhagic manifestations and changes in plasma fibrinogen and the fibrinolytic system in patients treated with recombinant tissue plasminogen activator and streptokinase. J Am Coll Cardiol 1988;11:1.
299. Collen D, Bounameaux H, DeCock F, et al. Analysis of coagulation and fibrinolysis during intravenous infusion of recombinant human tissue type plasminogen activator in patients with acute myocardial infarction. Circulation 1986;73:511.
300. Stump DC, Topol EJ, Chen AB, et al. Monitoring of hemostasis parameters during coronary thrombolysis with recombinant tissue type plasminogen activator. Thromb Haemost 1985;59:133.
301. Stump DC, Taylor FB, Nesheim ME, et al. Pathological fibrinolysis as a cause of clinical bleeding. Semin Thromb Hemost 1990;16:260.
302. Lawler CM, Bovill EG, Stump DC, et al. Fibrin fragment D-Dimer and fibrinogen B beta peptides in plasma as markers of clot lysis during thrombolytic therapy in acute myocardial infarction. Blood 1990;76:1341.
303. Tracy RP, Bovill EG. Fibrinolytic parameters and hemostatic monitoring: identifying and predicting patients at risk for major hemorrhagic events. Am J Cardiol 1992;69:52A.
304. Hirsh J. Heparin and low-molecular-weight heparins. Coronary Artery Dis 1992;3:990.
305. Lawson JH, Butenas S, Ribarik N, et al. Complex-dependent inhibition of factor VIIa by antithrombin III and heparin. J Biol Chem 1993;268:767.
306. Salzman EW. Low-molecular-weight heparin and other new antithrombotic drugs. N Engl J Med 1992;326:1017.
307. Micic M, Rauschenbach C, Breddin HK. The effects of recombinant hirudin on various platelet functions. Haemostasis 1991;1:107.
308. Friedberg RC, Hagen P-O, Pizzo SV. The role of endothelium in factor Xa regulation: the effect of plasma proteinase inhibitors and hirudin. Blood 1988;71:1321.
309. Theroux P, Waters D, Lam J, et al. Reactivation of unstable angina after the discontinuation of heparin. N Engl J Med 1992;327:141.
310. Verstraete M, Nurmohamed M, Kienast J, et al. Biologic effects of recombinant hirudin (CGP39393) in human volunteers: European Hirudin in Thrombosis Group. J Am Coll Cardiol 1993;22:1080.
311. Steering Committee. Final report on the aspirin component of the ongoing Physicians Health Study. N Engl J Med 1989;321:129.
312. Gimple LW, Gold HK, Leinbach RC, et al. Correlation between template bleeding times and spontaneous bleeding during treatment of acute myocardial infarction with recombinant tissue type plasminogen activator. Circulation 1989;80:581.
313. Kiyomoto A, Sasaki Y, Odawara A, et al. Inhibition of platelet aggregation by diltiazem. Circ Res 1983; 52(Suppl I):I-115.
314. Mehta J. Influence of calcium-channel blockers on platelet function and arachidonic acid metabolism. Am J Cardiol 1985;55(Suppl):158B.
315. Bayle ALJ. Traité des Maladies du Cerveau et de ses Membranes. Maladies Mentales. Paris: Gabon, 1826.
316. Labadie EL. Fibrinolysis in the Formation and Growth of Chronic Subdural Hematomas. In R Sawaya (ed), Fibrinolysis and the Central Nervous System. Philadelphia: Hanley-Belfus, 1990;141.
317. Labadie EL, Glover D. Local alterations of hemostatic-fibrinolytic mechanisms in reforming subdural hematomas. Neurology 1975;25:669.
318. Ito H, Yamamoto S, Komai T, et al. Role of local hyperfibrinolysis in the etiology of chronic subdural hematoma. J Neurosurg 1976;45:26.
319. Ito H, Komai T, Yamamoto S. Fibrinolytic enzyme in the lining walls of chronic subdural hematoma. J Neurosurg 1978;48:197.
320. Weir B, Gordon P. Factors affecting coagulation: fibrinolysis in chronic subdural fluid collections. J Neurosurg 1985;58:242.
321. Califf RM, Topol EJ, Kereiakes DJ, et al. Cardiac resuscitation should not be a contraindication to thrombolytic therapy for myocardial infarction. Circulation 1988;78(Suppl II):II-127.
322. Scholz KM, Tebbe U, Herrmann C, et al. Frequency of complications of cardiopulmonary resuscitation after thrombolysis during acute myocardial infarction. J Am Coll Cardiol 1992;69:724.
323. Harker LA, Malpass TW, Branson HE, et al. Mechanism of abnormal bleeding in patients undergoing cardiopulmonary bypass: acquired transient platelet dysfunction associated with selective (alpha) granule release. Blood 1980;56:824.
324. Kereiakes DJ, Topol EJ, George BS, et al. Emergency coronary artery bypass surgery preserves global and

regional left ventricular function after intravenous tissue plasminogen activator therapy for acute myocardial infarction. J Am Coll Cardiol 1988;11:899.
325. Harker LA. Bleeding after cardiopulmonary bypass. N Engl J Med 1986;314:1446.
326. Salzman EW, Weinstein MJ, Weintraub RM, et al. Treatment with desmopressin acetate to reduce blood loss after cardiac surgery. N Engl J Med 1986;314:1402.
327. Kase CS. Intracerebral hemorrhage: nonhypertensive causes. Stroke 1986;17:590.
328. Vinters HV. Cerebral amyloid angiopathy. A critical review. Stroke 1987;18:311.
329. Kalyan-Raman UP, Kalyan-Raman K. Cerebral amyloid angiopathy causing intracranial hemorrhage. Ann Neurol 1984;16:321.
330. Okazaki H, Regan TJ, Campbell RJ. Clinical pathologic studies of primary cerebral amyloid angiopathy. Mayo Clin Proc 1979;54:22.
331. Vonsattel JP, Hedley-Whyte ET, Ropper AH, et al. Coincidence of fibrinoid necrosis with amyloid angiopathy as the cause of cerebral hemorrhage. J Neuropathol Exp Neurol 1984;43:316.
332. Powers JM, Schlaepfer WW, Willingham MC, et al. An immunoperoxidase study of senile cerebral amyloidosis with pathogenetic considerations. J Neuropathol Exp Neurol 1981;40:598.
333. Greenberg SM, Rebeck GW, Vonsattel JPG, et al. Apolipoprotein E ε4 and cerebral hemorrhage associated with amyloid angiopathy. Ann Neurol 1995;38:254.
334. Greenberg SM, Briggs ME, Hyman BT, et al. Apolipoprotein E ε4 is associated with presence and earlier onset of hemorrhage in cerebral amyloid angiopathy. Stroke 1996;27:1333.
335. Graffagnino C, Herbstreith MH, Schmechel DE, et al. Cystatin mutation in an elderly man with sporadic amyloid angiopathy and intracerebral hemorrhage. Stroke 1995;26:2190.
336. Alberts MJ, Davis JP, Graffagnino C, et al. Endoglin gene polymorphism as a risk factor for sporadic intracerebral hemorrhage. Ann Neurol 1997;41:683.
337. Alberts MJ, Graffagnino C, McClenny C, et al. ApoE genotype and survival from intracerebral hemorrhage. Lancet 1995;346:575.
338. Rosenblum B. Pathophysiology of Arteriovenous Malformations: Recent Advances in Analysis and Therapy. In B Rosenblum (ed), State of the Art Reviews in Neurosurgery: Cerebral and Spinal Arteriovenous Malformations. Philadelphia: Hanley-Belfus, 1988;1.
339. Wright JO, Hiratzke LF, Brandt B, et al. Thrombosis of the Björk-Shiley prosthesis: illustrative cases and review of the literature. J Thorac Cardiovasc Surg 1982;84:138.
340. Charcot JM, Bouchard C. Nouvelles recherches sur la pathogénie de l'hémorragie cérébrale. Arch Physiol Norm Pathol 1868;1:110.
341. Green FHK. Miliary aneurysms in the brain. J Pathol Bacteriol 1930;33:71.
342. Ross Russell RW. Observations on intracerebral aneurysms. Brain 1963;86:425.
343. Cole FM, Yates P. Intracerebral microaneurysms and small cerebrovascular lesions. Brain 1967;90:759.
344. Cole FM, Yates PO. The occurrence and significance of intracerebral micro-aneurysms. J Pathol Bacteriol 1967;30:393.
345. Fisher CM. Pathological observations in hypertensive cerebral hemorrhage. J Neuropathol Exp Neurol 1971;30:536.
346. Cole FM, Yates PO. Pseudoaneurysms in relationship to massive cerebral hemorrhage. J Neurol Neurosurg Psychiatry 1967;30:61.
347. Weinrich DJ, Burke JF, Pauletto FJ. Left ventricular mural thrombi complicating acute myocardial infarction. Ann Intern Med 1984;100:789.
348. Johannessen K-A, Nordrehaug JE, von der Lippe G. Left ventricular thrombosis and cerebrovascular accident in acute myocardial infarction. Br Heart J 1984;51:553.
349. Asinger RW, Mikell FL, Elsperger J, et al. Incidence of left ventricular mural thrombosis after acute transmural myocardial infarction. Serial evaluation by two dimensional echocardiography. N Engl J Med 1981;305:297.
350. Stratton JR, Resnick AD. Increased embolic risk in patients with left ventricular thrombi. Circulation 1987;75:1004.
351. Gravlee GP, Hudspeth AS, Toole JF. Bilateral brachial paralysis from watershed infarction after coronary artery bypass. J Thorac Cardiovasc Surg 1984;88:742.
352. Amann FW, Kiowski W, Pfisterer M, et al. Fibrinolytic therapy in thrombotic obstruction of a tilting disc prosthesis. Am Heart J 1986;112:1084.
353. Gagnon RM, Beaudet R, Lemire J, et al. Streptokinase thrombolysis of a chronically thrombosed mitral prosthetic valve. Cath Cardiovasc Diagn 1984;10:5.
354. Kurzrok S, Singh AK, Most AS, et al. Thrombolytic therapy for prosthetic cardiac valve thrombosis. J Am Coll Cardiol 1987;9:592.
355. Ortuno F, Fontcuberta J, Pons-Llaurado G, et al. Successful treatment of prosthetic heart-valve thrombosis with high short-term doses of streptokinase. Lancet 1988;II:626.
356. Page A, Gateau P, Roudant R, et al. Traitement thrombolytique dans les thromboses de prothese valvulaires. Nouv Press Med 1980;42:3186.
357. Rabago R, Corrales M, Rey M, et al. Fibrinolytic therapy for prosthetic heart valve thrombosis. Circulation 1993;88(Suppl):I-342.
358. Horowitz SG, Zito JL, Donnarumma R, et al. Computed tomographic-angiographic findings within the first five hours of cerebral infarction. Stroke 1991; 22:1245.
359. Gomez CR, Burger SK, Puricelli M, et al. Early computed tomography demonstration of cerebral infarction does not correlate with clinical outcome. J Stroke Cerebrovas Dis 1992;2:146.

360. Toni D, Fiorelli M, Bastianello S, et al. Hemorrhagic transformation of brain infarct: predictability in the first 5 hours from stroke onset and influence on clinical outcome. Neurology 1996;46:341.
361. von Kummer R, Bozzao L, Bastianello S, et al. for the ECASS Group. Extent of ischemic brain edema and the response to plasminogen activator in acute hemispheric stroke. Stroke 1997;28:270.
362. Moulin T, Cattin F, Crépin-Leblond T, et al. Early CT signs in acute middle cerebral artery infarction: predictive value for subsequent infarct locations and outcome. Neurology 1996;47:366.
363. Ott BR, Zamani A, Kleefied J, et al. The clinical spectrum of hemorrhagic infarction. Stroke 1986;17:630.
364. Hart RG, Easton JD. Hemorrhagic infarcts. Stroke 1986;17:586.
365. Cerebral Embolism Study Group. Cardioembolic stroke, early anticoagulation, and brain hemorrhage. Arch Intern Med 1987;147:636.
366. Jorgensen L, Torvik A. Ischemic cerebrovascular diseases in an autopsy series, part 2. Prevalence, location, pathogenesis and clinical course of cerebral infarcts. J Neurol Sci 1969;9:285.
367. Furlan AJ, Cavalier SJ, Hobbs RE, et al. Hemorrhage and anticoagulation after nonseptic embolic brain infarction. Neurology 1982;32:280.
368. Koller RL. Recurrent embolic cerebral infarction and anticoagulation. Neurology 1982:32:283.
369. Weisberg LA. Nonseptic cardiogenic cerebral embolic stroke: clinical-CT correlations. Neurology 1985;35:896.
370. Lodder J, van der Lugt PJM. Evaluation of the risk of immediate anticoagulant treatment in patients with embolic stroke of cardiac origin. Stroke 1983;14:42.
371. Cerebral Embolism Study Group. Immediate anticoagulation of embolic stroke: a randomized trial. Stroke 1983;14:68.
372. Hakim AM, Ryder-Cooke A, Melanson D. Sequential computerized tomographic appearance of strokes. Stroke 1983;14:893.
373. Cerebral Embolism Study Group. Immediate anticoagulation of embolic stroke: brain hemorrhage and management options. Stroke 1984;15:779.
374. Lodder J. CT-detected hemorrhagic infarction: relation with the size of the infarct and the presence of midline shift. Acta Neurol Scand 1984;70:329.
375. Fisher M, Zito JL, Siva A, et al. Hemorrhagic infarction: a clinical and CT study. Stroke 1984;15:192.
376. Shields RW, Laureno R, Lachman T, et al. Anticoagulant-related hemorrhage in acute cerebral embolism. Stroke 1984;15:426.
377. Hornig CR, Dorndorf W, Agnoli AL. Hemorrhagic cerebral infarction: a prospective study. Stroke 1986;17:179.
378. Lodder J, Krijne-Kubat B, Broekman J. Cerebral hemorrhagic infarction at autopsy: cardiac embolic cause and the relationship to the cause of death. Stroke 1986;17:626.
379. Hart RG for the Cerebral Embolism Study Group. Timing of Hemorrhagic Transformation of Cardioembolic Stroke. In T Stober, K Schimrigk, D Ganten, et al. (eds), Central Nervous System Control of the Heart. Boston: Martinus Nijhoff, 1986;229.
380. Hart RG, Tegeler CH. Hemorrhagic infarction on CT in the absence of anticoagulant therapy. Stroke 1986; 17:558.
381. Sherman GB, Hart RG, et al. Brain Hemorrhage in Embolic Stroke. In R Stober, K Schimrigk, D Ganten, et al. (eds), Central Nervous System Control of the Heart. Boston: Martinus Nijhoff, 1986;249.
382. Laureno R, Shields RW, Narayan T. The diagnosis and management of cerebral embolism and hemorrhagic infarction with sequential computerized cranial tomography. Brain 1987;110:93.
383. Fisher CM, Adams RD. Observations on brain embolism with special reference to the mechanism of hemorrhagic infarction. J Neuropathol Exp Neurol 1951;10:92.
384. Beghi E, Bogliun G, Cavaletti G, et al. Hemorrhagic infarction: risk factors, clinical and tomographic features, and outcome. A case-control study. Acta Neurol Scand 1989;80:226.
385. Lodder J, Krijne-Kuhat B, van der Lugt PJM. Timing of autopsy-proven hemorrhagic infarction with reference to cardioembolic stroke. Stroke 1988;19:1482.
386. Pessin MS, del Zoppo GJ, Estol CJ. Thrombolytic agents in the treatment of stroke. Clin Neuropharm 1990;13:271.
387. del Zoppo GJ, Pessin MS, Mori E, et al. Thrombolytic intervention in acute thrombotic and embolic stroke. Semin Neurol 1991;11:368.
388. Zivin JA. A Perspective on the Future of Thrombolytic Stroke Therapy. In MD Ginsberg, WD Dietrich (eds), Cerebrovascular Diseases. New York: Raven, 1989;33.
389. Pessin MS. Hemorrhagic Transformation in the Natural History of Acute Embolic Stroke. In W Hacke, GJ del Zoppo, M Hirschberg (eds), Thrombolytic Therapy in Acute Ischemic Stroke. Berlin: Springer-Verlag, 1991;67.
390. Bozzoa L, Angeloni U, Bastianello S, et al. Early angiographic and CT findings in patients with hemorrhagic infarction in the distribution of the middle cerebral artery. Am J Neuroradiol 1991;12:1115.
391. Pessin MS, Teal PA, Caplan LR. Hemorrhagic infarction: guilt by association? Am J Neuroradiol 1991; 12:1123.
392. Faris AA, Hardin CA, Poser CM. Pathogenesis of hemorrhagic infarction of the brain. Arch Neurol 1963; 9:468.
393. Bruetman ME, Fields WS, Crawford ES, et al. Cerebral hemorrhage in carotid artery surgery. Arch Neurol 1963;9:458.
394. Ogata J, Yutani C, Imakita M, et al. Hemorrhagic infarct of the brain without a reopening of the occluded arteries in cardioembolic stroke. Stroke 1989;20:876.

395. Okada Y, Yamaguchi T, Minematsu K, et al. Hemorrhagic transformation in cerebral embolism. Stroke 1989;20:598.
396. Bogousslavsky J, Regli F, Uske A, et al. Early spontaneous hematoma in cerebral infarct: is primary cerebral hemorrhage overdiagnosed? Neurology 1991;41:837.
397. Caplan LR, Skillman J, Ojemann R, et al. Intracerebral hemorrhage following carotid endarterectomy: a hypertensive complication? Stroke 1978;9:457.
398. Sundt TM, Sharbrough FW, Piepgras DG, et al. Correlation of cerebral blood flow and electroencephalographic changes during carotid endarterectomy with results of surgery and hemodynamics of cerebral ischemia. Mayo Clin Proc 1981;56:533.
399. Petito CK. Early and late mechanisms of increased vascular permeability following experimental cerebral infarction. J Neurpathol Exp Neurol 1979;38:222.
400. Garcia JH. Experimental ischemic stroke: a review. Stroke 1983;14:5.
401. Kamijyo Y, Gureia JM, Cooper J. Temporary regional cerebral ischemia in the cat: a model of hemorrhagic and subcortical infarction. J Neuropathol Exp Neurol 1977;36:338.
402. Garcia JH, Lowry SL, Briggs L, et al. Brain capillaries expand and rupture in areas of ischemia and reperfusion. In M Reivich, HL Hurtig (eds), Cerebrovascular Diseases. New York: Raven, 1983;169.
403. Laurent JP, Molinari GF, Oakley JC. Primate model of cerebral hematoma. J Neuropathol Exp Neurol 1976; 35:560.
404. Globus JH, Epstein JA. Massive cerebral hemorrhage: spontaneous and experimentally induced. J Neuropathol Exp Neurol 1953;12:107.
405. Saku Y, Choki J, Waki R, et al. Hemorrhagic infarct induced by arterial hypertension in cat brain following middle cerebral artery occlusion. Stroke 1990;21:589.
406. Fisher CM, Adams RD. Observations on Brain Embolism with Special Reference to Hemorrhagic Infarction. In AJ Furlan (ed), The Heart and Stroke. Berlin: Springer-Verlag, 1987;17.
407. Lyden PD, Zivin JA, Soll M, et al. Intracerebral hemorrhage after experimental embolic infarction. Anticoagulation. Arch Neurol 1987;44:848.
408. Pessin MS, Estol CJ, Lafranchise F, et al. Safety of anticoagulation after hemorrhagic infarction. Neurology 1993;43:1298.
409. Sloan MA. Thrombolytic Therapy in Experimental Focal Cerebral Ischemia. In R Sawaya (ed), Fibrinolysis and the Central Nervous System. Philadelphia: Hanley and Belfus, 1990;177.
410. del Zoppo GJ. Relevance of focal cerebral ischemia models. Experience with fibrinolytic agents. Stroke 1990;21(Suppl IV):IV-155.
411. Hirschberg M. Update on Animal Model Experience with Recombinant Tissue Plasminogen Activator. In W Hacke, GJ del Zoppo, M Hirschberg (eds), Thrombolytic Therapy in Acute Ischemic Stroke. Berlin: Springer-Verlag, 1991;114.
412. Brott T. Thrombolytic therapy for stroke. Cerebrovasc Brain Metab Rev 1991;3:91.
413. Brott T. Thrombolytic therapy. Neurol Clin 1992; 10:219.
414. Slivka A, Pulsinelli W. Hemorrhagic complications of thrombolytic therapy in experimental stroke. Stroke 1987;18:1148.
415. Clark WM, Madden KP, Zivin JA, et al. Intracerebral hemorrhage: TPA versus streptokinase thrombolytic therapy. Neurology 1989;39(Suppl I):I-183.
416. Lyden PD, Madden KP, Clark WM, et al. Incidence of cerebral hemorrhage after antifibrinolytic treatment for embolic stroke in rabbits. Stroke 1990;21:1589.
417. Fisher M, Phillips DA, Davis MA, et al. Delayed treatment with a t-PA analogue and streptokinase in a rabbit embolism stroke model. Stroke 1990;21(Suppl I):I-135.
418. del Zoppo GJ, Copeland BR, Anderchele K, et al. Hemorrhagic transformation following tissue plasminogen activator in experimental cerebral infarction. Stroke 1990;21:596.
419. Lyden PD, Zivin JA, Clark W, et al. Tissue plasminogen activator-mediated thrombolysis of cerebral emboli and its effect on hemorrhagic infarction in rabbits. Neurology 1989;39:703.
420. del Zoppo GJ, Higashida RT, Furlan AJ, et al. and the PROACT Investigators. The Prolyse in Acute Cerebral Thromboembolism Trial (PROACT): results of 6 mg dose tier. Stroke 1996;27:164.
421. Matsumoto K, Kato A, Konmura E, et al. Acute cerebellar edema following intra-arterial tissue plasminogen activator thrombolysis for basilar artery occlusion—case report. Neurol Med Chir 1996;36:455.
422. Larrue V, von Kummer R, del Zoppo GJ, et al. Hemorrhagic transformation in acute ischemic stroke. Potential contributing factors in the European Cooperative Acute Stroke Study. Stroke 1997;28:957.
423. Ueda T, Hatakeyama T, Sasaki S, et al. Changes in coagulation and fibrinolytic system after local intra-arterial thrombolysis for acute ischemic stroke. Neurol Med Chir 1995;35:136.
424. Willig V, Pawelec D, Mau J. Heparin effects in the European Cooperative Acute Stroke Study. Stroke 1997;28:272.
425. Grond M, Rudolf J, Neveling M, et al. Immediate heparin after rt-PA therapy does not increase risk of hemorrhage. Stroke 1997;28:272.
426. The NINDS rt-PA Stroke Study Group. Symptomatic intracerebral hemorrhage after rt-PA for stroke. Stroke 1997;28:272.
427. Hommel M, Cornu C, Boutitie F for the Multicenter Acute Stroke Trial—Europe Study Group. Thrombolytic therapy in acute ischemic stroke. N Engl J Med 1997;336:66.
428. Ueda T, Hatakeyama T, Kumon Y, et al. Evaluation of risk of hemorrhagic transformation in local intra-arterial thrombolysis in acute ischemic stroke by initial SPECT. Stroke 1994;25:298.

429. Alexandrov AV, Black SE, Ehrlich LE, et al. Simple visual analysis of brain perfusion on HMPAO SPECT predicts early outcome in acute stroke. Stroke 1996; 27:1537.
430. Hanson SK, Grotta JC, Rhoades H, et al. Value of single-photon emission computed tomography in acute stroke therapeutic trials. Stroke 1993;24:1322.
431. Alexandrov AV, Grotta JC, Davis SM, et al. Brain SPECT and thrombolysis in acute ischemic stroke: time for a clinical trial. J Nucl Med 1996;37:1259.
432. Kaufmann AM, Firlik A, Yonas H, et al. Emergent stroke therapy and quantitative cerebral blood flow. Stroke 1997;28:253.
433. Alexandrov AV, Black SE, Devous MD, et al. SPECT Safe Thrombolysis Study (SSTS). Patients, methods, and study design. Neurology 1997;48(Suppl):A271.
434. Kanaya H, Kuroda K. Development in Neurosurgical Approaches to Hypertensive Intracerebral Hemorrhage in Japan. In HH Kaufman (ed), Intracerebral Hematomas. New York: Raven, 1992;197.
435. Segal R, Dujovny M, Nelson D, et al. Local urokinase treatment for spontaneous intracerebral hematoma. Clin Res 1982;30:412A.
436. Matsumoto K, Hondo H. CT-guided stereotactic evaluation of hypertensive intracerebral hematomas. J Neurosurg 1984;61:440.
437. Niizuma H, Suzuki J. Stereotactic aspiration of putaminal hemorrhage using a double track aspirator technique. Neurosurgery 1988;22:432.
438. Narayan RJ, Narayan TM, Katz DA, et al. Lysis of intracranial hematomas with urokinase in a rabbit model. J Neurosurg 1985;62:580.
439. Itakura T, Komai N, Nadai E, et al. Stereotactic evacuation of hypertensive intracerebral hematoma using plasminogen activator. American Association of Neurological Surgeons, Dallas, TX, May 3–7, 1987.
440. Niizuma H, Otsuki T, Johkura H, et al. CT-guided stereotactic aspiration of intracerebral hematoma: result of a hematoma-lysis method using urokinase. Appl Neurophysiol 1985;48:427.
441. Kaufmann HH, Schochet S, Koss W, et al. Efficacy and safety of tissue plasminogen activator. Neurosurgery 1987;20:403.
442. Mohadjer M, Eggert R, May J, et al. CT-guided stereotactic fibrinolysis of spontaneous and hypertensive cerebellar hemorrhage: long term results. J Neurosurg 1990;73:217.
443. Kaufmann HH. Stereotactic Aspiration with Fibrinolytic and Mechanical Assistance. In HH Kaufmann (ed), Intracerebral Hematomas. New York: Raven, 1992;181.
444. Pang D, Sclabassi RJ, Horton JA. Lysis of intraventricular blood clot with urokinase in a canine model: part I: canine intraventricular blood cast model. Neurosurgery 1986;19:540.
445. Pang D, Sclabassi RJ, Horton JA. Lysis of intraventricular blood clot with urokinase in a canine model: part II: in vivo safety study of intraventricular urokinase. Neurosurgery 1986;19:547.
446. Pang D, Sclabassi RJ, Horton JA. Lysis of intraventricular blood clot with urokinase in a canine model: part III: effects of intraventricular urokinase on clot lysis and posthemorrhagic hydrocephalus. Neurosurgery 1986;19:553.
447. Todo T, Usui M, Takakura K. Treatment of severe intraventricular hemorrhage by intraventricular infusion of urokinase. J Neurosurg 1991;74:81.
448. Findlay JM, Weir BKA, Stollery DE. Lysis of intraventricular hematoma with tissue plasminogen activator. J Neurosurg 1991;74:803.
449. Fisher CM, Kistler JP, Davis JM. Relation of cerebral vasospasm to subarachnoid hemorrhage visualized by computerized tomographic scanning. Neurosurgery 1980;6:1.
450. Kistler JP, Crowell RW, Davis KR, et al. The relation of cerebral vasospasm to the extent and location of subarachnoid blood visualized by CT scan. A prospective study. Neurology 1983;33:424.
451. Findlay JM, Macdonald RL, Weir BKA. Current concepts of pathophysiology and management of cerebral vasospasm following aneurysmal subarachnoid hemorrhage. Cerebrovasc Brain Metab Rev 1991;3:336.
452. Macdonald RL, Weir BKA. A review of hemoglobin and the pathogenesis of cerebral vasospasm. Stroke 1991;22:971.
453. Fodstad H, Nilsson IM. Coagulation and fibrinolysis in blood and cerebrospinal fluid after aneurysmal subarachnoid hemorrhage. Effect of tranexamic acid (AMCA) Acta Neurol Chir 1981;56:25.
454. Findlay JM, Weir BKA, Kanamaru K, et al. Intrathecal fibrinolytic therapy after subarachnoid hemorrhage: dosage study in a primate model and review of the literature. Can J Neurol Sci 1989;16:28.
455. Alksne JF, Branson PJ, Bailey M. Modification of experimental post-subarachnoid hemorrhage vasculopathy with intracisternal plasmin. Neurosurgery 1986;19:20.
456. Alksne JF, Branson PJ, Bailey M. Modification of experimental post-subarachnoid vasculopathy with intracisternal plasmin. Neurosurgery 1988;23:335.
457. Findlay JM, Weir BKA, Steinke D, et al. Effect of intrathecal thrombolytic therapy on subarachnoid clot and chronic vasospasm in a primate model of SAH. J Neurosurgery 1988;69:723.
458. Findlay JM, Weir BKA, Gordon P, et al. Safety and efficacy of intrathecal thrombolytic therapy in a primate model of cerebral vasospasm. Neurosurgery 1989;24:491.
459. Findlay JM, Weir BKA, Kanamaru K, et al. The effect of timing of intrathecal fibrinolytic therapy on cerebral vasospasm in a primate model of subarachnoid hemorrhage. Neurosurgery 1990;26:201.
460. Seifert V, Eisert WG, Stolke D, et al. Efficacy of single intracisternal injection of recombinant tissue plasminogen activator to prevent delayed cerebral vasospasm

after experimental subarachnoid hemorrhage. Neurosurgery 1989;25:590.

461. Brinker T, Seifert V, Stolke D. Effect of intrathecal fibrinolysis on cerebrospinal fluid absorption after experimental subarachnoid hemorrhage. J Neurosurg 1991; 74:784.

462. Findlay JM, Weir BKA, Kassell NF, et al. Intracisternal recombinant tissue plasminogen activator after aneurysmal subarachnoid hemorrhage. J Neurosurg 1991;75:181.

463. Öhman J, Servo A, Heiskanen O. Effect of intrathecal fibrinolytic therapy on clot lysis and vasospasm in patients with aneurysmal subarachnoid hemorrhage. J Neurosurg 1991;75:197.

464. Stolke D, Seifert V. Single intracisternal bolus of recombinant tissue plasminogen activator in patients with aneurysmal subarachnoid hemorrhage: preliminary assessment of efficacy and safety in an open clinical study. Neurosurgery 1992;30:877.

465. Mizoi K, Yoshimoto T, Fujiwara S, et al. Prevention of vasospasm by clot removal and intrathecal bolus injection of tissue-type plasminogen activator. Preliminary report. Neurosurgery 1991;28:807.

466. Zabramski JM, Spetzler RF, Lee KS, et al. Phase I trial of tissue plasminogen activator for the prevention of vasospasm in patients with aneursymal subarachnoid hemorrhage. J Neurosurg 1991;75:189.

467. Sasaki T, Ohta T, Kikuchi M, et al. A phase II clinical trial of recombinant human tissue-type plasminogen activator against cerebral vasospasm after aneurysmal subarachnoid hemorrhage. Neurosurgery 1994;35:597.

468. Findlay JM, Kassell NF, Weir BKA, et al. A randomized trial of intraoperative, intracisternal tissue plasminogen activator for the prevention of vasospasm. Neurosurgery 1995;37:168.

469. Shah M, Taylor RT. Low back pain associated with streptokinase. BMJ 1990;301:1219.

470. Dickinson RJ, Rosser A. Low back pain associated with streptokinase. BMJ 1991;302:111.

471. Fishwick D, Prasan A, Adams P. Thrombolysis and low back pain. BMJ 1995;310:504.

472. Lear J, Rajapakse R. Low back pain associated with anistreplase. BMJ 1993;306:896.

473. Segal L, Adair D. Compartment syndrome of the triceps as a complication of thrombolytic therapy. Orthopedics 1990;13:90.

474. Burnside J, Costello JM, Angelastro NJ, et al. Forearm compartment syndrome following thrombolytic therapy for acute myocardial infarction. Clin Cardiol 1994; 17:345.

475. Blankenship JC. Median and ulnar neuropathy after streptokinase infusion. Heart Lung 1991;20:221.

Chapter 20

Complications of Cardiovascular Drugs

James F. Meschia and José Biller

Objectives

- To appreciate that neurologic complications of cardiovascular drugs are protean but uncommon
- To understand that virtually all neurologic complications are reversible with discontinuation of the offending agent
- To recognize that many antihypertensives and antiarrhythmics can greatly exacerbate the weakness of myasthenia gravis
- To recognize that some drugs, such as hydralazine and cholestyramine, cause neurologic complications indirectly by causing hypovitaminosis
- To appreciate that the neurotoxicity of some drugs can be reversed by administration of specific antidotes, as in the cases of nitroprusside and digoxin
- To understand that the likelihood of neurotoxicity with a class of agents can be greatly increased by coadministration of other agents, as in HMG-CoA reductase inhibitors

Antihypertensive Medications

Cerebral Infarction Caused by Therapeutic Doses of Antihypertensives

Antihypertensive therapy is highly effective in the primary prevention of stroke. The estimated risk reduction derived from several prospective clinical trials is 38% for all types of stroke and 40% for fatal stroke. The relative risk reduction in stroke resulting from the use of antihypertensives diminishes with age from 4.0 at 50 years to 1.0 at 90 years.[1] Overall, benefits of treating hypertension extend to people between the ages of 60 and 80. In one large trial, no benefit was observed in treating hypertension in people older than 80.[2] Clinical experience over the past few decades, however, suggests that there may be risk factors for developing cerebral infarction from antihypertensive therapy. These potential risk factors for cerebral infarction include rapid reduction of blood pressure in hypertension, old age, preexisting large vessel occlusive disease, and complicated migraine.

Cortical blindness, paraplegia, and death have been reported after rapid lowering of extreme hypertension.[3–5] The pattern of infarction often follows a watershed vascular distribution. In one patient whose hypertension was caused by renal artery thrombosis, even gradual lowering of blood pressure over several days failed to prevent watershed infarctions.[6] Focal cerebral ischemia may be the result of medication-induced postural hypotension.[7] This possible link between focal cerebral ischemia and postural hypotension has led some physicians to discourage the use of prazosin and methyldopa as first-line agents in the elderly and in patients with a history of cerebral ischemia.[8]

Preexisting large-vessel high-grade stenosis or occlusion may predispose to cerebral ischemia in the setting of systemic hypotension. Clinical examples of ischemia distal to a stenosis or occlusion can be found for both the anterior[9–11] and posterior circulation.[12] In a neuropathologic series of 135 patients who were resuscitated after cardiac arrest and who died from 1 day to several weeks later with morphologic signs of systemic cerebral anoxia, 5.2% had strokes secondary to hypotension; but in these patients, there was no association with the degree of atherosclerosis.[13] The authors concluded that the combination of cerebral atherosclerosis and hypotension is not a major cause of brain infarction in the elderly.

Exacerbating Cerebral Infarction by Treating Hypertension in the First Few Days

Protein synthesis is inhibited when cerebral perfusion decreases below 0.55 ml per g per minute. Anaerobic glycolysis is stimulated when perfusion decreases below 0.35 ml per g per minute. Neurotransmitters are released and energy metabolism is disturbed when perfusion decreases below 0.20 ml per g per minute. Anoxic depolarization occurs at perfusion rates below 0.15 ml per g per minute.[14] Two zones have been defined within a cerebral infarction: the core and ischemic penumbra. Neural tissue within the core is irreversibly damaged by profound ischemia. Between the core of an infarct and surrounding normally perfused brain is a mantle of tissue known as the penumbra that is dysfunctional but maintains cellular energy metabolism. If no reperfusion occurs, the infarcted core engulfs the penumbra in the course of only a few hours. Because autoregulation of cerebral perfusion is disturbed in an infarction, the concern is that treating hypertension could foster the conversion of ischemic penumbral tissue to infarcted tissue.[15, 16] There are several reports of worsening neurologic deficit in patients with acute stroke who were being treated for hypertension.[17, 18] In one prospective case-control study of 868 patients with acute stroke, high systolic blood pressure on admission was related to a lower frequency of early stroke progression.[19] In the only placebo-controlled trial of the use of antihypertensive medications in the setting of acute stroke, no difference was observed in neurologic outcome in the six patients given placebo as compared with the 10 given antihypertensive medications.[20]

Cerebral Infarction Due to Intentional Antihypertensive Overdose

At least two cases of cerebral infarction have been reported in patients after intentional verapamil overdose.[21, 22] Surprisingly, no other well-documented case of antihypertensive overdose survivors sustaining cerebral infarction has been reported.[23–27] The apparent infrequence of watershed infarctions in the overdose population may partly be due to the relative youth of those attempting suicide. They may have well-preserved autoregulation of cerebral blood flow. Patients with antihypertensive overdose who present in coma often make a complete neurologic recovery with aggressive therapy.[23–27] Some have suggested that beta-adrenergic blocker drugs may be neuroprotective.

Neurologic Complications Reported with Specific Antihypertensive Agents

Beta-Adrenergic Blockers

Acebutolol. There is one report of anti-acetylcholine receptor antibody–positive myasthenia gravis developing in a woman 2 weeks after starting acebutolol for hypertension.[28] Her disease fatally progressed despite discontinuation of the drug. One patient developed a reversible perioral and acral anesthesia with paresthesias with acebutolol.[29]

Atenolol. This drug may rarely induce encephalopathy in the elderly. Arber and others describe inducing a reversible delirium in an 85-year-old woman when her atenolol was increased from 50 to 100 mg twice a day.[30] There is one report of a 77-year-old woman with a history of recurrent depression who developed a reversible delirium while receiving electroconvulsive therapy and atenolol.[31] The author suggested that electroconvulsive therapy may increase permeability of the blood-brain barrier to atenolol. There is one report of atenolol promoting scotoma and scintillations without headache in a migraineur.[32] One patient with a history of encephalitis had seizures precipitated by atenolol.[33]

Carteolol. Seventy-eight patients were enrolled in a prospective study comparing beta-blockers with and without intrinsic sympathetic activity. The investigators found mild elevation in creatine kinase (CK) and significant nocturnal leg cramps to be associated with the intrinsic sympathetic activity plus the beta-blockers pindolol and carteolol.[34]

Esmolol. The ultrashort-acting water-soluble beta-adrenoreceptor antagonist esmolol has been reported to cause seizures in the absence of hypoglycemia, hypotension, or electrolyte disturbance.[35]

Labetalol. A reversible myopathy has been reported with labetalol. An 11-year-old patient and a 14-year-old patient developed proximal weakness and markedly elevated CK levels during labetalol therapy. Muscle biopsies performed in both patients were consistent with rhabdomyolysis. The patients' strength returned to normal within 2 months of stopping the drug.[36] Circumoral and scalp paresthesias have been reported with labetalol.[37–39]

Metoprolol. A reversible carpal tunnel syndrome has been reported with metoprolol and other beta-blockers. After more than 9 years of therapy with metoprolol, a man developed the signs, symptoms, and nerve conduction abnormalities of carpal tunnel syndrome in the right hand. Complete relief of symptoms was reported 10 weeks after stopping metoprolol.[40] Metoprolol has also been reported to cause delirium. A 41-year-old man developed progressive delirium 2 days after starting metoprolol.[41] The delirium persisted while the patient's physician had him taper the metoprolol and start propafenone. The delirium cleared within 24 hours after stopping both the metoprolol and propafenone. Propafenone was thought to have prolonged the delirium by reducing the rate of clearance of metoprolol. A 60-year-old man taking metoprolol developed a polymyalgia-like illness consisting of bilateral proximal leg myalgias, livedo reticularis, anemia, and an elevated erythrocyte sedimentation rate to 132 mm per hour.[42] The patient was thought to have had a polymyalgia rheumatica–like illness due to metoprolol. Within 1 month of stopping metoprolol, the patient became asymptomatic; within 2 months, the livedo reticularis cleared and the hematocrit and erythrocyte sedimentation rate normalized.

Nadolol. One man developed diplopia after the first dose of nadolol. After four doses, he developed bilateral blurry vision. On examination he had bilateral papilledema and constricted visual fields.[43]

Pindolol. Pindolol can induce muscle cramps as can carteolol. In one series this complaint developed in 14 of 300 patients treated for hypertension with this drug.[44] The time between starting the drug and the onset of muscle cramps ranged between 3 and 34 months. Many beta-blockers are used to treat essential tremor, yet pindolol seems uniquely able to induce tremor.[45, 46] When pindolol was compared with atenolol in a randomized study, the only important difference in side effects was a higher incidence of sleep disturbances with pindolol.[47] This difference was attributed to the greater lipophilicity of pindolol.

Propranolol. Clinical myotonia was precipitated in at least three cases.[48–50] The ages of the patients ranged from 20 to 57 years. All of the patients had myotonia on electromyography (EMG). Clinical myotonia completely resolved in all of the cases, with the length of time to recovery ranging from 6 weeks to 3 months. One of the patients had a persistently myotonic EMG even after drug withdrawal.[48] Rechallenge with propranolol was done in two cases, and in both cases symptoms recurred.[48, 50] Muscle biopsy was abnormal in all of the cases. One of the patients had frontal balding, and his brother had EMG evidence of myotonia, strongly suggesting that he had had asymptomatic myotonia that was made manifest clinically by propranolol.[48] It is not known how propranolol might induce myotonia, but one study on isolated muscle preparation shows that propranolol can cause contractures through a site of action outside the neuromuscular junction.[51]

Forfar et al. reported on a patient taking sotalol who developed severe painless proximal weakness in her arms and legs along with a mild elevation in her erythrocyte sedimentation rate.[52] The weakness continued when sotalol was replaced with propranolol. During the 6 months of propranolol therapy, her CK ranged from 700 to 2,200. Withdrawal and rechallenge of propranolol led to resolution and recurrence, respectively, of weakness and CK elevation. Muscle biopsy on propranolol was normal. Propranolol, like metoprolol, can cause a reversible carpal tunnel syndrome.[53]

There is one report of intermittent generalized dystonia with high doses of propranolol.[54] The patient also had schizoaffective disorder and neuroleptic exposure "some months" earlier. Her posturing ceased with discontinuation of propranolol. Propranolol, like many other beta-blockers, can induce or worsen clinical signs of myasthenia gravis.[55, 56]

Numerous reports describe propranolol causing agitated delirium that rarely progresses to coma. The encephalopathy is rarely seen with doses of less than 240 mg per day and is reversible.[57] The cases described usually had factors predisposing to drug-induced encephalopathy. One patient was 71 years old and had hyperthyroidism.[58] A 12-year-old girl who lapsed into a reversible coma with propranolol also had systemic lymphoma treated with chemotherapy and an ill-defined right parietal lesion on head computed tomography.[59] Some patients carried psychiatric diagnoses and had concomitant exposure to antipsychotics, anticholinergics, or antidepressants.[60–62] Propranolol may cause confusion in some patients by altering the pharmacokinetics of coadministered neurotropic drugs. Propranolol is known to increase blood levels of some neuroleptics, including chlorpromazine.[63] At least two patients developed acute confusion with the combination of the tetracyclic antidepressant maprotiline and propranolol.[60, 64] In one of the cases propranolol was found to increase maprotiline to toxic levels.[63] Three cases have been reported of an agitated delirium developing after propranolol withdrawal.[65, 66]

Timolol. Timolol eye drops used to treat glaucoma in a known myasthenic patient was said to precipitate generalized weakness.[67]

Potential Class-Specific Side Effects of Beta-Adrenoreceptor Antagonists. Diplopia constituted only 0.25% of total suspected adverse reactions to beta-blockers notified to the Committee on Safety of Medicines (UK) over 16 years. Reports of diplopia occurred with propranolol, practolol, atenolol, oxprenolol, pindolol, nadolol, acebutolol, metoprolol, sotalol, and timolol. Diplopia was reversible in all cases. It is suspected that beta-blockers can as a group unmask underlying myasthenia gravis in these patients.[68]

Calcium Channel Blockers

Diltiazem. There are few reports of significant neurologic complications with diltiazem. There is one report of three patients with reversible myoclonus. Electroencephalography done in two of the three showed no epileptiform activity.[69] One patient developed a painful myopathy severe enough to impair walking. His CK was 4,000 U per liter (100% CK-MM isoform). Withdrawal and rechallenge led to resolution and recurrence, respectively, of the myalgias and elevated CK level.[70] One man developed the clinical, pharmacologic, and electrodiagnostic criteria for Lambert-Eaton syndrome with the use of diltiazem. The syndrome appeared and disappeared with the increase and decrease of serum diltiazem concentration. The patient lacked antibodies to the voltage-operated calcium channel, and an extensive search for malignancy was unrevealing.[71] Diltiazem-induced parkinsonism has rarely been reported.[72, 73]

Diltiazem has been reported to increase carbamazepine levels by 40%, resulting in clinical carbamazepine toxicity.[74]

Isradipine. Concerns over the relative safety of isradipine were raised after the MIDAS study comparing isradipine with hydrochlorothiazide in their ability to prevent progression of intima-media thickness of the carotid arteries.[75] An unexplained insignificant trend toward more vascular events including stroke was seen with isradipine.

Nicardipine. A case of severe generalized hyperkinesia has been reported with the long-acting preparation.[76]

Nifedipine. Myoclonic dystonia has been described in two patients taking nifedipine.[77, 78] In one patient the myoclonus involved the face and bilateral upper extremities, and in the other patient the legs were also affected. The movements were symmetric and occurred at rest and with action. Symptoms resolved within 1–3 days of discontinuation of the medicine. Nifedipine can dramatically potentiate the neuromuscular blockade seen with magnesium sulfate given for tocolysis or treatment of preeclampsia.[79, 80]

Verapamil. Weakness due to preexisting neuromuscular disease (myasthenia gravis, Lambert-Eaton syndrome) or Duchenne's muscular dystrophy can be made considerably worse by administration of verapamil.[81–83] This is thought to be due to an impairment in excitation-contraction coupling. Clinical and electrographic fasciculations were caused by verapamil in one patient with a preexisting idiopathic polyneuropathy.[84] One man developed myoclonic dystonia 10 months after starting verapamil, and the symptoms took 3 weeks to resolve after discontinuing the medication.[85] A few cases of verapamil-induced parkinsonism have been reported.[86, 87] A bipolar man with mild haloperidol-induced tardive dyskinesia developed choreoathetosis when he was treated with lithium and verapamil. The movements stopped when verapamil was discontinued.[88] There is one report of delirium caused by verapamil; however, this patient had bipolar disorder and claimed to be sensitive to drugs.[89] Verapamil can increase carbamazepine levels into a clinically toxic range.[90–93]

Angiotensin-Converting Enzyme Inhibitors

Captopril. Peripheral neuropathy has been described with captopril.[94–96] Some have had a Guillain-Barré syndrome, with cerebrospinal fluid (CSF) showing albuminocytologic dissociation. Captopril may predispose to autoimmune neuropathy because, like D-penicillamine, it has a sulfhydryl group. Ageusia or dysgeusia occurs in 0.1–3.0% of patients taking captopril.[97–100] The dysgeusia is often described as foul, salty, or metallic.[98] The problem may resolve with substitution of angiotensin-converting enzyme inhibitor.[101] Zinc supplementation is ineffective in treating the taste impairment. Exacerbation of chorea after cardiopulmonary bypass and induction of parkinsonism have been reported.[102, 103]

Renal and cerebral circulation in chronically hypertensive premature infants may be particularly vulnerable to reductions in blood pressure. Such patients often have hyperreninemia. Captopril may excessively lower blood pressure in such patients. In their series of nine premature neonates, oliguria and seizures often accompanied rapid reduction in blood pressure with captopril.[104]

Rarely, encephalopathy may occur with captopril.[105–107] Naloxone reversed the encephalopathy in one patient.[106] It has been suggested that captopril confusion may be the result of inhibition of enkephenyl dipeptidyl carboxypeptidase by the drug.

Enalapril. Paresthesias are uncommonly associated with enalapril,[108] and there are rare reports of enalapril causing distal polyneuropathy.[109, 110] Enalapril has also caused polymyalgia rheumatica.[111] There is one report of enalapril-induced psychosis.[112]

Diuretics

The neurologic complications stemming from diuretics are almost entirely due to alterations in electrolytes. Diuretic-induced hyponatremia can lead to seizures, stupor, coma, extensor plantar responses, and death.[113–115] Many diuretics lower serum potassium and thus may induce quadriparesis in patients with hypokalemic periodic paralysis.[116] Hyperkalemic paralysis has been reported with the use of spironolactone.[117, 118] Diuretics may so grossly alter serum magnesium as to cause seizures.[119, 120] There is one report of myalgias caused by hydrochlorothiazide being severe enough to make a patient bed bound.[121] Loop diuretics, including furosemide and bumetanide, have been implicated in ototoxicity.[122]

Other Antihypertensives

Clonidine. Myalgias have been noted.[123] They are usually most troublesome in the femoral adductors. Delirium, sometimes with vivid frightening dreams and visual hallucinations, is a rare complication.[124–126]

Hydralazine. Hydralazine can cause pyridoxine deficiency and thereby a sensorimotor polyneuropathy that resolves with pyridoxine replacement and drug withdrawal.[127] This hydralazine-induced peripheral neuropathy may be more likely to occur in patients who are slow acetylators of isoniazid.[128] Hydralazine rarely causes peripheral neuropathy at a dose of 100–200 mg per day.[129]

Methyldopa. The centrally acting antihypertensive methyldopa has long been known to produce a reversible parkinsonism or aggravate preexisting parkinsonism.[130–132] It inhibits L-amino acid decarboxylase and is successively decarboxylated and hydroxylated to form the false neurotransmitter alpha-methylnorepinephrine, which displaces norepinephrine.[133] There are two reports of generalized choreiform movements caused by methyldopa.[134, 135] One patient had bilateral cerebral infarcts, and the other had renal failure, a condition that could increase the serum concentration of methyldopa.

Minoxidil. Bilateral optic neuritis was attributed to minoxidil administration in one patient who had undergone renal transplantation and was taking prednisone and azathioprine as well.[136]

Nitroprusside. Thiocyanate and cyanide are metabolites of the potent parenteral antihypertensive nitroprusside.[137] Signs of mild thiocyanate neurotoxicity include tinnitus, miosis, and hyperreflexia.[138] Signs suggesting cyanide poisoning include hypotension, bradycardia, bright red venous blood, metabolic acidosis, and almond odor of breath or gastric contents.[139] Encephalopathy, coma, and death can result from severe thiocyanate and cyanide toxicity. Cyanide poisoning due to nitroprusside has resulted in bilateral globus pallidus necrosis.[140] The principal pathway for metabolizing cyanide is through the enzyme rhodanese, which is found mostly in the liver. Rhodanese converts cyanide to thiocyanate, which is then renally excreted. Therefore, hepatic or renal insufficiency predisposes to cyanide or thiocyanate toxicity. It is important to recognize and diagnose cyanide poisoning because there are specific antidotes, including sodium thiosulfate and sodium nitrite.[141]

Prazosin. This $alpha_1$-adrenoreceptor antagonist is contraindicated in patients with narcolepsy because it can induce status cataplecticus.[142, 143] This finding has also been made in a canine model of cataplexy.

Antiarrhythmic Medications

Adenosine

Migraineurs may have headache triggered by adenosine.[144]

Amiodarone

A vast array of neurologic symptoms have been attributed to amiodarone. Ten percent to 50% of patients taking amiodarone develop some combination of tremor, ataxia, and peripheral neuropathy.[145–150] Nystagmus is not a typical associated finding.[145] These neurologic side effects improve or resolve within 2 days to 4 weeks of decreasing or discontinuing amiodarone. Neurologic side effects can be disabling and lead to decreasing or discontinuing amiodarone in approximately 5% of patients.[151]

In one series of 151 prospectively studied patients taking antiarrhythmic medications, 25% had electrophysiologic evidence of polyneuropathy, and 3% had clinical evidence of polyneuropathy.[152] Numerous cases have been described of a distal generalized sensorimotor polyneuropathy induced by amiodarone.[153–157] Distal paresthesias, gait disorder, and weakness are usually the first symptoms noted. Cranial nerves are not involved. Autonomic neuropathy has been reported once.[158] CSF protein is usually normal or slightly elevated. EMG shows distal muscle denervation. Nerve conduction velocities can be normal to markedly reduced. Nerve biopsy often shows lysosomal inclusions in Schwann's cells, fibroblasts, and capillary epithelial cells, suggesting a drug-induced neurolipidosis.

Amiodarone has been implicated as a cause of optic neuropathy.[159–161] The incidence of optic neuropathy is significantly greater in patients treated with amiodarone than age-matched controls. However, no study has been done with a control group matched for cardiovascular disease. The optic disk typically shows swelling or pallor. There may be significant cup-to-disk ratio, a finding opposite that seen in ischemic optic neuropathy. In one pathologic study of an asymptomatic man taking amiodarone, lamellar inclusions were selectively found in large axons of the optic nerve.[162] There are a few reports of pseudotumor cerebri with amiodarone.[163–166] Acute intracranial hypertension can occur during intravenous infusion of amiodarone.[167]

A myopathy with or without neuropathy can be seen with amiodarone use.[168–170] Involvement of spinal cord or cerebellum has been seen in patients with amiodarone peripheral neuropathy.[171, 172]

Amiodarone rarely causes delirium.[173] Amiodarone can increase both free and protein-bound phenytoin (Dilantin).[174]

Movement disorders described with amiodarone include myoclonus, hemiballism, orofacial and generalized dyskinesias, and parkinsonism.[175, 176] The reversibility of amiodarone-induced parkinsonism appears to be related to duration of therapy. Complete reversal is likely if patients have been exposed for 12 days or less.[176]

Disopyramide

A dysesthetic slowly reversible lower extremity peripheral neuropathy has been reported with disopyramide.[177]

Encainide

A single case of fevers, chills, and myalgias in the calves has been reported. All symptoms resolved with discontinuation of encainide.[178]

Flecainide

Dizziness and visual disturbances occur in slightly less than one-third of patients taking flecainide.[179] Flecainide can induce a symmetric distal peripheral neuropathy.[180] Dystonia and acute weakness in a patient with fiber type disproportion have both been reportedly due to flecainide.[181, 182] Generalized seizures occurred in a 12-year-old patient with a flecainide level of more than 4 μg per ml.[183] Dysarthria and visual hallucinations were seen in a 65-year-old patient with a flecainide level of 2.5 μg per ml.[184]

Lidocaine

Intravenous lidocaine can produce diplopia, dysarthria, and more seriously, encephalopathy and partial or generalized seizures.[185, 186] Seizures precipitated by lidocaine usually occur when plasma levels exceed 9 μg per ml.[183] In one study of six normal volunteers, the total convulsant dose was 6–9 mg per kg. All induced seizures were accompanied by spikes on ictal electroencephalography recordings.[187] The Boston Collaborative Drug Surveillance Program found a convulsion rate of 5.7 per 1,000 treated with intravenous lidocaine for arrhythmias.[188] As part of their delirium, patients may experience "doom anxiety," an apprehension of death that can reach delusional proportions.[189] Use of additional antiarrhythmics may predispose to delirium.[190] One patient who was taking propafenone and mexiletine developed generalized myoclonus after the administration of a therapeutic dose of intravenous lidocaine. The myoclonus resolved with discontinuation of the lidocaine and administration of diazepam.[191]

Mexiletine

This primary amine is structurally related to lidocaine. Commonly reported neurologic side effects include tremor, ataxia, slurred speech, blurred vision, impaired memory, and diplopia. Approximately 5% of patients need to discontinue the drug because of such side effects.[192, 193] Patients may experience visual hallucinations that start 2–3 days after initiation of therapy and resolve 8–12 hours after drug discontinuation. Patients are typically fully oriented during the hallucinations.[194, 195]

Procainamide

The neurologic complications of procainamide usually relate to the nerve, muscle, or neuromuscular junction. The nervous system may be one of the target organs in the lupus-like reaction seen in approximately 10% of patients taking procainamide. Patients with procainamide-induced lupus-like reaction can develop a distal sensorimotor polyneuropathy. There have been reports of improvement in neuropathy both with drug discontinuation and corticosteroids.[196, 197] Rarely, procainamide can produce a myopathy.[198–200] Muscle biopsy may show a necrotizing myositis or simply perivascular inflammation. The CK can be normal or greater than 10,000 IU per liter. Procainamide can unmask and aggravate myasthenic symptoms in myasthenia gravis.[201–203] High doses of procainamide can cause severe bulbar, limb, and respiratory weakness in nonmyasthenic patients, especially if there is a preexisting peripheral neuropathy.[204–206]

Propafenone

A reversible generalized myoclonus has been reported with propafenone.[207] One patient with ocular myasthenia became generally weak after taking propafenone.[208] One patient developed a small fiber peripheral neuropathy. The symptoms of jabbing and crushing pain resolved on discontinuation of the medication.[209] One patient developed a transient global amnesia with propafenone.[210]

Quinidine

Quinidine causes a neurologic syndrome known as *cinchonism*, named after cinchona bark, which was the original crude preparation of quinidine. Cinchonism occurs in approximately 1% of patients taking quinidine.[211] Cinchonism includes, to a varying degree, headache, flushing, mydriasis, delirium, and visual changes. The visual disturbances may rarely be confused with retinal transient ischemic attacks.[212] When taken with digoxin, quinidine can produce delirium even when the serum concentration is in the therapeutic range.[213] Some suggest that quinidine-induced delirium is an anticholinergic syndrome that can be reversed with physostigmine.[214] As with many antiarrhythmics, quinidine can exacerbate weakness in patients with myasthenia gravis.[202, 215]

Sotalol

One patient developed hemifacial edema followed by atrophy when exposed to cold weather and sotalol.[216]

Tocainide

The neurologic side effects of tocainide are dose related and typically disappear with discontinuation of the drug.[217] These side effects include tremors, restlessness, and confusion. Seizures have been reported after ingestion of 16 g of tocainide.[218]

Inotropes

Cardiac Glycosides

Delirium was reported with digitalis as early as 1874.[219] The patients are often combative and disoriented.[220–223] Delirium typically occurs with levels of digoxin above the therapeutic range; however, a level within the therapeutic range does not exclude the diagnosis of digoxin delirium.[224] Symptoms resolve over 1–2 weeks after stopping the medication. Rapid reversal of delirium can be done with digoxin immune Fab (Digibind), the Fab fragment of an antibody that binds digoxin.[225] Ophthalmic symptoms of digoxin toxicity include xanthopsia or other dyschromatopsia, blurry vision, scintillating scotomata, diplopia, and pain with ocular movement. The color defects can be detected with Ishihara's or AOH-R-R plates or the Farnsworth-Munsell 100-Hue test. The defects usually clear with decreasing digoxin serum levels.[226, 227] Trigeminal neuralgia may also be caused by digitalis toxicity.[228, 229]

Nitrates

It was recognized at the turn of the century that nitroglycerine could induce debilitating headaches. The headaches were referred to as "dynamite headaches" because they occurred among factory workers manufacturing explosives.[230] The same headache occurs in 50% of patients who receive 0.3–0.4 mg of nitroglycerine for angina pectoris. The headaches are pulsatile and bifrontal or bitemporal. They are made worse by bending forward or physical exertion. They rarely last more than 20 minutes.[231] Migraineurs and patients with cluster headaches can have headaches triggered by either nitroglycerine or isosorbide dinitrate.[232, 233] There are isolated reports of intracranial hypertension and reversible abducens nerve palsy with nitroglycerine.[234, 235] Visual hallucinations were attributed to isosorbide dinitrate in one depressed 87-year-old woman.[236]

Antilipemic Medications

Cholestyramine

This bile acid sequestrant can lead to the malabsorption of fat-soluble vitamins, especially above doses of 24 g per day.[237] Vitamin K deficiency can cause hypoprothrombinemia. A fetus developed subdural hematoma after the mother was prescribed cholestyramine without vitamin K supplements.[238] There is one report of rhabdomyolysis in the setting of concomitant lovastatin and cholestyramine use.[239]

Fibrates

Clofibrate

Approximately 1–5% of patients need to discontinue clofibrate secondary to side effects, most of which are gastrointestinal.[240, 241] Rarely, patients develop a myopathy syndrome of myalgias, weakness, stiffness, malaise, and an elevated CK level.[242–246] The syndrome is far less common than the 10–20% occurrence of CK elevation. Rush et al. reviewed 78 patients with clofibrate myopathy and found the treatment duration premyopathy to be between 3 and 730 days, with a mean of 56 days.[247] Elevated CK level was found in all 78 patients. Weakness was reported in 32 of 45. Myalgia was reported in 43 of 64. The time to recovery ranged from 2–65 days, with a mean of 35 days. EMG may be normal or myopathic. Some patients may have myocardial involvement as well as skeletal muscle involvement.[248] Clofibrate is rapidly hydrolyzed to p-chlorophenoxyisobutyric acid (CPIB) which is 92–97% protein bound. Forty percent to 70% of an oral dose of clofibrate is recovered in urine as the glucuronide conjugate of CPIB. States that impair protein binding or excretion of CPIB, such as renal failure and the nephrotic syndrome, predispose to the myositis syndrome.[249–251] Myopathology includes breakdown of contractile material, deranged mitochondria, membrane-bound dense bodies, and discontinuities in sarcolemma. Macrophages invade severely affected fibers.[252, 253] There is one report of a man with diabetes and subclinical neuropathy who developed a reversible whole-body myokymia with clofibrate.[254]

Gemfibrozil

A congener of clofibrate, gemfibrozil rarely causes neurologic side effects by itself. One man developed pain in his legs so severe that it impaired walking. His CK level revealed a high of 540 U per liter. His symptom resolved and the CK level normalized secondarily after stopping gemfibrozil. His symptoms and CK elevation recurred with rechallenge.[255] One patient developed a compartment syndrome of her left calf that required emergency fasciotomy.[256] There is a 5% chance of myositis with the combination of gemfibrozil and lovastatin.[257, 258] Rhabdomyolysis with renal failure has been seen with this combination.[259] Muscle biopsy of gemfibrozil and lovastatin myopathy shows multiple foci of mononuclear cell infiltration with myophagocytosis. Electron microscopy shows subsarcolemmal accumulations of autophagic lysosomes.[260]

A frontotemporal throbbing headache associated with dry mouth can be caused by gemfibrozil. In the cases described, the headache would recur approximately 1 hour after each dose.[261, 262] A reversible decreased libido has also been attributed to gemfibrozil.[263, 264]

HMG-CoA Reductase Inhibitors

Lovastatin

Side effects of lovastatin leading to drug withdrawal occur in less than 5% of patients.[257] Clinical myopathy occurs in 0.2% of all patients taking lovastatin, 5% of patients taking gemfibrozil with lovastatin, and 30% of patients taking cyclosporine and other immunosuppressants with lovastatin.[265] Many patients in the latter high-risk group had recently undergone cardiac transplantation.[266, 267] Rhabdomyolysis may occur in patients taking lovastatin and gemfibrozil.[268] Some authors suggest that myalgias and elevated serum CK levels reported with many lipid-lowering agents may be the result of lowering the cholesterol content of the sarcolemmal phospholipid bilayer, thereby increasing membrane fluidity.[269] Other drugs that are claimed to increase the risk of rhabdomyolysis with lovastatin include macrolide antibiotics, nicotinic acid, and itraconazole.[270–274]

A mild reversible sensorimotor or sensory polyneuropathy has been reported.[275] There is one report of lovastatin unmasking Parkinson's disease in two patients.[276] Withdrawal of the drug may lead to improvement in parkinsonian symptoms over several months. The authors speculate that lovastatin may lead to accumulation of HMG-CoA and its metabolite acetyl-CoA in the brain and that high levels of acetyl-CoA may stimulate synthesis of acetylcholine. In one study, however, measured metabolites of lovastatin in human CSF were of insufficient concentration to inhibit HMG-CoA reductase in a sensitive bioassay.[277]

Pravastatin

As with other HMG-CoA reductase inhibitors, pravastatin can in rare instances cause a myopathy. Symptoms of myalgias and CK elevation seem to occur no more frequently with pravastatin than with lovastatin or simvastatin.[278, 279] An increase of CK level of at least fourfold was seen in 1.4% of patients taking pravastatin alone and in 4% of patients taking the combination of pravastatin and gemfibrozil. Musculoskeletal pains were seen in 1.4% of patients taking pravastatin alone and in 9.3% of patients taking gemfibrozil and pravastatin.[280] Muscle biopsy data are limited and conflicting. One patient who had been taking pravastatin for 5 months developed the myopathologic features of dermatomyositis. The authors do not report that the myopathy cleared with discontinuation of the drug.[281] A report from England and other reports describe patients who developed microscopic and biochemical features of a mitochondrial myopathy as a result of treatment with pravastatin.[282] Interestingly, despite rapid resolution of symptoms with drug discontinuation and reemergence of symptoms with rechallenge, the microscopic and biochemical abnormalities were still present 1 year after stopping the drug.

Simvastatin

As many as 13% of patients taking simvastatin complain of myalgias.[283] The majority of them do not have elevations in CK level. Some patients do experience massive rhabdomyolysis with the drug.[284, 285] Hypothyroidism may present with hypercholesterolemia that is correctable with thyroid replacement therapy. Treating such a case of secondary hypercholesterolemia with an HMG-CoA reductase inhibitor may bring out a subclinical myopathy.[286] It is also important to exclude nephrotic syndrome as a cause of hypercholesterolemia before treating with HMG-CoA reductase inhibitor because renal insufficiency may predispose to the myotoxicity of the drug.

As with pravastatin, simvastatin myopathy has been shown in some cases to have microscopic and chemical features of a mitochondrial myopathy.[282] A case of simvastatin-induced rhabdomyolysis followed by the mitochondrial encephalopathy with lactic acidosis and stroke-like episodes syndrome (MELAS) has been described.[287] The patient did not have the point mutation known to be responsible for 80% of MELAS. She had low muscle CoQ_{10} levels while symptomatic. Her symptoms resolved with discontinuation of simvastatin and CoQ_{10} replacement therapy. Inhibition of HMG-CoA reductase leads to a deficiency in mevalonate. Mevalonate is required for the synthesis of CoQ_{10}, an important compound in the mitochondrial respiratory chain.

Simvastatin can cause distal sensorimotor polyneuropathy that has the electrophysiologic and pathologic features of axonal degeneration. It is often reversible with medication discontinuation.[288]

Conclusion

Debilitating neurologic side effects from cardiovascular drugs occur uncommonly. The importance in recognizing that a neurologic condition is drug induced is that discontinuation of the offending agent results in resolution of symptoms in nearly all cases. There are numerous examples of host susceptibility to drug-induced complications. Patients with myasthenia gravis or Lambert-Eaton syndrome may become acutely weak with the administration of calcium channel antagonists. Patients with myasthenia gravis or myotonic dystrophy may experience worsening weakness or myotonia with the administration of beta-adrenergic antagonists. Patients with an inherited periodic paralysis can have attacks precipitated by diuretics. Narcoleptics experience status cataplecticus with prazosin. Patients who suffer from migraines or cluster headaches may be intolerant to nitrates.

In a few instances, the pathophysiology of drug-induced neurotoxicity has been established, and specific therapies are available. Hydralazine can cause a polyneuropathy by depleting pyridoxine. Cholestyramine can predispose to intracranial hemorrhages by preventing the adequate absorption of vitamin K and thereby causing a hypoprothrombinemia. Nitroprusside can cause irreversible central nervous system dysfunction through the generation of the metabolites thiocyanate and cyanide.

An otherwise well-tolerated drug may cause adverse effects in combination with other drugs. For example, the likelihood of developing myopathy from HMG-CoA reductase inhibitors is increased with the coadministration of fibrates, and general paresis in women receiving tocolytic doses of magnesium sulfate may be potentiated by the coadministration of nifedipine.

References

1. Whisnant JP. Effectiveness and efficacy of treatment of hypertension for stroke. Neurology 1996;46:301.
2. Amery A, Brixko P, Clement D, et al. Mortality and morbidity results from the European Working Party on High Blood Pressure in the Elderly. Lancet 1985;1:1349.
3. Graham DI. Ischemic brain damage of cerebral perfusion failure type after treatment of severe hypertension. BMJ 1975;2:739.
4. Cove DH, Seddon M, Fletcher RF, et al. Blindness after treatment for malignant hypertension. BMJ 1979;2:245.
5. Ledingham JG, Rajagopalan B. Cerebral complications in the treatment of accelerated hypertension. Q J Med 1979;48:25.
6. Haas DC, Streeten DHP, Kim RC, et al. Death from cerebral hypoperfusion during nitroprusside treatment of acute angiotensin-dependent hypertension. Am J Med 1983;75:1071.
7. Hankey G, Gubbay SS. Focal cerebral ischemia and infarction due to antihypertensive therapy. Med J Aust 1987;146:412.
8. Moulds RFW. Strokes and hypertension—the effect of treatment. Med J Aust 1987;146:406.
9. Ruff RL, Talman WT, Petito F. Transient ischemic attacks associated with hypotension in hypertensive patients with carotid artery stenosis. Stroke 1981;12:353.
10. Somerville ER. Orthostatic transient ischemic attacks: a symptom of large vessel occlusion. Stroke 1984;15:1066.
11. Dobkin BH. Orthostatic hypotension as a risk factor for symptomatic occlusive cerebrovascular disease. Neurology 1989;39:30.
12. Fagan SC, McCormick PW, Diaz FG. Hemodynamic vertebrobasilar insufficiency as an adverse effect of antihypertensive therapy. DICP 1989;23:238.
13. Torvik A, Skullerud K. How often are brain infarcts caused by hypotensive episodes? Stroke 1976;7:255.
14. Hossmann K-A. Viability thresholds and the penumbra of focal ischemia. Ann Neurol 1994;36:557.
15. Powers WJ. Acute hypertension after stroke: the scientific basis for treatment decisions. Neurology 1993; 43:461.
16. Yatsu FM, Zivin J. Hypertension in acute strokes: not to treat. Arch Neurol 1985;42:999.
17. Lavin P. Management of hypertension in patients with acute stroke. Arch Intern Med 1986;146:66.
18. Britton M, de Faire U, Helmers C. Hazards of therapy for excessive hypertension in acute stroke. Acta Med Scand 1980;207:253.
19. Jorgensen HS, Nakayama H, Raaschou HO, et al. Effect of blood pressure and diabetes on stroke in progression. Lancet 1994;344:156.
20. Lisk DR, Grotta JC, Lamki LM, et al. Should hypertension be treated after acute stroke? A randomized controlled trial using single photon emission computed tomography. Arch Neurol 1993;50:855.
21. Samniah N, Schlaeffer F. Cerebral infarction associated with oral verapamil overdose. Clin Toxicol 1988;26:365.
22. Shah AR, Passalacqua BR. Case report: sustained-release verapamil overdose causing stroke: an unusual complication. Am J Med Sci 1992;304:357.
23. Lip GYH, Ferner RE. Poisoning with antihypertensive drugs: calcium antagonists. J Hum Hypertens 1995; 9:155.
24. Lip GYH, Ferner RE. Poisoning with antihypertensive drugs: alpha adrenoreceptor antagonists. J Hum Hypertens 1995;9:523.
25. Lip GYH, Ferner RE. Poisoning with antihypertensive drugs: beta adrenoreceptor blocker drugs. J Hum Hypertens 1995;9:213.
26. Lip GYH, Ferner RE. Poisoning with antihypertensive drugs: angiotensin converting enzyme inhibitors. J Hum Hypertens 1995;9:711.
27. Zarifis J, Lip GYH, Ferner RE. Poisoning with antihypertensive drugs: methyldopa and clonidine. J Hum Hypertens 1995;9:787.
28. Confavreux C, Charles N, Aimard G. Fulminant myasthenia gravis soon after initiation of acebutolol therapy. Eur Neurol 1990;30:279.
29. Logan R, Holmden RH. Subjective anesthesia with acebutalol. N Z Med J 1978;87:403.
30. Arber N. Delirium induced by atenolol. BMJ 1988; 297:1048.
31. Kramer BA. Severe confusion in a patient receiving electroconvulsive therapy and atenolol. J Nerv Ment Dis 1986;174:562.
32. Kumar KL, Cooney TG. Visual symptoms after atenolol therapy for migraine. Ann Intern Med 1990;112:712.
33. Russell D, Veger T, Bunaes VB, et al. Epileptic seizures precipitated by atenolol. J Neurol Neurosurg Psychiatry 1979;42:484.
34. Imai Y, Watanabe N, Hashimoto J, et al. Muscle cramps and elevated serum creatinine phosphokinase levels induced by beta-adrenoreceptor blockers. Eur J Clin Pharmacol 1995;48:29.
35. Das G, Ferris JC. Generalized convulsions in a patient receiving ultrashort-acting beta-blocker infusion. Drug Intell Clin Pharm 1988;22:484.
36. Willis JK, Tilton AH, Harkin JC, et al. Reversible myopathy due to labetalol. Pediatr Neurol 1990;6:275.

37. Gabriel R. Circumoral paraesthesias and labetalol. BMJ 1978;1:580.
38. Bailey RR. Scalp tingling and difficulty in micturition in patients on labetalol. Lancet 1977;2:720.
39. Hua ASP, Thomas GW, Kincaid-Smith P. Scalp tingling in patients on labetalol. Lancet 1977;2:295.
40. Emara MK, Saadah AM. The carpal tunnel syndrome in hypertensive patients treated with beta-blockers. Postgrad Med J 1988;64:191.
41. Ahmad S. Metoprolol-induced delirium perpetuated by propafenone. Am Fam Physician 1991;44:1142.
42. Snyder S. Metoprolol-induced polymyalgia-like syndrome. Ann Intern Med 1991;114:96.
43. Kaul S, Wong M, Singh BN, et al. Nadolol and papilledema. Ann Intern Med 1982;97:454.
44. Zimlichman R, Krauss S, Paran E. Muscle cramps induced by beta blockers with intrinsic sympathomimetic activity properties: hint of a possible mechanism. Arch Intern Med 1991;151:1021.
45. Koller W, Orebaugh C, Lawson L, et al. Pindolol-induced tremor. Clin Neuropharmacol 1987;10:449.
46. Hod H, Kaplinsky N, Har-Zahav J, et al. Pindolol-induced tremor. Postgrad Med J 1980;56:346.
47. Foerster E-Ch, Greminger P, Siegenthaler W, et al. Atenolol versus pindolol: side-effects in hypertension. Eur J Clin Pharmacol 1985;28(Suppl):89.
48. Blessing W, Walsh JC. Myotonia precipitated by propranolol therapy. Lancet 1977;1:73.
49. Satya-Murti S, Heiman T, Martinez LB. Possible propranolol-myotonin association. N Engl J Med 1977; 297:223.
50. Turkewitz LJ, Sahgal V, Spiro A. Propranolol-induced myotonia. Mt Sinai J Med 1984;51:207.
51. Acharya SRK, Rao S. Propranolol and myotonia. Lancet 1977;1:1208.
52. Forfar JC, Brown GJ, Cull RE. Proximal myopathy during beta-blockade. BMJ 1979;2:1331.
53. Lipponi G, Lucantoni C, Antonicelli R, et al. Clinical and electromyographic evidence of carpal tunnel syndrome in a hypertensive patient with chronic beta-blocker treatment. Ital J Neurol Sci 1992;13:157.
54. Crawford JP. Dystonic reaction to high dose propranolol. BMJ 1977;2:1156.
55. Choi KL, Wat MS, Ip TP, et al. Phaeochromocytoma associated with myasthenia gravis precipitated by propranolol treatment. Aust N Z J Med 1995;25:257.
56. Herishanu Y, Rosenberg P. Letter: beta-blockers and myasthenia gravis. Ann Intern Med 1975;83:834.
57. Kuhr BM. Prolonged delirium with propranolol. J Clin Psychiatry 1979;40:194.
58. Topliss D, Bond R. Acute brain syndrome after propranolol treatment. Lancet 1977;2:1133.
59. Helson L, Duque L. Acute brain syndrome after propranolol. Lancet 1978;1:98.
60. Saiz-Ruiz J, Moral L. Delirium induced by the association of propranolol and maprotiline. J Clin Psychopharmacol 1988;8:77.
61. Lima BR, Vanneman D. Propranolol, benztropine, fluphenazine decanoate, and delirium. Am J Psychiatry 1983;140:659.
62. Miller FA, Rampling D. Adverse effects of combined propranolol and chlorpromazine therapy. Am J Psychiatry 1982;139:1198.
63. Peet M, Middlemiss DN, Yates RA. Propranolol in schizophrenia. II: clinical and biochemical aspects of combining propranolol with chlorpromazine. Br J Psychiatry 1981;138:112.
64. Tollefson G, Lesar T. Effect of propranolol on maprotiline clearance. Am J Psychiatry 1984;141:148.
65. Golden RN, Hoffman J, Falk D, et al. Psychoses associated with propranolol withdrawal. Biol Psychiatry 1989;25:351.
66. Patterson JR. Psychosis following discontinuation of a long-acting propranolol preparation. J Clin Psychopharmacol 1985;5:125.
67. Shaivitz SA. Timolol and myasthenia gravis. JAMA 1979;242:1611.
68. Weber JCP. Beta-adrenoreceptor antagonists and diplopia. Lancet 1982;2:826.
69. Jeret JS, Somasundaram M, Asaikar S. Diltiazem-induced myoclonus. NY State J Med 1992;92:447.
70. Ahmad S. Diltiazem myopathy. Am Heart J 1993; 126:1494.
71. Ueno S, Hara Y. Lambert-Eaton myasthenic syndrome without anti-calcium channel antibody: adverse effect of calcium antagonist diltiazem. J Neurol Neurosurg Psychiatry 1992;55:409.
72. Dick RS, Barold SS. Diltiazem-induced parkinsonism. Am J Med 1989;87:95.
73. Graham DF, Stewart-Wynne EG. Diltiazem-induced acute parkinsonism. Aust N Z J Med 1994;24:70.
74. Brodie MJ, Macphee GJA. Carbamazepine neurotoxicity precipitated by diltiazem. BMJ 1986;292:1170.
75. Borhani NO, Mercuri M, Borhani PA, et al. Final outcome of the Multicenter Isradipine Diuretic Atherosclerosis Study (MIDAS). JAMA 1996;276:785.
76. Das G. Severe generalized hyperkinesia to nicardipine SR therapy. Int J Clin Pharmacol Ther 1994;32:612.
77. Medina AD, Biasini O, Rivera A, et al. Nifedipine and myoclonic dystonia. Ann Intern Med 1986;104:125.
78. Pedro-Botet ML, Caralps BA. Nifedipine and myoclonic disorders. Nephron 1989;51:218.
79. Snyder SW, Cardwell MS. Neuromuscular blockade with magnesium sulfate and nifedipine. Am J Obstet Gynecol 1989;161:35.
80. Ben-Ami M, Giladi Y, Shalev E. The combination of magnesium sulfate and nifedipine: a cause of neuromuscular blockade. Br J Obstet Gynecol 1994;101:262.
81. Swash M, Ingram DA. Adverse effect of verapamil in myasthenia gravis. Muscle Nerve 1992;15:396.
82. Krendel DA, Hopkins LC. Adverse effect of verapamil in a patient with the Lambert-Eaton syndrome. Muscle Nerve 1986;9:519.
83. Zalman F, Durant NN, Campion DS. Acute respiratory

failure following intravenous verapamil in Duchenne's muscular dystrophy. Am Heart J 1983;105:510.
84. Thömke F, Vogt T, Röder R, et al. Fasciculations due to verapamil in a patient with neuropathy. J Neurol 1990;237:448.
85. Hicks CB, Abraham K. Verapamil and myoclonic dystonia. Ann Intern Med 1985;103:154.
86. Garcia-Albea E, Jiménez-Jiménez FJ, Ayuso-Peralta L, et al. Parkinsonism unmasked by verapamil. Clin Neuropharm 1993;16:263.
87. Padrell MD, Navarro M, Faura CC, et al. Verapamil-induced parkinsonism. Am J Med 1995;99:436.
88. Helmuth D, Ljaljevic Z, Ramirez L, et al. Choreoathetosis induced by verapamil and lithium treatment. J Clin Psychopharmacol 1989;9:454.
89. Jacobsen FM, Sack DA, James SP. Delirium induced by verapamil. Am J Psychiatry 1987;144:248.
90. Macphee GJA, McInnes GT, Thompson GG, et al. Verapamil potentiates carbamazepine neurotoxicity: a clinically important inhibitory interaction. Lancet 1986;1:700.
91. Beattie B, Biller J, Mehlhaus B, et al. Verapamil-induced carbamazepine neurotoxicity. Eur Neurol 1988;28:104.
92. Eimer M, Carter BL. Elevated serum carbamazepine concentrations following diltiazem initiation. Drug Intell Clin Pharm 1987;21:340.
93. Maoz E, Grossman E, Thaler M, et al. Carbamazepine neurotoxic reaction after administration of diltiazem. Arch Intern Med 1992;152:2503.
94. Chakraborty TK, Ruddell WSJ. Guillain-Barré neuropathy during treatment with captopril. Postgrad Med J 1987;63:221.
95. Atkinson AB, Brown JJ, McAreavey, et al. Neurologic dysfunction in two patients receiving captopril and cimetidine. Lancet 1980;2:36.
96. Samanta A, Burden AC. Peripheral neuropathy due to captopril. BMJ 1985;291:1172.
97. Zazgornik J, Kaiser W, Biesenbach G. Captopril-induced dysgeusia. Lancet 1993;341:1542.
98. Chia HM, Kalra L, Lakhani AK, et al. Captopril-induced taste disturbance. Lancet 1993;342:304.
99. Vlasses PH, Ferguson RK. Temporary ageusia related to captopril. Lancet 1979;2:526.
100. McNeil JJ, Anderson A, Christophidis N. Taste loss associated with oral captopril treatment. BMJ 1979; 2:1555.
101. Mauersberger H, Witte PU. Disappearance of captopril-induced taste disturbance after substitution with angiotensin-converting-enzyme inhibitor HOE498. Lancet 1985;1:517.
102. Blackburn MEC, Gibbs JL, Dickinson DF. Chorea after cardiopulmonary bypass: exacerbation by captopril. Int J Cardiol 1991;30:236.
103. Sandyk R. Parkinsonism induced by captopril. Clin Neuropharm 1985;8:197.
104. Perlman JM, Volpe JJ. Neurologic complications of captopril treatment of neonatal hypertension. Pediatrics 1989;83:47.
105. Haffner CA, Smith BS, Pepper C. Hallucinations as an adverse effect of angiotensin converting enzyme inhibition. Postgrad Med J 1993;69:240.
106. Gillman MNA, Sandyk R. Reversal of captopril induced psychosis with naloxone. Am J Psychiatry 1985;142:270.
107. Rapoport S, Zyman P. Captopril and central nervous system effects. Ann Intern Med 1983;98:1023.
108. Inman WHW, Rawson NSB, Wilton LV, et al. Postmarketing surveillance of enalapril. BMJ 1988;297:826.
109. Ahmad S. Enalapril and peripheral neuropathy. J Am Geriatr Soc 1995;43:1182.
110. Hormigo A, Alves M. Peripheral neuropathy in a patient receiving enalapril. BMJ 1992;305:1332.
111. Leloet X, Moore N, Deshayes P. Pseudopolymyalgia rheumatica during treatment with enalapril. BMJ 1989;298:325.
112. Ahmad S. Enalapril-induced acute psychosis. Ann Pharmacother 1991;25:558.
113. Hirschl MM, Seidler D, Laggner AN. Spironolactone-associated hyponatremic coma. Nephron 1994;67:503.
114. Emsley RA. Thiazides, compulsive water drinking and hyponatremic encephalopathy. J Neurol Neurosurg Psychiatry 1984;47:886.
115. Ashraf N, Locksley R, Arieff AI. Thiazide-induced hyponatremia associated with death or neurologic damage in outpatients. Am J Med 1981;70:1163.
116. Boulton AJM, Hardisty CA. Hypokalemic periodic paralysis precipitated by diuretic therapy and minor surgery. Postgrad Med J 1982;58:106.
117. Udezue EO, Harrold BP. Hyperkalemic paralysis due to spironolactone. Postgrad Med J 1980;56:254.
118. Kalbian VV. Iatrogenic hyperkalemic paralysis with electrocardiographic changes. South Med J 1974;67:342.
119. Fitzgerald MX, Brennan NJ. Muscle cramps, collapse, and seizures in two patients taking metolazone. BMJ 1976;1:1381.
120. Gunson GH. Seizures and metolazone. BMJ 1976; 2:476.
121. Kavi NG, Mengel CE. Hydrochlorothiazide and myalgias. Ann Intern Med 1988;109:84.
122. Rybak LP. Ototoxicity of loop diuretics. Otolaryngol Clin North Am 1993;26:829.
123. Schwarz KO. Clonidine-induced myalgias. Med J Aust 1987;147:365.
124. Hoffmann WF, Ladogana L. Delirium secondary to clonidine therapy. NY State J Med 1981;81:382.
125. Allen RM, Flemenbaum A. Delirium associated with combined fluphenazine-clonidine therapy. J Clin Psychiatry 1979;40:236.
126. Brown MJ, Salmon D, Rendell M. Clonidine hallucinations. Ann Intern Med 1980;93:456.
127. Raskin NH, Fishman RA. Pyridoxine-deficiency neuropathy due to hydralazine. N Engl J Med 1965; 273:1182.

128. Tsujimoto G, Horai Y, Ishizaki T, et al. Hydralazine-induced peripheral neuropathy seen in a Japanese slow acetylator patient. Br J Clin Pharmacol 1981;11:622.
129. Burley D, Steen J. Drug-induced peripheral neuropathies. BMJ 1979;1:1082.
130. Groden BM. Parkinsonism occurring with methyldopa treatment. BMJ 1963;1:1001.
131. Peaston MJT. Parkinsonism associated with alpha-methyldopa therapy. BMJ 1963;2:168.
132. Strang RR. Parkinsonism occurring during methyldopa therapy. Can Med Assoc J 1966;95:928.
133. Ross RT. Drug-induced parkinsonism and other movement disorders. Can J Neurol Sci 1990;17:155.
134. Yamadori A, Albert ML. Involuntary movement disorder caused by methyldopa. N Engl J Med 1972; 286:610.
135. Neil EM, Waters AK. Generalized choreiform movements as a complication of methyldopa therapy in chronic renal failure. Postgrad Med J 1981;57:732.
136. Gombos GM. Bilateral optic neuritis following minoxidil administration. Ann Ophthal 1983;15:259.
137. Palmer RF, Lasseter KC. Sodium nitroprusside. N Engl J Med 1975;292:294.
138. Harmon C, Wohlreich MM. Sodium nitroprusside-induced delirium. Psychosomatics 1995;36:83.
139. Kulig KW, Ballantyne B, Becker C, et al. Cyanide toxicity. Am Fam Physician 1993;48:107.
140. Kim YH, Foo M, Terry RD. Cyanide encephalopathy following therapy with sodium nitroprusside: report of a case. Arch Pathol Lab Med 1982;106:392.
141. Robin ED, McCauley R. Nitroprusside-related cyanide poisoning: time (long past due) for urgent, effective interventions. Chest 1992;102:1842.
142. Guilleminault C, Mignot E, Aldrich M, et al. Prazosin contraindicated in patients with narcolepsy. Lancet 1988;2:511.
143. Aldrich MS, Rogers AE. Exacerbation of human cataplexy by prazosin. Sleep 1989;12:254.
144. Brown SGA, Waterer GW. Migraine precipitated by adenosine. Med J Aust 1995;162:389.
145. Charness ME, Morady F, Scheinman MM. Frequent neurologic toxicity associated with amiodarone therapy. Neurology 1984;34:669.
146. Palakurthy PR, Iyer V, Meckler RJ. Unusual neurotoxicity associated with amiodarone therapy. Arch Intern Med 1987;147:881.
147. Raeder EA, Podird PJ, Lown B. Side effects and complications of amiodarone therapy. Am Heart J 1985; 109:975.
148. Fogoros RN, Anderson KP, Winkle RA, et al. Amiodarone: clinical efficacy and toxicity in 96 patients with recurrent, drug-refractory arrhythmias. Circulation 1983;68:88.
149. Greene HL, Graham EL, Werner JA. Toxic and therapeutic effects of amiodarone in the treatment of cardiac arrhythmias. J Am Coll Cardiol 1983;2:1114.
150. Coulter DM, Edwards IR, Savage RL. Survey of neurologic problems with amiodarone in the New Zealand Intensive Medicines Monitoring Program. N Z Med J 1990;103:98.
151. Anderson NE, Lynch NM, O'Brien KP. Disabling neurologic complications of amiodarone. Aust N Z J Med 1985;15:300.
152. The Collaborative Group for the Study of Polyneuropathy. Antiarrhythmic drugs and polyneuropathy. J Neurol Neurosurg Psychiatry 1994;57:340.
153. Pellissier JF, Pouget J, Cros D, et al. Peripheral neuropathy induced by amiodarone chlorhydrate. J Neurol Sci 1984;63:251.
154. Lemaire JF, Autret A, Biziere K, et al. Amiodarone neuropathy: further arguments for human drug-induced neurolipidosis. Eur Neurol 1982;21:65.
155. Fraser AG, McQueen INF, Watt AH, et al. Peripheral neuropathy during longterm high-dose amiodarone therapy. J Neurol Neurosurg Psychiatry 1985;48:576.
156. Martinez-Arizala A, Sobol SM, McCarty GE, et al. Amiodarone neuropathy. Neurology 1983;33:643.
157. Jacobs JM, Costa-Jussà FR. The pathology of amiodarone neurotoxicity. Brain 1985;108:753.
158. Manolis AS, Tordjman T, Mack KD, et al. Atypical pulmonary and neurologic complications of amiodarone in the same patient. Arch Intern Med 1987;147:1805.
159. Gittinger JW, Asdourian GK. Papillopathy caused by amiodarone. Arch Ophthalmol 1987;105:349.
160. Feiner LA, Younge BR, Kazmier FJ, et al. Optic neuropathy and amiodarone therapy. Mayo Clin Proc 1987;62:702.
161. Nazarian SM, Jay WM. Bilateral optic neuropathy associated with amiodarone therapy. J Clin Neuro-Ophthamol 1988;8:25.
162. Mansour AM, Puklin JE, O'Grady R. Optic nerve ultrastructure following amiodarone therapy. J Clin Neuro-Ophthalmol 1988;8:231.
163. Borruat F-X, Regli F. Pseudotumor cerebri as a complication of amiodarone therapy. Am J Ophthalmol 1993;116:776.
164. Fikkers BG, Bogousslavsky J, Regli F, et al. Pseudotumor cerebri with amiodarone. J Neurol Neurosurg Psychiatry 1986;49:606.
165. Zandijcke MV, Dewachter A. Pseudotumor cerebri with amiodarone. J Neurol Neurosurg Psychiatry 1986; 49:1463.
166. Grogan WA, Narkun DM. Pseudotumor cerebri with amiodarone. J Neurol Neurosurg Psychiatry 1987; 50:651.
167. Lopez AC, Lopez AM, Jimenez SF, et al. Acute intracranial hypertension during amiodarone infusion. Crit Care Med 1985;13:688.
168. Clouston PD, Donnelly PE. Acute necrotizing myopathy associated with amiodarone therapy. Aust N Z Med 1989;19:483.
169. Meier C, Krauer B, Muller U, et al. Neuromyopathy during chronic amiodarone treatment: a case report. J Neurol 1979;220:231.

170. Roth RF, Itabashi H, Louie J, et al. Amiodarone toxicity: myopathy and neuropathy. Am Heart J 1990;119:1223.
171. Abarbanel JM, Osiman A, Frisher S, et al. Peripheral neuropathy and cerebellar syndrome associated with amiodarone therapy. Israel J Med Sci 1987;23:893.
172. Hugon J, Vallat JM, Dumas M, et al. Myeloneuropathy, neurologic toxicity, and amiodarone. Neurology 1985;35:282.
173. Trohman RG, Castellanos D, Castellanos A, et al. Amiodarone-induced delirium. Ann Intern Med 1988;108:68.
174. Gore JM, Haffajee CI, Alpert JS. Interaction of amiodarone and diphenylhydantoin. Am J Cardiol 1984; 54:1145.
175. Dotti MT, Federico A. Amiodarone-induced parkinsonism: a case report and pathogenetic discussion. Mov Disord 1995;10:233.
176. Werner EG, Olanow CW. Parkinsonism and amiodarone therapy. Ann Neurol 1989;25:630.
177. Dawkins KD, Gibson J. Peripheral neuropathy with disopyramide. Lancet 1978;1:329.
178. Goli-Bijanki R, Nair CK, Nair N, et al. Previously unreported adverse reaction to encainide. Chest 1989; 96:688.
179. Grentzkow GD, Sullivan JY. Extracardiac adverse effects of flecainide. Am J Cardiol 1984;53:101B.
180. Palace J, Shah R, Clough C. Flecainide induced peripheral neuropathy. BMJ 1992;305:810.
181. Miller LG, Jankovic J. Persistent dystonia possibly induced by flecainide. Mov Disord 1992;7:62.
182. Ferrick KJ, Power M. Profound exacerbation of neuromuscular weakness by flecainide. Am Heart J 1990; 119:414.
183. Kennerdy A, Thomas P, Sheridan DJ. Generalized seizures as the presentation of flecainide toxicity. Eur Heart J 1989;10:950.
184. Ramhamadany E, Mackenzie S, Ramsdale DR. Dysarthria and visual hallucinations due to flecainide toxicity. Postgrad Med J 1986;62:61.
185. Bedynek J, Weinstein N, Kah RE, et al. Ventricular tachycardia: control by intermittent, intravenous administration of lidocaine hydrochloride. JAMA 1966; 198:139.
186. Crampton RS, Oriscello RG. Petit and grand mal convulsions during lidocaine hydrochloride treatment of ventricular tachycardia. JAMA 1968;204:109.
187. Usubiaga JE, Wikinski J, Ferrero R, et al. Local anesthetic-induced convulsions in man: an electroencephalographic study. Anesth Analg 1966;45:611.
188. Boston Collaborative Drug Surveillance Program. Drug-induced convulsions. Lancet 1972;2:677.
189. Saravay SM, Marke J, Steinberg MD, et al. "Doom anxiety" and delirium in lidocaine toxicity. Am J Psychiatry 1987;144:159.
190. Ilyas M, Owens D, Kvasnicka G. Delirium induced by a combination of antiarrhythmic drugs. Lancet 1969; 2:1368.
191. Christie JM, Valdes C, Markowsky SJ. Neurotoxicity of lidocaine combined with mexiletine. Anesth Analg 1993;77:1291.
192. Campbell RWF. Mexiletine. N Engl J Med 1987; 316:29.
193. Nygaard TW, Sellers TD, Cook TS, et al. Adverse reactions to antiarrhythmic drugs during therapy for ventricular arrhythmias. JAMA 1986;256:55.
194. Holt P. Visual hallucinations. N Z Med J 1988;101:29.
195. Campbell NPS, Chaturvedi NC, Kelly JG, et al. Mexiletine [KO 1173] in the management of ventricular dysrhythmias. Lancet 1973;2:404.
196. Ahmad S. Procainamide and peripheral neuropathy. South Med J 1981;74:509.
197. Sahenk Z, Mendell JR, Rossio JL, et al. Polyradiculopathy accompanying procainamide-induced lupus erythematosus: evidence for drug-induced enhanced sensitization to peripheral nerve myelin. Ann Neurol 1977;1:378.
198. Venkayya RV, Poole RM, Pentz WH. Respiratory failure from procainamide-induced myopathy. Ann Intern Med 1993;119:345.
199. Fontiveros ES, Cumming WJK, Hudgson P. Procainamide-induced myositis. J Neurol Sci 1980;45:143.
200. Taylor JA. Procainamide toxicity. Lancet 1968;1:978.
201. Drachman DA, Skom JH. Procainamide—a hazard in myasthenia gravis. Arch Neurol 1965;13:316.
202. Kornfield P, Horowitz SH, Genkins G, et al. Myasthenia gravis unmasked by antiarrhythmic agents. Mt Sinai J Med 1976;43:10.
203. Godley PJ, Morton TA, Karboski JA, et al. Procainamide-induced myasthenic crisis. Ther Drug Monit 1990;12:411.
204. Oh SJ, Elmore RS, Sarala PK, et al. Procainamide-induced myasthenia-like syndrome. Muscle Nerve 1986;9:670.
205. Miller B, Skupin A, Rubenfire M, et al. Respiratory failure produced by severe procainamide intoxication on a patient with preexisting neuropathy caused by amiodarone. Chest 1988;94:663.
206. Niakan E, Bertorini TE, Acchiardo SR, et al. Procainamide-induced myasthenia-like weakness in a patient with peripheral neuropathy. Arch Neurol 1981;38:378.
207. Chua TP, Farrell T, Lipkin DP. Myoclonus associated with propafenone. BMJ 1994;308:113.
208. Lecky BRF, Weir D, Chong E. Exacerbation of myasthenia by propafenone. J Neurol Neurosurg Psychiatry 1991;54:377.
209. Galasso PJ, Stanton MS, Vogel H. Propafenone-induced peripheral neuropathy. Mayo Clin Proc 1995;70:469.
210. Jones RJ, Brace SR, Tuin ELV. Probable propafenone-induced transient global amnesia. Ann Pharmacother 1995;29:586.
211. Cohen IS, Jick H, Cohen SI. Adverse reactions to quinidine in hospitalized patients: findings based on data from the Boston Collaborative Drug Surveillance Program. Prog Cardiovasc Dis 1977;20:151.

212. Fisher CM. Visual disturbances associated with quinidine and quinine. Neurology 1981;31:1569.
213. Eiseman DP, McKegney FP. Delirium at therapeutic serum concentrations of digoxin and quinidine. Psychosomatics 1994;35:91.
214. Summers WK, Allen RE, Pitts FN. Does physostigmine reverse quinidine delirium? West J Med 1981;135:411.
215. Stoffer SS, Chandler JH. Quinidine-induced exacerbation of myasthenia gravis in patient with Graves' disease. Arch Intern Med 1980;140:283.
216. Aho K, Haapa K. Facial atrophy during sotalol treatment. J Neurol Neurosurg Psychiatry 1982;45:179.
217. Horn HR, Hadidian Z, Johnson JL, et al. Safety evaluation of tocainide in the American Emergency Use Program. Am Heart J 1980;100:1037.
218. Clark CWF, El-Mahdi EO. Fatal oral tocainide overdosage. BMJ 1984;288:760.
219. Durozier P. De délire et du coma digitaliques. Gaz Hebdo Med Chir 1874;11:780.
220. Marriott HJL. Delirium from digitalis toxicity. JAMA 1968;203:178.
221. Shear MK, Sacks MH. Digitalis delirium: report of two cases. Am J Psychiatry 1978;135:109.
222. King JT. Digitalis delirium. Ann Intern Med 1950; 33:1360.
223. Gregory DW. Digitalis delirium: a reminder. So Med J 1980;73:371.
224. Eisendrath SJ, Sweeny MA. Toxic neuropsychiatric effects of digoxin at therapeutic serum concentrations. Am J Psychiatry 1987;144:506.
225. Varriale P, Mossavi A. Rapid reversal of digitalis delirium using digoxin immune Fab therapy. Clin Cardiol 1995;18:351.
226. Piltz JR, Wertenbaker C, Lance SE, et al. Digoxin toxicity: recognizing the varied visual presentations. J Clin Neuro-Ophthalmol 1993;13:275.
227. Chuman MA, LeSage J. Color vision deficiencies in two cases of digoxin toxicity. Am J Ophthalmol 1985; 100:682.
228. Bernat JL, Sullivan JK. Trigeminal neuralgia from digitalis intoxication. JAMA 1979;241:164.
229. Wedzicha JA, Gibb WR, Lees AJ, et al. Chorea in digoxin toxicity. J Neurol Neurosurg Psychiatry 1984; 47:419.
230. Laws GC. The effects of nitroglycerine upon those who manufacture it. JAMA 1898;31:793.
231. Raskin NH. Chemical headaches. Ann Rev Med 1981; 32:63.
232. Bernat JL. Cluster headaches from isosorbide dinitrate. Ann Neurol 1979;6:554.
233. Mueller RA, Meinenberg O. Hemicrania with oculosympathetic paresis from isosorbide dinitrate. N Engl J Med 1983;308:458.
234. Ahmad S. Nitroglycerin and intracranial hypertension. Am Heart J 1991;121:1850.
235. Alexander J, Kaplan K, Davidson R, et al. Intravenous nitroglycerine-induced abducens nerve palsy. Am Heart J 1983;106:1159.
236. Rosenthal R. Visual hallucinations and suicidal ideation attributed to isosorbide dinitrate. Psychosomatics 1987;28:555.
237. Steiner A, Weisser B, Vetter W. A comparative review of the adverse effects of treatments for hyperlipidaemia. Drug Saf 1991;6:118.
238. Sadler LC, Lane M, North R. Severe fetal intracranial haemorrhage during treatment with cholestyramine for intrahepatic cholestasis of pregnancy. Br J Obstet Gynecol 1995;102:169.
239. Chrysanthopoulos C, Kounis N. Rhabdomyolysis due to combined treatment with lovastatin and cholestyramine. BMJ 1992;304:1225.
240. Committee of Principle Investigators (WHO). A cooperative trial in the primary prevention of heart disease using clofibrate. Br Heart J 1978;40:1069.
241. Coronary Drug Research Group. Clofibrate and niacin in coronary heart disease. JAMA 1975;231:360.
242. Langer T, Levy RI. Acute muscular syndrome associated with administration of clofibrate. N Engl J Med 1968;279:856.
243. Rumpf KW, Albers R, Scheler F. Clofibrate-induced myopathy syndrome. Lancet 1976;1:249.
244. Katsilambros N, Braaten J, Ferguson BD, et al. Muscular syndrome after clofibrate. N Engl J Med 1972;286:1110.
245. Sekowski I, Samuel P. Clofibrate-induced acute muscular syndrome. Am J Cardiol 1972;30:572.
246. Smith AF, Macfie WG, Oliver MF. Clofibrate, serum enzymes, and muscle pain. BMJ 1970;2:86.
247. Rush P, Baron M, Kapusta M. Clofibrate myopathy: a case report and a review of the literature. Semin Arthritis Rheum 1986;15:226.
248. Smals AGH, Beex LVAM, Kloppenborg PWC. Clofibrate-induced muscle damage with myoglobinuria and cardiomyopathy. N Engl J Med 1977;296:942.
249. Knodel LC, Talbert RL. Adverse effects of hypolipidaemic drugs. Med Toxicol 1987;2:10.
250. Pierides AM, Alvarez-Ude F, Kerr DNS, et al. Clofibrate-induced muscle damage in patients with chronic renal failure. Lancet 1975;2:1279.
251. Rimon D, Ludatscher R, Cohen L. Clofibrate-induced muscular syndrome: case report with ultrastructural findings and review of the literature. Israel J Med Sci 1984;20:1082.
252. Abourizk N, Khalil BA, Bahuth N, et al. Clofibrate-induced muscular syndrome. J Neurol Sci 1979;42:1.
253. Bardosi A, Scheidt P, Goebel HH. Mitochondrial myopathy—a result of clofibrate/etofibrate treatment? Acta Neuropathol 1985;68:164.
254. Teravainer H, Makitie J. Myokymia, unusual side-effect of clofibrate. Lancet 1976;2:1298.
255. Magarian GJ, Lucas LM, Colley C. Gemfibrozil-induced myopathy. Arch Intern Med 1991;151:1873.
256. Chow LT, Chow W-H. Acute compartment syndrome: an unusual presentation of gemfibrozil induced myositis. Med J Aust 1993;158:48.
257. Bradford RH, Shear CL, Chremos AN, et al. Expanded

clinical evaluation of lovastatin (EXCEL) study results. Arch Intern Med 1991;151:43.
258. Pierce LR, Wysowski DK, Gross TP. Myopathy and rhabdomyolysis associated with lovastatin-gemfibrozil combination therapy. JAMA 1990;264:71.
259. Marais GE, Larson KK. Rhabdomyolysis and acute renal failure induced by combination lovastatin and gemfibrozil therapy. Ann Intern Med 1990;112:228.
260. Chucrallah A, DeGirolami U, Freeman R, et al. Lovastatin/gemfibrozil myopathy: a clinical, historical, and ultrastructural study. Eur Neurol 1992;32:293.
261. Arellano F, DeCos MA, Valiente R, et al. Gemfibrozil-induced headache. Lancet 1988;1:705.
262. Alvarez-Sabin J, Codina A, Rodriguez C, et al. Gemfibrozil-induced headache. Lancet 1988;2:1246.
263. Bain SC, Lemon M, Jones AF. Gemfibrozil-induced impotence. Lancet 1990;336:1389.
264. Pizarro S, Bargay J, D'Agosto P. Gemfibrozil-induced impotence. Lancet 1990;336:1135.
265. Tobert JA. Rhabdomyolysis in patients receiving lovastatin after cardiac transplantation. N Engl J Med 1988;318:47.
66. Norman DJ, Illingworth DR, Munson J, et al. Myolysis and acute renal failure in a heart transplant recipient receiving lovastatin. N Engl J Med 1988;318:46.
267. East C, Alivizatos PA, Grundy SM, et al. Rhabdomyolysis in patients receiving lovastatin after cardiac transplantation. N Engl J Med 1988;318:47.
268. Kogan AD, Orenstein S. Lovastatin-induced acute rhabdomyolysis. Postgrad Med J 1990;66:294.
269. London SF, Gross KF, Ringel SP. Cholesterol-lowering agent myopathy (CLAM). Neurology 1991;41:1159.
270. Suki WN. Myopathic effects of lovastatin. West J Med 1991;154:223.
271. Lees RS, Lees AM. Rhabdomyolysis from the coadministration of lovastatin and the antifungal agent itraconazole. N Engl J Med 1995;333:664.
272. Reaven P, Witztum JL. Lovastatin, nicotinic acid, and rhabdomyolysis. Ann Intern Med 1988;109:597.
273. Spach DH, Bauwens JE, Clark CD, et al. Rhabdomyolysis associated with lovastatin and erythromycin use. West J Med 1991;154:213.
274. Ayanian JZ, Fuchs CS, Stone RM. Lovastatin and rhabdomyolysis. Ann Intern Med 1988;109:682.
275. Ahmad S. Lovastatin and peripheral neuropathy. Am Heart J 1995;130:1321.
276. Muller T, Kuhn W, Pohlau D, et al. Parkinsonism unmasked by lovastatin. Ann Neurol 1995;37:685.
277. Botti RE, Trisari J, Pan HY, et al. Evaluation of pravastatin and lovastatin in the cerebrospinal fluid of healthy subjects. Clin Neuropharmacol 1991;14:256.
278. The Lovastatin Pravastatin Study Group. A multicenter comparative trial of lovastatin and pravastatin in the treatment of hypercholesterolemia. Am J Cardiol 1993;71:810.
279. The Simvastatin Pravastatin Study Group. Comparison of the efficacy, safety and tolerability of simvastatin and pravastatin for hypercholesterolemia. Am J Cardiol 1993;71:1408.
280. Wiklund O, Bergman M, Bondjers G, et al. Pravastatin and gemfibrozil alone and in combination for the treatment of hypercholesterolemia. Am J Med 1993;94:13.
281. Schalke BB, Schmidt B, Toyka K, et al. Pravastatin-associated inflammatory myopathy. N Engl J Med 1992;327:649.
282. England J, Walsh JC, Stewart P, et al. Mitochondrial myopathy developing on treatment with the HMG-CoA reductase inhibitors—simvastatin and pravastatin. Aust N Z J Med 1995;25:374.
283. Scott RS, Lintott CJ, Wilson MJ. Simvastatin and side effects. N Z Med J 1991;104:493.
284. Deslypere JP, Vermeulen A. Rhabdomyolysis and simvastatin. Ann Intern Med 1991;114:342.
285. Bizzaro N, Bagolin E, Milani L, et al. Massive rhabdomyolysis and simvastatin. Clin Chem 1992;38:1504.
286. Al-Jubouri MA, Briston PG, Sinclar D, et al. Myxoedema revealed by simvastatin induced myopathy. BMJ 1994;308:588.
287. Chariot, P, Abadia R, Danan C, et al. Simvastatin-induced rhabdomyolysis followed by a MELAS syndromes Am J Med 1993;94:109.
288. Phan T, McLeod JG, Pollard JD, et al. Peripheral neuropathy associated with simvastatin. J Neurol Neurosurg Psychiatry 1995;58:625.

Chapter 21

Complications of Anticonvulsant Drugs and Ketogenic Diet

John P. Phillips

Objectives

- To appreciate that the side effect profile is often what determines the choice of antiepileptic drug (AED)
- To differentiate between common and rare risks of antiepileptic treatment
- To recognize dose-responsive side effects so that appropriate dose adjustments may be made without discontinuing therapy
- To understand rational laboratory monitoring of chronic AED treatment
- To recognize clinical signs of serious drug toxicity and know when drug discontinuation is indicated
- To appreciate the potential cognitive and behavioral complications of AED treatment that may affect academic or vocational performance

General Considerations

AEDs profoundly affect the practice of neurology. Approximately 2.5 million people in the United States have epilepsy, which in perhaps 70% of cases is controlled with a single drug. This is an enormous improvement since the days when seizures were uncontrollable and patients suffered the effects of "treatment" such as leeches, arsenic, and starvation. Today's AEDs do have potential side effects; however, most are minor and do not require drug withdrawal. These side effects can generally be divided into two groups. Idiosyncratic, often severe hypersensitive reactions usually occur within the initial phase of drug treatment. They are not dose responsive and require AED withdrawal to prevent serious complications. More common reactions are toxic effects of the drug, which are often temporary, dose-related, and usually do not require stopping treatment. Because efficacy of the major AEDs (phenobarbital [PB], phenytoin [PHT], carbamazepine [CBZ], valproic acid [VPA]) is equal for generalized convulsive seizures or partial seizures with or without generalization, the choice of which drug to use is often based on the side effect profile.[1, 2] This chapter reviews side effects of the major AEDs in use today, the newer medications lamotrigine (LTG), gabapentin (GBN), and topiramate (TPM), as well as side effects of the ketogenic diet. Felbamate (FBM) is discussed only briefly because of its limited clinical use.

Carbamazepine

CBZ inhibits voltage-dependent sodium channels and is used for treatment of partial seizures with or without secondary generalization, as well as primary generalized tonic-clonic seizures. Reported side effects with CBZ have ranged from 33 to 50%, although serious side effects requiring discontinuation of CBZ occur in only approximately 5% of patients.[3] As is the case with other AEDs, polytherapy carries a higher risk of side effects than monotherapy.[4] More side effects occur at the onset of treatment because CBZ induces its own metabolism through stimulation of hepatic microsomal enzymes.[5–7] For this reason, the manufacturer suggests gradual dose increases.[8]

The most common side effects with CBZ are neurologic. In a series of 220 children treated with CBZ, 43% had drowsiness, 20% had incoordination, and 5.9% had vertigo.[3] Another 15% had slurred speech, tremor, headache, diplopia, or movement disorders. In all cases, the symptoms were transient and dose related, often occurring at initiation of therapy or with dose increases. In no instance did CBZ need to be withdrawn because of these neurologic side effects. Similar findings have been reported by other authors.[4, 5, 9–11]

Benign transient leukopenia is the most common hematologic reaction associated with CBZ, occurring in 2–12% of patients.[3, 12–14] A more significant leukopenia may occur within the first several weeks of therapy. It is more common in patents with low baseline white blood counts (WBCs)[14] and resolves after stopping CBZ.[13] Isolated thrombocytopenia is rare and also responds to discontinuation of CBZ.[15–17] Minor platelet depression occurs in approximately 2% of patients, often within the first month of therapy and does not require stopping CBZ.[18, 19] Anemia, eosinophilia, lymphocytosis, leukocytosis, and macrocytosis have been rarely reported.[20]

Aplastic anemia is a rare but often fatal reaction associated with CBZ. In reviewing 27 reported cases of aplastic anemia (16 fatal), Sobotka et al. noted that average duration of treatment with CBZ was 4.4 months, with a range of 4–1,500 days.[18] Most cases involved confounding variables such as polytherapy or intercurrent illness, and no relationship to dose was found. Pellock estimated a CBZ-associated aplastic anemia prevalence rate of less than 1 per 50,000, with 2.2 deaths per million exposures from either aplastic anemia or agranulocytosis.[3]

Hematologic monitoring to prevent serious blood dyscrasias is of unclear benefit, because serious hematologic side effects occur rapidly.[18] Total WBC of less than 2,500–3,000 or an absolute neutrophil count of less than 1,000 is of concern and warrants decreasing or stopping CBZ if clinically feasible.[3, 18] Careful discussion with patients of symptoms of bone marrow failure is probably more important than routine laboratory monitoring, emphasizing that the physician should be contacted immediately if petechiae, pallor, fever, infection, or undue weakness occurs.[13]

The incidence of cutaneous eruptions secondary to CBZ ranges from 3 to 12%.[3, 21, 22] Mild rashes are the most common, although life-threatening reactions do occur, including Stevens-Johnson syndrome and toxic epidermal necrolysis.[22] The rash usually occurs within the first several months of treatment.[23] Most authors recommend immediately stopping CBZ with the development of any rash, although Murphy et al. reported that 16 of 20 patients with CBZ-associated skin eruptions were able to remain on CBZ with corticosteroid treatment.[24] They cautioned against this approach in patients with constitutional symptoms; these suggest a more serious reaction unlikely to respond to corticosteroids.

Mild transient elevations in liver function test results occur in approximately 5–10% of those treated with CBZ.[3] Serious liver disease is much rarer, and fatal hepatitis has been reported.[25, 26] Symptoms include lethargy, rash, and fever.[27] Promptly discontinuing CBZ is essential if symptoms of hepatic failure occur, which is usually associated with liver function test results increasing at least threefold.[3] The risk for liver damage is highest within the first month of treatment.[28, 29]

Hyponatremia is a well-described complication of CBZ, more commonly seen in the elderly and in those taking high doses.[30, 31] The mechanism of action is unclear but may include a direct hypothalamic effect and action at the antidiuretic hormone receptor.[32] In most patients, CBZ-induced hyponatremia is clinically asymptomatic, although cases of seizure exacerbation from hyponatremia have been reported.[33, 34] Concomitant phenytoin administration may correct CBZ-associated hyponatremia.[30, 35]

Cardiac side effects of CBZ are uncommon and do not occur in children or young adults without underlying heart disease.[36, 37] Cardiac conduction defects, atrioventricular block, sick sinus syndrome, and asystole have been reported in the elderly.[38–41] Other side effects include congestive heart failure, increased cholesterol levels, and myocarditis.[42–44]

Cardiac function should be monitored periodically in elderly patients or those with underlying heart disease who are treated with CBZ.[40, 45]

Movement disorders are a rare side effect of CBZ therapy. Dystonia may occur within the first month of therapy and resolves on discontinuation of CBZ.[46, 47] In some cases dystonia resolves spontaneously, and it is possible to continue CBZ. Tics, choreoathetosis, and myoclonus have also occurred as complications of CBZ.[48–50]

Pulmonary toxicity from CBZ is presumably part of a hypersensitivity reaction. It usually occurs within the first several months of treatment, is not dose dependent, and is often associated with a skin rash.[51–53] Bronchial biopsies have demonstrated granulomatous inflammation and eosinophilia.[54–56] Prompt clinical improvement occurs with discontinuation of CBZ.

Case reports of clinically significant renal disease from CBZ therapy are uncommon.[57–60] In several series of children and adults on CBZ, no clinical findings of renal failure were identified despite laboratory evidence of mild renal tubular dysfunction.[61, 62] CBZ has been implicated in urinary retention in a patient with diabetes and in overflow urinary incontinence.[63, 64]

The effect of any AED on sexual function is difficult to prove. Confounding variables are the underlying epilepsy itself, concomitant brain dysfunction, and psychosocial factors. In patients taking CBZ, some studies have demonstrated increased sex hormone–binding globulin, which decreases free testosterone concentration.[65] Sexual desire and function have corresponded to testosterone levels in men.[66] It therefore seems possible that CBZ may affect a patient's sexual function, although this has not been adequately studied.

Seizure exacerbation as a consequence of CBZ has been well described in children[67–70] and less commonly in adults.[71, 72] At greatest risk are younger patients, those with generalized spike and polyspike and wave discharges on electroencephalography,[70] and those with atypical absence epilepsy.[67] Toxic levels of CBZ and carbamazepine-10-11-epoxide may also be risk factors for seizure exacerbation.[71, 72]

Rarely reported side effects of CBZ are hair loss and pancreatitis.[73, 74] CBZ may be associated with biochemical and histologic evidence of osteomalacia; however, this is not clinically significant.[75, 76] Systemic lupus crythematosus with and without antinuclear antibodies rarely occurs with CBZ; this resolves after discontinuation of CBZ.[77–79] No effect on the peripheral nervous system was found in a series of 12 patients on CBZ monotherapy; all had normal nerve conduction velocities and electromyographic findings.[80] Clinical evidence also suggests normal peripheral nerve and muscle function in patients on monotherapy.[3]

Phenytoin

As with CBZ, PHT inhibits voltage-dependent sodium channels and is used for treatment of partial seizures with or without secondary generalization, as well as most primary generalized epilepsies. Acute dose-related neurologic side effects are the most common. Nystagmus occurs more frequently with levels of more than 20 μg per ml, ataxia at levels of more than 30 μg per ml, and overt mental status changes at levels of more than 40 μg per ml.[81]

Transient cerebellar dysfunction is commonly seen with PHT intoxication, and permanent cerebellar abnormalities can also occur with chronic therapy or even after a single episode of toxicity.[82–84] Patients on long-term treatment with PHT may be at higher risk for cerebellar damage, although how much the underlying epilepsy may be involved is unclear.[85, 86] Cases of PHT-associated cerebellar degeneration in patients who never had seizures suggests that the drug alone may be toxic to the cerebellum.[82, 87] The pathophysiology is unclear; Purkinje cell loss in patients on chronic PHT therapy has been reported.[88, 89]

Dysmorphic facies may develop in patients on chronic PHT therapy. This includes hirsutism, acromegalic facial features, and gingival hypertrophy. The gingival hypertrophy can cause significant dental problems. It occurs in approximately 50% of those on chronic PHT therapy and is more common with poor oral hygiene and high drug levels.[90, 91] At times, gingival overgrowth may be so severe as to cover the teeth entirely. Treatment involves encouraging good oral hygiene, decreasing the dose if possible, or surgically resecting the gums in severe cases.

Decreased bone density has been reported with PHT,[92] although clinically significant bone disease such as rickets or osteomalacia is rare.[93] The mechanism of PHT-induced bone disease is unknown.

Vitamin D therapy should be considered in patients on chronic PHT therapy with biochemical or radiologic evidence of altered bone metabolism.[93] Paradoxically, an osteogenic effect of PHT has been suggested by in vitro and in vivo studies.[94, 95]

Peripheral neuropathy is a common complication of long-term PHT therapy, although it is usually asymptomatic. Up to 71% of patients on long-term PHT therapy show abnormal electrodiagnostic study results, most often slowed nerve conduction velocities.[96] Peripheral neuropathy is more often seen with long-term therapy or prolonged high drug levels.[97] Biopsy of peripheral nerve has demonstrated segmental demyelination and axonal shrinkage.[98] Clinical and electrophysiologic findings may improve after PHT is discontinued.[98, 99]

Mild elevations in liver function test results may occur during PHT treatment. They occur in approximately 2% of patients, are transient, and affect just the aspartate aminotransferase level.[100] Significant hepatotoxicity is rare but potentially life-threatening. It is seen as part of a hypersensitivity syndrome and usually occurs within the first 2 months of therapy.[101] Systemic signs occur before hepatitis.[102] Associated features are skin rash (either desquamating or pruritic), fever, eosinophilia, lymphadenopathy, hepatomegaly, and sometimes coagulopathy or splenomegaly.[101] Treatment is supportive. Corticosteroids have been successfully used in some cases.[103] Patients may recover if PHT is stopped immediately; however, 25–38% suffer fatal hepatic necrosis.[101, 102] Pathologic lesions include hepatocellular degeneration, necrosis, granulomatous reactions, vasculitis, and infiltration by malignant reticuloendothelial cells.[104]

Other rare hypersensitivity reactions include pseudolymphoma,[105] pseudo-mycosis fungoides,[106] toxic epidermal necrolysis,[107] multiple myeloma,[108] disseminated intravascular coagulation,[109] renal failure, polymyositis,[110] thrombocytopenia, pancytopenia, red cell aplasia, and vasculitis.[93] The most common hypersensitivity reaction is a maculopapular skin rash that occurs in approximately 7% of patients.[111] In all cases of hypersensitivity reactions, PHT must be discontinued to avoid systemic complications.

Immunosuppression occurs occasionally in patients treated with PHT and may relate to the genesis of pseudolymphoma. IgG, IgE, and IgA concentrations are significantly decreased in some patients while on PHT therapy.[112–114] Cellular immunity can also be depressed.[113, 115] Although PHT-associated immune suppression is often asymptomatic, specific IgG subtype deficiencies have been reported in a patient with recurrent upper respiratory tract infections that resolved after PHT therapy was discontinued.[116]

Folate deficiency and megaloblastic anemia have been long recognized as potential complications of PHT therapy.[117, 118] Mild macrocytosis occurs in up to 50% of patients on PHT and is clinically insignificant. Frank anemia is rare but responds to oral folate therapy.[93] The mechanism of folate deficiency is unclear; abnormal absorption has been suggested.[119, 120]

Vitamin K–dependent clotting factors may be deficient in infants born to mothers taking PHT.[121] Severe hemorrhagic complications occur rarely. Routine administration of vitamin K to pregnant mothers in the last month of gestation prevents this problem.

Bone marrow depression is a rare and potentially fatal complication of PHT therapy. Aplastic anemia, leukopenia, thrombocytopenia, and agranulocytosis have been reported.[117, 122] Treatment includes prompt cessation of PHT. Human recombinant granulocyte macrophage colony-stimulating factor has been used in a case of agranulocytosis.[123] Treatment of thrombocytopenia using intravenous immune globulin has also been reported.[124] Several reports of PHT and cimetidine causing thrombocytopenia exist, suggesting a possible synergistic role in megakaryocyte suppression.[125–127]

A benign leukopenia is commonly seen with PHT. The WBC count remains stable, between 3,000 and 4,000 per ml, and progression to agranulocytosis does not occur despite continuing therapy.[122] Absolute neutrophil counts of persistently less than 1,000 per ml are more ominous; careful monitoring with discontinuation of PHT should be considered.[128]

Movement disorders are uncommon side effects seen with most anticonvulsant drugs. Chorea, dystonia, asterixis, athetosis, dyskinesias, and hemiballism have been described in patients taking PHT.[129–133] Sometimes the movements are dose responsive.[93]

Serum thyroid hormone levels are sometimes altered by PHT and CBZ, both of which are enzyme-inducing anticonvulsants. Accelerated metabolism of thyroid hormones may occur due to hepatic microsomal enzyme induction by these anticonvulsants.[134] Significant thyroid disease due to PHT is very rare: In a series of 317 patients on PHT monotherapy, none were found to have clinically significant PHT-induced thyroid function abnormalities.[100]

Sex hormone abnormalities are also seen with PHT. Impotence and hyposexuality are rare clinical problems that may in part be due to increased sex hormone–binding globulin, which decreases free testosterone serum levels.[135, 136]

Hyperglycemia rarely occurs with PHT therapy, but may be clinically significant in patients with diabetes. PHT decreases pancreatic insulin secretion and stimulates glucagon release.[137,138] In patients without diabetes, there are no problems with carbohydrate metabolism and glucose tolerance test results remain normal.[139]

Other side effects include inhibition of antidiuretic hormone release by PHT, which may be used to treat the hyponatremia associated with CBZ therapy.[140] Impotence has also been reported.[141]

Valproic Acid

VPA is a branched-chain fatty acid used in the past as an organic solvent. It has a broad spectrum of anticonvulsant activity, effective in most types of focal and generalized seizures. The mechanism of action is unclear. VPA appears to enhance gamma-aminobutyric acid and block voltage-sensitive sodium channels, although other anticonvulsant actions may also occur.[142]

Benign side effects from VPA are common, often dose responsive, and transient. More bothersome side effects necessitating treatment withdrawal are reported in 4–8% of those on monotherapy.[143] Life-threatening reactions are rare in patients without specific risk factors.

The most common side effects from VPA are gastrointestinal. Abdominal pain, nausea, and vomiting are reported in approximately 12% of patients on monotherapy.[141] Enteric-coated preparations are more easily tolerated, and taking the medication with meals or starting at a low dose and gradually increasing can help. Weight gain can be a troublesome problem for some patients, particularly adolescent girls. Weight gain is reported in 11–50% of those on monotherapy.[144] The mechanism of weight gain is unclear, but may be due to increased appetite or impaired beta oxidation of fatty acids.[145] Caloric restriction, although difficult, usually helps.

Dose-related tremor is also commonly seen. It occurs in approximately 10% of patients and is similar to essential tremor.[146] The tremor may be annoying but seldom requires dose reduction or treatment withdrawal. Propranolol, amantadine, and acetazolamide (AZM) have been successfully used as treatment but are rarely necessary.[146, 147]

Alopecia occurs in some patients. An incidence of 4–6% has been reported.[148] Regrowth usually occurs after discontinuing or decreasing VPA, although the new hair may be of different texture or color.[149]

An advantage of VPA is that although neurologic side effects do occur, they are less common than with the other major AEDs. Sedation occurs in 2–10% but is rarely persistent and does not require medication withdrawal.[150] Transient sedation or confusion has been reported after a single therapeutic dose in healthy volunteers,[151] with high doses,[152] in patients after brain surgery,[153] and in patients on polypharmacy.[154]

Cognitive and behavioral effects of VPA are subtle. Children have not been studied as well as adults.[155] Some authors report minor deficits in attention, visuomotor skills, learning, and psychomotor speed in patients taking VPA.[156–158] Aggressive behavior is seen rarely.[148]

A mild elevation in liver function test results occurs in up to 44% of patients taking VPA.[159] It is generally asymptomatic and responds to dose reduction,[160] although in many cases no dose adjustment is necessary.[161] Distinguishing this minor laboratory abnormality from impending liver disease is essential. Fatal hepatotoxicity from VPA usually occurs within the first 6 months of treatment. It is often accompanied by nausea, vomiting, lethargy, anorexia, or seizure exacerbation.[160, 162] Acute elevations of ammonia and liver function test results occur, although in 25% of cases the ammonia concentrations are normal.[163] Immediately withdrawing VPA is essential,[164] and carnitine administration may help.[165]

Isolated hyperammonemia occurs in approximately 35% of patients taking VPA.[166] Lethargy, stupor, or coma may result from marked ammonia elevations. Carnitine supplementation in symptomatic patients helps decrease ammonia levels.[166]

The incidence of fatal hepatotoxicity is approximately 1 per 50,000,[162] although it is much higher in patients younger than 2 years old on polytherapy (1 per 600).[167] Patients with undiagnosed metabolic abnormalities are at substantial risk of hepatic disease.[164, 168–170] The role of carnitine in preventing VPA hepatotoxicity has been extensively reviewed.[165, 171, 172] Underlying carnitine deficiency may predispose patients to liver disease when treated with VPA,[173] but there is no evidence that carnitine supplementation prevents liver disease in normal patients. Indeed, fatalities have occurred despite normal serum carnitine levels[174] and appropriate carnitine supplementation.[175]

The most common hematologic side effect is dose-responsive thrombocytopenia and prolonged bleeding time.[176, 177] In most cases this is of no clinical significance[178]; however, platelet counts should be closely monitored with high-dose therapy. Rare cases of myelodysplasia,[179–181] neutropenia,[182, 183] and fibrinogen depletion[184] have been reported in association with VPA. Macrocytosis without anemia is also seen,[185] as well as an idiosyncratic decrease in factor VIII complex.[186]

Asymptomatic amylase elevations occur in approximately 20% of patients taking VPA and usually normalize without dose adjustment.[187] Life-threatening pancreatitis is quite rare. It is more common in the first several months of therapy. Patients at higher risk include those on polytherapy, patients with developmental delay, and children.[188] Survival is more likely if VPA is abruptly withdrawn as soon as any clinical or laboratory indication of pancreatitis develops. Complications may include pseudocyst formation, hemorrhagic pancreatitis, and coagulopathies.[188]

There are rare reports of miscellaneous side effects with VPA. Several patients on chronic VPA therapy have developed transient, dose-related chorea.[147] Hearing loss, both reversible and irreversible, has been reported.[189, 190] Reversible dementia,[191, 192] parkinsonism,[193] and systemic lupus erythematosus[194] have also been described.

Phenobarbital

PB is the oldest of the commonly used AEDs. It is most useful in generalized tonic-clonic seizures, but is also effective in focal seizures and remains the drug of choice for neonatal epilepsy.[195] Serious side effects are rarer than with the other AEDs, with the exception of neurologic reactions. Overt sedation occurs, as well as more subtle cognitive and behavioral problems. Because of its easy dosing, low cost, and availability, it remains a preferred drug for all seizure types in many developing countries.[196]

Neurologic side effects of PB include sedation, behavior problems, mood disorders, and cognitive problems. These are common complications of PB therapy and occurred in 64% of patients on monotherapy in a large pediatric study.[197] Most of these side effects are temporary, and the reported incidence of those requiring treatment withdrawal varies from 4% to 20%.[197–199]

Temporary sedation is extremely common with PB: Two-thirds of adults experience sedation at some point in the treatment course.[200] Irritability, oppositional behavior, hyperactivity, and poor attention are often seen in children on PB. The incidence was 42% in a series of children treated with PB for febrile seizures.[198] In some patients, this behavior can be temporary and dose responsive.[198] PB may also cause fussiness, sleep disturbance,[201] and hyperactivity that in one study did not fully resolve after withdrawal of PB.[202] Depression is also more commonly seen in patients taking PB.[203, 204] In children, 40% of those with a family history of major affective disorder were depressed if treated with PB versus only 4% for those treated with CBZ.[204]

The influence of PB on learning and cognition is of particular concern. Investigators have shown PB affecting comprehension,[201] motor coding,[205] learning,[206] memory,[201, 207] and attention.[208] These effects are usually reversible after treatment discontinuation, although one study of PB in children with febrile seizures demonstrated an IQ loss of 5 points even 6 months after stopping PB.[209] This study analyzed data based on intention to treat, however, and may have yielded different results had analysis been done only on patients who actually followed treatment protocol. Multiple in vitro studies of PB have also demonstrated a deleterious effect on spinal cord neurons,[210] sympathetic neurons,[211] cortical neurons,[212] and fetal spinal cord neurons.[213]

Hematologic complications of PB therapy are extremely rare and are usually part of an allergic reaction. A large, multicentered VA study of adult antiepileptic treatment showed no significant hematologic effects during 2 years of follow-up.[214] Neonatal coagulopathy, similar to vitamin K deficiency, may rarely cause serious hemorrhagic disease in the newborn.[215] It is prevented by administration of vitamin K.

A mild skin rash occurs in 4% of those taking PB.[22] Serious skin eruptions such as toxic epidermal necrolysis, exfoliative dermatitis, and Stevens-Johnson syndrome are also reported. When rash is part of a hypersensitivity reaction, systemic effects often include fever, adenopathy, eosinophilia, hepatitis, and hematologic abnormalities.[216] Immediate withdrawal of PB is essential, particularly if any signs of systemic involvement are present; the risk of precipitating status epilepticus is actually very low.[217] Corticosteroids are used in treating serious hypersensitivity reactions.

Connective tissue reactions including frozen shoulder, Dupuytren's contractures, and general joint pain have been associated in the past with AEDs. The multicenter VA study demonstrated a small risk (6%) for such connective tissue disorders in patients taking barbiturates, but not other AEDs.[218]

Primidone

Primidone (PRM) is effective in the treatment of focal and generalized seizures including myoclonic epilepsy. Several studies have shown PRM to be as effective as PB for generalized and focal seizures.[214, 219] It is metabolized to PB (25%) and phenylethylmalonamide.[220] At usual therapeutic doses in animals, phenylethylmalonamide itself has little anticonvulsant activity or few side effects but may potentiate the antiepileptic action of PB.[221] PRM, on the other hand, does have anticonvulsant action independent of PB.[222]

The incidence of acute neurologic side effects ranges from 43% to 100%.[223–225] Drowsiness, dizziness, and gastrointestinal upset may be severe but are usually transient. Tolerance to these effects develops rapidly, often over the first several days of therapy.[225] To improve compliance, many clinicians begin with a low dose and increase over several weeks. Although the incidence of acute side effects is high, because of the rapid tolerance, only 8% actually require discontinuation of treatment.[197]

Hematologic side effects of PRM are unusual. Several patients with megaloblastic anemia while taking PRM have been described.[226–228] This may respond to folate treatment. There are also reports of thrombocytopenia and systemic lupus erythematosus.[229, 230]

No isolated hepatic or renal effects have been reported, although they can be seen as part of the hypersensitivity syndrome.[231] An allergic rash is seldom reported.[232] As with PB, frozen shoulder and Dupuytren's contractures have been described.[218] In the multicenter VA study, it was clearly shown that impotence and decreased libido were more often seen with PRM than other major AEDs.[214]

Because PRM is a barbiturate that is partially metabolized to PB, it likely has similar cognitive effects. PRM has not been studied nearly as well as PB but is associated with increased depression, poorer neuropsychometric test scores, and an increase on the psychopathic deviant scale of the Minnesota Multiphasic Personality Inventory when compared with CBZ.[233]

Ethosuximide

Ethosuximide (ESM) is the drug of choice for typical absence epilepsy and is therefore commonly used in children. It can also be used for atypical absence seizures but has no effect in focal epilepsies.[234] The anticonvulsant action of ESM is through inhibition of low-voltage calcium channels.

ESM is generally well tolerated. Incidence of side effects ranges up to 44%,[235] the most common of which are self-limited gastrointestinal upset and drowsiness. In a series of 39 previously untreated patients on monotherapy, 23% developed nausea and 13% had sedation.[236] Headache also occurs. These side effects are usually transient and dose responsive. Rarely is treatment withdrawal necessary. Skin rash is a less common reaction and usually requires treatment withdrawal to avoid systemic complications. Exanthemas, urticaria, erythema multiforme, and Stevens-Johnson syndrome have been reported in association with ESM.[237]

Multiple reports exist of ESM-induced systemic lupus erythematosus.[238–240] Fever, rash, arthritis, and lymphadenopathy are common symptoms.[241] Pericarditis and pleural effusions may also occur. The syndrome usually abates with discontinuation of ESM; however, extended corticosteroid treatment is sometimes necessary.[242] Rarely, systemic lupus erythematosus with nephritis persists despite discontinuation of ESM.[241] Asymptomatic induction of antinuclear antibodies by ESM is more common than clinical systemic lupus erythematosus.[241]

Hematologic reactions to ESM are rare but potentially life-threatening. Fatal aplastic anemia and agranulocytosis have been reported.[243] Severe aplastic anemia has been successfully treated with corticosteroids.[244] Bone marrow transplantation was also successfully used in a child who had an allogenic twin donor.[245] It is unclear whether periodic blood counts in the absence of clinical symptoms can detect serious dyscrasias early enough to affect outcome. The manufacturer recommends periodic blood counts, and some authors suggest monthly complete blood counts (CBCs)[246] for the entire treatment duration or at least for the initial phase, followed by less frequent CBCs thereafter.[234] As is the case with CBZ, PHT, and VPA, a mild granulocytopenia may occur that responds to dose reduction.[246] Certainly, any clinical indication of bone marrow suppression should be immediately evaluated.

Movement disorders associated with ESM are exceedingly rare. Acute dyskinesias and akathisia have been described, in both cases resolving after intravenous diphenhydramine administration.[247, 248] A parkinsonian syndrome has also been reported.[249]

Exacerbation of seizures with ESM therapy has been described. This includes worsening of underlying absence and myoclonic seizures.[250, 251]

Cases of ESM inducing psychosis, anxiety, depression, and hallucinations in adolescents or young adults with mental illness have been reported.[252] The symptoms usually abate with withdrawal of ESM, and in one case rechallenging with ESM caused a recurrence of symptoms.[253] Cognitive function in general improves while taking the drug. In the series of Browne et al. of 39 patients taking ESM, neuropsychometric testing improved in 17.[236] Better absence seizure control would certainly improve cognitive function, but ESM was also found to improve IQ scores in nonepileptic children.[254] Neuropsychometric and tissue culture evidence suggests that ESM should not cause significant cognitive dysfunction, unless perhaps overt sedation or exacerbation of an underlying emotional disorder occurs.[255]

Other organ system toxicity from ESM is unusual. A child was reported with elevated liver function test results that resolved after discontinuing ESM, but no other reports of significant liver disease were found in the available literature.[256] This is in contrast to the hepatotoxicity occasionally seen with other major AEDs. One case of thyroid disease clearly related to ESM was reported by Nishiyama et al.[257]

Lamotrigine

Lamotrigine (LTG) is one of several recent additions to the antiepileptic armamentarium. It is chemically unrelated to other established AEDs.[258] As with PHT and CBZ, the anticonvulsant action includes inhibition of excitatory neurotransmitter release via blocking voltage-sensitive sodium channels. Seizure types effected by LTG include primarily generalized seizures (tonic-clonic, absence, atonic) and partial seizures with or without secondarily generalization.[259] The most common side effects are neurologic, gastrointestinal, and dermatologic. Treatment withdrawal is necessary most often because of rash, occurring in 2–12% of patients.[259–261]

Neurologic side effects are the most common. Some might be dose related, but rarely do they result in treatment withdrawal. A large multicenter study of LTG versus placebo as add-on therapy found significant problems with dizziness (50%), diplopia (33%), ataxia (24%), blurred vision (23%), and sedation (14%).[262] Dizziness and diplopia may occur more frequently when LTG is combined with CBZ.[263] Better mood may also be an effect of LTG in some patients.[264]

LTG may cause an allergic skin rash that typically occurs within the first several weeks of therapy. It is an erythematous, maculopapular eruption that resolves after stopping medication. Rarely, the rash progresses to Stevens-Johnson syndrome, which has been reported with monotherapy as well as polytherapy.[265] Fatal Stevens-Johnson syndrome occurred in a patient taking LTG and CBZ.[266] Because a rash is more frequent with rapid dose escalation, the manufacturer recommends beginning LTG at a low dose and increasing slowly.[8] Significant hepatic or hematologic reactions are extremely rare.

Gabapentin

GBN is another new AED that was designed to mimic the action of gamma-aminobutyric acid

(GABA, a major central nervous system inhibitory neurotransmitter). Although GBN may increase GABA levels in human brain, its mechanism of anticonvulsant action remains largely unknown.[267, 268] It is effective as adjuvant therapy in partial complex seizures with and without secondary generalization. Several features of GBN metabolism are unique: GBN does not undergo hepatic metabolism, it is excreted unchanged in the urine, and it has no significant protein binding.[269] Therefore, drug-drug interactions do not exist, and there is no hepatic toxicity.

Side effects from GBN are most commonly neurologic. As add-on therapy, approximately 10% of patients complain about nystagmus, somnolence, diplopia, tremor, ataxia, or dizziness.[270] Fatigue is reported in up to 20% of patients, but is usually transient and seen at the onset of therapy.[271] More problematic side effects occur in children with underlying developmental delay and attention deficit hyperactivity disorder; exacerbation of hyperactivity, aggression, and temper tantrums often require dose reduction or treatment withdrawal.[272–275]

Weight gain[276] and movement disorders[277, 278] are rare effects of GBN. Increased seizures have been reported.[279] Significant hepatic or renal toxicity has not been described, and hematopoietic reactions are extremely rare.[280]

Acetazolamide

AZM is a carbonic anhydrase inhibitor that is most effective in treating absence and catamenial epilepsy. Because of the frequent development of tolerance, it is usually not as effective as other AEDs and therefore is not first-line therapy.

Side effects from AZM rarely occur. The most commonly reported is hypercalciuria. Although often asymptomatic, this may be associated with renal stones and osteomalacia.[281–284] Other dose-related side effects have occasionally been described, including gastritis,[285–287] alteration of taste,[288] hypokalemia,[289] hirsutism,[290] impotence,[291] and mental status changes associated with electrolyte imbalance.[292]

Serious hypersensitivity reactions have been reported, including anaphylaxis,[293] Stevens-Johnson syndrome,[294] and aplastic anemia.[295] In Sweden, 11 cases of possible AZM-associated aplastic anemia were reported during a 17-year period, giving an incidence of 1 in 18,000 patient-years.[296] Ten of these cases were fatal, and most occurred within several months of treatment onset.

Topiramate

TPM is the most recent addition to the AED armamentarium. It is approved by the Food and Drug Administration (FDA) for use as add-on therapy for partial seizures with or without secondary generalization. Serious side effects are rare. Nine percent to 21% of those treated with TPM have treatment-limiting side effects, usually occurring at high doses or with rapid dose escalation.[297, 298] Drug interaction with the traditional AEDs is not of clinical significance except with CBZ and PHT; these potent enzyme inducers increase TPM clearance by approximately 50%.[299] Plasma drug levels should therefore be carefully monitored when these medications are added or discontinued.

The most common side effects of TPM are headache, somnolence, fatigue, dizziness, impaired concentration, paresthesias, and mild weight loss.[300] Nephrolithiasis occurs in approximately 1.5%, but usually does not require surgery.[300] Significant hepatic, bone marrow, or renal effects have not been reported.

Ketogenic Diet

It has been known since at least the 1800s that seizure control improves with starvation, although the mechanism for this still is not known. The ketogenic diet was devised in 1921 as a way of maintaining ketosis typical of starvation but with careful attention to the patient's nutritional needs. It is used for all seizure types, with generalized epilepsies responding best. The diet is most effective in children.[301] A high-fat, low-carbohydrate ratio is strictly maintained; "cheating" may precipitate status epilepticus.

Short-term side effects are common. Fifty percent of patients starting the ketogenic diet have gastrointestinal upset, nausea, or vomiting.[301] Corn oil as the fat source is better tolerated in some patients.[302] Transient drowsiness and metabolic derangements may occur.[303] At our institution, several patients have required hospitalization due to hypernatremic dehydration and severe constipation. Poor neutrophil function may occur, but is rarely of clinical significance.[304] Urolithiasis occurs in up to 5% of patients on the ketogenic diet, and periodic screening for hematuria is recommended.[305] Optic neuropathy has been reported in patients not on adequate vitamin supplementation.[306] In a review of 58 epileptic patients treated with the ketogenic diet, three developed renal stones, two had hyperuricemia, one had acidosis, one had hypocalcemia, one suffered recurrent infections, and one refused to eat.[307] Only the patients with renal stones, infections, and refusal to eat had to be taken off the diet.

Despite the extremely high fat intake, serum cholesterol and triglyceride levels are usually only modestly elevated. Occasional patients (some with familial hyperlipidemias) may have markedly elevated fasting lipid levels.[308] Very long-chain fatty acid concentrations are high, suggesting peroxisomal dysfunction, which may cause diagnostic confusion in patients who have not been fully evaluated for the etiology of seizures.[309] The long-term cardiovascular effects have not been adequately studied. Livingston et al. evaluated a number of adults who had been treated with the ketogenic diet as children and found no evidence of hypertension, atherosclerosis, or elevated lipid levels.[310]

Felbamate

Felbamate (FBM) was approved by the FDA in August 1993 for treatment of partial seizures in adults and as add-on therapy for generalized seizures in children with Lennox-Gastaut syndrome. As more patients were exposed to FBM after FDA approval, an alarming incidence of aplastic anemia was noted. One year later, in August 1994, a warning was jointly issued by the FDA and the drug manufacturer suggesting that FBM use be limited to only those patients in whom the medication was absolutely necessary.

The incidence of aplastic anemia associated with FBM is approximately 1 in 2,000 patients per year.[311] Thrombocytopenia and fatal hepatitis have also been reported.[312, 313] Although it is not clear that laboratory monitoring prevents serious side effects, the manufacturer has recommended blood counts with liver function tests every 1–2 weeks for the duration of treatment. More common side effects include insomnia, weight loss, stomach upset, dizziness, fatigue, headache, and ataxia.[311, 314, 315] FBM has a number of drug interactions that require dose adjustment when used as add-on therapy. At this point FBM is used primarily by epileptologists for patients with seizures intractable to all other AEDs, for those who understand the substantial risk involved, and for those who are willing to maintain close follow-up with their physicians.

Conclusion

Physicians are frequently asked to treat patients with seizures. Because many AEDs are equally effective in decreasing seizure frequency, the choice of which drug to use is often based on side effect profile. Rational follow-up of patients taking AEDs also depends on side effect profile; liver function tests, CBCs, or electrolytes may need to be monitored periodically. Patients taking barbiturates should be questioned about possible cognitive side effects. In all cases, the "cure" should be no worse than the disease. A "no treatment" option can be considered in those with rare or mild seizures.

Serious drug reactions are rare but require prompt recognition and treatment to avoid life-threatening complications. Much more common are temporary, dose-responsive side effects that may require a dose adjustment but not treatment withdrawal. Differentiating between these two types of side effects is essential. As new medications and anticonvulsant treatments become available, clinicians will need to evaluate potential side effects as well as efficacy to arrive at the best treatment option for patients.

Acknowledgment

The author would like to thank Michael J. Phillips for thoughtful comments and editing, and Jorge J. Asconapé M.D. for critical review of this manuscript.

References

1. de Silva M, MacArdle B, McGowan M, et al. Randomised comparative monotherapy trial of phenobarbitone, phenytoin, carbamazepine, or sodium valproate

for newly diagnosed childhood epilepsy. Lancet 1996; 347:709.
2. Heller AJ, Chesterman P, Elwes RD, et al. Phenobarbitone, phenytoin, carbamazepine, or sodium valproate for newly diagnosed adult epilepsy: a randomised comparative monotherapy trial. J Neurol Neurosurg Psychiatry 1995;58:44.
3. Pellock JM. Carbamazepine side effects in children and adults. Epilepsia 1987;28(Suppl 3):S64.
4. Schoeman JF, Elyas AA, Brett EM, et al. Correlation between plasma carbamazepine-10, 11-epoxide concentration and drug side-effects in children with epilepsy. Dev Med Child Neurol 1984;26:756.
5. Schain RJ, Ward JW, Guthrie D. Carbamazepine as an anticonvulsant in children. Neurology 1977;27:476.
6. Davis EH. Clinical trials of tegretol in trigeminal neuralgia. Headache 1969;9:77.
7. Pippenger CE. Clinically significant carbamazepine drug interactions: an overview. Epilepsia 1987;28(Suppl 3):S71.
8. Physician's Desk Reference (51st ed). Oradell, NJ: Medical Economics Co, 1997.
9. Herranz JL, Armijo JA, Arteaga R. Clinical side effects of phenobarbital, primidone, phenytoin, carbamazepine, and valproate during monotherapy in children. Epilepsia 1988;29:794.
10. Okuno T, Ito M, Nakano S, et al. Carbamazepine therapy and long-term prognosis in epilepsy of childhood. Epilepsia 1989;30:57.
11. Keranen T, Sivenius J. Side effects of carbamazepine, valproate and clonazepam during long-term treatment of epilepsy. Acta Neurol Scand 1983;97(Suppl):69.
12. Livingston S, Villamater C, Sakata Y, et al. Use of carbamazepine in epilepsy. Results in 87 patients. JAMA 1967;200:204.
13. Hart RG, Easton JD. Carbamazepine and hematological monitoring. Ann Neurol 1982;11:309.
14. Killian JM, Fromm GH. Carbamazepine in the treatment of neuralgia. Use and side effects. Arch Neurol 1968;19:129.
15. Baciewicz G, Yerevanian BI. Thrombocytopenia associated with carbamazepine: case report and review. J Clin Psychiatry 1984;45:315.
16. Pearce J, Ron MA. Thrombocytopenia after carbamazepine. Lancet 1968;2:223.
17. Rutman JY. Effect of carbamazepine on blood elements. Ann Neurol 1978;3:373.
18. Sobotka JL, Alexander B, Cook BL. A review of carbamazepine's hematologic reactions and monitoring recommendations. DICP Annals of Pharmacotherapy 1990;24:1214.
19. Cereghino JJ, Brock JT, Van Meter JC, et al. Carbamazepine for epilepsy. A controlled prospective evaluation. Neurology 1974;24:401.
20. Monaco F, Riccio A, Benna P, et al. Further observations on carbamazepine plasma levels in epileptic patients. Relationships with therapeutic and side effects. Neurology 1976;26:936.
21. Kramlinger KG, Phillips KA, Post RM. Rash complicating carbamazepine treatment. J Clin Psychopharmacol 1994;14:408.
22. Chang DK, Shear NH. Cutaneous reactions to anticonvulsants. Semin Neurol 1992;12:329.
23. Pelekanos J, Camfield P, Camfield C, et al. Allergic rash due to antiepileptic drugs: clinical features and management. Epilepsia 1991;32:554.
24. Murphy JM, Mashman J, Miller JD, et al. Suppression of carbamazepine-induced rash with prednisone. Neurology 1991;41:144.
25. Hopen G, Nesthus I, Laerum OD. Fatal carbamazepine-associated hepatitis. Report of two cases. Acta Med Scand 1981;210:333.
26. Zucker P, Daum F, Cohen MI. Fatal carbamazepine hepatitis. J Pediatr 1977;91:667.
27. Holmes GL. Carbamazepine Toxicity. In RH Levy, RH Mattson, BS Meldrum (eds), Antiepileptic Drugs (4th ed) New York: Raven, 1995;567.
28. Levy M, Goodman MW, Van Dyne BJ, et al. Granulomatous hepatitis secondary to carbamazepine. Ann Intern Med 1981;95:64.
29. Mitchell MC, Boitnott JK, Arregui A, et al. Granulomatous hepatitis associated with carbamazepine therapy. Am J Med 1981;71:733.
30. Sordillo P, Sagransky DM, Mercado RM, et al. Carbamazepine-induced syndrome of inappropriate antidiuretic hormone secretion. Reversal by concomitant phenytoin therapy. Arch Intern Med 1978;138:299.
31. Lahr MB. Hyponatremia during carbamazepine therapy. Clin Pharmacol Ther 1985;37:693.
32. Ringel RA, Brick JF. Perspective on carbamazepine-induced water intoxication: reversal by demeclocycline. Neurology 1986;36:1506.
33. Kalff R, Houtkooper MA, Meyer JW. Carbamazepine and serum sodium levels. Epilepsia 1984;25:390.
34. Koivikko MJ, Valikangas SL. Hyponatraemia during carbamazepine therapy in children. Neuropediatrics 1983;14:93.
35. Perucca E, Richens A. Water intoxication produced by carbamazepine and its reversal by phenytoin. Br J Clin Pharmacol 1980;9:302P.
36. Matteoli S, Trappolini M, Curione M, et al. Effects of carbamazepine on heart conduction in young patients: a serial study using ambulatory ECG. Giornale Italiano di Cardiologia 1994;24:391.
37. Kenneback G, Bergfeldt L, Tomson T. Electrophysiological evaluation of the sodium-channel blocker carbamazepine in healthy human subjects. Cardiovasc Drugs Ther 1995;9:709.
38. Beermann B, Edhag O, Vallin H. Advanced heart block aggravated by carbamazepine. Br Heart J 1975;37:668.
39. Byrne E, Wong CH, Chambers DG, et al. Carbamazepine therapy complicated by nodal bradycardia and water intoxication. Aust N Z J Med 1979;9:295.
40. Boesen F, Andersen EB, Jensen EK et al. Cardiac conduction disturbances during carbamazepine therapy. Acta Neurol Scand 1983;68:49.

41. Benassi E, Bo GP, Cocito L, et al. Carbamazepine and cardiac conduction disturbances. Ann Neurol 1987;22: 280.
42. Terrence CF, Fromm G. Congestive heart failure during carbamazepine therapy. Ann Neurol 1980;8:200.
43. Isojarvi JI, Pakarinen AJ, Myllyla VV. Serum lipid levels during carbamazepine medication. A prospective study. Arch Neurol 1993;50:590.
44. Taliercio CP, Olney BA, Lie JT. Myocarditis related to drug hypersensitivity. Mayo Clin Proc 1985;60:463.
45. Weig SG, Pollack P. Carbamazepine-induced heart block in a child with tuberous sclerosis and cardiac rhabdomyoma: implications for evaluation and follow-up. Ann Neurol 1993;34:617.
46. Bradbury AJ, Bentick B, Todd PJ. Dystonia associated with carbamazepine toxicity. Postgrad Med J 1982; 58:525.
47. Soman P, Jain S, Rajsekhar V, et al. Dystonia—a rare manifestation of carbamazepine toxicity. Postgrad Med J 1994;70:54.
48. Robertson PL, Garofalo EA, Silverstein FS, et al. Carbamazepine-induced tics. Epilepsia 1993;34:965.
49. Tariot PN, Erb R, Leibovici A, et al. Carbamazepine treatment of agitation in nursing home patients with dementia: a preliminary study. J Am Geriatr Soc 1994; 42:1160.
50. Bimpong-Buta K, Froescher W. Carbamazepine-induced choreoathetoid dyskinesias. J Neurol Neurosurg Psychiatry 1982;45:560.
51. De Swert LF, Ceuppens JL, Teuwen D, et al. Acute interstitial pneumonitis and carbamazepine therapy. Acta Paediatr Scand 1984;73:285.
52. Stephan WC, Parks RD, Tempest B. Acute hypersensitivity pneumonitis associated with carbamazepine therapy. Chest 1978;74:463.
53. Fernandez AR, Gullon BJA, Riesgo AC, et al. Acute pulmonary toxicity caused by carbamazepine: apropos of a case. Archivos de Bronconeumologia 1994;30:471.
54. Lewis IJ, Rosenbloom L. Glandular fever-like syndrome, pulmonary eosinophilia and asthma associated with carbamazepine. Postgrad Med J 1982;58:1001.
55. Lee T, Cochrane GM, Amlot P. Pulmonary eosinophilia and asthma associated with carbamazepine. BMJ Clinical Research Edition 1981;282:440.
56. King GG, Barnes DJ, Hayes MJ. Carbamazepine-induced pneumonitis. Med J Aust 1994;160:126.
57. Jubert P, Almirall J, Casanovas A, et al. Carbamazepine-induced acute renal failure. Nephron 1994;66:121.
58. Hogg RJ, Sawyer M, Hecox K, et al. Carbamazepine-induced acute tubulointerstitial nephritis. J Pediatr 1981;98:830.
59. Hegbrant J, Kurkus J, Oqvist B. Carbamazepine-related acute renal failure. Neurology 1993;43:446.
60. Lambert M, Fournier A. Acute renal failure complicating carbamazepine hypersensitivity. Rev Neurol 1992; 148:574.
61. Korinthenberg R, Wehrle L, Zimmerhackl LB. Renal tubular dysfunction following treatment with antiepileptic drugs. Eur J Pediatr 1994;153:855.
62. Otsuka T, Sunaga Y, Hikima A. Urinary N-acetyl-beta-glucosaminidase and guanidinoacetic acid levels in epileptic patients treated with anti-epileptic drugs. Brain Dev 1994;16:437.
63. Steiner I, Birmanns B. Carbamazepine-induced urinary retention in long-standing diabetes mellitus. Neurology 1993;43:1855.
64. Anders RJ, Wang E, Radhakrishnan J, et al. Overflow urinary incontinence due to carbamazepine. J Urol 1985;134:758.
65. Isojarvi JI, Pakarinen AJ, Myllyla VV. A prospective study of serum sex hormones during carbamazepine therapy. Epilepsy Research 1991;9:139.
66. Herzog AG. Reproductive endocrine considerations and hormonal therapy for men with epilepsy. Epilepsia 1991;32(Suppl 6):S34.
67. Snead OC III, Hosey LC. Exacerbation of seizures in children by carbamazepine. N Engl J Med 1985;313: 916.
68. Dhuna A, Pascual-Leone A, Talwar D. Exacerbation of partial seizures and onset of nonepileptic myoclonus with carbamazepine. Epilepsia 1991;32:275.
69. Shields WD, Saslow E. Myoclonic, atonic, and absence seizures following institution of carbamazepine therapy in children. Neurology 1983;33:1487.
70. Talwar D, Arora MS, Sher PK. EEG changes and seizure exacerbation in young children treated with carbamazepine. Epilepsia 1994;35:1154.
71. So EL, Ruggles KH, Cascino GD, et al. Seizure exacerbation and status epilepticus related to carbamazepine-10, 11-epoxide. Ann Neurol 1994;35:743.
72. Neufeld MY. Exacerbation of Focal Seizures Due to Carbamazepine Treatment in an Adult Patient. In Clinical Neuropharmacology. New York: Raven, 1993;359.
73. Shuper A, Stahl B, Weitz R. Carbamazepine-induced hair loss. Drug Intell Clin Pharm 1985;19:924.
74. Soman M, Swenson C. A possible case of carbamazepine-induced pancreatitis. Drug Intell Clin Pharm 1985;19:925.
75. O'Hare JA, Duggan B, O'Driscoll D, et al. Biochemical evidence for osteomalacia with carbamazepine therapy. Acta Neurol Scand 1980;62:282.
76. Hoikka V, Alhava EM, Karjalainen P, et al. Carbamazepine and bone mineral metabolism. Acta Neurol Scand 1984;70:77.
77. Oner A, Topaloglu R, Besbas N, et al. Carbamazepine induced systemic lupus erythematosus. Another warning. Clin Neurol Neurosurg 1990;92:261.
78. De Giorgio CM, Rabinowica AL, Olivas RD. Carbamazepine-induced antinuclear antibodies and systemic lupus erythematosus-like syndrome. Epilepsia 1991; 32:128.
79. Drory VE, Yust I, Korczyn AD. Carbamazepine-Induced Systemic Lupus Erythematosus. In Clinical Neuropharmacology. New York: Raven, 1989;115.

80. Luhdorf K, Nielsen CJ, Orbaek K, et al. Motor and sensory conduction velocities and electromygraphic findings in man before and after carbamazepine treatment. Acta Neurol Scand 1983;67:103.
81. Kutt H, Winters W, Kokenge R, et al. Diphenylhydantoin metabolism, blood levels, and toxicity. Arch Neurol 1964;11:642.
82. Lindvall O, Nilsson B. Cerebellar atrophy following phenytoin intoxication. Ann Neurol 1984;16:258.
83. Masur H, Fahrendorf G, Oberwittler C, et al. Cerebellar atrophy following acute intoxication with phenytoin. Neurology 1990;40:1800.
84. Imamura T, Ejima A, Sahara M, et al. Cerebellar atrophy and persistent cerebellar ataxia after acute intoxication of phenytoin. Brain Nerve 1992;44:149.
85. Ney GC, Lantos G, Barr WB, et al. Cerebellar atrophy in patients with long-term phenytoin exposure and epilepsy. Arch Neurol 1994;51:767.
86. McLain LW, Martin JT, Allen JH. Cerebellar degeneration due to chronic phenytoin therapy. Ann Neurol 1980;7:18.
87. Rapport RL, Shaw CM. Phenytoin-related cerebellar degeneration without seizures. Ann Neurol 1977;2:437.
88. Dam M. The density and ultrastructure of the Purkinje cells following diphenylhydantoin treatment in animals and man. Acta Neurol Scand 1972;49(Suppl):3.
89. Ghatak NR, Santoso RA, McKinney WM. Cerebellar degeneration following long-term phenytoin therapy. Neurology 1976;26:818.
90. Roehrich N, Cimasoni G. Gingival hyperplasia of drug origin. A review of the literature. Schweizer Monatsschrift fur Zahnmedizin 1994;104:1471.
91. Nishikawa S, Nagata T, Morisaki I, et al. Pathogenesis of drug-induced gingival overgrowth. A review of studies in the rat model. Journal of Periodontology 1996;67:463.
92. Chung S, Ahn C. Effects of anti-epileptic drug therapy on bone mineral density in ambulatory epileptic children. Brain Dev 1994;16:382.
93. Bruni J. Phenytoin Toxicity. In RH Levy, RH Mattson, BS Meldrum (eds), Antiepileptic Drugs. New York: Raven, 1995;345.
94. Lau KH, Nakade O, Barr B, et al. Phenytoin increases markers of osteogenesis for the human species in vitro and in vivo. J Clin Endocrinol Metab 1995;80:2347.
95. Nakade O, Baylink DJ, Lau KH. Phenytoin at micromolar concentrations is an osteogenic agent for human-mandible-derived bone cells in vitro. Journal of Dental Research 1995;74:331.
96. Mochizuki Y, Suyehiro Y, Tanizawa A, et al. Peripheral neuropathy in children on long-term phenytoin therapy. Brain Dev 1981;3:375.
97. So EL, Penry JK. Adverse effects of phenytoin on peripheral nerves and neuromuscular junction: a review. Epilepsia 1981;22:467.
98. Ramirez JA, Mendell JR, Warmolts JR, et al. Phenytoin neuropathy: structural changes in the sural nerve. Ann Neurol 1986;19:162.
99. Dobkin BH. Reversible subacute peripheral neuropathy induced by phenytoin. Arch Neurol 1977;34:189.
100. Verma NP, Haidukewych D. Differential but infrequent alterations of hepatic enzyme levels and thyroid hormone levels by anticonvulsant drugs. Arch Neurol 1994;51:381.
101. Aaron JS, Bank S, Ackert G. Diphenylhydantoin-induced hepatotoxicity. Am J Gastroenterol 1985; 80:200.
102. Parker WA, Shearer CA. Phenytoin hepatotoxicity: a case report and review. Neurology 1979;29:175.
103. Chopra S, Levell NJ, Cowley G, et al. Systemic corticosteroids in the phenytoin hypersensitivity syndrome. Br J Dermatol 1996;134:1109-1112.
104. Mullick FG, Ishak KG. Hepatic injury associated with diphenylhydantoin therapy. A clinicopathologic study of 20 cases. Am J Clin Pathol 1980;74:442.
105. Braddock SW, Harrington D, Vose J. Generalized nodular cutaneous pseudolymphoma associated with phenytoin therapy. Use of T-cell receptor gene rearrangement in diagnosis and clinical reveiw of cutaneous reactions to phenytoin. J Am Acad Dermatol 1992;27:337.
106. Wolf R, Kahane E, Sandbank M. Mycosis fungoides-like lesions associated with phenytoin therapy. Arch Dermatol 1985;121:1181.
107. Gately LE, Lam MA. Phenytoin-induced toxic epidermal necrolysis. Ann Intern Med 1979;91:59.
108. Kanoh T, Dobashi H, Inada T. Multiple myeloma associated with phenytoin (diphenylhydantoin) therapy. Rinsho Ketsueki—Japanese Journal of Clinical Hematology 1996;37:239.
109. Hanukoglu A, Fried D, Gotlieb A. Dyphenylhydantoin induced hypersensitivity reaction with an unusal purpuric skin lesion. Eur J Pediatr 1980;134:177.
110. Haruda F. Phenytoin hypersensitivity: 38 cases. Neurology 1979;29:1480.
111. Chadwick D, Shaw MD, Foy P, et al. Serum anticonvulsant concentrations and the risk of drug induced skin eruptions. J Neurol Neurosurg Psychiatry 1984;47:642.
112. Bardana EJ, Gabourel JD, Davies GH, et al. Effects of phenytoin on man's immunity. Evaluation of changes in serum immunoglobulins, complement, and antinuclear antibody. Am J Med 1983;74:289.
113. Basaran N, Hincal F, Kansu E, et al. Humoral and cellular immune parameters in untreated and phenytoin- or carbamazepine-treated epileptic patients. Int J Immunopharmacol 1994;16:1071.
114. Ruff ME, Pincus LG, Sampson HA. Phenytoin-induced IgA depression. Am J Dis Child 1987;141:858.
115. Sorrell TC, Forbes IJ, Burness FR, et al. Depression of immunological function in patients treated with phenytoin sodium (sodium diphenylhydantoin). Lancet 1971;2:1233.
116. Ishizaka A, Nakanishi M, Kasahara E. Phenytoin-induced IgG2 and IgG4 deficiencies in a patient with epilepsy. Acta Paediatr 1992;81:646.
117. Pisciotta AV. Phenytoin Hematological Toxicity. In DM

Woodbury, JK Penry, CE Pippenger (eds), Antiepileptic Drugs. New York: Raven, 1982;257.
118. Kendle E. Megalogblastic anemia during anticonvulsant therapy. Del Med J 1969;41:147.
119. Rosenberg IH, Godwin HA, Streiff RR, et al. Impairment of intestinal deconjugation of dietary folate. A possible explanation of megaloblastic anaemia associated with phenytoin therapy. Lancet 1968;2:530.
120. Carl GF, Smith ML. Phenytoin-folate interactions: differing effects of the sodium salt and the free acid of phenytoin. Epilepsia 1992;33:372.
121. Solomon GE, Hilgartner MW, Kutt H. Coagulation defects caused by diphenylhydantoin. Neurology 1972;22:1165.
122. Iivanainen M, Savolainen H. Side effects of phenobarbital and phenytoin during long-term treatment of epilepsy. Acta Neurol Scand 1983;68(Suppl 97):49.
123. Rawanduzy A, Sarkis A, Rovit RL. Severe phenytoin-induced bone marrow depression and agranulocytosis treated with human recombinant granulocyte-macrophage colony-stimulating factor. Case Report. J Neurosurg 1993;79:121.
124. Howrie DL, Schwinghammer TL, Wollman M. Use of i.v. immune globulin for treatment of phenytoin-induced thrombocytopenia. Clinical Pharmacy 1989;8:734.
125. Yue CP, Mann KS, Chan KH. Severe thrombocytopenia due to combined cimetidine and phenytoin therapy. Neurosurgery 1987;20:963.
126. Wong YY, Lichtor T, Brown FD. Severe thrombocytopenia associated with phenytoin and cimetidine therapy. Surg Neurol 1985;23:169.
127. Arbiser JL, Goldstein AM, Gordon D. Thrombocytopenia following administration of phenytoin, dexamethasone and cimetidine: a case report and a potential mechanism. J Intern Med 1993;234:91.
128. O'Connor CR, Schraeder PL, Kurland AH, et al. Evaluation of the mechanisms of antiepileptic drug-related chronic leukopenia. Epilepsia 1994;35:149.
129. Micheli F, Lehkuniec E, Gatto M, et al. Hemiballism in a patient with partial motor status epilepticus treated with phenytoin. Functional Neurology 1993;8:103.
130. Chadwick D, Reynolds EH, Marsden CD. Anticonvulsant-induced dyskinesias: a comparison with dyskinesias induced by neuroleptics. J Neurol Neurosurg Psychiatry 1976;39:1210.
131. Zinsmeister S, Marks RE. Acute athetosis as a result of phenytoin toxicity in a child. Am J Dis Child 1976;130:75.
132. Harrison MB, Lyons GR, Landow ER. Phenytoin and dyskinesias: a report of two cases and review of the literature. Mov Disord 1993;8:19.
133. Shulman LM, Singer C, Weiner WJ. Phenytoin-induced focal chorea. Mov Disord 1996;11:111.
134. Isojarvi JI, Pakarinen AJ, Myllyla VV. Thyroid function with antiepileptic drugs. Epilepsia 1992;33:142.
135. Isojarvi JI, Repo M, Pakarinen AJ. Carbamazepine, phenytoin, sex hormones, and sexual function in men with epilepsy. Epilepsia 1995;36:366.
136. Murialdo G, Galimberti CA, Fonzi S, et al. Sex hormones, gonadotropins and prolactin in male epileptic subjects in remission: role of the epileptic syndrome and of antiepileptic drugs. Neuropsychobiology 1994; 30:29.
137. Malherbe C, Burrill KC, Levin SR, et al. Effect of diphenylhydantoin on insulin secretion in man. N Engl J Med 1972;286:339.
138. Tamburrano S, Luyckx AS, Lefebvre PJ. Studies on the hyperglycemic effect of diphenylhydantoin in normal golden hamsters. Horm Metab Res 1976;6(Suppl):74.
139. Perry-Keene DA, Larkins RG, Heyma P, et al. The effect of long-term diphenylhydantoin therapy on glucose tolerance and insulin secretion: a controlled trial. Clin Endocrinol 1980;12:575.
140. Fichman MP, Kleeman CR, Bethune JE. Inhibition of antidiuretic hormone secretion by diphenylhydantoin. Arch Neurol 1970;22:45.
141. Wilder BJ, Ramsay RE, Murphy JV, et al. Comparison of valproic acid and phenytoin in newly diagnosed tonic-clonic seizures. Neurology 1983;33:1474.
142. Dean J. Valproate. In E Wyllie (ed), The Treatment of Epilepsy. Principles and Practice. Philadelphia: Lea & Febiger, 1993;915.
143. Dreifuss FE, Langer DH. Side effects of valproate. Am J Med 1988;84:39.
144. Isojarvi JIT, Laatikainen TJ, Knip M, et al. Obesity and endocrine disorders in women taking valproate for epilepsy. Ann Neurol 1996;39:579.
145. Breum L, Astrup A, Gram L, et al. Metabolic changes during treatment with valproate in humans: implication for untoward weight gain. Metabolism: Clinical & Experimental 1992;41:666.
146. Karas BJ, Wilder BJ, Hammond EJ, et al. Treatment of valproate tremors. Neurology 1983;33:1380.
147. Lancman ME, Asconape JJ, Penry JK. Choreiform movements associated with the use of valproate. Arch Neurol 1994;51:702.
148. Egger J, Brett EM. Effects of sodium valproate in 100 children with special reference to weight. BMJ Clinical Research Education 1981;283:577.
149. Herranz JL, Arteaga R, Armijo JA. Change in hair colour induced by valproic acid. Dev Med Child Neurol 1981;23:386.
150. Jeavons PM, Clark JE. Sodium valproate in treatment of epilepsy. BMJ 1974;2:584.
151. Boxer CM, Herzberg JL, Scott DF. Has sodium valproate hypnotic effects? Epilepsia 1976;17:367.
152. Chadwick DW, Cumming WJ, Livingstone I, et al. Acute intoxication with sodium valproate. Ann Neurol 1979;6:552.
153. Landau J, Baulac M, Durand G, et al. Impairment of consciousness induced by valproate treatment following neurosurgical operation. Acta Neurochir 1993; 125:92.
154. Sackellares JC, Lee SI, Dreifuss FE. Stupor following administration of valproic acid to patients receiving other antiepileptic drugs. Epilepsia 1979;20:697.
155. Legarda SB, Booth MP, Fennell EB, et al. Altered cog-

nitive functioning in children with idiopathic epilepsy receiving valproate monotherapy. J Child Neurol 1996; 11:321.

156. Prevey ML, Delaney RC, Cramer JA, et al. Effect of valproate on cognitive functioning. Arch Neurol 1996; 53:1008.
157. Gallassi R, Morreale A, Lorusso S, et al. Cognitive effects of valproate. Epilepsy Research 1990;5:160.
158. Aldenkamp AP, Alpherts WCJ, Blennow G, et al. Withdrawal of antiepileptic medication in children—effects on cognitive function. Neurology 1993;43:41.
159. Sussman NM, McLain LW. A direct hepatotoxic effect of valproic acid. JAMA 1979;242:1173.
160. Gram L, Bentsen KD. Hepatic toxicity of antiepileptic drugs: a review. Acta Neurol Scand 1983;68(Suppl):81.
161. Murphy JV, Marquardt K. Asymptomatic hyperammonemia in patients receiving valproic acid. Arch Neurol 1982;39:591.
162. Dreifuss FE, Langer DH, Moline KA, et al. Valproic acid hepatic fatalities. II. U.S. experience since 1984. Neurology 1989;39:201.
163. Scheffner D, Konig S, Rauterberg-Ruland I, et al. Fatal liver failure in 16 children with valproate therapy. Epilepsia 1988;29:530.
164. Konig SA, Siemes H, Blaker F, et al. Severe hepatotoxicity during valproate therapy: an update and report of eight new fatalities. Epilepsia 1994;35:1005.
165. Coulter DL. Carnitine deficiency in epilepsy: risk factors and treatment. J Child Neurol 1995;10(Suppl):2S32.
166. Bohles H, Sewell AC, Wenzel D. The effect of carnitine supplementation in valproate induced hyperammonaemia. Acta Paediatr 1996;85:446.
167. Bryant AE, Dreifuss FE. Valproic acid hepatic fatalities. III. U.S. experience since 1986. Neurology 1996;46:465.
168. Appleton RE, Farrell K, Applegarth DA, et al. The high incidence of valproate hepatotoxicity in infants may relate to familial metabolic defects. Can J Neurol Sci 1990;17:145.
169. Verbiest HB, Straver JS, Colombo JP, et al. Carbamyl phosphate synthetase-1 deficiency discovered after valproic acid induced coma. Acta Neurol Scand 1992;86:275.
170. Tokatli A, Coskun T, Cataltepe S, et al. Valproate-induced lethal hyperammonaemic coma in a carrier of ornithine carbamoyltransferase deficiency. J Inherit Metab Dis 1991;14:836.
171. Coulter DL. Carnitine, valproate, and toxicity. J Child Neurol 1991;6:7.
172. Kossak BD, Schmidt Sommerfeld E, Schoeller DA, et al. Impaired fatty acid oxidation in children on valproic acid and the effect of L-carnitine. Neurology 1993;43: 2362.
173. Triggs WJ, Bohan TP, Lin SN, et al. Valproate induced coma with ketosis and carnitine insufficiency. Arch Neurol 1990;47:1131.
174. Laub MC, Paetzke-Brunner I, Jaeger G. Serum carnitine during valproic acid therapy. Epilepsia 1986;27:559.
175. Murphy JV, Groover RV, Hodge C. Hepatotoxic effects in a child receiving valproate and carnitine. J Pediatr 1993;123:318.
176. Gidal B, Spencer N, Maly M, et al. Valproate mediated disturbances of hemostasis. Neurology 1994;44:1418.
177. Delgado MR, Riela AR, Mills J. Thrombocytopenia secondary to high valproate levels in children with epilepsy. J Child Neurol 1994;9:311.
178. Ward M, Barbaro NM, Laxer KD, et al. Preoperative valporate administration does not increase blood loss during temporal lobectomy. Epilepsia 1996;37:98.
179. Smith FR, Boots M. Sodium valproate and bone marrow suppression. Ann Neurol 1980;8:197.
180. Ganick DJ, Sunder T, Finley JL. Severe hematologic toxicity of valproic acid. Am J Pediatr Hematol Oncol 1990;12:80.
181. Kishi T, Fujita N, Kawaguchi H, et al. Bone marrow suppression induced by high dose valproic acid. Arch Dis Child 1994;71:153.
182. Jaeken J, van Goethem C, Casaer P, et al. Neutropenia during sodium valproate treatment. Arch Dis Child 1979;54:986.
183. Symon DN, Russell G. Sodium valproate and neutropenia. Arch Dis Child 1983;58:235.
184. Majer RV, Green PJ. Neonatal afibrinogenaemia due to sodium valproate. Lancet 1987;2:740.
185. Ozkara C, Dreifuss OC, Hansen AC. Changes in red blood cells with valproate therapy. Acta Neurol Scand 1993;88:210.
186. Kreuz W, Linde R, Funk M, et al. Valproate therapy induces von Willebrand disease type I. Epilepsia 1992;33:178.
187. Bale JF, Gay PE, Madsen JA. Monitoring of serum amylase levels during valproic acid therapy. Ann Neurol 1982;11:217.
188. Asconapé JJ, Penry K, Dreifuss FE, et al. Valproate associated pancreatitis. Epilepsia 1993;34:177.
189. Armon C, Brown E, Carwile S, et al. Sensorineural hearing loss: a reversible effect of valproic acid. Neurology 1990;40:1896.
190. Asconapé JJ, Lancman ME, Dibert SW, et al. Sensorineural hearing loss associated with the use of valproate. Ann Neurol 1993;34:263.
191. Papazian O, Canizales E, Alfonso I, et al. Reversible dementia and apparent brain atrophy during valproate therapy. Ann Neurol 1995;38:687.
192. Vaquerizo J, Gomez-Martin H, Gonzalez IE, et al. Reversible neuropsychological deterioration associated with valproate. Revista de Neurologia 1995;23:148.
193. Armon C, Shin C, Miller P, et al. Reversible parkinsonism and cognitive impairment with chronic valproate use. Neurology 1996;47:626.
194. Asconapé JJ, Manning KR, Lancman ME. Systemic lupus erythematosus associated with use of valproate. Epilepsia 1994;35:162.
195. Painter MJ, Gaus LM. Phenobarbital. In E Wyllie (ed), The Treatment of Epilepsy, Principles & Practice. Philadelphia: Lea & Febiger, 1993;900.
196. Ismael S. The efficacy of phenobarbital in controlling

epilepsy in children. Paediatrica Indonesiana 1990; 30:97.
197. Herranz JL, Armijo JA, Arteaga R. Clinical side effects of phenobarbital, primidone, phenytoin, carbamazepine, and valproate during monotherapy in children. Epilepsia 1988;29:794.
198. Wolf SM, Forsythe A. Behavior disturbance, phenobarbital, and febrile seizures. Pediatrics 1978;61:728.
199. Heller AJ, Chesterman P, Elwes RD. Phenobarbitone, phenytoin, carbamazepine, or sodium valproate for newly diagnosed adult epilepsy: a randomised comparative monotherapy trial. J Neurol Neurosurg Psychiatry 1995;58:44.
200. Cramer JA, Mattson RH. Phenobarbital Toxicity. In RH Levy, RH Mattson, BS Meldrum (eds), Antiepileptic Drugs (4th ed). New York: Raven, 1995;409.
201. Camfield CS, Chaplin S, Doyle AB, et al. Side effects of phenobarbital in toddlers; behavioral and cognitive aspects. J Pediatr 1979;95:361.
202. Burd L, Kerbeshian J, Fisher W. Does the use of phenobarbital as an anticonvulsant permanently exacerbate hyperactivity? Canadian Journal of Psychiatry-Revue Canadienne de Psychiatrie 1987;32:10.
203. Robertson MM, Trimble MR, Townsend HR. Phenomenology of depression in epilepsy. Epilepsia 1987;28:354.
204. Brent DA, Crumrine PK, Varma RR, et al. Phenobarbital treatment and major depressive disorder in children with epilepsy. Pediatrics 1987;80:909.
205. Meador KJ, Loring DW, Huh K, et al. Comparative cognitive effects of anticonvulsants. Neurology 1990;40:391.
206. Calandre EP, Dominguez-Granados R, Gomez-Rubio M, et al. Cognitive effects of long term treatment with phenobarbital and valproic acid in school children. Acta Neurol Scand 1990;81:504.
207. Macleod CM, Dekabian AS, Hunt E. Memory impairment in epileptic patients: selective effects of phenobarbital concentration. Science 1978;202:1102.
208. Riva D, Devoti M. Discontinuation of phenobarbital in children: effects on neurocognitive behavior. Pediatr Neurol 1996;14:36.
209. Farwell JF, Lee YJ, Hirtz DG, et al. Phenobarbital for febrile seizures—effects on intelligence and on seizure recurrence. 1990;322:364.
210. Serrano EE, Kunis DM, Ransom BR. Effects of chronic phenobarbital exposure on cultured mouse spinal cord neurons. Ann Neurol 1988;24:429.
211. Johnson MI, Rueger D, Loegering MB, et al. Therapeutic levels of phenobarbital inhibit development and maintenance of dendrites induced by osteogenic protein 1. Ann Neurol 1996;40:286
212. Neale EA, Sher PK, Graubard BI, et al. Differential toxicity of chronic exposure to phenytoin, phenobarbital, or carbamazepine in cerebral cortical cell cultures. Pediatr Neurol 1985;1:143.
213. Bergey GK, Swaiman KF, Schrier BK, et al. Adverse effects of phenobarbital on morphological and biochemical development of fetal mouse spinal cord neurons in culture. Ann Neurol 1981;9:584.
214. Mattson RH, Cramer JA, Collins JF, et al. Comparison of carbamazepine, phenobarbital, phenytoin, and primidone in partial and secondarily generalized tonic clonic seizures. N Engl J Med 1985;313:145.
215. Mountain KR, Hirsh J, Gallus AS. Neonatal coagulation defect due to anticonvulsant drug treatment in pregnancy. Lancet 1970;1:265.
216. Shear NH, Spielberg SP. Anticonvulsant hypersensitivity syndrome. In vitro assessment of risk. J Clin Invest 1988;82:1826.
217. Pelekanos J, Camfield P, Camfield C, et al. Allergic rash due to antiepileptic drugs: clinical features of managment. Epilepsia 1991;32:554.
218. Mattson RH. Barbiturate related connective tissue disorders. Arch Intern Med 1989;149:911.
219. White PT, Plott D, Norton J. Relative anticonvulsant potency of primidone; a double blind comparison. Arch Neurol 1966;14:31.
220. Olesen OV, Dam M. The metabolic conversion of primidone (Mysoline) to phenobarbitone in patients under long term treatment. An attempt to estimate the independent effect of primidone. Acta Neurol Scand 1967;43:348.
221. Baumel IP, Gallagher BB, Mattson RH. Phenylethylmalonamide (PEMA). An important metabolite of primidone. Arch Neurol 1972;27:34.
222. Bourgeois BF, Dodson WE, Ferrendelli JA. Primidone, phenobarbital, and PEMA: I. Seizures protection, neurotoxicity, and therapeutic index of individual compounds in mice. Neurology 1983;33:289.
223. Smith BH, McNaughton FL. Mysoline, a new anticonvulsant drug. Can Med Assoc J 1953;68:464.
224. Sciarra D, Carter S, Vicale CT. Clinical evaluation of primidone (mysoline), new anticonvulsant drug. JAMA 1954;154:827.
225. Leppik IE, Cloyd JC, Miller K. Development of tolerance to the side effects of primidone. Ther Drug Monit 1984;6:189.
226. Baker H, Frank O, Hutner SH, et al. Lesions in folic acid metabolism induced by primidone. Experientia 1962;18:224.
227. Chalmers J. Megaloblastic anemia and anticonvulsant therapy. Lancet 1954;47:920.
228. Fuld H, Moorhouse EH. Observations on megaloblastic anaemias after primidone. BMJ 1956;1:1021.
229. Parker WA. Primidone thrombocytopenia. Ann Intern Med 1974;81:559.
230. Ahuja GK, Schumacher GA. Drug induced systemic lupus erythematosus. Primidone as a possible cause. JAMA 1966;198:669.
231. Leppik IE, Cloyd JC. Primidone Toxicity. In RH Levy, RH Mattson, BS Meldrum (eds), Antiepileptic Drugs (4th ed). New York: Raven, 1995;487.
232. Gabriel RM. Delayed reaction to primidone in pregnancy. BMJ 1957;1:344.
233. Rodin EA, Rim CS, Kitano H, et al. A comparison of the effectivness of primidone versus carbamazepine in epileptic outpatients. J Nerv Ment Dis 1976;163:41.
234. Sherwin AL. Ethosuximide. In E Wyllie (ed), The

Treatment of Epilepsy. Principles & Practice. Philadelphia: Lea & Febiger, 1993;923.

235. Weinstein AW, Allen RJ. Ethosuximide treatment of petit mal seizures. A study of 87 pediatric patients. Am J Dis Child 1966;111:63.
236. Browne TR, Dreifuss FE, Dyken PR, et al. Ethosuximide in the treatment of absence (petit mal) seizures. Neurology 1975;25:515.
237. Almeyda J, Levantine A. Drug reactions XX. Cutaneous reactions to anticonvulsants. Br J Dermatol 1972;87:646.
238. Livingston S, Rodriguez H, Greene CA, et al. Systemic lupus erythematosus. Occurrence in association with ethosuximide therapy. JAMA 1968;203:731.
239. Dabbous IA, Idriss HM. Occurrence of systemic lupus erythematosus in association with ethosuximide therapy—case report. J Pediatr 1970;76:617.
240. Beernink DH, Miller JJ. Anticonvulsant induced antinuclear antibodies and lupus like disease in children. J Pediatr 1973;82:113.
241. Singsen BH, Fishman L, Hanson V. Antinuclear antibodies and lupus like syndromes in children receiving anticonvulsants. Pediatrics 1976;57:529.
242. Ansell BM. Drug induced systemic lupus erythematosus in a nine year old boy. Lupus 1993;2:193.
243. Spittler JF. Agranulocytosis due to ethosuximide with a fatal outcome. Klinische Padiatrie 1974;186:364.
244. Seip M. Aplastic anemia during ethosuximide medication. Treatment with bolus methylprednisolone. Acta Paediatr Scand 1983;72:927.
245. Massey GV, Dunn NL, Heckel JL, et al. Aplastic anemia following therapy for absence seizures with ethosuximide. Pediatr Neurol 1994;11:59.
246. Dreifuss FE. Ethosuximide Toxicity. In RH Levy, RH Mattson, BS Meldrum (eds), Antiepileptic Drugs (4th ed). New York: Raven, 1995;675.
247. Kirschberg GJ. Dyskinesia an unusual reaction to ethosuximide. Arch Neurol 1975;32:137.
248. Ehyai A, Kilroy AW, Fenichel GM, et al. Dyskinesia and akathisia induced by ethosuximide. Am J Dis Child 1978;132:527.
249. Goldensohn ES, Hardie J, Borea ED, et al. Ethosuximide in the treatment of epilepsy. JAMA 1962; 180:840.
250. Todorov AB, Lenn JN, Gabor AJ. Exacerbation generalized nonconvulsive seizures with ethosuximide therapy. Arch Neurol 1978;35:389.
251. Gordon N. Treatment of epilepsy with a-ethyl-a-methylsuccinimide (P.M. 671). Neurology 1961;11:266.
252. Roger J, Grangeon H, Gueyj J, et al. Psychiatric and psychologic effects of ethosuximide treatment of epileptics. Encephale 1968;57:407.
253. Fischer M, Korskjaer G, Pedersen E. Psychotic episodes in zarondan treatment. Epilepsia 1965;6:325.
254. Smith WL, Philippus MJ, Guard HL. Psychometric study of children with learning problems and 14-6 positive spike EEG patterns, treated with ethosuximide (Zarontin) and placebo. Arch Dis Child 1968;43:616.
255. Sher PK, Neale EA, Graubard BI, et al. Differential neurochemical effects of chronic exposure of cerebral cortical cell culture to valproic acid, diazepam, or ethosuximide. Pediatr Neurol 1985;1:232.
256. Coulter DL. Ethosuximide induced liver dysfunction. Arch Neurol 1983;40:393.
257. Nishiyama S, Matsukura M, Fujimoto S, et al. Reports of two cases of autoimmune thyroiditis while receiving anticonvulsant therapy. Eur J Pediatr 1983;140:116.
258. Rambeck B, Wolf P. Lamotrigine clinical pharmacokinetics. Clin Pharmacokinet 1993;25:433.
259. Fitton A, Goa KL. Lamotrigine. An update of its pharmacology and therapeutic use in epilepsy. Drugs 1995;50:691.
260. Messenheimer JA. Lamotrigine. Epilepsia 1995; 36(Suppl 2):S87.
261. Besag FM, Wallace SJ, Dulac O, et al. Lamotrigine for the treatment of epilepsy in childhood. J Pediatr 1995;127:991.
262. Schachter SC, Leppik IE, Matsuo F, et al. A multicentre placebo controlled evaluation of the safety of lamotrigine (Lamictal) as add-on therapy in patients with partial seizures. Epilepsia 1993;33:S119.
263. Richens A. Lamotrigine Toxicity. In RH Levy, RH Mattson, BS Meldrum (eds), Antiepileptic Drugs (4th ed). New York: Raven, 1995;897.
264. Smith D, Baker G, Davies G, et al. Outcomes of add on treatment with lamotrigine in partial epilepsy. Epilespia 1993;34:312.
265. Dooley J, Camfield P, Gordon K, et al. Lamotrigine-induced rash in children. Neurology 1996;46:240.
266. Sterker M, Berrouschot J, Schneider D. Fatal course of toxic epidermal necrolysis under treatment with lamotrigine. Int J Clin Pharmacol Ther 1995;33:595.
267. Honmou O, Oyelese AA, Kocsis JD. The anticonvulsant gabapentin enhances promoted release of GABA in hippocampus: a field potential analysis. Brain Res 1995;692:273.
268. Petroff OA, Rothman DL, Behar KL, et al. The effect of gabapentin on brain gamma-aminobutyric acid in patients with epilepsy. Ann Neurol 1996;39:95.
269. McLean MJ. Gabapentin. Epilepsia 1995;36(Suppl 2):S73.
270. U.S. Gabapentin Study Group. The long-term safety and efficacy of gabapentin (Neurontin) as add-on therapy in drug-resistant partial epilepsy. Epilepsy Research 1994;18:67.
271. Morris GL. Efficacy and tolerability of gabapentin in clinical practice. Clin Ther 1995;17:891.
272. Lee DO, Steingard RJ, Cesena M, et al. Behavioral side effects of gabapentin in children. Epilepsia 1996;37:87.
273. Khurana DS, Riviello J, Helmers S, et al. Efficacy of gabapentin therapy in children with refractory partial seizures. J Pediatr 1996;128:829.
274. Wolf SM, Shinnar S, Kang H, et al. Gabapentin toxicity in children manifesting as behavioral changes. Epilepsia 1995;36:1203.
275. Tallian KB, Nahata MC, Lo W, et al. Gabapentin asso-

ciated with aggressive behavior in pediatric patients with seizures. Epilepsia 1996;37:501.
276. Gidal BE, Maly MM, Nemire RE, et al. Weight gain and gabapentin therapy. Ann Pharmacother 1995;29:1048.
277. Buetefisch CM, Gutierrez A, Gutmann L. Choreoathetotic movements. A possible side effect of gabapentin. Neurology 1996;46:851.
278. Reeves AL, So EL, Sharbrough FW, et al. Movement disorders associated with the use of gabapentin. Epilepsia 1996;37:988.
279. Vossler DG. Exacerbation of seizures in Lennox-Gastaut syndrome by gabapentin. Neurology 1996;46:852.
280. Ramsay RE. Gabapentin Toxicity. In RH Levy, RH Mattson, BS Meldrum (eds), Antiepileptic Drugs (4th ed). New York: Raven, 1995;857.
281. Stafstrom CE, Gilmore HE, Kurtin PS. Nephrocalcinosis complicating medical treatment of posthemorrhagic hydrocephalus. Pediatr Neurol 1992;8:179.
282. Tawil R, Moxley RT, Griggs RC. Acetazolamide-induced nephrolithiasis: implications for treatment of neuromuscular disorders. Neurology 1993;43:1105.
283. Ahlstrand C, Tiselius HG. Urine composition and stone formation during treatment with acetazolamide. Scand J Urol Nephrol 1987;221:225.
284. Mallette LE. Acetazolamide-accelerated anticonvulsant osteomalacia. Arch Intern Med 1977;137:1013.
285. Cho CH, Chen SM, Chen SW, et al. Pathogenesis of gastric ulceration produced by acetazolamide in rats. Digestion 1984;29:5.
286. Woodbury DM. Carbonic Anhidrase Inhibitors. In GH Glaser, JK Penny, DM Woodbury (eds), Antiepileptic Drugs: Mechanisms of Action. New York: Raven, 1980;167.
287. Herman J, Nassar F, Dalli N. Endoscopically proved erosive gastritis due to acetazolamide. Isr J Med Sci 1980;16:866.
288. Miller LG, Miller SM. Altered taste secondary to acetazolamide therapy. J Fam Pract 1990;31:199.
289. Davis AR, Diggory P, Seward HC. Prevalance of chronic hypokalaemia amongst elderly patients using acetozolamide and diuretics. Eye 1995;9:381.
290. Weiss IS. Hirsutism after chronic administration of acetazolamide. Am J Ophthalmol 1974;78:327.
291. Epstein RJ, Allen RC, Lunde MW. Organic impotence associated with carbonic anhydrase inhibitor therapy for glaucoma. Ann Ophthalmol 1987;19:48.
292. Rowe TO. Acetazolamide delirium. Am J Psychiatry 1977;134:587.
293. Peralta J, Abelairas J, Fernandez-Guardiola J. Anaphylactic shock and death after oral intake of acetazolamide. Am J Ophthalmol 1992;114:367.
294. Sud RN, Grewal SS. Stevens Johnson syndrome due to Diamox. Indian J Ophthalmol 1981;29:101.
295. Shapiro S, Fraunfelder FT. Acetazolamide and aplastic anemia. Am J Ophthalmol 1992;113:328.
296. Keisu M, Wiholm BE, Ost A, et al. Acetazolamide-associated aplastic anaemia. J Intern Med 1990;228:627.
297. Faught E, Wilder BJ, Ramsay RE, et al. Topiramate placebo-controlled dose-ranging trial in refractory partial epilepsy using 200-, 400-, and 600-mg daily dosages. Topiramate YD Study Group. Neurology 1996;46:1684.
298. Ben-Menachem E, Henriksen O, Dam M, et al. Double-blind, placebo-controlled trial of topiramate as add-on therapy in patients with refractory partial seizures. Epilepsia 1996;37:539.
299. Bourgeois BF. Drug interaction profile of topiramate. Epilepsia 1996;37(Suppl 2):S14.
300. Shorvon SD. Safety of topiramate: adverse events and relationships to dosing. Epilepsia 1996;37(Suppl 2):S18.
301. Prasad AN, Stafstrom CF, Holmes GL. Alternative epilepsy therapies: the ketogenic diet, immunoglobulins, and steroids. Epilepsia 1996;37(Suppl):S81.
302. Woody RC, Brodie M, Hampton DK, et al. Corn oil ketogenic diet for children with intractable seizures. J Child Neurol 1988;3:21.
303. Schwartz RH, Eaton J, Bower BD, et al. Ketogenic diets in the treatment of epilepsy: short-term clinical effects. Dev Med Child Neurol 1989;31:145.
304. Woody RC, Steele RW, Knapple WL, et al. Impaired neutrophil function in children with seizures treated with the ketogenic diet. J Pediatr 1989;115:427.
305. Herzberg GZ, Fivush BA, Kinsman SL, et al. Urolithiasis associated with the ketogenic diet. J Pediatr 1990;117:743.
306. Hoyt CS, Billson FA. Optic neuropathy in ketogenic diet. Br J Ophthalmol 1979;63:191.
307. Kinsman SL, Vining EPG, Quaskey SA, et al. Efficacy of the ketogenic diet for intractable seizure disorders: review of 58 cases. Epilepsia 1992;33:1132.
308. Dekaban AS. Plasma lipids in epileptic children treated with the high fat diet. Arch Neurol 1966;15:177.
309. Theda C, Woody RC, Naidu S, et al. Increased very long chain fatty acids in patients on a ketogenic diet: a cause of diagnostic confusion. J Pediatr 1993;122:724.
310. Livingston S, Pauli LL, Pruce I. Ketogenic diet in the treatment of childhood epilepsy. Dev Med Child Neurol 1977;19:833.
311. Leppik IE. Felbamate. Epilepsia 1995;36(Suppl 2):S66.
312. O'Neil MG, Perdun CS, Wilson MB, et al. Felbamate-associated fatal acute hepatic necrosis. Neurology 1996;46:1457.
313. Ney GC, Schaul N, Loughlin J, et al. Thrombocytopenia in association with adjunctive felbamate use. Neurology 1994;44:980.
314. Bergen DC, Ristanovic RK, Waicosky K, et al. Weight loss in patients taking felbamate. Clin Neuropharmacol 1995;18:23.
315. Ettinger AB, Jandorf L, Berdia A, et al. Felbamate-induced headache. Epilepsia 1996;37:503.

Chapter 22

Complications of Psychostimulants

Kelda Harris Walsh and David W. Dunn

Objectives

- To appreciate the shared complications of the three classic psychostimulants: methylphenidate, dextroamphetamine, and pemoline
- To recognize the impact of the classic psychostimulants on movement disorders, particularly Tourette's disorder
- To understand the unique side effects of each of the classic psychostimulants
- To recognize the potential neurologic and psychiatric adverse effects of the sympathomimetics from either therapeutic or recreational uses
- To appreciate the withdrawal effects of amphetamines, caffeine, and cocaine
- To recognize the various neurologic and psychiatric complications of amphetamine and cocaine abuse
- To understand the potential neonatal complications of in utero exposure to amphetamines and cocaine

General Considerations

Stimulants have a long history of both therapeutic and recreational use. The current indications for methylphenidate, pemoline, and dextroamphetamine are narcolepsy and attention deficit hyperactivity disorder (ADHD). These medications may also have a limited role in the treatment of depression and obesity.[1] The sympathomimetics are present in a variety of cold preparations, and caffeine is a component of many pain remedies. In addition to the therapeutic uses, all these drugs have been abused. Cocaine and the amphetamines are the stimulants frequently consumed by recreational drug users.[2] In this chapter, we review the neurologic and neuropsychiatric effects of stimulants used either therapeutically or recreationally.

Most Common Side Effects Secondary to Therapeutic Doses of Classic Psychostimulants

The classic psychostimulants—methylphenidate, dextroamphetamine, and pemoline—have been widely used for ADHD, narcolepsy, and major depressive disorder. Presently, methylphenidate and dextroamphetamine are first-line agents. Because of a 4- to 17-fold increase in the rate of hepatic failure with pemoline, this drug is considered a second-line agent for ADHD.[3,4] The stimulants' six most common side effects, in order of descending frequency, are insomnia, anorexia, irritability and agitation, weight loss, abdominal pain, and headache.[5–7] These side effects are often time limited and respond to dose reduction.[6] Clinicians have written little about abdominal pain and headache, except to note their prevalence, focusing on the other four symptoms instead.

Insomnia and other sleep changes secondary to the psychostimulants have been studied in adults and children. Although psychostimulant treatment often appears to improve the sleep of children with ADHD (they comply better with bedtime and appear to be less restless in their sleep), nocturnal activity monitoring and sleep studies have shown that even single morning doses of methylphenidate at 0.3–0.4 mg per kg decrease sleep duration significantly in ADHD children compared with normal controls.[8] Children with ADHD who take evening doses of dextroamphetamine are less oppositional and defiant in the evening and appear to parents to wake up less frequently, but in fact sleep less efficiently.[9] The duration of stages 1, 2, and rapid eye movement (REM) sleep decrease, as do the number of REM episodes and percentage of REM sleep. These children may appear to sleep better because they complain of fewer nightmares secondary to the decrease in REM sleep. Similar dose-dependent findings have been reported with pemoline in normal adults.[10] The relative sleep impairment of the three medications has not been well studied, although therapeutic doses of pemoline may trigger fewer sleep problems than dextroamphetamine.[11] Although sleep returns to normal after discontinuation of the psychostimulants, the return to normal sleep architecture may take as long as 2 months.[7]

The second most common psychostimulant side effect, anorexia, and its complication of weight loss (or failure to gain weight at the expected rate in children) have been the focus of several nutrition studies. Decreased appetite is significantly related to dose, with ratings of anorexia as much as doubled when children increase their methylphenidate doses from 0.3 to 0.5 mg per kg.[12, 13] This anorectic effect not only decreases total food intake,[7] but, as shown in one small study of adult volunteers, higher doses (30 mg per 70 kg) also result in reductions in fat and protein intake, with relative sparing of carbohydrate consumption.[14] In the latter study, for all doses studied (10–30 mg per 70 kg), doses relatively modest compared with those frequently used clinically in hyperactive children, subjects reduced calorie consumption by 24–30%. However, one study of depressed adults treated with low-dose psychostimulants (averaging 9 mg per day of dextroamphetamine and 11 mg per day of methylphenidate) demonstrated little to no anorexia, or even improvement in appetite with treatment.[15] The resolution of depression, a disease that can cause profound anorexia, may in these cases outweigh the mild, transient anorexic effects of low-dose stimulant use.

When stimulants cause anorexia, it occurs early in the course of treatment; sustained or late-onset anorexia should raise clinical suspicion of other contributing factors. Chewing regular or sustained-release methylphenidate has been reported by two authors to trigger severe gastrointestinal distress, anorexia, and, in one case, behavioral problems.[16, 17] Late-onset anorexia and gastrointestinal distress in patients using pemoline mandates further investigation for evidence of liver toxicity. Complicating anorexia, particularly in the psychostimulant treatment of children, is weight loss or slowed weight gain. This weight loss occurs frequently, but the duration and severity of weight loss is controversial. Much of this is likely due to variations in growth studies with inconsistencies in which doses are used and how they are reported (absolute dose, cumulative dose, or milligram per kilogram), inconsistent verification of compliance, and varying length of treatment.[18] Studies assessing weight gain in children have not consistently applied the same growth norms, which have included matched normal controls, matched untreated ADHD controls, and various growth charts. The most frequently used norms—the Boston and Iowa growth charts—are based on measurements obtained in the 1930s and may not provide true normative data for children studied 40–50 years later, thus underestimating stimulant impact.[18] Additionally, Tanner stages in children are often not reported, despite findings that stimulants affect height much less during postpuberty than during prepuberty[19] and that stimulant metabolism and half-life change markedly in puberty, at least for pemoline.[20]

Even with these factors limiting study comparison, several findings have been consistent. Weight gain in the initial months of stimulant treatment is significantly less than expected, even after absolute weight loss stops. Children may not return to normal weight gain velocity for 6 months (on pemoline, using unspecified norms),[21] 12 months (using Iowa norms),[22] or even 24 months (using newer National Center for Health Statistics norms)[23] of treatment. Weight decrements are dose dependent for methylphenidate, with several studies reporting that doses of 20 mg per day produce weight gain comparable to norms,[24–26] whereas high-dose methylphenidate (30–40 mg per day) appears to have a particularly adverse effect on weight gain, comparable with the growth impairment of dextroamphetamine.

The benefit of summer medication holidays for children with impaired weight gain is controversial. Most consistently, summer dextroamphetamine breaks appear to significantly improve weight gain.[25, 26] Methylphenidate studies have shown less impact from summer medication breaks. Safer et al. found that although children taking methylphenidate improved weight gain over the first summer break, the change was not significant.[25] Satterfield et al. reported similar findings in a group of 72 ADHD children treated with methylphenidate: a nonsignificant trend for less weight loss over the first summer break, with a statistically significant improvement in weight gain for children who spent two consecutive summers off medication.[22] A third study found children randomly assigned to take summer breaks (most studies allow families to make this decision) from methylphenidate treatment were comparable in weight to year-round controls after the second summer, but weighed significantly more after the first summer break.[27] It appears that some children persistently failing to gain weight normally benefit from summer medication holidays from psychostimulants, particularly dextroamphetamine.

Although impact on weight is controversial in the psychostimulant literature, irritability and agitation secondary to therapeutic doses are not. Although many parents and teachers of children treated with psychostimulants report irritability and agitation, placebo-controlled studies have found that a high percentage of children show these symptoms at similar levels under placebo conditions and may in fact improve when treated.[12] Many of the affective symptoms attributed to stimulants at therapeutic doses may in fact be symptoms of the illness being treated.[13] Changes in mood or activity level occurring in adolescence after years of stable good response may reflect decreasing body clearance with age and need for dose adjustment.[28, 29]

Less Commonly Reported Adverse Effects Shared by the Classic Psychostimulants

Cardiovascular

Cardiovascular effects of psychostimulants, when found, are generally benign and may include small changes in blood pressure or pulse, palpitations, and dizziness.[7] A series of 154 medically ill, depressed adults treated with dextroamphetamine and 44 treated with methylphenidate revealed few cardiovascular effects.[15] Complications reported included two cases of significant blood pressure elevation, one case of atrial fibrillation, and three cases of sinus tachycardia. In adults, subcutaneous methylphenidate has produced dose-dependent increases in blood pressure and heart rate,[30] whereas lower doses (0.3 mg per kg) in children have not done so consistently.[31] Regular monitoring of blood pressure and heart rate should be part of the follow-up for patients taking stimulant medication.

Neurologic

The stimulants' tendency to cause or unmask movement disorders is more often a problem than the cardiovascular adverse effects. Tics, Tourette's disorder, and choreoathetoid movements have been reported frequently.

Tics and Tourette's Disorder

In 1974, Golden reported the first case of Tourette's disorder developing in a child who had received methylphenidate for 8 weeks.[32] The onset of symptoms in this case was unusually rapid, suggesting induction by the medication. Later authors, reporting large series of Tourette's disorder cases appearing during stimulant treatment, noted that patients had a high rate of premorbid tics, positive family history of tics or Tourette's disorder, or both. Presence of these apparent risk factors became contraindications to stimulant use.[17] Because of the high comorbidity of ADHD and Tourette's disorder, these contraindications were problematic for clinicians seeking to manage ADHD symptoms in Tourette patients, especially because the relative risks of tic development were not known.

Denckla et al. reviewed 1,520 charts of children with minimal brain dysfunction treated with stimulants.[33] They found that 1.3% of children developed tics de novo during treatment, 13.3% with premorbid tics had exacerbations with stimulant treatment, and one child developed Tourette's disorder. Of those with new-onset tics, more than half had resolution of their symptoms when they stopped using stimulants, and four patients rechallenged with stimulants did not develop tics. Another large series of 122 stimulant-treated patients showed a 9% rate of tic development and 0.8% rate of Tourette's disorder onset, with no significant relationship to positive personal or family history of tics, stimulant type, or dose demonstrated in those developing tics or Tourette's disorder.[34] This compares with the survey by Comings et al. of the general untreated population in a school study, identifying prevalence of tics at 1.25%, and Tourette's disorder at 0.036% in 3,034 5–15 year olds.[35]

Many of the initial assumptions made about stimulant use in Tourette's disorder have since been challenged. The pattern of swift onset that Golden believed demonstrated a drug effect occurs in many patients with Tourette's disorder naïve to stimulants and is not universal in those treated with stimulants.[36] Tourette's disorder appearing after years of stimulant use may reflect the natural course of the illness, which is typically preceded by ADHD by years, rather than stimulant induction.[37] A study of 250 Tourette's disorder patients revealed a 5.3-year average lag in Tourette's disorder development after stimulant treatment was initiated; family histories for tics were as likely to be positive in Tourette's disorder patients exposed to stimulants as those not exposed to stimulants.[22]

It appears likely that Tourette's disorder appearing during stimulant treatment may not necessarily be induced by the stimulants. Its more frequent occurrence in ADHD treatment may reflect more the high frequency of premorbid ADHD in patients who eventually develop Tourette's disorder, with or without stimulant exposure. Tics may be transient and resolve on withdrawal of psychostimulants, and Tourette's disorder onset likely is no faster on stimulants than off. Other questions remain. Although it is widely accepted that stimulants are helpful for the spectrum of ADHD symptoms seen frequently in Tourette's disorder, their impact on the tics themselves has not been consistently demonstrated in the literature. Psychostimulants have been shown to improve motor tics[38] or vocal tics[39] in some patients. The conclusion of Erenberg et al. that cautious use of stimulants may help some children seems more appropriate currently than a blanket contraindication to their use in children with tic or Tourette histories.[40]

Chorea

New-onset choreoathetoid movements have been reported in patients taking each of the three classic psychostimulants and have been attributed to the dopamine agonist properties of the drugs.[41–45] Dextroamphetamine (10-mg dose) has been shown to exacerbate chorea in patients with premorbid Sydenham's chorea, Huntington's disease, and systemic lupus erythematosus.[46] A patient withdrawn from perphenazine, but continued on dextroamphetamine, developed severe dyskinesias, including choreoathetosis that interfered with his ability to feed himself, which resolved promptly on the cessation of the dextroamphetamine. The authors hypothesized that long-term perphenazine therapy caused the patient to develop dopamine-receptor supersensitivity. When perphenazine was withdrawn, the sensitive receptors were bombarded with the dopamine agonist effects of dextroamphetamine, leading to the movement disorder.[47]

Choreoathetosis induction appears to be most frequent and problematic with pemoline. One prospective study demonstrated severe choreoathetoid movements in five of 20 ADHD children given a single 2 mg per kg dose of pemoline.[45] The movements began near the time of peak plasma levels and persisted up to 8 hours. The children who developed choreoathetoid movements did not differ significantly in their peak pemoline plasma levels from those who did not, but the total amount of body pemoline in affected children was doubled. Patients with slower elimination half-lives (a 600% variability has been reported) may be at greater risk for chorea and other types of neurotoxicity.[28]

Metabolic

Many researchers have studied the failure of psychostimulant-treated children to gain height as quickly as their peers, evaluating impact of dose, dose duration, and summer medication holidays. Slowed linear growth velocity has been reported with use of all of the classic psychostimulants,[18, 21, 23, 24] although time to onset and duration have varied. Pemoline appears to have its most significant impact on height in the first 12–18 months of treatment, with return to normal National Center for Health Statistics height velocity by 24 months of sustained treatment.[21, 23] High-dose methylphenidate (30 mg per day or more) significantly decreases height velocity, an effect found in two studies to be ameliorated by at least one summer off medication during long-term treatment.[24, 27]

Another study found that although methylphenidate did not adversely affect linear growth until the second year of treatment, linear growth continually decelerated in prepubertal children treated for up to 4 years, with a mean height percentile loss of 18.1% after the fourth year of treatment.[18] Significant risk factors for slowed linear growth included being taller at the initiation of treatment and having a larger cumulative lifetime dosage. Even so, it was estimated at the end of the study that less than 2% of variation in final height was accounted for by stimulant dosage. The authors concluded that if 2% of height were lost permanently secondary to long-term stimulant use, that this loss would be acceptable to at least some children and their families.

Longer-term outcome studies suggest that even that small variation in final height may be regained in adolescence. The study by Vincent et al. of 31 adolescents (12.5 years of age or older) treated for at least 6 months with stimulants demonstrated no variation from National Center for Health Statistics height norms.[19] Klein and Mannuzza's follow-up study of adolescents and young adults who had lost height velocity during childhood stimulant treatment, with a mean daily dose of 45 mg per day of methylphenidate exposure for an average of 2 years, found the subjects no longer differed from normal controls or U.S. Public Health Service means for height.[48] The studies are small and limited: Neither of these studies controlled for variation in cumulative stimulant dose, which appeared to vary widely, and required only 6 months of treatment for study inclusion. These studies, although promising, do not guarantee that all children with large cumulative stimulant exposure will ultimately achieve their expected heights.

Psychiatric

Behavioral rebound has been reported in children taking short-acting forms of dextroamphetamine and methylphenidate. The very existence of behavioral rebound is controversial and consists of worsening of ADHD symptoms as medication effects wear off late in the day, to the point that children are more inattentive, distractible, or defiant than they were before medication administration.[49] Criteria used in studies as to what constitutes rebound vary and have included objective machine measurement of motor activity and ratings scales by parents and teachers. Rebound effects have been demonstrated in normal children 5 hours after single dextroamphetamine doses.[50] At 8 hours after a single dose of dextroamphetamine, ADHD children escalated their motor activity beyond that of untreated ADHD controls and maintained that escalation, even in sleep, until their dextroamphetamine dose the next morning.[50] Another study of twice-daily dosing of methylphenidate showed a significant increase in affective and ADHD symptoms with a 0.3-mg but not a 0.6-mg dose.[51] Longer-acting preparations or more frequent dosing may ameliorate this problem in some children.

Psychosis, including psychotic mania, has been reported with use of all the psychostimulants. The rate appears low, with six reports of psychosis in the 4,200 child side effect cases reviewed by Barkley in the 1970s,[6] and a total of 20 child cases reported by 1992.[49] Visual and auditory hallucinations, bizarre preoccupations, and paranoid delusions have been reported, occurring days to months after treatment initiation.[14, 52, 53] Some episodes labeled "mania" or "hypomania" failed duration criteria from the *Diagnostic and Statistical Manual of Mental Disorders,* 4th edition (DSM-IV) and resolved promptly after drug discontinuation.[54] Three of the eight "hypomania/mania" patients in the literature to date[10, 15, 54, 55] had positive family histories for bipolar disorder, and one patient appeared to have been hallucinating before stimulant use.[10]

Complications Reported with Specific Psychostimulants

Methylphenidate

Single cases of stuttering (on trials of both methylphenidate and pemoline)[56] and paroxysmal kinesigenic dystonia[38] have been reported. Although the stuttering resolved promptly with medication discontinuation, the dystonia resolved only with carbamazepine treatment.

Wroblewski et al. evaluated 30 adults with active seizure disorders, most secondary to traumatic brain injury, and found that treatment with methylphenidate tended to reduce seizure frequency.[57] Although four patients had more frequent seizures on methylphenidate, three had recently started or increased doses of tricyclic antidepressants.

Methylphenidate has been diverted from children with ADHD and abused by parents or caretakers. Opiate and methadone users inject methylphenidate intravenously for its stimulant effect. Approximately 20% of these users develop tachycardia, tachypnea, sweating, and chills. Panic attacks and paranoid ideations have also occurred.[58] The abuse of methylphenidate has also been associated with choreoathetosis and other hyperkinetic movement disorders.[59]

The repeated intravenous injection of methylphenidate may cause foreign body granulomas in the lungs and on heart valves. This seems to be the result of talc and cornstarch filler in the methylphenidate hydrochloride (Ritalin) preparation. Repeated intravenous injection has led to yellow-white retinal emboli in small vessels clustering around the macula.[60, 61] There have been several case reports of accidental intracarotid injection of methylphenidate with resultant transient and permanent hemipareses.[62] Wolf et al. have reported an eosinophilic syndrome with low-grade fever, arthralgia, and myalgia in patients who had injected crushed methylphenidate tablets intravenously.[63]

Pemoline

Pemoline seems to be less often abused. It has caused paranoia and hallucinations in chronic users.[64] There is a report of chorea after an accidental ingestion of pemoline by a toddler.[65]

Dextroamphetamine

Apparent new-onset of spasticity[15] and exacerbation of the spasticity of amyotrophic lateral sclerosis with dextroamphetamine treatment have been reported.[66] Stereotypies developed in an adolescent with ADHD after increase in dextroamphetamine dose.[67]

Caffeine

Caffeine is probably the most commonly used stimulant medication. It is present in coffee, tea, many soft drinks, both prescription and over-the-counter pain medications, and nonprescription stimulants. Caffeine is a methylated xanthine related to theophylline. It is a competitive antagonist at the adenosine receptor. Caffeine stimulates the cerebral cortex and the medullary respiratory centers and, at high doses, can increase reflex excitability in the spinal cord. Caffeine is a vasodilator by its effect on vascular musculature. It also stimulates cardiac muscle, relaxes smooth muscle, and promotes diuresis.[68]

With an appropriate dose there may be improved reaction time, decreased fatigue, jitters, and a decrease in hand steadiness.[69] In prepubertal children caffeine can reduce errors of omission and improve variability of response on continuous performance measures of attention and can improve manual dexterity in the dominant hand.[70] Caffeine intoxication can follow ingestion of 100 mg of caffeine, the amount present in one cup of coffee. It is more often seen after more than 250 mg, but because of tolerance may not occur even at high doses. Symptoms of intoxication include restlessness, anxiousness, excitation, trouble sleeping, flushing, diuresis, abdominal cramps, muscle twitching, tachycardia, and a hypomanic state of rapid speech and thought, agitation, and excessive energy. At significantly elevated plasma levels, more than 30 mg per liter, caffeine intoxication can cause seizures. Caffeine has been shown to be an antagonist at benzodiazepine receptors, a potential explanation for its ability to cause seizures.[71]

Caffeine-induced sleep disorder occurs with excess nighttime use of coffee, tea, or caffeine-containing soft drinks. Caffeine also has been found to contribute to insomnia in people taking caffeine-containing analgesics or cold and allergy medications. In a series of 2,885 adults, 5.4% were found to be taking medications containing caffeine.[72] When questioned about sleep habits, the people consuming caffeine-containing medications reported significantly more trouble falling asleep.

Psychiatric manifestations of anxiety and nervousness, or caffeine-induced anxiety disorder, may be a particular problem for those individuals at risk for anxiety or panic attacks. In one survey, patients with panic attacks had increased sensitivity to a single cup of coffee, had more often stopped drinking coffee because of adverse effects, and by self-report questionnaire, had an association between anxiety and depression scores and caffeine consumption.[73]

This correlation between anxiety and depression scores and caffeine was not observed in normal controls or in individuals with mood disorders.

A withdrawal syndrome consisting of headache, depression, anxiety, and fatigue has been documented after cessation of use of even low to moderate amounts of caffeine.[74] The decrease in wakefulness, depressed mood, and headaches are transient, but the reduction in motor activity is more persistent. In one series of pregnant women working in health care professions, the cessation of caffeine was suggested as one contributing cause of the "encephalopathy" of pregnancy, a feeling of increased fatigue and slowness of thought occurring during pregnancy.[75] An increase in alpha and theta voltage bifrontally has been seen on analog electroencephalography during caffeine abstinence.[76] Similarly, individuals who have a baseline diffuse paroxysmal slowing on electroencephalography had an increased firing rate of this pattern during abstinence from caffeine.[77] The authors postulated a chronic vasoconstriction with caffeine use with a subsequent vasodilatation during withdrawal.

Nicotine

Nicotine is a ganglionic stimulating agent. It can cause release of catecholamine and is a central nervous system (CNS) stimulant. Through its effect on chemoreceptors in the carotid and aortic body, nicotine stimulates respiration. It can cause tremors and, with marked overdose, seizures. Nicotine additionally acts as a peripheral vasoconstrictor.[78] Nicotine intoxication is rare and is not included as a DSM-IV diagnosis.[79]

The two main psychiatric disorders associated with nicotine are nicotine dependence and nicotine withdrawal. The features of dependence seen with nicotine include tolerance, as shown by increasing use without adverse effects, withdrawal symptoms on cessation of use, and difficulty in stopping use of tobacco, even after knowing the serious health problems related to its use. Nicotine withdrawal is characterized by nervousness, irritability, difficulty sleeping, trouble concentrating, depressed mood, weight gain, and decreased heart rate.[79]

A syndrome of tobacco-alcohol amblyopia may occur after prolonged use of both substances, often combined with poor nutrition. The disorder begins with decreased color perception and a centrocecal scotoma. A moderate, often asymmetric, loss of visual acuity follows. If the individual is able to abstain from tobacco and alcohol, there may be improvement in vision.[80] There also appears to be a pure tobacco amblyopia not associated with poor nutrition or alcohol. It is not known whether the nicotine or another substance present in tobacco smoke is the cause of this syndrome.[81]

Amphetamines

Amphetamine causes both increased release of and increased extracellular concentration of norepinephrine and dopamine and probably serotonin. Euphoria is secondary to its effect on dopaminergic neurons, as are the movement disorders seen with amphetamine use. Attention, motor activity, and systemic cardiovascular effects are mediated by norepinephrine.[7, 82] The dextro isomer of amphetamine and methamphetamine are the main agents abused. D-Amphetamine is usually taken orally, and methamphetamine ("ice" or "crystal") is either smoked or injected intravenously. The half-life of amphetamine is approximately 4 hours. Because of this longer half-life, amphetamines are taken less often than cocaine. Like cocaine, they are used either repeatedly or episodically.[83] Amphetamine use may have increased more recently. Baberg et al. found that in 1995, 15.6% of patients seen by psychiatric consultants on a university general hospital service were users of amphetamine or methamphetamine, as compared with 4.5% in 1992.[84]

Acute effects of amphetamines are increased alertness, hyperactivity, and a sense of well-being. Headaches, anxiety, and confusion may also occur. Additional complications of amphetamine intoxication are chest pain, respiratory depression, and psychomotor agitation or retardation. Violence, repetitive behaviors, and dysphoria may also occur. There is elevation of the systemic blood pressure, and the pupils are minimally dilated. Tolerance to the acute effects of amphetamine develops quickly.[79] Acute poisoning causes fever, tremor, flushing, elevated blood pressure, delirium, seizures, and coma. Death may follow as a consequence of cardiovascular shock, disseminated intravascular coagulation, and severe hyperthermia. Benzodiazepines can be used to treat the acute effects of amphetamine, if sedation is needed. The rate of excretion can be enhanced by acidification of the urine with ammonium chloride, unless the patient has developed myoglobinuria and potential renal failure.[2]

Amphetamine withdrawal is characterized by a dysphoric mood that begins within hours to a few days of cessation of use. It is usually accompanied by changes in sleep patterns, vivid dreams, increased appetite, and fatigue. During the period of depression there is often severe drug craving, and relapses are common. Amphetamine withdrawal is not physiologically dangerous but may be associated with suicidal ideation. The main depressive state may last days to a few weeks. This depressive state may be severe enough to warrant use of antidepressants such as desipramine.[79, 85]

Seizures

Seizures occur less often with amphetamine than with cocaine. Dextroamphetamine has been suggested as the stimulant of choice in children with both ADHD and epilepsy because of its reported ability to increase the seizure threshold.[86] Nevertheless, seizures have followed intravenous, intranasal, and oral use of amphetamines. These seizures have followed use by both novice and long-term abusers of amphetamines. Most amphetamine-induced seizures occur within 24 hours of drug exposure.[87] These seizures are typically generalized tonic-clonic convulsions with no long-term neurologic sequelae. Most are brief seizures, although status epilepticus has occurred.[88] Unless there is additional neurologic damage, long-term therapy with an antiepileptic drug is not needed.

Stroke

Stroke is the other main neurologic complication. This may follow either acute or chronic amphetamine use. Stroke may follow respiratory, oral, or intravenous administration of amphetamine. Both ischemic and hemorrhagic infarcts have been reported, independent of the frequency or route of administration.[89, 90] As one example, Yen et al. reported five patients with intracerebral hemorrhages (three lobar, one caudate, and one putaminal) and two patients with middle cerebral infarcts after inhalation of methamphetamine.[91] Mechanisms for amphetamine-induced stroke are embolism, elevation of systemic blood pressure, and changes in cerebral vasculature.[90, 92] Endocarditis has followed intravenous use of amphetamine, with subsequent embolic stroke.[90] Amphetamine may cause transient hypertension. This has not been consistently documented in those patients with amphetamine-associated intracerebral or subarachnoid hemorrhage, perhaps because of delay in seeking medical attention.[92] Subarachnoid hemorrhage from aneurysms and intracerebral hemorrhage from vascular malformations have been temporally associated with the use of amphetamine. The presumed mechanism is either an increase in blood pressure or changes in vasculature.[93] Amphetamine-induced vasculitis results in both ischemic and hemorrhagic infarcts.[93, 94] Amphetamine-induced vasculitis has been seen on angiography after both oral and intravenous use. The arteries have a characteristic beaded appearance with segmental changes in vessel size.[95] Rumbaugh et al. demonstrated reduced size of small cerebral arteries and reduced blood flow in Rhesus monkeys given intravenous methamphetamine, suggesting this is an effect of amphetamine and not an effect of contaminants in street drugs.[96] Vasculitis has also been found on pathologic examination. Citron et al. described fibrinoid necrosis of the media and intima of arteries and a perivascular infiltrate similar to that seen in periarteritis nodosa.[97] Caplan et al. conclude that immunologic mechanisms are the most common explanations for strokes in those abusing drugs.[89]

Psychiatric Complications

Chronic amphetamine use can cause hallucinations and paranoid delusions during the period of intoxication. Hallucinations usually clear within 24 hours, but the paranoid ideations may last for a week or more. When these hallucinations and delusions persist beyond that seen with intoxication or withdrawal, a diagnosis of amphetamine-induced psychotic disorder is made. The patient should be placed in a nonstimulating environment. Intramuscular haloperidol can be used for sedation.[79, 85]

Chronic amphetamine use can precipitate the onset of schizophrenia and may be the etiology for a schizophrenia-like psychotic illness. Initially, it may be impossible to distinguish a transient drug-induced psychosis from schizophrenia. If chronic amphetamine use does lead to the maintenance of chronic psychosis, the presumed mechanism is a depleted dopaminergic state resulting from permanent damage to dopaminergic brain terminals.[98]

Pediatric Complications

Maternal amphetamine use during pregnancy can have an adverse effect on the infant, although these adverse effects occur less frequently with amphetamines than with narcotics or cocaine. There is an increased incidence of placental hemorrhage, and the infants have an increased risk of prematurity and intrauterine growth retardation. Oro and Dixon described neonatal withdrawal symptoms, including abnormal sleep patterns, jitters, hypertonia, and poor feeding.[99] Eriksson et al. noted lethargy extreme enough to require tube feeding in two infants.[100] This lethargy might represent a withdrawal syndrome similar to the depression seen in adults withdrawing from amphetamine. As with cocaine, the adverse effect of amphetamine on the infant is complicated by the frequent use of other drugs, the risk of maternal infection, and the environmental difficulties to which the child may be exposed.

Other Amphetamines: MDMA and MDEA

Other amphetamines that have been implicated in neurologic dysfunction include 3,4-methylenedioxymethamphetamine (MDMA; "ecstasy") and 3,4-methylenedioxyethyamphetamine (MDEA; "eve"). Both drugs are usually taken orally, and both cause hallucinations, anxiety, paranoia, and psychosis. Cerebral edema associated with hyponatremia has followed ingestion of MDMA.[101] Henry et al. reported seven deaths after MDMA use.[102] Clinical features included seizures, hyperthermia, coma, disseminated intravascular coagulation, and renal failure.

Sympathomimetics

Phenylpropanolamine and ephedrine are sympathomimetic amines with effects similar to but weaker than amphetamine. They affect both the sympathetic nervous system and the CNS, stimulate both alpha and beta receptors, and cause the release of norepinephrine. They are available in many over-the-counter cold remedies and have been used in combination with caffeine as appetite suppressants and "legal" stimulants. They are sold on the streets as look-alike or substitutes for amphetamines.[83]

Neurologic Complications

Adverse effects have occurred with both appropriate doses and overdoses of phenylpropanolamine, although CNS toxic effects are much more common with elevated levels. Lake et al., reviewing 142 case reports of adverse effects from phenylpropanolamine, found that in one-third of reports, patients had taken an overdose of phenylpropanolamine.[103] Hypertension is the main and most serious adverse effect of phenylpropanolamine and appears to be a major factor in the etiology of the CNS adverse effects. Lake et al. found 45 reports of hypertensive crisis, including 24 with intracranial hemorrhage and 15 with hypertensive encephalopathy or seizures.[103] CNS side effects include headache, dizziness, anxiety, and confusion. Severe complications are seizures and stroke. Mueller reported adverse effects necessitating an emergency room visit in 11 patients, most of whom had taken phenylpropanolamine thinking it was amphetamine.[104] Five patients developed severe headaches after phenylpropanolamine use, four experienced the new onset of psychiatric symptoms, and two suffered generalized seizures. Fallis and Fisher described a patient who experienced an intracerebral hemorrhage and had angiographic evidence of vasculitis associated with use of a diet pill containing phenylpropanolamine.[105] In the series by Lake et al., there were eight deaths associated with phenylpropanolamine. In six of the eight cases, intracranial hemorrhage was documented. In two of the eight cases, death followed the use of an appropriate dosage of phenylpropanolamine.[103]

Psychiatric Complications

Anxiety, confusion, agitation, mania, hallucinations, and paranoid psychosis have all been reported. Lake et al. found 30 reports of psychiatric symptoms associated with phenylpropanolamine.[103] Risk factors for adverse psychiatric events are past history of mood disorder or psychosis and a family history of psychiatric disorder.[106]

Ephedrine, pseudoephedrine, and oxymetazoline are similar to phenylpropanolamine in actions, although the incidence of adverse reactions is less. They may cause an increase in blood pressure and heart rate and have been implicated as a cause of headaches, anxiety, seizures, and paranoid psychosis.[107, 108]

Cocaine

Cocaine is a centrally acting stimulant and a local anesthetic. It blocks the reuptake of dopamine, norepinephrine, and serotonin, thus increasing the activity of catecholamines and serotonin. The euphoria is presumed to be related to activation of mesolimbic and mesocortical dopaminergic pathways. The half-life of cocaine is approximately 45–60 minutes, with cocaine metabolized by cholinesterases. Benzoylecgonine, one of the main breakdown products, is also a stimulant and has a much longer half-life. Cocaine hydrochloride is inhaled nasally or injected intravenously and can be absorbed through mucous membranes. The alkaloid form, "crack," is not destroyed by high temperatures and is usually smoked. The peak action occurs within minutes after intravenous injection or smoking of cocaine. The peak effect is seen 30–60 minutes after nasal use and 60–90 minutes after oral ingestion. Because of the short half-life, users need frequent doses to maintain the euphoric state. The cocaine sold on the streets is often adulterated with caffeine, phenylpropanolamine, ephedrine, lidocaine, or strychnine.[2, 85, 109]

The acute effects of cocaine include euphoria, excitement, disinhibition, and a heightened sense of confidence and self-esteem. With cocaine intoxication, there are changes in blood pressure and heart rate, pupillary dilation, chills, respiratory impairment, chest pain, confusion, and coma. Weight loss may occur during prolonged use. Cocaine dependence may develop after only a brief period of use. An exaggerated manic response may lead to impulsive, destructive actions and excessive psychomotor agitation. Cocaine withdrawal is similar to amphetamine withdrawal and consists of a dysphoric state with fatigue, sleep disturbance, and increased appetite.[79, 85]

During cocaine intoxication and cocaine withdrawal, the sensorium is usually clear. At higher doses, there can be generalized anxiety and panic reactions, listed in the DSM-IV as cocaine-induced anxiety disorder.[79] This may be followed by hallucinations and paranoid delusions, which usually resolve within several days but may linger for a few weeks, creating confusion between cocaine-induced psychotic disorder and schizophrenia. Emergency room visits are prompted by cardiopulmonary, neurologic, or psychiatric symptoms. Brody et al. described 233 hospital visits by 216 cocaine-using patients.[110] Chest pain was a complaint in 39.5% of patients, shortness of breath in 21.9%, and palpitations in 20.6%. Two patients died, one from cardiac arrest after a seizure and the second from a cardiac arrest in the emergency room. Deaths have also occurred both from overdose followed by seizures and respiratory depression and from agitated delirium similar to the malignant neuroleptic syndrome. These latter patients developed hyperthermia, delirium with agitation and psychosis, respiratory arrest, and death.[111] The acute effects of cocaine do not usually require therapy because the half-life of the drug is less than 60 minutes. Benzodiazepines can be used if sedation is necessary. Increased blood pressure has been treated with nitroprusside or phentolamine, and nitroglycerin and calcium channel blockers have been used for vasoconstriction causing chest pain.[2]

Seizures

The most common neurologic complaints in cocaine use are dizziness and headaches.[110] Seizures occurred in 0.6–16.7% of cocaine users who subsequently were seen in a hospital or clinic.[112, 113] This is probably an underestimate of the true incidence of seizures that occur after cocaine use. Seizures have followed nasal, intravenous, and oral administration and can occur after smoking crack cocaine.[114] Seizures have been described as a preterminal event that occurs after ingestion of an overdose of cocaine.[115] Single, brief primarily generalized seizures are associated with typical acute cocaine use.[116] Seizures usually occur within 90 minutes of use of intravenous or crack cocaine.[113] Status epilepticus has followed acute exposure to cocaine in individuals with no other predisposing factors for seizures. In addition to acute symptomatic seizures after cocaine use, cocaine may lower seizure threshold and precipitate focal or secondarily generalized seizures in individuals with preexisting seizures, stroke, focal neurologic deficits, or concurrent alcohol or other drug use. In one recent series, 21% of cocaine-related seizures were thought to be acute symptomatic, and 79% occurred in patients predisposed to a seizure disorder.[117]

Children are also at risk from seizures from environmentally acquired cocaine. Seizures have occurred in an 11-day-old infant exposed to cocaine from a powder used to treat breast soreness and in toddlers who found cocaine after parties in their parents' home.[118, 119] Children younger than 8 years of age may have either focal or generalized seizures without evidence of structural neurologic damage.[120] Other neurologic symptoms and signs seen in children exposed to cocaine include dizziness, lethargy, obtundation, and delirium.

Movement Disorders

In addition to seizures, patients who use cocaine may present with movement disorders. Dystonia has been related to cocaine withdrawal and has occurred frequently enough in patients using cocaine and who receive neuroleptics that it is assumed that cocaine lowers the threshold for neuroleptic-induced dystonia.[121] Cocaine may cause a new onset of multifocal tics and can lead to exacerbation of symptoms of Tourette's disorder.[122] Daras et al. have described choreoathetosis, akathisia, and parkinsonism with tremor after use of cocaine.[123] These movement disorders seem to resolve spontaneously within a week of abstinence from cocaine.

Stroke

Stroke is the most serious neurologic complication of cocaine. Strokes have been temporally related to cocaine use and have been seen after all routes of cocaine administration. The type of agent used may be important. Levine et al. found that cocaine hydrochloride tended to cause hemorrhagic infarctions, whereas the alkaloid cocaine caused either ischemic or hemorrhagic stroke.[124, 125] In contrast, a study from Grady Hospital Atlanta using a retrospective case-control method did not show any significant association between alkaloid cocaine use and stroke.[126] Patients have developed transient ischemic attacks, ischemic infarctions, intracerebral hemorrhages, and subarachnoid hemorrhages. These strokes may occur within a few hours of cocaine use or after an overnight binge. In addition to cerebral infarctions, thalamic, brain stem, and spinal cord infarctions have occurred.[127–129]

Several different mechanisms have been suggested as possible causes of cocaine-induced strokes. Cocaine has significant effects on the systemic circulation. Sudden elevation in blood pressure may be responsible for strokes. Patients have been described who developed subarachnoid and intracerebral hemorrhages in association with underlying aneurysms and arteriovenous malformations.[130–132] Presumably, the sudden increase in blood pressure caused the rupture of these lesions.

Cocaine may cause cardiomyopathy, myocardial infarction, and cardiac arrhythmias. Intravenous cocaine users are also at risk for endocarditis. These cardiac problems can in turn lead to embolic strokes.[90, 133–136]

Cocaine may have a direct effect on the cerebral circulation.[137] Konzen et al. found angiographic or histopathologic evidence of vasospasm in three patients with cocaine-associated infarctions in the territory of the internal carotid artery.[138] Both angiographic and pathologic evidence of cerebral vasculitis has been found in some series, but not in others.[124, 139–142] In the majority of reports, vasculitis associated with cocaine use does not seem to be a factor. Cocaine appears to be much less likely to cause arteritis than amphetamine or methamphetamine. Kibayashi et al. suggest an interactive process in which cocaine reduces the upper limit of cerebrovascular autoregulation to lower blood pressure levels, which, in the individual with hypertension, may result in vasodilation and increased blood flow with subsequent rupture of vessel walls.[143]

Cocaine has hematologic effects that increase the risk of thrombus formation. It has been associated with increased levels of activated platelets, which are present intermittently and in only some individuals,[144, 145] and has also been shown to cause an increase in plasminogen activator inhibitor. No change in levels of fibrinogen, plasminogen, or lipoprotein has been associated with cocaine administration.[146] Cocaine use may lead to reduced levels of protein C and antithrombin III. This may have an interactive effect, increasing the risk of stroke after cocaine use.[147]

Withdrawal and Psychiatric Complications

Cocaine apparently causes true withdrawal syndromes. Gawin and Kleber describe a sequence of phases of abstinence symptoms.[148] Initially, there is agitation, depression, and insomnia, followed by exhaustion and hypersomnolence. During this phase noradrenergic dysregulation may increase vulnerability to panic attacks. A second phase, occurring 1–10 weeks after abstinence, is characterized by waxing and waning dysphoria. During the third phase, there is normal mood but episodic craving for cocaine prompted by environmental reminders of cocaine use. Chronic users of cocaine may develop a syndrome of cocaine-induced paranoia and hypervigilance during intoxication. In the series by Rosse et al., this syndrome was reported in 68% of chronic users.[149] This may be followed by cocaine-induced compulsive foraging, a persistent picking through the environment for overlooked drug. This latter syndrome has been seen in half of chronic users. Therapy to prevent relapse involves behavioral and supportive therapies. Antidepressants, particularly desipramine, have been shown to be helpful during the dysphoric stage of abstinence.

Pediatric Complications

Does maternal cocaine use during pregnancy imperil the infant? The recent media portrayal of the "crack baby" suggests dire problems for society, but the literature is less convincing. Methodologic issues include difficulties in assessing frequency and dose of drug use; the additional effects of alcohol, marijuana, tobacco, and other drug use; and the potential effects of infections, malnutrition, and poverty. There does seem to be a definite association between cocaine use during pregnancy and both abruptio placenta and premature labor, possibly due to catecholamines released by cocaine increasing uterine contracture or possibly due to a direct effect of cocaine on uterine musculature. Cocaine-exposed infants are smaller, but this may be the effect of shorter gestation. Jacobson et al., studying 417 inner city black infants, found that the reduction in birth size seen in infants exposed to cocaine was best explained by poor maternal nutrition and shorter gestation and that the combined effect of alcohol and tobacco was a stronger predictor of reduced birth weight and length.[150] Kliegman et al. found that cocaine use documented by toxicology at the time of delivery predicted prematurity, but had only a weak predictive effect for intrauterine growth retardation.[151]

Cocaine may be a teratogen with effects on the CNS. Microcephaly, midline prosencephalic anomalies, disorders of neuronal migration and differentiation, and neural tube defects have all been reported after in utero exposure to cocaine.[152] Hoyme et al. described limb reduction defects and intestinal atresia or infarction presumed to be due to a fetal vascular disruption secondary to in utero cocaine exposure.[153] The prenatal onset of cerebral infarction has been seen in cocaine-exposed infants, possibly because of fluctuations in maternal blood pressure and uterine blood flow. The reports of an increased incidence of intraventricular hemorrhage have been less consistent. Gestational age is a major complicating factor. With an increased incidence of premature births, intraventricular hemorrhage may be more a phenomenon of the gestational age of the infant and not a direct toxic effect of cocaine.

There does seem to be a withdrawal syndrome associated with in utero cocaine exposure. Chiriboga et al. described hypertonia, tremor, and gaze abnormalities in cocaine-exposed infants.[154] King et al. did not note tone changes, but found behavioral abnormalities consistent with withdrawal.[155]

Other reported associations of in utero exposure to cocaine are movement disorders and seizures. Beltran and Coker reported dystonia in four infants exposed to cocaine in utero.[156] One infant had generalized dystonia, and three had torticollis. The dystonia resolved over the first year of life. These infants seem to have an increased risk of neonatal seizures, as would be expected from the effect of cocaine on adults. Electroencephalographic abnormalities consisting of discontinuity and bursts of sharp waves and spikes were seen in 17 of 38 infants exposed to cocaine in utero. By 3–12 months of age, 9 of 10 infants with previously abnormal electroencephalograms had normal tracings.[157]

The long-term effect of in utero cocaine exposure has been difficult to determine. Initial studies suggested significant delays in development. Singer et al. found lower cognitive and motor development scores in cocaine-exposed infants even after controlling for intraventricular hemorrhage and chronologic age.[158] Azuma and Chasnoff also found cognitive delays at 3 years of age in these infants, but noted that head circumference, home environment, and perseverance of the child were mediating factors.[159] Snodgrass suggests that the effect of cocaine is but one of several factors adversely affecting the infant.[160] Other major contributors include poor nutrition of the mother, the use of alcohol and other drugs by the mother, and a suboptimal home environment. Zuckerman and Frank recommend assessment during the school-age years for potential deficits in attention, language, and social skills that might result from neurotransmitter changes secondary to prenatal cocaine exposure.[161]

Conclusion

The adverse effects of the therapeutic use of psychostimulants are reasonably well established. Insomnia, anorexia, irritability, and hyperkinetic movement disorders are known complications of the use of methylphenidate, pemoline, and dextroamphetamine at appropriate dosages. The effect on growth is probably limited. In contrast, the adverse effects of stimulant abuse are more controversial. Methodologic problems of these studies include lack of certainty about dose of agent, frequency of use, and the extent of contamination of drug. In addition, the complicating factors of poor nutrition, infections, repeated trauma, and poverty limit our ability to define exact mechanisms of damage in natural population studies. Nevertheless, the extent of health-related problems from these agents is impressive. Seizures and strokes are probable complications of stimulant abuse and dependency, and withdrawal and psychotic reactions occur. This combined with the violence and financial burdens of these agents make them a formidable public health concern.

References

1. Fawcett J, Busch KA. Stimulants in Psychiatry. In AF Schatzberg, CB Nemeroff (eds), The American Psychiatric Press Textbook of Psychopharmacology. Washington, DC: American Psychiatric Press, 1995;417.
2. Brust JCM. Neurological Aspects of Substance Abuse. Boston: Butterworth–Heinemann, 1993;60.
3. Physicians' Desk Reference (50th ed). Montvale, NJ: Medical Economics Company, 1996.
4. Tolman KG, Freston JW, Berenson MM, et al. Hepatotoxicity due to pemoline: report of two cases. Digestion 1973;9:532.
5. Holmes VF. Medical use of psychostimulants: an overview. Int J Psychiatry Med 1995;25:1.
6. Barkley RA. A review of stimulant drug research with hyperactive children. J Child Psychol Psychiatry 1977; 18:137.
7. Hoffman BB, Lefkowitz RJ. Catecholamines, Sympathomimetic Drugs, and Adrenergic Receptor Antagonists. In JG Hardman, LE Limbird (eds), Goodman and Gilman's The Pharmacological Basis of Therapeutics (9th ed). New York: McGraw-Hill, 1996;199.
8. Tirosh E, Sadeh A, Munvez R, et al. Effects of methylphenidate on sleep in children with attention-deficit hyperactivity disorder. Am J Dis Child 1993;147: 1313.
9. Chatoor I, Well KC, Conners CK, et al. The effects of nocturnally administered stimulant medication on EEG sleep and behavior in hyperactive children. J Am Acad Child Adolesc Psychiatry 1983;22:337.
10. Sternbach H. Pemoline-induced mania. Biol Psychiatry 1981;16:987.
11. Pratt DS, Dubois RS. Hepatotoxicity due to pemoline (Cylert): a report of two cases. J Pediatr Gastroenterol Nutr 1990;10:239.
12. Ahmann PA, Waltonen SJ, Olson KA, et al. Placebo-controlled evaluation of Ritalin side effects. Pediatrics 1993;91:1101.
13. Barkley RA, McMurray MB, Edelbrock CS, et al. Side effects of methylphenidate in children with attention deficit hyperactivity disorder: a systemic, placebo-controlled evaluation. Pediatrics 1990;86:184.
14. Foltin RW, Kelly TH, Fischman MW. Effect of amphetamine on human macronutrient intake. Physiol Behav 1995;58:899.
15. Masand P, Pickett P, Murray GB. Psychostimulants for secondary depression in medical illness. Psychosomatics 1992;32:203.
16. Rosse RB, Licamele WL. Slow-release methylphenidate: problems when children chew tablets. J Clin Psychiatry 1984;45:525.
17. Pleak RR. Adverse effects of chewing methylphenidate. Am J Psychiatry 1995;152:811.
18. Mattes JA, Gittelman R. Growth of hyperactive children on maintenance regimen of methylphenidate. Arch Gen Psychiatry 1983;40:317.
19. Vincent J, Varley CK, Leger P. Effects of methylphenidate on early adolescent growth. Am J Psychiatry 1990;147:501.
20. Collier CP, Soldin SJ, Swanson JM, et al. Pemoline pharmacokinetics and long-term treatment in children with attention-deficit disorder and hyperactivity. Clin Pharmacokinet 1985;10:269.
21. Dickinson LC, Lee J, Ringdahl IC, et al. Impaired growth in hyperkinetic children receiving pemoline. J Pediatr 1979;94:538.
22. Satterfield JH, Cantwell DP, Schell A, et al. Growth of

hyperactive children treated with methylphenidate. Arch Gen Psychiatry 1979;36:212.
23. Friedmann M, Thomas J, Carr R, et al. Effect on growth in pemoline-treated children with attention-deficit disorder. Am J Dis Child 1981;135:329.
24. Safer DJ, Allen RP. Factors influencing the suppressant effects of two stimulant drugs on the growth of hyperactive children. Pediatrics 1973;51:660.
25. Safer D, Allen R, Barr E. Depression of growth in hyperactive children on stimulant drugs. N Engl J Med 1972;287:217.
26. Anonymous. Growth of children given stimulant drugs. Nutr Rev 1973;31:91.
27. Klein RG, Landa B, Mattes JA, et al. Methylphenidate and growth in hyperactive children, a controlled withdrawal study. Arch Gen Psychiatry 1988;45:1127.
28. Sallee F, Stiller R, Perel J, et al. Oral pemoline kinetics in hyperactive children. Clin Pharmacol Ther 1985;37:606.
29. Waltz G. Change in response to pemoline at puberty. Am J Psychiatry 1990;147:368.
30. Martin WR, Sloan JJW, Sapira JD, et al. Physiologic, subjective, and behavioral effects of amphetamine, methamphetamine, ephedrine, phenmetrazine, and methylphenidate in man. Clin Pharmacol Ther 1971; 12:245.
31. Brown RT, Wynne ME, Slimmer LW. Attention deficit disorder and the effect of methylphenidate on attention, behavioral and cardiovascular functioning. J Clin Psychiatry 1984;45:473.
32. Golden GS. Gilles de la Tourette's syndrome following methylphenidate administration. Dev Med Child Neurol 1974;16:76.
33. Denckla MB, Bemporad JR, MacKay MD. Tics following methylphenidate administration: a report of 20 cases. JAMA 1976;235:1349.
34. Lipkin PH, Goldstein IJ, Adesman AR. Tics and dyskinesias associated with stimulant treatment in attention-deficit hyperactivity disorder. Arch Pediatr Adolesc Med 1994;148:859.
35. Comings DE, Hines JA, Comings BG. An epidemiological study of Tourette's syndrome in a single school district. J Clin Psychiatry 1990;51:463.
36. Shapiro AK, Shapiro E. Do stimulants provoke, cause, or exacerbate tics and Tourette syndrome. Comp Psychiatry 1988;22:265.
37. Gadow KD, Sverd J. Stimulants for ADHD in child patients with Tourette's syndrome: the issue of relative risk. Dev Behav Pediatr 1990;11:269.
38. Gay CT, Ryan SG. Paroxysmal kinesigenic dystonia after methylphenidate administration. J Child Neurol 1994;9:45.
39. Gadow KD, Nolan E, Sprafkin J, et al. School observations of children with attention-deficit hyperactivity disorder and comorbid tic disorder: effects of methylphenidate treatment. Dev Behav Pediatr 1995; 16:167.
40. Erenberg G, Cruse RP, Rothner AD. Gilles de la Tourette's syndrome: effects of stimulant drugs. Neurology 1985;35:1346.
41. Weiner WJ, Nausieda PA, Klawans HL. Methylphenidate induces chorea: case report and pharmacologic implications. Neurology 1978;28:1041.
42. Mattson FJ, Calverley JF. Dextroamphetamine-sulfate-induced dyskinesias. JAMA 1968;204:108.
43. Case Q, McAndrew JB. Dexedrine dyskinesia: an unusual iatrogenic tic. Clin Pediatr 1974;13:71.
44. Singh BK, Singh A, Chusid E. Chorea in long-term use of pemoline. Ann Neurol 1983;13:218.
45. Sallee FR, Stiller RL, Perel JM, et al. Pemoline-induced abnormal involuntary movements. J Clin Psychopharmacol 1989;9:125.
46. Klawans HL, Weiner WJ. The effect of D-amphetamine on choreiform movement disorders. Neurology 1974; 24:312.
47. Connor DF, Benjamin S, Ozbayrak KR. Case study: neuroleptic withdrawal dyskinesia exacerbated by ongoing stimulant treatment. J Am Acad Child Adolesc Psychiatry 1995;34:1490.
48. Klein RG, Mannuzza S. Hyperactive boys almost grownup. III. Methylphenidate effects upon ultimate height. Arch Gen Psychiatry 1988;45:1131.
49. Wilens TE, Biederman J. The stimulants. Psychiatr Clin North Am 1992;15:191.
50. Rapoport JL, Buchsbaum MS, Zahn TP, et al. Dextroamphetamine: cognitive and behavioral effects in normal prepubertal boys. Science 1978;199:560.
51. Johnston C, Pelham WE, Hoza J, et al. Psychostimulant rebound in attention deficit disordered boys. J Am Acad Child Adolesc Psychiatry 1988;27:806.
52. Bloom AS, Russell LJ, Weisskopf B, et al. Methylphenidate-induced delusional disorder in a child with attention deficit disorder with hyperactivity. J Am Acad Child Adolesc Psychiatry 1988;27:88.
53. Lucas AR, Weiss M. Methylphenidate hallucinosis. JAMA 1971;217:1079.
54. Masand PS, Pickett P, Murray GB. Hypomania precipitated by psychostimulant use in depressed medically ill patients. Psychosomatics 1995;36:145.
55. Koehler-Troy C, Strober M, Malenbaum R. Methylphenidate-induced mania in a prepubertal child. J Clin Psychiatry 1986;47:566.
56. Burd L, Kerbeshian J. Stuttering and stimulants. J Clin Psychopharmacol 1991;11:72.
57. Wroblewski BA, Leary JM, Phelan AM, et al. Methylphenidate and seizure frequency in brain injured patients with seizure disorders. J Clin Psychiatry 1992;53:86.
58. Haglund RMJ, Howerton LL. Ritalin: consequences of abuse in a clinical population. Int J Addict 1982;17:349.
59. Extein I. Methylphenidate-induced choreoathetosis. Am J Psychiatry 1978;135:252.
60. AtLee WE. Talc and cornstarch emboli in eyes of drug abusers. JAMA 1972;219:49.

61. Schatz H, Drake M. Self-injected retinal emboli. Ophthalmology 1979;86:468.
62. Chillar RK, Jackson AL, Alaan L. Hemiplegia after intracarotid injection of methylphenidate. Arch Neurol 1982;39:598.
63. Wolf J, Fein A, Fehrenbacher L. Eosinophilic syndrome with methylphenidate abuse. Ann Intern Med 1978; 89:224.
64. Polchert SE, Morse RM. Pemoline abuse. JAMA 1985;254:946.
65. Nausieda PA, Koller WC, Weiner WJ, et al. Pemoline-induced chorea. Neurology 1981;31:356.
66. Rundell JR, Cassem EH, Murray GB. Exacerbation by dextroamphetamine of spasticity in a patient with motor neuron disease. J Clin Psychopharmacol 1988;8:146.
67. Koizumi HM. Obsessive-compulsive symptoms following stimulants. Biol Psychiatry 1985;20:1332.
68. Sawynok J. Pharmacological rationale for the clinical use of caffeine. Drugs 1995;49:37.
69. Richardson NJ, Rogers PJ, Elliman NA, et al. Mood and performance effects of caffeine in relation to acute and chronic caffeine deprivation. Pharm Biochem Behav 1995;52:313.
70. Bernstein GA, Carroll ME, Crosby RD, et al. Caffeine effects on learning, performance, and anxiety in normal school-age children. J Am Acad Child Adolesc Psychiatry 1994;33:407.
71. Pentel P. Toxicity of over-the-counter stimulants. JAMA 1984;252:1898.
72. Brown SL, Salive ME, Pahor M, et al. Occult caffeine as a source of sleep problems in an older population. J Am Geriatr Soc 1995;43:860.
73. Boulenger J, Uhde TW, Wolff EA, et al. Increased sensitivity to caffeine in patients with panic disorders. Preliminary evidence. Arch Gen Psychiatry 1984;41:1067.
74. Silverman K, Evans SM, Strain EC, et al. Withdrawal syndrome after the double-blind cessation of caffeine consumption. N Engl J Med 1992;327:1109.
75. Purvin VA, Dunn DW. Caffeine and the benign encephalopathy of pregnancy. Acta Neurol Scand 1987;75:76.
76. Reeves RR, Struve FA, Patrick G, et al. Topographic quantitative EEG measures of alpha and theta power changes during caffeine withdrawal: preliminary findings from normal subjects. Clin Electroenceph 1995;26:154.
77. Patrick G, Reeves RR, Struve FA. Does caffeine cessation increase firing rates of diffuse paroxysmal slowing dysrhythmia? A serendipitous observation. Clin Electroenceph 1996;27:78.
78. Taylor P. Agents Acting at the Neuromuscular Junction and Autonomic Ganglia. In JG Hardman, LE Limbird (eds), Goodman & Gilman's The Pharmacological Basis of Therapeutics (9th ed). New York: McGraw-Hill, 1996;177.
79. Diagnostic and Statistical Manual of Mental Disorders (4th ed). Washington, DC: American Psychiatric Association, 1994.
80. Krumsiek J, Krüger C, Patzold U. Tobacco-alcohol amblyopia neuro-ophthalmological findings and clinical course. Acta Neurol Scand 1985;72:180.
81. Rizzo JF, Lessell S. Tobacco amblyopia. Am J Ophthal 1993;116:84.
82. Holman RB. Biological effects of central nervous system stimulants. Addiction 1994;89:1435.
83. Lake CR, Quirk RS. CNS stimulants and the look-alike drugs. Psychiatric Clin North Am 1984;7:689.
84. Baberg HT, Nelesen RA, Dimsdale JE. Amphetamine use: return of an old scourge in a consultation psychiatry setting. Am J Psychiatry 1996;153:789.
85. Gawin FH, Khalsa ME, Ellinwood E. Stimulants. In M Galanter, HD Kleber (eds), The American Psychiatric Press Textbook of Substance Abuse Treatment. Washington, DC: American Psychiatric Press, 1994;111.
86. Green WH. Child and Adolescent Clinical Psychopharmacology (2nd ed). Baltimore: Williams & Wilkins, 1995.
87. Alldredge BK, Lowenstein DH, Simon RP. Seizures associated with recreational drug abuse. Neurology 1989;39:1037.
88. Lowenstein DH, Allredge BK. Status epilepticus at an urban public hospital in the 1980s. Neurology 1993; 43:483.
89. Caplan LR, Hier DB, Banks G. Current concepts of cerebrovascular disease—stroke: stroke and drug abuse. Stroke 1982;13:869.
90. Kaku DA, Lowenstein DH. Emergence of recreational drug abuse as a major risk factor for stroke in young adults. Ann Intern Med 1990;113:821.
91. Yen DJ, Wang SJ, Ju TH, et al. Stroke associated with methamphetamine inhalation. Eur Neurol 1994;34:16.
92. Delaney P, Estes M. Intracranial hemorrhage with amphetamine abuse. Neurology 1980;30:1125.
93. Matick H, Anderson D, Brumlik J. Cerebral vasculitis associated with oral amphetamine overdose. Arch Neurol 1983;40:253.
94. Harrington H, Heller HA, Dawson D, et al. Intracerebral hemorrhage and oral amphetamine. Arch Neurol 1983;40:503.
95. Rumbaugh CL, Bergeron RT, Fang HCH, et al. Cerebral angiographic changes in the drug abuse patient. Radiology 1971;101:335.
96. Rumbaugh CL, Bergeron RT, Scanlan RL, et al. Cerebral vascular changes secondary to amphetamine abuse in the experimental animal. Radiology 1971;101:345.
97. Citron BP, Halpern M, McCarron M, et al. Necrotizing angiitis associated with drug abuse. N Engl J Med 1970;283:1003.
98. Flaum M, Schultz SK. When does amphetamine-induced psychosis become schizophrenia? Am J Psychiatry 1996;153:812.
99. Oro AS, Dixon SD. Perinatal cocaine and methamphetamine exposure: maternal and neonatal correlates. J Pediatr 1987;111:571.
100. Eriksson M, Larsson G, Winbladh B, et al. The influ-

ence of amphetamine addiction on pregnancy and the newborn infant. Acta Paediatr Scand 1978;67:95.
101. Matthai SM, Davidson DC, Sills JA, et al. Cerebral oedema after ingestion of MDMA ("ecstasy") and unrestricted intake of water. BMJ 1996;312:1359.
102. Henry JA, Jeffreys KJ, Dawling S. Toxicity and deaths from 3,4-methylenedioxymethamphetamine. Lancet 1992;340:384.
103. Lake CR, Gallant S, Masson E, et al. Adverse drug effects attributed to phenylpropanolamine: a review of 142 case reports. Am J Med 1990;89:195.
104. Mueller SM. Neurologic complications of phenylpropanolamine. Neurology 1983;33:650.
105. Fallis RJ, Fisher M. Cerebral vasculitis and hemorrhage associated with phenylpropanolamine. Neurology 1985;35:405.
106. Marshall RD, Douglas CJ. Phenylpropanolamine-induced psychosis. Potential predisposing factors. Gen Hosp Psychiatry 1994;16:358.
107. Pentel P. Toxicity of over-the-counter stimulants. JAMA 1984;252:1898.
108. Ticoll B, Shugar G. Paranoid psychosis induced by oxymetazoline nasal spray. Can Med Assoc J 1994; 150:375.
109. Farrar HC, Kearns GL. Cocaine: clinical pharmacology and toxicity. J Pediatr 1989;115:665.
110. Brody SL, Slovis CM, Wrenn KD. Cocaine-related medical problems: consecutive series of 233 patients. Am J Med 1990;88:325.
111. Wetli CV, Mash D, Karch SB. Cocaine-associated agitated delirium and the neuroleptic malignant syndrome. Am J Emerg Med 1996;4:425.
112. Harden CL, Daras M, Tuchman AJ. Cocaine causing convulsions in a large municipal hospital population. J Epilepsy 1992;5:175.
113. Pascual-Leone A, Dhuna A, Altafullah I, et al. Cocaine-induced seizures. Neurology 1990;40:404.
114. Choy-Kwong M, Lipton RB. Seizures in hospitalized cocaine users. Neurology 1989;39:425.
115. Mittleman RE, Wetli CV. Death caused by recreational cocaine use. An update. JAMA 1984;252:1889.
116. Myers JA, Earnest MP. Generalized seizures and cocaine abuse. Neurology 1984;34:675.
117. Koppel BS, Samkoff L, Daras M. Relation of cocaine use to seizures and epilepsy. Epilepsia 1996;37:875.
118. Chaney NE, Franke J, Wadlington WB. Cocaine convulsions in a breast-feeding baby. J Pediatr 1988; 112:134.
119. Rivkin M, Gilmore HE. Generalized seizures in an infant due to environmentally acquired cocaine. Pediatrics 1989;84:1100.
120. Mott SH, Packer RJ, Soldin SJ. Neurologic manifestations of cocaine exposure in childhood. Pediatrics 1994;93:557.
121. Choy-Kwong M, Lipton RB. Dystonia related to cocaine withdrawal: a case report and pathogenic hypothesis. Neurology 1989;39:996.
122. Pascual-Leone A, Dhuna A. Cocaine-associated multifocal tics. Neurology 1990;40:999.
123. Daras M, Koppel BS, Atos-Radzion E. Cocaine-induced choreoathetoid movements ("crack dancing"). Neurology 1994;44:751.
124. Levine SR, Brust JCM, Futrell N, et al. Cerebrovascular complications of the use of the "crack" form of alkaloidal cocaine. N Engl J Med 1990;323:699.
125. Levine SR, Brust JCM, Futrell N, et al. A comparative study of the cerebrovascular complications of cocaine: alkaloidal versus hydrochloride—a review. Neurology 1991;41:1173.
126. Qureshi AI, Akbar MS, Czander E, et al. Crack cocaine use and stroke in young patients. Neurology 1997; 48:341.
127. Lowenstein DH, Massa SM, Rowbotham MC, et al. Acute neurologic and psychiatric complications associated with cocaine abuse. Am J Med 1987;83:841.
128. Mody CK, Miller BL, McIntyre HB, et al. Neurologic complications of cocaine abuse. Neurology 1988;38:1189.
129. Rowley HA, Lowenstein DH, Rowbotham MC, et al. Thalamomesencephalic strokes after cocaine abuse. Neurology 1989;39:428.
130. Lichtenfeld PJ, Rubin DB, Feldman RS. Subarachnoid hemorrhage precipitated by cocaine snorting. Arch Neurol 1984;41:223.
131. Klonoff DC, Andrews BT, Obana WG. Stroke associated with cocaine use. Arch Neurol 1989;46:989.
132. Daras M, Tuchman AJ, Koppel BS, et al. Neurovascular complications of cocaine. Acta Neurol Scand 1994; 90:124.
133. Petty GW, Brust JCM, Tatemichi TK, et al. Embolic stroke after smoking "crack" cocaine. Stroke 1990; 21:1632.
134. Sauer CM. Recurrent embolic stroke and cocaine-related cardiomyopathy. Stroke 1991;22:1203.
135. Daras M, Tuchman AJ, Marks S. Central nervous system infarction related to cocaine abuse. Stroke 1991;22:1320.
136. Sloan MA, Mattioni TA. Concurrent myocardial and cerebral infarctions after intranasal cocaine use. Stroke 1992;23:427.
137. Nolte KB, Gelman BB. Intracerebral hemorrhage associated with cocaine abuse. Arch Pathol Lab Med 1989; 113:812.
138. Konzen JP, Levine SR, Garcia JH. Vasospasm and thrombus formation as possible mechanisms of stroke related to alkaloidal cocaine. Stroke 1995;26:1114.
139. Krendel DA, Ditter SM, Frankel MR, et al. Biopsy-proven cerebral vasculitis associated with cocaine abuse. Neurology 1990;40:1092.
140. Gradon JD, Wityk R. Diagnosis of probable cocaine-induced cerebral vasculitis by magnetic resonance angiography. South Med J 1995;88:1264.
141. Aggarwal SK, Williams V, Levine SR, et al. Cocaine-associated intracranial hemorrhage: absence of vasculitis in 14 cases. Neurology 1996;46:1741.

142. Nolte KB, Brass LM, Fletterick CF. Intracranial hemorrhage associated with cocaine abuse: a prospective study. Neurology 1996;46:1291.
143. Kibayashi K, Mastri AR, Hirsch CS. Cocaine induced intracerebral hemorrhage: analysis of predisposing factors and mechanisms causing hemorrhagic strokes. Hum Pathol 1995;26:659.
144. Kugelmass AD, Oda A, Monahan K, Cabral C, et al. Activation of human platelets by cocaine. Circulation 1993;88:876.
145. Rinder HM, Ault KA, Jatlow PI, et al. Platelet alpha-granule release in cocaine users. Circulation 1994; 90:1162.
146. Moliterno DJ, Lange RA, Gerard RD, et al. Influence of intranasal cocaine on plasma constituents associated with endogenous thrombosis and thrombolysis. Am J Med 1994;96:492.
147. Martínez N, Díez-Tejedor E, Frank A. Vasospasm/thrombus in cerebral ischemia related to cocaine abuse. Stroke 1996;27:147.
148. Gawin FH, Kleber HD. Abstinence symptomatology and psychiatric diagnosis in cocaine abusers. Arch Gen Psychiatry 1986;43:107.
149. Rosse RB, Fay-McCarthy M, Collins JP, et al. The relationship between cocaine-induced paranoia and compulsive foraging: a preliminary report. Addiction 1994;89:1097.
150. Jacobson JL, Jacobson SW, Sokol RJ, et al. Effects of alcohol use, smoking, and illicit drug use on fetal growth in black infants. J Pediatr 1994;124:757.
151. Kliegman RM, Madura D, Kiwi R, et al. Relation of maternal cocaine use to the risks of prematurity and low birth weight. J Pediatr 1994;124:751.
152. Volpe JJ. Neurology of the Newborn (3rd ed). Philadelphia: Saunders, 1995;824.
153. Hoyme HE, Jones KL, Dixon SD, et al. Prenatal cocaine exposure and fetal vascular disruption. Pediatrics 1990;85:743.
154. Chiriboga CA, Bateman DA, Brust JCM, et al. Neurologic findings in neonates with intrauterine cocaine exposure. Pediatr Neurol 1993;9:115.
155. King TA, Perlman JM, Laptook AR, et al. Neurologic manifestations of in utero cocaine exposure in near-term and term infants. Pediatrics 1995;96:259.
156. Beltran RS, Coker SB. Transient dystonia of infancy, a result of intrauterine cocaine exposure? Pediatr Neurol 1995;12:354.
157. Doberczak TM, Shanzer S, Senie RT, et al. Neonatal neurologic and electroencephalographic effects of intrauterine cocaine exposure. J Pediatr 1988;113: 354.
158. Singer LT, Yamashita TS, Hawkins S, et al. Increased incidence of intraventricular hemorrhage and developmental delay in cocaine-exposed, very low birth weight infants. J Pediatr 1994;124:765.
159. Azuma SD, Chasnoff IJ. Outcome of children prenatally exposed to cocaine and other drugs: a path analysis of three-year data. Pediatrics 1993;92:396.
160. Snodgrass SR. Cocaine babies: a result of multiple teratogenic influences. J Child Neurol 1994;9:227.
161. Zuckerman B, Frank DA. Prenatal cocaine exposure: nine years later. J Pediatr 1994;124:731.

Chapter 23

Complications of Botulinum Toxin

Allison Brashear

Objectives

- To review the mechanism of action of botulinum toxin (BTX) type A in the treatment of patients with movement disorders, spasticity, and other neurologic disorders
- To become familiar with the many uses of BTX in clinical practice
- To recognize the common side effects associated with the use of BTX in clinical practice
- To understand the relationship between possible side effects of BTX to the site treated and dosage of drug used
- To appreciate the role of immunity in the use of BTX
- To appreciate the role of BTX in benefiting many patients with chronic neurologic disorders

Mechanism of Action of Botulinum Toxin

Clostridium botulinum, long feared as the world's deadliest toxin, capable of killing those ingesting a trace amount, is now a medical treatment for many patients. First introduced in 1979 as a treatment for strabismus,[1] BTX provides clinical benefits to individuals with movement disorders, spasticity, and other disorders caused by increased muscle tone.[2] The source of the toxin is the organism *C. botulinum*, capable of synthesizing seven unique toxin serotypes, labeled A–G.[3] Although only type A has been approved for clinical use in the United States, research is continuing into the clinical use of serotypes B and F.

Each serotype of BTX is synthesized as a single chain polypeptide, and later nicked by a protease enzyme to form a dichain held together by a single disulfide bond. The disulfide bond is reduced, separating to form light and heavy chains. The heavy chain binds to high affinity receptors on the presynaptic nerve terminals at the neuromuscular junction; the light chain enters the cytosol and blocks the neurotransmitter release of acetylcholine.[3] Thus, nerve impulses from the nerve cell body are unable to trigger acetylcholine release from the presynaptic nerve terminal and activate the postsynaptic muscle fibers.

The BTX injected locally acts at the neuromuscular junctions to cause muscle weakness and atrophy. However, the toxin has an effect elsewhere in the nervous system.[4] Radionucleotide studies in animals have documented retrograde transmission of the toxin to the anterior horn cells as well as nearby segments of the spinal cord.[3, 5]

Electromyographic studies in eight patients treated with small doses of BTX in the neck demonstrated subclinical electrical changes on single-fiber needle examination in the neuromuscular junction in distant foot muscles.[6] Such changes on single-fiber electromyography suggest spread of the toxin to distant muscles by blood flow or retrograde axonal transport.[6] Although these studies demonstrate remote changes in the motor unit, no findings of clinical weakness have been identified in those individuals studied. To date, young children and elderly adults have been treated with BTX with no long-term side effects reported.[7–10]

The clinical effects of BTX may last 8 weeks to 6 months, depending on the site of injection, dose used, and the individual response of the patient treated.[2] All clinical effects of BTX resolve with time, and symptoms of spasm recur, unless further injections of BTX are administered. Within 1–2 weeks of the injection, the affected nerve terminal resprouts new neuromuscular junctions. Large denervated terminal branches spread out to reinnervate the nearby denervated muscle.[11] Although repair from BTX injection begins microscopically within weeks, the weakness and atrophy of the injected muscle may last for months. Gradually, 2–4 months after a BTX treatment, resprouting of the nerve terminals results in increased muscle strength, resolution of atrophy, and recurrence of spasm in the overactive muscle.

The current accepted clinical indications of BTX include focal dystonia, spasticity, and hemifacial spasm. Each indication has side effects related to the dose of BTX used and the site injected.

Clinical Indications

Focal Dystonia

Dystonia is an involuntary movement disorder with uncontrollable twisting and turning spasms that are often painful and disabling. Dystonia may affect the entire body (generalized) or one anatomic area (focal). Types of focal dystonia include twisting and turning of the neck (torticollis), uncontrollable blinking (blepharospasm), limb dystonia (including writer's cramp), vocal dystonia (spasmodic dysphonia), and oromandibular dystonia (spasms with the jaw open or closed).

Torticollis

Torticollis, a painful involuntary twisting and turning of the neck muscles, may present at any age. Localized injections of BTX to the overactive agonist muscles of the neck cause localized weakness. Thus, the underactive antagonist muscles are allowed to function normally. Benefits of periodic BTX injections include improved range of motion and decreased pain.[2] Generally, improvement is noted in 3–7 days after injections, and benefits last anywhere from 2 to 6 months.[2, 8, 12–21]

Iatrogenic side effects from localized injections to the neck for torticollis include dysphagia, neck weakness, and difficulty opening the jaw.[8, 12–21] Comella et al. studied 18 patients with torticollis before and after treatment with BTX and reported 33% of individuals studied described new dysphagia and 50% had abnormal radiologic swallowing studies.[22] Those who complained of swallowing difficulties always had accompanying radiologic abnormalities. Neither the dose of BTX injected nor the muscles injected predicted which individuals would develop swallowing problems.[22] Rarely, an exacerbation of an underlying radiculopathy[23] or plexopathy[24] has been reported after injections of BTX in neck muscles. Few patients report systemic effects of fever or malaise for a few days after the injections.[2] All of the side effects of injections for torticollis begin several days after the injections and last for 1–2 weeks. Dysphagia can usually be managed by eating slowly or changing to a thick liquid diet while symptoms persist. Rarely, individuals require brief treatment with a nasogastric feeding tube.

Blepharospasm

Blepharospasm, an uncontrollable blinking of the eyelids, may result in functional blindness. Until the introduction of BTX, the only available treatments were oral medication and surgery, with neither providing substantial relief. Injections of BTX for blepharospasm are given subcutaneously to the orbicularis oris to the overactive muscle causing excessive blinking and allow the eye to remain open.[2, 25–27]

Side effects of BTX injections for blepharospasm include ptosis due to spread of the BTX to the nearby levator palpebrae muscle located on the middle of the eyelid. Weakness of this eye opening muscle may result in drooping of the eyelid. Typically, if ptosis develops, it lasts 1–2 weeks. Patients may find this to be of concern for cosmetic reasons, and excessive drooping of the lid may result in visual problems. An excessive weakness of the orbicularis oris may result in difficulty closing the eyelid. The patient may report seeing light when the eye has been closed for sleep, or soap may enter the closed eyelid while bathing. Neither side effect is severely disabling and can be managed with patching the eye closed when needed. While injections of BTX may result in less frequent eye blinking, some patients may complain of dry eye. This is easily managed with frequent administration of artificial tears. Last, a few individuals treated with BTX may report a brief period of double vision due to extension of the BTX injections into the nearby inferior oblique muscle.

Limb Dystonia

Limb dystonia, including writer's cramp, may be the most under-reported form of focal dystonia.[2, 28–31] Involuntary spasms occur when an individual initiates use of the arm or hand. Typically, these occur with writing, but may follow other movements, such as typing or playing a musical instrument. Until the use of BTX, treatment of limb dystonia was limited to adaptive instruments for writing and retraining to write with the other hand.[2, 28, 29]

Side effects of BTX injections for limb dystonia include transient, reversible arm and hand weakness.[28–31] Weakness may occur in nearby muscles, not targeted for injection, due to diffusion of toxin through muscle planes.[30] Weakness generally lasts 1–2 weeks and resolves, but during that time the patient may find the hand or arm difficult to use. Pullman et al. noted excessive weakness in one-third of dystonia patients treated with BTX.[30] In most cases they noted excessive weakness in the finger extensors after injection of the wrist extensors.[30] Similarly, Yoshimura et al. treated 17 patients with limb dystonia with BTX, and although 82% of the patients treated noted subjective improvement, 53% noted focal weakness after treatment.[31] More significant weakness was noted in those individuals who received higher doses, but improvement was also more likely in this group. Sheehan et al. reported a localized pain resembling neuralgic amyotrophy in two patients treated with BTX for limb dystonia.[32] Based on their experience, Sheehan et al. believe that severe unexplained pain in the upper arm or shoulder after BTX injections in that limb is a contraindication to further BTX treatment.[32] More mild side effects of bruising, transient pain at the injection site, and atrophy of the muscles injected have also been reported.[29] Despite the improvement reported in many studies with BTX injections for limb dystonia, patients may still complain of a loss of coordination from the dystonic movements. In professional musicians, BTX improves the abnormal movement, but is often insufficient to return them to a professional level of playing.[33] A long-term study from the National Institutes of Health of 37 patients with focal hand dystonia who were treated for 2 years with periodic BTX injections noted that 24 individuals discontinued treatment because of inadequate response, inaccessibility to a qualified provider, or expense of the treatment.[29]

Spasmodic Dysphonia

Spasmodic dysphonia is an involuntary spasm of the vocal chords causing tight spastic speech.[34] Patients often describe voice breaks (periods of no speech) and a tightness in the throat while attempting to talk. Symptoms of spasmodic dysphonia are made worse by stress, such as public speaking, talking on the telephone, and fatigue.[34, 35] Until the use of BTX, treatment of spasmodic dysphonia was limited to surgical sectioning of the recurrent laryngeal nerve.[26]

Side effects of BTX injections into the vocal chord for spasmodic dysphonia include a breathy, soft voice and dysphagia.[36] The voice changes are due to the excessive weakness of the vocalis resulting in poor adduction or closure of the chords. Breathiness may last up to a month and always resolves spontaneously.[37, 38] The dysphagia described by patients occurs when BTX spreads to nearby pharyngeal muscles. Symptoms may be managed conservatively by changing to a thick liquid diet and tucking the chin when swallowing. Dysphagia generally resolves within 2–4 weeks after the injections.[36]

Oromandibular Dystonia

Oromandibular dystonia may present as difficulty opening or closing the jaw when eating or talking. The overactive muscles in the jaw-opening dystonia include overactivity of the muscles of mastication, masseters, medial pterygoids, and temporalis. The more rare form of jaw-closing dystonia involves spasm of the lateral pterygoid muscles and occasionally the digastric muscles located below the jaw.

Side effects of the injections of either set of muscles may result in excessive weakness of the jaw.

The transient excessive weakness resolves spontaneously after 1–2 weeks and does not need further treatment. A few patients report mild dysphagia, but changes in diet are rarely needed.

Spasticity

BTX has recently been shown to be efficacious in the treatment of spasticity associated with cerebral palsy and stroke.[7, 9, 10] Injections in lower limbs in children with hypertonia and a nonfixed joint contracture demonstrated improved range of motion and functional gait assessment and decreased muscle tone.[7, 9] A preliminary study in patients with upper limb spasticity after stroke demonstrated reduced muscle tone after treatment with BTX. Benefits of the injections peaked at 2 weeks, with return of spasticity 10 weeks after injections.[10] Side effects of injection in both the upper and lower extremity for spasticity include soreness at the injection site and occasional weakness of the injected limb.[7, 9] Benefits of the injections last 2–6 months and may be enhanced when combined with continued physical therapy. The need for repeat injections, particularly in children, should be reevaluated periodically. Young children with cerebral palsy treated early may not require continued serial injections if the treatments are combined with appropriate orthopedic care and physical therapy.

Immunity to Botulinum Toxin

Rarely, individuals treated with repeated BTX injections may spontaneously develop a lack of response to the treatment after previously receiving benefit from the injections. An acquired nonresponse to BTX injections may be explained by injection technique, a lack of potency of the particular vial of toxin, an incorrect choice of muscles to be injected, or an immunogenetic response to BTX. Botulinum toxin antibodies have been demonstrated in some patients who lose their clinical response to the treatments. Recent studies have shown that such nonresponders who had two consecutive injections without a clinical response were younger and treated with a higher dose.[39] The presence of the BTX antibody may be detected by a bioassay. The results of the assay are reported as positive if a patient's blood acts to protect a mouse subsequently injected with the toxin. If the mouse survives a lethal dose of BTX, the patient's serum is presumed to have antibodies that were passed on to the mouse. However, the mouse bioassay has a low sensitivity and a negative result does not dismiss the presence of antibodies.[40] Other biochemical techniques, such as the enzyme-linked immunosorbent assay, need to be further studied before they can be used in clinical practice. Regardless of antibody status, those patients who do not respond to BTX may be candidates for treatment with other serotypes of BTX currently under development.

References

1. Scott AB. Botulinum toxin injections into extraocular muscles as an alternative to strabismus surgery. Ophthalmology 1980;87:1044.
2. Jankovic J, Brin M. Therapeutic uses of botulinum toxin. N Engl J Med 1994;324:1186.
3. Oguma K, Fujinaga Y, Inoue K. Structure and function of *Clostridium botulinum* toxins. Microbiology Immunology 1995;39:161.
4. Simpson LL. Botulinum Neurotoxin and Tetanus. San Diego: Academic, 1989.
5. Williams RS, Tse CK, Dolly JO, et al. Radioiodination of botulinum neurotoxin type A with retention of biological activity and its binding to brain synaptosomes. Eur J Biochem 1983;131:437.
6. Garner CG, Straube A, Witt TN, et al. Time course of distant effects of local injections of botulinum toxin. Mov Disord 1993;8:33.
7. Koman LA, Mooney JF, Smith B, et al. Management of cerebral palsy with botulinum-A toxin: preliminary investigation. J Pediatr Orthop 1993;13:489.
8. Koay CE, Alun-Jones T. Pharyngeal paralysis due to botulinum toxin. J Laryngol Otol 1989;103:698.
9. Calderon-Gonzalez R, Calderon-Sepulveda R, Rincon-Reyes M, et al. Botulinum toxin A in management of cerebral palsy. Pediatr Neurol 1994;10:284.
10. Simpson DM, Alexander MD, O'Brien C, et al. Botulinum toxin type A in the treatment of upper extremity spasticity. Neurology 1996;46:1306.
11. Hamjian JA, Walker FO. Serial neuropsychological studies of intramuscular botulinum-A toxin in humans. Muscle & Nerve 1994;17:1385.
12. Brin MF, Fahn S, Moskowitz C, et al. Localized injections of botulinum toxin for the treatment of focal dystonia and hemifacial spasm. Mov Disord 1987;2:237.
13. Tsui JKC, Fross RD, Calne S, et al. Local treatment of spasmodic torticollis with botulinum toxin. Can J Neurol Sci 1987;14:533.

14. Stell R, Thompason PD, Marsden CD. Botulinum toxin in spasmodic torticollis. J Neurol Neurosurg Psychiatry 1988;51:920.
15. Borodic GE, Joseph M, Fay L, et al. Botulinum A toxin for the treatment of spasmodic torticollis: dysphagia and regional toxin spread. Head Neck 1990;12:392.
16. Gelb DJ, Lowenstein DH, Aminoff MJ. Controlled trial of botulinum toxin injections in the treatment of spasmodic torticollis. Neurology 1989;39:80.
17. Greene P, Kane U, Fan S, et al. Double-blind, placebo-controlled trial of botulinum toxin injections for the treatment of spasmodic torticollis. Neurology 1990; 40:1213.
18. Blackie JD, Lees AJ. Botulinum toxin treatment in spasmodic torticollis. J Neurol Neurosurg Psychiatry 1990;53:640.
19. Peowe W, Wagner M, Kleedorfer B, et al. Botulinum toxin A on the treatment of spasmodic torticollis: a one year follow-up study [abstract]. Mov Disord 1990;5:74.
20. Comella CL, Buchman AS, Tanner CM. Frequency of dysphagia following Botox injection for spasmodic torticollis [abstract]. Mov Disord 1990;5:75.
21. Jankovic J, Schwartz K. Botulinum toxin injections for cervical dystonia. Neurology 1990;40:277.
22. Comella CL, Tanner CM, DeFoor-Hill L, et al. Dysphagia after botulinum toxin injections for spasmodic torticollis. Neurology 1992;42:1307.
23. Defazio G, Lepore V, Cataldo M, et al. Cervical radiculopathy following botulinum toxin therapy for cervical dystonia. Func Neurol 1993;8:193.
24. Sampaio C, Castro-Caldas A, Sales-Luis ML, et al. Brachial plexopathy after Botulinum toxin administration for cervical dystonia [letter]. J Neurol Neurosurg Psychiatry 1993;56:220.
25. Assessment: the clinical usefulness of botulinum toxin-A in treating neurologic disorders. Report of the Therapeutics and Technology Assessment Subcommittee of the American Academy of Neurology. Neurology 1990;40:1332.
26. Clinical use of botulinum toxin. NIH Consensus Development Conference Consensus Statement, Vol 8. Bethesda, MD: National Institutes of Health, 1990;1.
27. American Academy of Ophthalmology. Botulinum toxin therapy of eye muscle disorders. Safety and effectiveness. Ophthalmology 1989;2:37.
28. Cohen LG, Hallett M, Geller BD, et al. Treatment of focal dystonias of the hand with botulinum toxin injections. J Neurol Neurosurg Psychiatry 1989;52:355.
29. Karp BI, Cole RA, Cohen LG, et al. Long-term botulinum toxin treatment of focal hand dystonia. Neurology 1994;44:70.
30. Pullman S, Greene P, Fahn S, et al. Approach to the treatment of limb disorders with botulinum toxin A: experience with 187 patients. Arch Neurol 1996; 53:617.
31. Yoshimura DM, Aminoff MJ, Olney RK. Botulinum toxin therapy for limb dystonias. Neurology 1992;42: 627.
32. Sheehan GL, Murray NMF, Marsden CD. Pain and remote weakness in limbs injected with botulinum toxin A for writer's cramp. Lancet 1995;346:154.
33. Cole RA, Cohen LG, Hallett M. Treatment of musician's cramp with botulinum toxin. Med Prob Perf Art 1991;6:137.
34. Blitzer A, Brin MF, Fahn S, et al. Clinical and laboratory characteristics of focal laryngeal dystonia: study of 110 cases. Laryngoscope 1988;98:636.
35. Ludlow CL, Connor NP. Dynamic aspects of phonatory control in spasmodic dysphonia. J Speech Hear Res 1987;30:197.
36. Sedory-Holzer SE, Ludlow CL. The swallowing side effects of botulinum toxin type A injection in spasmodic dysphonia. Laryngoscope 1996;106:86.
37. Ludlow CL, Nauton RF, Sedory SE, et al. Effects of botulinum toxin injections on speech in adductor spasmodic dysphonia. Neurology 1988;38:1220.
38. Ludlow CL, Bagley JA, Yin SG, et al. A comparison of different injection techniques in the treatment of spasmodic dysphonia with botulinum toxin. J Voice 1992; 6:380.
39. Jankovic J, Schwartz K. Response and immunoresistance to botulinum toxin injections. Neurology 1995; 45:1743.
40. Borodic G, Johnson E, Goodnough M, et al. Botulinum toxin therapy, immunologic resistance, and problems with available materials. Neurology 1996;46:26.

Chapter 24
Complications of Chemotherapy

Nina A. Paleologos

Objectives

- To understand the common and dose-limiting neurologic toxicities of many antineoplastic agents
- To appreciate the less common, but sometimes life-threatening, neurologic toxicities of some antineoplastic agents
- To understand that antineoplastic drugs in the same class are likely to cause similar neurotoxicities
- To understand that the neurotoxicity of some agents can be greatly increased when combined with cranial or spinal radiotherapy
- To recognize the unique neurotoxic syndromes that some agents cause when combined with other drugs
- To recognize the neurologic complications of the biologic modifiers frequently used in patients with neoplastic disease

Neurotoxicity is a common complication of antineoplastic agents and can be dose limiting. Symptoms can occur during treatment, shortly after treatment, or can be delayed by weeks to months following treatment. Disability may be mild and easily reversible and therefore acceptable, or it can be fatal. In some patients, significant disability can persist long after they are successfully treated for the underlying malignancy. The diagnosis may be difficult and needs to be differentiated from symptoms caused by metastatic disease, opportunistic infection, metabolic derangements, and toxicities of other agents frequently taken by cancer patients, such as anticonvulsants, antibiotics, antiemetics, and pain medications. High-dose therapy, combination chemotherapy, and intracarotid or intrathecal administration are usually associated with neurotoxicities more severe than that seen with standard oral or intravenous therapy. Some drugs work synergistically with other drugs or with radiotherapy, causing more serious neurotoxicity or unique syndromes.

Both the peripheral nervous system and central nervous system (CNS) can be affected by chemotherapy. Diffuse peripheral neuropathy is common. An often painful, pure sensory or sensorimotor neuropathy is routinely seen with the microtubule agents and cis-platinum. At times, the neuropathy can present acutely or subacutely mimicking Guillain-Barré syndrome. Focal neuropathies are less common but can also occur, at times associated with intra-arterial therapy.

CNS complications are also common. Acute encephalopathy often is accompanied by seizures and is frequently reversible. Chronic encephalopathy can be a severely debilitating complication, characterized by dementia, apraxia, and seizures. It is usually seen in patients who have also had cranial radiation and is usually irreversible, at times with progressive symptoms and changes on neuroimaging studies. Specific focal syndromes include cerebellar disorders, myelopathy, visual deficits, aseptic meningitis, headache, stroke-like episodes, and extrapyramidal disorders.

Antimetabolites

The antifolates, cytidine analogues, fluorinated pyrimidines, purine analogues, and other miscellaneous antimetabolites are commonly used antineoplastic agents. Most have some degree of neurotoxicity.

Antifolates

Folate-dependent enzymes play a critical role in the synthesis of the nucleotide precursors of DNA. The antifolate drugs inhibit these enzymes, particularly dihydrofolate reductase, depleting reduced folates and causing inhibition of purine and thymidine biosynthesis.

Methotrexate

The neurotoxicity of methotrexate (MTX) is dose and route dependent. Neurotoxicity is also determined by prior or concurrent use of other therapies with overlapping or synergistic neurotoxicity. MTX has little neurotoxicity when used orally or in lower intravenous doses unless cranial irradiation has also been given. Multimodality therapy with prior or concurrent cranial radiotherapy is more likely to produce neurotoxicity than MTX alone.[1] MTX crosses the blood-brain barrier poorly, limited by low lipid solubility and slow passive diffusion. Cerebrospinal fluid (CSF) pharmacokinetics have been studied; however, blood-to-brain and CSF-to-brain pharmacokinetics are not well understood in humans.[2–4] High-dose intravenous MTX (more than 1 g per m^2) and intrathecal MTX (IT-MTX) are associated with acute (within 24–48 hours), subacute (days to weeks after treatment), and chronic (3 months or more) encephalopathy. The acute encephalopathy associated with high-dose intravenous MTX and IT-MTX presents with seizures, confusion, lethargy or stupor, and headache. It usually resolves without residual deficit and does not necessarily recur on re-treatment. A subacute encephalopathy characterized by stroke-like episodes resulting in multifocal deficits, including hemiparesis, aphasia, dysarthria, seizures, and confusion or delirium, typically occurs several days after the second or third weekly intravenous dose and usually resolves spontaneously within 2–3 days.[5–7] Retreatment is possible in most patients, although subsequent episodes can occur. Acute to subacute encephalopathy has been reported in as many as 22% of breast cancer patients.[7] Computed tomographic (CT) scan results and CSF analysis are normal; however, electroencephalography usually shows diffuse or focal slowing.[6] A chronic delayed leukoencephalopathy can follow repeated doses of intravenous high-dose MTX or IT-MTX. A few cases have been reported following standard dose intravenous MTX.[8, 9] It is characterized by progressive personality change, dementia, focal neurologic signs, and sometimes seizures. Symptoms can appear months to years after therapy. White matter changes, including astrocytosis, axonal swelling, demyelination, and frank necrosis and angiopathy, are seen pathologically. The risk of delayed leukoencephalopathy increases with cumulative doses and with prior or concurrent cranial radiation.[2] CT may show focal hypodensities, calcification, and atrophy. White matter changes can be seen on magnetic resonance imaging (MRI) before neurologic symptoms occur.[10] Neurologic deficits are usually permanent. Some patients can improve somewhat or stabilize. Some continue to progress to a state of severe dementia, apraxias, and quadriparesis, followed by coma or death.

IT-MTX frequently causes an acute chemical meningitis characterized by headache, fever, nuchal rigidity, neck or back pain, nausea, vomiting, and dizziness. Onset of symptoms is usually within a few hours of treatment. Symptoms usually resolve spontaneously over 12–72 hours. CSF usually shows pleocytosis and elevated protein levels. The syndrome can be mistaken for bacterial meningitis, but the onset of symptoms after instillation of drug is usually too rapid to be due to growth from bacterial contamination. Rarely, IT-MTX may produce an acute or delayed myelopathy with paraplegia.[11] Recovery is variable. Cranial nerve injuries and hemiparesis are other rare complications of IT-MTX.[12, 13] The acute, subacute, delayed, and chronic encephalopathies seen with intravenous MTX can also occur associated with IT-MTX. Risk factors for IT-MTX neurotoxicity include prior or concurrent radiotherapy, conditions that decrease CSF clearance of MTX such as hydrocephalus and meningeal tumor, and MTX solutions containing preservatives.[2] IT-MTX overdose can cause encephalopathy and ascending myelopathy and can be lethal.[14]

Sterile, preservative-free solutions of MTX with added hydrocortisone have been used to reduce the neurotoxicity of IT-MTX. Treatment of MTX neurotoxicity other than IT-MTX overdose has been attempted with corticosteroids, folate, and intravenous leucovorin. Reports of success in patients have been anecdotal.[1, 15] There is no known effective treatment for the chronic leukoencephalopathy. Treatment of IT-MTX overdose has included CSF drainage, ventriculolumbar perfusion, CSF exchange, systemic corticosteroids, and systemic leucovorin.[16–18] Treatment of IT-MTX overdose with intrathecal carboxypeptidase-G2, an enzyme that hydrolyzes MTX into inactive metabolites, has been shown to be helpful in a rhesus monkey model.[19]

Many mechanisms have been postulated as underlying the neurotoxicity of MTX, including depletion of reduced cerebral folates, inhibition of cerebral protein or glucose metabolism, inhibition of catecholamine synthesis, and increased blood-brain barrier permeability.[2]

Edatrexate and Trimetrexate

Both edatrexate and trimetrexate are investigational antifolate drugs that are not thought to have neurotoxicity.

Cytidine Analogues

Cytosine Arabinoside (Cytarabine, Ara-C)

Ara-C inhibits DNA polymerase α, is incorporated into DNA, and terminates DNA chain elongation, thus inhibiting DNA synthesis. It is used primarily against leukemia and lymphoma. Neurotoxicity increases with increasing dose, increasing age, subsequent courses of treatment, and the route of administration. The mechanism of Ara-C neurotoxicity is not well understood. There is little neurotoxicity with usual intravenous doses (100–200 mg per m^2). High-dose intravenous therapy (2–24 g per m^2) can cause a subacute encephalopathy characterized by lethargy, confusion, aphasia, and seizures.[20] Cerebellar dysfunction starting with nystagmus and a mild gait ataxia, and sometimes progressing to severe ataxia with dysarthria, can also occur. Symptoms usually peak in severity 2–3 days after onset.[21, 22] Most patients recover within 1–2 weeks after treatment has been stopped. Cerebellar neurotoxicity at doses totaling less than 18 g per m^2 is usually mild to moderate and usually reversible. At higher doses, severe cerebellar dysfunction is a major dose-limiting toxicity. Age appears to be an important factor. In one study of 418 patients, no patient younger than 20 years of age had significant cerebellar symptoms. Three percent of patients between the ages of 20 and 50 and 19% of patients older than 50 developed severe neurotoxicity.[22] Neuroimaging may show cerebellar atrophy and reversible white matter abnormalities.[23] CSF study results are usually normal. Nonspecific slowing can be seen on electroencephalography. Neuropathologic studies show Purkinje cell loss predominantly in the deep primary and secondary cerebellar sulci. The molecular and granular layers of the cerebellum are relatively spared. The rest of the CNS is usually spared.[24]

Less commonly seen with intravenous Ara-C is peripheral neuropathy, reported almost exclusively with multidrug regimens usually including vincristine. Although Ara-C may potentiate the peripheral neurotoxicity of other agents, it is believed unlikely to be capable of producing peripheral neuropathy on its own.[2]

Visual symptoms can also complicate intravenous Ara-C treatment, including photophobia, blurred vision, blindness, eye pain, and oculomotor paresis.[25–27] Extrapyramidal symptoms have also been reported.[28, 29]

Intrathecal Ara-C is capable of causing an aseptic chemical meningitis similar to that seen with IT-MTX. Myelopathy and cauda equina syndrome have also been reported with intrathecal Ara-C and are also similar to that seen with IT-MTX.[30, 31] Symptoms can occur from several days to several weeks after intrathecal treatment and can be severe. Improvement is seen over weeks after discontinuance of treatment; however, in some patients the paraplegia or quadriplegia is incompletely reversible. Demyelination, microvacuolization of the white matter, and axonal dystrophic changes are seen pathologically.[31] Encephalopathy with or without seizures, and sometimes seizures alone, can be seen with intrathecal Ara-C.[32, 33] Encephalopathy seems to be less common and less severe than that seen with IT-MTX. Prior radiation or IT-MTX treatment may increase the risk of intrathecal Ara-C neurotoxicity.[32, 34]

The pathophysiologic mechanism of Ara-C neurotoxicity is not known. There is no specific treatment other than discontinuation of the drug. Patients with mild to moderate resolving cerebellar dysfunction can be successfully re-treated.[2]

5-Azacytidine

The cytidine analogue 5-azacytidine has little significant neurotoxicity compared with Ara-C. It can cause an encephalopathy, which can rarely progress to coma.[35] Muscle weakness, pain, and tenderness can also be seen.[35]

Fluorinated Pyrimidines

5-Fluorouracil

5-Fluorouracil (5-FU) is an analogue of the pyrimidine uracil with a fluorine atom substitution in place of hydrogen on the fifth carbon of the pyrimidine ring. It interferes with DNA synthesis by inhibiting thymidylate synthetase. The primary route of administration is intravenous by bolus or prolonged infusion. It also can be given intraperitoneally or intra-arterially. Patients with a congenital dihydropyrimidine dehydrogenase deficiency may develop neurotoxicity at lower doses.[36] 5-FU produces a cerebellar syndrome consisting of truncal and limb ataxia, nystagmus, and dysarthria similar to that seen with Ara-C.[37, 38] The syndrome is usually reversible after discontinuation of the drug. An encephalopathy characterized by confusion, headache, lethargy, and seizures can also occur.[39–41] An acute parkinsonian syndrome with cerebellar dysfunction has been reported.[42] Oculomotility disturbances including disturbance of conversion and divergence can also occur but are uncommon.[43] 5-FU treatment has also been associated with cerebrovascular events.[44] The neurotoxicity of 5-FU is increased when it is used in combination with allopurinol, N-phosphonoacetyl-L-aspartate (PALA), alpha-interferon, and thymidine.[45–49] The characteristics of the neurotoxicities seen are similar to those seen with 5-FU alone. The combination of 5-FU and levamisole has been associated with a multifocal inflammatory leukoencephalopathy.[50, 51] Symptoms begin within 3–5 months of beginning chemotherapy and include mental status changes and focal neurologic signs. MRI scans show multiple gadolinium-enhancing white matter lesions that can be confused with metastases or infection. Biopsies have shown demyelination and perivascular inflammation similar to that seen in patients with multiple sclerosis.[50] Patients have improved with discontinuation of the drug and with corticosteroid administration.

Floxuridine

The neurotoxicity of floxuridine (FUDR) is similar to that seen with 5-FU.

Ftorafur

A prodrug that is metabolized to 5-FU, ftorafur has more neurotoxicity than 5-FU. It causes an acute or subacute encephalopathy, sometimes with coma.[49] High concentrations of the drug are found in CSF.[49] Neurotoxicity can be dose limiting. Interestingly, cerebellar toxicity is not as prominent as it is with 5-FU, but ataxia can be seen in some patients with encephalopathy.[49]

Doxifluridine

Dizziness, ataxia, and alterations of consciousness and behavior are caused by doxifluridine, an antineoplastic drug used in breast and colon cancer.[49] A Wernicke-Korsakoff–like syndrome with confusion, unsteadiness, and diplopia can also be seen and seems to be associated with higher doses and shorter infusion times.[49, 52]

Carmofur

Used primarily in Japan, carmofur causes a subacute leukoencephalopathy that is incompletely reversible. Patients can be left with severe neurologic disability.[53, 54]

Miscellaneous Antimetabolites

6-Mercaptopurine and 6-Thioguanine

The purine analogues 6-mercaptopurine and 6-thioguanine have no appreciable neurotoxicity.

Fludarabine

Fludarabine is an adenosine analogue that inhibits DNA polymerase, inhibits RNA synthesis, and is a DNA chain terminator. In low doses it can cause transient confusion, visual changes, and somnolence.[55, 56] Transient visual hallucinations have been reported in one patient.[57] Peripheral neuropathy can also be seen.[58] On occasion, even with lower doses and particularly in older patients, a reversible syndrome characterized by focal CNS signs can also be seen.[59] MRI scans reveal foci of hyperintensity on the T2-weighted images.[59] At higher doses (more than 40 mg per m^2 per day for 5 days) a delayed and irreversible progressive encephalopathy is seen. Confusion, lethargy, cortical blindness, and seizures occur, sometimes progressing to coma and death.[49, 56, 60, 61] Postmortem examinations have demonstrated focal or diffuse necrotizing demyelination in the brain, particularly in the occipital lobes and in the posterior columns of the spinal cord.[56, 61] The development of neurotoxicity appears to be a function of both the dose and the rate of drug administration. The total cumulative dose may not be a factor as long as drug administration is kept to low doses given in short courses over an extended time period.[62]

Pentostatin (Deoxycoformycin)

Mild to moderate lethargy can be seen with lower doses of the adenosine analogue pentostatin. At higher doses a more severe encephalopathy occurs, characterized by confusion, lethargy, seizures, and sometimes coma.[49, 63, 64]

2-Chlordeoxyadenosine (2CdA, Cladribine, Leustatin)

No significant neurotoxicity is seen with 2-chlordeoxyadenosine at conventional doses. A delayed irreversible motor weakness with paraparesis has developed in some patients treated with high-dose 2-chlordeoxyadenosine.[49]

Hydroxyurea

Hydroxyurea inhibits ribonucleotide reductase and is principally used in the myeloproliferative syndromes. It also has been used as a radiation sensitizer in patients with primary brain tumors. It is generally administered orally, but more recently high-dose continuous infusion regimens have been evaluated. It readily enters the CSF.[49] Headache, drowsiness, confusion, and dizziness have been reported, but symptoms are not usually severe.[49]

N-*Phosphonoacetyl*-L-*Aspartate*

PALA inhibits aspartate transcarbamoylase, which in turn inhibits pyrimidine biosynthesis. It is used primarily as a modulator of 5-FU. Up to 41% of patients treated with PALA experience acute perioral paresthesias, mild lethargy, weakness, or dizziness.[65] An encephalopathy can also occur that improves after discontinuation of the drug. Seizures are associated with PALA treatment in patients with or without underlying focal structural brain lesions.[65] These seizures seem to have a predisposition for patients with structural brain lesions, are multiple, and progress to status epilepticus in some patients. The seizures frequently recur despite anticonvulsant therapy.[65] When combined with 5-FU the cerebellar neurotoxicity of 5-FU appears to be increased.[49]

Antimicrotubule Agents

Vinca *Alkaloids*

The *Vinca* alkaloids include vincristine, vindesine, vinorelbine, and vinblastine, and all cause similar neurotoxicities. Vincristine appears to be the most neurotoxic of the four. These agents bind tubulin, thereby preventing microtubule formation, which results in mitotic arrest. They also affect microtubules involved in chemotaxis and directional migration (intracellular transport). The effects on chemotaxis and directional transport are thought to be underlying the neurotoxicity of these agents.

Peripheral neuropathy is the principal toxicity of vincristine. It occurs, to some degree, in almost all patients and is the usual dose-limiting toxicity.[66] The severity of peripheral neuropathy is related to both total dose and duration of treatment. It initially presents with distal paresthesias and distal symmetric sensory loss with loss of ankle reflexes. Motor weakness with footdrops, muscular atrophy, and then hand and wrist weakness occur with continued treatment. Neuritic pain can also occur. Symptoms and signs are usually symmetric and if severe are incompletely reversible even with cessation of the drug. Most patients improve significantly after the drug is stopped, but recovery can take up to several months. Electrophysiologic testing may show normal or near normal motor and sensory nerve conduction velocities and often demonstrates diminished amplitudes of motor and sensory action potentials, suggesting axonal degeneration.[67] Risk factors include preexistent neuropathy, age, nutritional state, irradiation of peripheral nerves, and combination with other agents such as etoposide, teniposide, and cyclosporine.[68–73] A mild autonomic neuropathy with constipation occurs commonly. More severe symptoms, including ileus, orthostatic hypotension, hypertension, impotence, and urinary retention, can also occur due to autonomic neuropathy.[39, 74, 75] Mononeuropathies of the femoral nerve and contralateral peroneal nerve temporally related to intravenous vincristine have been reported in a child.[76] Ptosis, ophthalmoplegia, facial weakness, hearing loss and tinnitus, vocal cord paralysis, and optic neuropathy secondary to unilateral or bilateral cranial neuropathies have been reported.[77–80]

Relief or prevention of vincristine-induced peripheral neuropathy in cancer patients has been observed with treatment using various agents including glutamic acid, pyridoxine, folinic acid, isaxonine, prednisone, and Org 2766 (a corticotropin [4-9] analogue).[69, 81–85] Gangliosides have been used to attenuate vincristine neurotoxicity in dorsal root ganglion cell cultures and in rabbits.[86, 87] Clinical trials are not yet completed.

In addition to peripheral neurotoxicity, vincristine can also occasionally cause CNS toxicity. Encephalopathy and coma, at times with seizures, can occur.[88, 89] Transient cortical blindness, ataxia, and extrapyramidal symptoms, including parkinsonism and athetosis, and other focal neurologic symptoms, can occur; usually resolving after the drug is discontinued.[90–92]

Intracarotid vincristine used to treat primary brain tumors is associated with transient ipsilateral ophthalmoplegia, ipsilateral optic neuropathy, and transient hemiparesis.[93]

A number of cases of inadvertent intrathecal vincristine administration have been observed. An almost universally fatal encephalopathy and ascending flaccid paralysis occurs. Seizures are sometimes noted.[94] One patient, treated with CSF drainage, dexamethasone, folinic acid, vitamin B_{12}, thiamine, and pyridoxine in an attempt to counter the effects of the vincristine, lived almost 1 year, but never regained consciousness.[94] Survival of another patient treated with immediate CSF drainage, ventriculolumbar perfusion with fresh frozen plasma in lactated Ringer's solution, and intravenous glutamic acid has also been reported.[95] Pathology has shown necrosis, demyelination, and widespread neuronal loss.

Paclitaxel (Taxol) and Docetaxel (Taxotere)

The taxanes stabilize microtubules, inhibiting proliferation of cells by inducing a sustained mitotic block at the metaphase-anaphase boundary.[49] They cause a predominantly sensory neuropathy. A combined sensorimotor neuropathy can also occur.[96] Numbness and paresthesias can start within days of treatment in up to 55% of patients treated with doses of paclitaxel of more than 200 mg per m^2.[96] The neuropathy caused by Docetaxel can occur at cumulative doses as low as 50 mg per m^2. Twenty percent of patients receiving cumulative doses of more than 600 mg per m^2 developed a moderate neuropathy.[97] Severe neuropathy interfering with function can also occur.[97] The predominantly sensory neuropathies produced by both paclitaxel and docetaxel appear to be dose dependent and, although mild in most patients, can be disabling.[97] Most patients improve with discontinuation of therapy. Some can stabilize or improve even with continuation of therapy.[98] Electrophysiologic studies done in patients treated with paclitaxel suggest both axonal degeneration and demyelination.[96] Nerve growth factor (NGF) can attenuate the neurotoxic effect of paclitaxel in animal models and is currently being evaluated in clinical trials.

Estramustine

Estramustine is an estradiol molecule linked to a nor-nitrogen mustard. It produces metaphase arrest through inhibitory and dissociative effects on microtubules. It was developed specifically for the treatment of advanced prostate carcinoma. It can enhance the effects of radiation in vitro.[99–101] It has been associated with cerebrovascular events.[49]

Platinum Analogues

The platinum analogues covalently bond to DNA, disrupting its function. The types of DNA lesions responsible for cytotoxicity are not clearly known. Some toxicities may be related to protein binding.[49]

Cis-platinum

Neurotoxicity with cis-platinum is commonly seen and can be dose limiting. Most frequently encountered is peripheral neurotoxicity. Peripheral neuropathy is dose related and cumulative, occasionally seen after cumulative doses of as little as 200 mg per m^2 and almost always seen after 400 mg per m^2.[102] Single-dose intensity also appears important.[103] The neuropathy is usually sensory, starting with distal tingling in the feet and then hands, followed by loss of vibratory sensation, and then a loss of position sense and ankle jerks. While pain and temperature sensitivity are relatively spared and motor strength is usually normal, some patients develop such a severe proprioceptive loss that they are unable to eat, write, or manipulate objects with their hands and can develop a severe sensory ataxia. Autonomic neuropathy can occur but is much less frequent.[104, 105] At times symptoms are delayed, beginning only after completion of therapy.[106] Symptoms can also continue to progress after cessation of therapy.[102, 107] Usually symptoms improve after completion of therapy and can continue to improve for many months.[106] Some patients do not recover completely. Electrophysiologic studies show decreased sensory nerve action potential amplitudes and prolonged sensory latencies.[108] Axonal loss of large myelinated fibers is seen pathologically.[109] It has been postulated that the dorsal root ganglia are the primary target of peripheral cis-platinum neurotoxicity.[110, 111] Prevention of cis-platinum–induced neuropathy has been shown in mice by concomitant administration of NGF and glutathione ester.[112, 113] Reversal of already developed neuropathy has been shown with neurotrophin-3 in rats.[114] Org 2766 was shown in one study to prevent or attenuate cis-platinum–induced neuropathy in women treated for ovarian cancer.[115]

Ototoxicity is another common peripheral neurotoxicity seen with cis-platinum. It is due to hair cell loss in the cochlea.[116] It is characterized by tinnitus and hearing loss in the high-frequency range (4.0–8.0 kHz) and progresses to lower frequencies.[116] Ototoxicity is more severe with higher cumulative and individual doses.[117] Concomitant or previous cranial irradiation may lead to enhanced ototoxicity.[118] Other risk factors include other ototoxic drugs such as the aminoglycoside antibiotics, ifosfamide, and furosemide.[116, 119] Uncommonly, cis-platinum can cause retrobulbar neuritis and papilledema.[120, 121]

CNS neurotoxicity can also occur with cis-platinum therapy. Lhermitte's sign occurs transiently in many patients, suggesting spinal cord toxicity involving the posterior columns.[102, 122] Somatosensory evoked responses have suggested spinal cord involvement.[103] Dorsal column myelopathy with demyelination has been seen pathologically.[121] Encephalopathy can occur rarely after intravenous cis-platinum administration and is characterized by confusion and seizures.[123–127] Focal visual symptoms, including homonymous hemianopia and cortical blindness, are sometimes associated with the encephalopathy.[127, 128] Hyponatremia secondary to the syndrome of inappropriate secretion of antidiuretic hormone (SIADH) can occur and is also a cause of encephalopathy and seizures in patients treated with cis-platinum.[129, 130]

Cis-platinum has also been implicated as causing the cerebrovascular toxicities associated with certain multidrug regimens.[131–133] Bleomycin is commonly included in these regimens and may be responsible. Another possibility is a combined toxicity between more than one agent. Intra-arterial cis-platinum is used primarily against primary brain and head and neck cancers. Intracarotid infusions are associated with encephalopathy, seizures, and single or multiple cranial neuropathies, including optic neuropathy.[134–137] Internal or external iliac intra-arterial cis-platinum has been associated with ipsilateral lumbosacral plexopathy or mononeuropathy.[138]

Carboplatin

Carboplatin is thought to be less neurotoxic than cis-platinum, but in high doses has been associated with ototoxicity, peripheral neuropathy, and cortical blindness.[49, 139] A case of thrombotic microangiopathy associated with encephalopathy, episodic aphasia, and finally coma and death has been reported. Neuroimaging was not reported but brain pathology showed microthrombi and multiple hemorrhagic infarcts.[140]

Alkylating Agents

Alkylating agents are antineoplastic drugs that act by covalent bonding of alkyl groups to DNA.

Nitrosoureas

The nitrosoureas affect the O_6 position of guanine and include BCNU [1,3-bis(2-chloroethyl)-1-nitrosourea, carmustine], CCNU (lomustine), methyl CCNU (semustine), ACNU, HECNU, streptozocin, and chlorozotocin. They are highly lipid soluble and cross the blood-brain barrier relatively easily. They have little neurotoxicity when used intravenously at conventional doses. In one study, high-dose intravenous BCNU was reported to cause an encephalomyelopathy characterized by altered mental status, diplopia, ataxia, seizures, and, in one patient, progressive quadriparesis.[141] None of the patients reported had cranial irradiation or known CNS metastatic disease. The total dose of BCNU received ranged from 1,500 to 2,850 mg per m^2.[141] Pathology demonstrated swollen axons; myelin vacuolization; areas of necrosis and edema; and fibrinoid necrosis and fibrin microthrombi, suggesting a vasculopathy. Visual loss has also been associated with high-dose intravenous BCNU.[142] Oral CCNU has been rarely associated with sudden blindness in patients who have been treated with whole brain irradiation.[143]

Intra-arterial and particularly intracarotid BCNU used in patients with intracerebral tumors has a high risk of neurotoxicity. Delayed ocular toxicity occurring ipsilateral to the side of the infusion is common.[142] Symptoms begin 2–14 weeks after treatment. Visual loss is subacute and can be severe.[142] Funduscopic examinations show arterial narrowing, nerve fiber-layer infarcts, and intraretinal hemorrhages. It has been suggested that the ocular toxicity of intra-arterial BCNU is related to a segmental intraretinal vasculitis, obstruction, or both.[142]

In addition to the ocular toxicity, an immediate transient or delayed and frequently fatal necrotizing encephalopathy has also been caused by intra-arterial BCNU.[144] It is characterized by confusion, seizures, and multifocal neurologic signs and symptoms.[2, 145] Cranial irradiation either before or concurrent with the BCNU may increase the risk.[2, 144, 145] Onset of symptoms can be delayed by several months.[144] CT scans may be normal but usually show ipsilateral hypodensities with edema and gyral enhancement. Microcalcifications can also be seen.[144, 145] Toxicity increases with increasing dose.[2] Supraophthalmic infusions seem to have a higher risk of encephalopathy than do infraophthalmic infusions.[146] Necrotizing encephalopathy has also been reported with intra-arterial ACNU.[147] Intra-arterial PCNU has been associated with ipsilateral blindness, focal seizures, and focal neurologic symptoms.[148]

Mustards

Mechlorethamine (Nitrogen Mustard)

The first nitrogen mustard to be used extensively was mechlorethamine. A necrotizing encephalopathy and ophthalmoplegia has been seen after intracarotid infusion.[2] Intravenous therapy can cause hearing loss and encephalopathy with hyperpyrexia.[149, 150]

Cyclophosphamide (Cytoxan)

Other than transient visual blurring and occasional confusion seen with high doses, cyclophosphamide is essentially free of neurotoxicity.[151, 152]

Ifosfamide

Of all the mustards, ifosfamide is probably the most neurotoxic. It is similar in structure and pharmacology to cyclophosphamide, which has little if any neurotoxicity. This implies the possibility that a metabolite of ifosfamide may be responsible for its neurotoxicity. Chloracetaldehyde, an oxidation product of ifosfamide produced in much greater quantities than with metabolism of cyclophosphamide, has been suggested as playing a causative role.[153, 154] Ifosfamide (both intravenous and oral) causes an encephalopathy that usually begins within 1–4 days of treatment and lasts for several days. Confusion, lethargy, hallucinations, and seizures are usually seen. Ataxia, cranial neuropathies, extrapyramidal signs, delirium, and coma can also occur.[155, 156] Risk factors may include renal insufficiency, high dosage, previous treatment with cisplatinum, impaired hepatic function, low serum albumin, age, prior cranial irradiation, and other CNS disease.[155–157] Barbiturates can induce phase I oxidative liver enzymes that may produce reactive intermediates in the breakdown of ifosfamide, thereby increasing neurotoxicity.[49] Electroencephalography initially shows slowing of the baseline rhythm and then high-voltage rhythmic delta discharges. These changes can be seen even in patients who do not develop clinical neurotoxicity.[154] Intravenous methylene blue has been used as an antidote for ifosfamide-induced encephalopathy.[158] A transient syndrome of painful paresthesias in patients with underlying peripheral neuropathy has been reported with ifosfamide treatment.[159]

Other Mustards

Melphalan and chlorambucil are other mustards that do not cause neurotoxicity in conventional intravenous dosages.

Miscellaneous Alkylating Agents

Thiotepa

Thiotepa is an aziridine that is metabolized to TEPA and other alkylating species. It is used both intravenously against solid tumors and intrathecally against leptomeningeal tumor. CSF penetration with systemic therapy is excellent.[160] In high intravenous doses it can cause inappropriate behavior, confusion, and somnolence. The lowest dose at which neurologic toxicity occurs appears to be 900 mg per m^2, with an incidence of 5%. The incidence is 10–15% at higher doses.[161] Preexistent CNS disease or previous radiotherapy may increase the risk of thiotepa-induced encephalopathy (personal observation).

Lumbar intrathecal injections of thiotepa have been associated with a myelopathy similar to that seen with intrathecal methotrexate.[162]

Busulfan

The alkylating agent busulfan is used primarily against myeloid leukemias and, in high doses, with bone marrow transplantation. Busulfan is lipophilic and penetrates into CSF easily.[163] The most commonly seen neurotoxicity associated with busulfan is seizures.[163–165] Seizures can be focal or generalized. Myoclonic jerks can be seen associated with the seizures or preceding seizures by up to several days.[165, 166] Phenytoin or clonazepam can be used successfully to prevent the seizures.[163, 165] There is a report of a case of myasthenia gravis complicating busulfan therapy.[167] The patient described tested negative for antibodies, continued to worsen after the busulfan was discontinued, and responded to thymectomy. No electromyographic results were reported.

Dacarbazine (DTIC)

The exact mechanism of action of dacarbazine is unknown. It is usually not neurotoxic, but has been associated with seizures (when used with doxorubicin Adriamycin), cerebral hemorrhage not related to thrombocytopenia (when used with dactinomycin [Actinomycin D]), and encephalopathy.[168–170]

Mitotane

Transient cognitive impairment, ataxia, and extrapyramidal symptoms have been seen with mitotane.[171]

Procarbazine

Procarbazine is a weak monoamine oxidase inhibitor. Its cytotoxic mechanism is not well understood. Neurotoxicity is more severe and more commonly seen when procarbazine is used intravenously. Oral procarbazine can also cause significant neurotoxicity. Peripheral neuropathy with paresthesias and depressed muscle stretch reflexes can occur in as many as 20% of patients. It is usually reversible or abates even with continued treatment.[172, 173] Alterations in consciousness, including lethargy, agitation, and psychosis, can occur. Electroencephalography reveals diffuse slow wave activity.[173] There may be synergy between procarbazine and the sedative effects of other medications.[172]

Hexamethylmelamine

Used primarily against advanced ovarian cancer, hexamethylmelamine's demethylated metabolites are found in high concentrations in the CNS. They may be responsible for centrally mediated anorexia, nausea, and vomiting. Other neurotoxicities seen include lethargy, agitation, psychosis, and sometimes coma. Peripheral neuropathy is less commonly seen.[174]

Antineoplastic Antibiotics

Doxorubicin (Adriamycin)

Doxorubicin is an anthracycline antibiotic used primarily against the hematopoietic malignancies. Mechanisms of action may be by inhibition of topoisomerase II, activation of protein kinase C–mediated signal transduction pathways, stimulation of apoptosis, and generation of free radicals. Doxorubicin causes both acute and chronic cardiac toxicity, including arrhythmias, pericarditis, and myocarditis that causes cardiomyopathy and congestive heart failure. Cardiac thrombi associated with the cardiac toxicity can lead to transient cerebral ischemia and infarction.[175] The combination of doxorubicin and cyclosporine has been reported to cause coma and death by increasing levels of doxorubicin in the brain.[176] One mechanism for this is postulated to be cyclosporine-induced inhibition of P-glycoprotein, the protein product of the multidrug-resistance gene.[177] P-glycoprotein is expressed in the luminal surfaces of capillary endothelial cells and may play a role in the competence of the blood-brain barrier.[178]

Inadvertent intrathecal administration of doxorubicin causes an acute severe encephalomyelopathy that can be fatal.[179, 180] Intracarotid doxorubicin administration after osmotic blood-brain barrier disruption caused delayed onset seizures, hemorrhage, and necrosis of ipsilateral brain in a canine model.[181]

Mitoxantrone

A doxorubicin analogue, mitoxantrone does not appear to have neurotoxicity when given intravenously, but when used intrathecally it causes myelopathy and severe nerve root damage.[182–184] Intrathecal mitoxantrone is therefore not recommended for use.

Bleomycin

A mixture of peptides that acts by oxidative cleavage of DNA, bleomycin is used against lymphomas, germ cell tumors, and head and neck cancers. Cerebral infarction has been associated with bleomycin, usually when it has been used in combination with cis-platinum with or without vincristine, etoposide, or vinblastine.[185]

Mitomycin C

The mechanism of action of mitomycin C is alkylation of DNA. Used against solid tumors it has little neurotoxicity. An encephalopathy thought to be due to thrombotic microangiopathy can occur.[185]

Other Antineoplastic Antibiotics

Daunorubicin, idarubicin, epirubicin, dactinomycin (Actinomycin D), and mithramycin have no appreciable neurotoxicity.

Topoisomerase Inhibitors

Topoisomerase I Inhibitors

The camptothecin analogues are a newer and promising family of drugs that inhibit the DNA-unwinding enzyme topoisomerase I. They include topotecan, irinotecan (CPT-II), 9-aminocamptothecin, and GG211. They are still being evaluated in broad-ranging clinical trials. Neurotoxicity has not yet been appreciated except perhaps with CPT-II, which is discussed in the section on experimental agents.

Topoisomerase II Inhibitors

Etoposide (VP-16) and teniposide (VM-26) are semisynthetic podophyllotoxin derivatives that inhibit DNA topoisomerase II. High-dose VP-16 can cause a peripheral neuropathy, confusion, and seizures.[186] VM-26 does not have any significant neurologic toxicity. Amsacrine (m-Amsa) is a synthetic aminoacridine that can also cause a transient neuropathy.[187] It has also been associated with seizures.[188]

Suramin is a polysulfonated napthylurea that also inhibits topoisomerase II. It is frequently associated with a severe predominantly motor peripheral polyneuropathy that can lead to a flaccid paralysis.[189] It is sometimes associated with bulbar and respiratory muscle weakness that may require mechanical intubation. Autonomic involvement can be associated with the weakness and can cause wide fluctuations in blood pressure and heart rate.[189] The syndrome, which appears similar to Guillain-Barré, evolves over several weeks. CSF shows elevated protein levels, normal cell counts, and normal cytology. Electrodiagnostic studies demonstrate blocks at multiple sites, suggesting a demyelinating process. Treatment with plasmapheresis does not seem to be helpful. The syndrome appears to be dose related, with an estimated 40% risk in patients whose plasma levels exceed 350 μg per ml.[189] Recovery may be incomplete with severe residual deficit remaining. Neuritic inhibition by suramin (via inhibition of binding by NGF to the NGF receptor) can be inhibited in vitro by NGF, suggesting that inhibition of NGF may have a role in this neurotoxicity and suggests a possible therapy.[190]

Miscellaneous Chemotherapeutic Drugs

L-Asparaginase is an enzyme that depletes the essential amino acid asparagine by catalyzing its hydrolysis to acetic acid and ammonia, leading to inhibition of protein synthesis. Encephalopathy characterized by confusion, stupor, seizures, and sometimes coma occurs in up to one-third of patients treated with high doses.[191, 192] Some have postulated that the encephalopathy is due to elevated serum ammonia levels, whereas others believe it to be due to low concentrations of L-asparagine or L-glutamine in the brain.[49, 192] L-Asparaginase has also been associated with thrombotic and hemorrhagic cerebrovascular events that occur in 1–2% of patients treated.[193, 194] Thrombosis of cerebral veins or dural sinuses with or without associated infarction or hemorrhage is probably more common than was previously recognized before the advent of MRI and MR angiography. Headache, mental status changes, and focal neurologic signs occur. Seizures frequently occur in patients with any type of cerebrovascular complication; however, their presence, especially when associated with headache, is most typical of patients with cortical vein or dural sinus thrombosis, hemorrhage, or both.[193] Inhibition and depletion of plasma proteins involved in coagulation (primarily antithrombin III, protein C, and protein S) and fibrinolysis is believed to be underlying the pathogenesis of these thromboses and hemorrhages.[193] A shift in the equilibrium between fibrinolysis and coagulation has been postulated to occur from the time of actual treatment to later as recovery from treatment occurs. Thrombotic complications appear to occur later than hemorrhage, supporting the theory of a hypercoagulable state during recovery.[193] Multiple treatment measures have been proposed, including anticoagulation, fresh frozen plasma, or both to replace antithrombin III and fibrinogen.[193]

Endocrine Therapies

Glucocorticoids

Prednisone, prednisolone, dexamethasone, and methylprednisolone are used as antineoplastic agents primarily against hematologic malignancies. Glucocorticoids are also used to control pain, edema, nausea, and vomiting and to improve appetite. Neurologic complications can occur with all of the glucocorticoids. Opportunistic infection in the nervous system occurring as a complication of corticosteroid treatment is a serious complication, discussion of which is outside the scope of this chapter. The most common neurologic complication seen in patients taking corticosteroids is probably myopathy. Weakness begins proximally in the hip girdle, progresses to the proximal arm muscles, and in serious cases, can become diffuse. Sensation, the extraocular muscles, and muscle stretch reflexes are preserved.[195] It appears to be dose dependent (although susceptibility among individuals may vary) and may occur with increased frequency with use of fluorinated corticosteroids such as dexamethasone.[196] Rarely, an acute severe quadriplegic myopathy can be seen with high-dose intravenous corticosteroids.[196, 197] Muscle atrophy occurs, which is seen histologically as affecting primarily type IIB fibers.[198] Electromyography reveals nonspecific myopathy with an increase in polyphasic potentials. Pathogenesis is probably related to inhibition of protein synthesis and increased protein catabolism. Treatment consists of reducing or, if possible, discontinuing the drug. Recovery can take weeks to months.[199]

Encephalopathy can also occur with glucocorticosteroid treatment. This can range from mild mood and behavioral alterations to severe affective disorders (mania or depression) and psychosis.[200] True corticosteroid psychosis with hallucinations has become rare with the use of synthetic corticosteroids. Insomnia is common.[201] Blurred vision is also common and thought to be due to changes in refraction. Tremor is a particularly distressing side effect of corticosteroids and occurs fairly frequently. Hiccups can also occur on occasion.[202]

Androgens

Danazol can cause lethargy, irritability, headache, and muscle cramps.[49]

Estrogens

Estrogens such as diethylstilbestrol and ethenyl estradiol are used in prostate and breast cancer. They can cause dizziness, headache, and depression.[49]

Antiestrogens

Tamoxifen, used in breast cancer and primary brain tumors, can cause reversible visual changes due to ocular toxicity. Rarely, patients can develop an acute reversible encephalopathy with confusion, delusions, and hallucinations.[203] Ataxia has also been reported.[204] The addition of tamoxifen to multidrug regimens in patients with breast cancer is associated with an increase in arterial thrombotic events, including cerebrovascular accidents.[205] The antiprogesteronal agent mifepristone is used to treat meningioma and, at times, patients with breast cancer and pituitary tumors. It has no known neurologic toxicity.[206]

Biologic Modifiers

Interferon-alpha

Used primarily against the hematologic malignancies, interferon-alpha has also been used against various solid tumors. Despite extensive knowledge regarding effects of interferon-alpha on cellular and molecular systems, the precise antineoplastic mechanisms are not well understood. Significant acute and delayed neurotoxicity can be seen. Encephalopathy can occur acutely or be delayed and is the most serious neurotoxicity seen. Acutely, behavioral changes can be seen including lethargy, confusion, depression, and impaired memory.[207–209] The symptoms usually are reversible with discontinuation of the treatment. Persistent encephalopathy can be seen weeks to years after discontinuation of treatment and may be more common than previously thought.[209] Parkinsonism, sometimes severe, can also develop.[209] Neuroimaging in these patients is normal except for atrophy. Electroencephalography can reveal diffuse slow activity. The mechanism for persistent encephalopathy and parkinsonism is unknown. Length of treatment does not appear to be related to neurotoxicity; however, dose and schedule of treatment do appear to be related to the severity of persistent symptoms.[209] Patients who received daily injections have worse acute and delayed neurotoxic symptoms.[209] Bilateral brachial plexopathy and lumbosacral root irritation have been reported, with symptoms resolving almost completely over 2 years.[210] Oculomotor nerve paralysis and hearing loss have also been described.[211, 212]

Interleukins

Interleukin-2 (IL-2) is a lymphokine used in patients with solid tumors, primarily malignant melanoma and renal carcinoma. It can cause acute or chronic encephalopathy, characterized by agitation, disorientation, and somnolence. Occasionally, a more severe encephalopathy progressing to coma can occur.[213] An increase in brain edema, thought to be due to an increase in capillary permeability (as part of the "vascular leak syndrome" seen systemically), has been postulated as a mechanism underlying the encephalopathy.[214] In one study, the patients with severe neurologic deterioration all had intracranial tumors and showed an increase in peritumoral edema. Other patients with extracranial tumors had minor transient mental status changes and were also thought to have an increase in cerebral water content.[214] Differences in the two groups may be due to differences in the integrity of the blood-brain barrier.

Multiple brief episodes of visual loss resembling transient ischemic attacks have been reported.[215] A syndrome of focal and multifocal deficits can also be caused by IL-2. Aphasia, hemiparesis, cortical blindness, hemisensory defects, and ataxia have been associated with encephalopathy and seizures.[216, 217] MRI scans show multiple hyperintense cortical, subcortical, and cerebellar lesions on T2-weighted images. These lesions have sometimes shown enhancement. Lesions seen on MRI can resolve over time.[216, 218] CSF is usually normal.[216] Most patients recover to normal or near normal function.[216, 218] The mechanism for this syndrome is unknown but may be secondary to induction of other cytokines such as tumor necrosis factor (TNF) or to direct toxicity of IL-2. An acute fatal leukoencephalopathy with demyelination seen pathologically has been reported in one patient.[219] Intrathecal IL-2 has been associated with a delayed dementia and cerebellar syndrome seen 3 months after treatment, with multiple white matter lesions seen on MRI.[220] Reversible brachial plexopathy thought to be immune-mediated has been reported with intravenous IL-2, as has carpal tunnel syndrome.[221, 222]

Interleukin-1 can cause headache, encephalopathy, and rarely seizures.[223] Interleukin-4 has been associated with headache. Experience with interleukin-1 and interleukin-4 is more limited than with IL-2, and further neurotoxicity may be seen over time.

Tumor Necrosis Factor

Transient aphasia and other focal neurologic deficits can be seen in patients treated with TNF.[224, 225] Encephalopathy can also occur.[226]

Levamisole

An antihelminthic drug, levamisole is used as an immune enhancer. In addition to the multifocal leukoencephalopathy seen when it is used with 5-FU (see previous section on 5-FU), levamisole alone can cause insomnia, headache, and dizziness.[227] Aseptic meningitis and seizures can also occur.[228]

Radiation Sensitizers

The nitromidazoles misonidazole, metronidazole, and etanidazole are radiosensitizers that cause an axonal, primarily sensory, peripheral neuropathy that can be dose limiting.[229–231]

Experimental Agents

Pentamethylmelamine

An *s*-triazene derivative similar to hexamethylmelamine, pentamethylmelamine (PMM) has significant neurotoxicity. For that reason and because only scattered responses were seen during clinical trials, further clinical investigations of this drug are on hold.[49] The neurotoxicity includes diarrhea, nausea, and vomiting and is thought to be centrally mediated by demethylated metabolites in the CNS.[49] Lethargy, depression, hallucinations, agitation, coma, and peripheral neuropathy can also be seen.[232]

Pyrazoloacridine

Pyrazoloacridine (PZA) has preclinical activity against solid tumor cell lines. In phase I clinical trials, neurotoxicity was dose limiting. Neuropsychiatric symptoms, motor symptoms, and dizziness were seen.[49] PZA is being evaluated further in phase II trials.

Acivisin

Acivisin is an amino acid antitumor antibiotic that inhibits carbamoylphosphate synthetase, which inhibits de novo pyrimidine biosynthesis. It is used alone or to promote use of preformed pyrimidines such as 5-FU. It has dose-limiting neurotoxicity. It is believed to cross the blood-brain barrier into brain via the large neutral amino acid transport system. Acivisin causes an encephalopathy characterized by somnolence, personality changes, hallucinations, and ataxia.[233, 234] It has been used against primary malignant glioma and non–small cell lung cancer. In an animal model, giving a continuous intravenous infusion of an amino acid mixture before, during, and after treatment with acivisin decreased entry of acivisin into the brain, preventing neurotoxicity.[233] There was also an increase in total body clearance of the drug, decreasing levels of drug in other tissues; however, the systemic antitumor effects did not seem to be altered.[233]

Retinoids

All-trans-retinoic acid and 9-cis-retinoic acid are differentiation agents that can cause headache and pseudotumor cerebri.[235]

CI-980

CI-980 is a synthetic mitotic inhibitor thought to be cytotoxic due to binding to the colchicine-binding site of tubulin. A phase I clinical trial revealed its neurotoxicity to be dose limiting.[236] Reversible confusion, lethargy, and disorientation occurred in two of three patients at the highest dose tested.[236]

Antibody-Based Immunotherapy

Monoclonal antibodies can be used to direct an inflammatory response against a target cell and be directly cytotoxic, or they may be used as carriers to deliver another molecule or radionuclide to a specific site. Some have neurotoxicity. 3F8, an antiganglioside monoclonal antibody, targets GD2 on neuroblastoma cells, but also binds GD2 on peripheral nerves and dorsal root ganglion cells, causing a severe pain syndrome.[237] Seizures, lethargy, confusion, stupor, and peripheral neuropathy have also been reported in patients with ovarian and breast cancers treated with monoclonal antibodies.[238, 239]

CPT-II (Irinotecan)

CPT-II is a topoisomerase I inhibitor. It is converted to a metabolite, SN-38, which appears to contribute greatly to its antitumor effect. It has activity against solid tumors and is currently being evaluated in multiple clinical trials. Severe neurotoxicity has not yet been appreciated. Transient visual disturbances, diaphoresis, diarrhea, abdominal cramps, salivation, lacrimation, miosis, bradycardia, hypotension, and piloerection are frequently seen and thought to be due to a cholinergic syndrome. Symptoms are usually mild to moderate and treated with atropine sulfate.[240]

Conclusion

Significant and frequent transient or permanent neurologic symptoms, disability, or both can be seen in patients with cancer. Neurotoxicity caused by medication, particularly agents used to treat cancer and its complications must be high on the differential list of causes of neurologic symptoms in patients with cancer. As new agents are developed, biologic treatments explored, and novel ways of using existing agents tried, new neurologic toxicities will be seen and will need to be appreciated, as will the important clinical problems they pose.

References

1. Bleyer WA. Neurologic sequelae of methotrexate and ionizing radiation: a new classification. Cancer Treat Rep 1981;65(Suppl I):89.
2. Rottenberg DA (ed). Neurological Complications of Cancer Treatment. Boston: Butterworth–Heinemann, 1991.
3. Bode U, Magrath IT, Bleyer WA, et al. Active transport of methotrexate from cerebrospinal fluid in humans. Cancer Res 1980;40:2184.
4. Shapiro WR, Young DF, Mehta BM. Methotrexate: distribution in cerebrospinal fluid after intravenous, ventricular and lumbar injections. N Engl J Med 1975; 293:161.
5. Martino RL, Benson AB III, Merritt JA, et al. Transient neurologic dysfunction following moderate-dose methotrexate for undifferentiated lymphoma. Cancer 1984;54:2003.
6. Walker RW, Allen JC, Rosen G, et al. Transient cerebral dysfunction secondary to high-dose methotrexate. J Clin Oncol 1986;4:1845.
7. Yap H-Y, Blumenschein GR, Yap BS, et al. High-dose methotrexate for advanced breast cancer. Cancer Treat Rep 1979;63:757.
8. Prince RA, Jamieson PA. The central nervous system in childhood leukemia. II. Subacute leukoencephalopathy. Cancer 1975;35:306.

9. Rubinstein LJ, Herman MM, Long TG, et al. Disseminated necrotizing leukoencephalopathy: a complication of treated central nervous system leukemia and lymphoma. Cancer 1975;35:291.
10. Lien HH, Blomlie V, Saeter G, et al. Osteogenic sarcoma: MR signal abnormalities of the brain in asymptomatic patients treated with high-dose methotrexate. Radiology 1991;179:547.
11. McLean DR, Clink HM, Enst P, et al. Myelopathy after intrathecal chemotherapy. A case report with unique magnetic resonance imaging changes. Cancer 1994;73:3037.
12. Boogerd W, Moffie D, Smets LA. Early blindness and coma during intrathecal chemotherapy for meningeal carcinomatosis. Cancer 1990;65:452.
13. Yim YS, Mahoney DH Jr, Oshman DG. Hemiparesis and ischemic changes of the white matter after intrathecal therapy for children with acute lymphocytic leukemia. Cancer 1991;67:2058.
14. Ettinger LJ. Pharmacokinetics and biochemical effects of a fatal intrathecal methotrexate overdose. Cancer 1982;50:444.
15. Fritch G, Urban C. Transient encephalopathy during the late course of treatment with high-dose methotrexate. Cancer 1984;53:1849.
16. Addiego JE, Ridgway D, Bleyer WA. The acute management of intrathecal methotrexate overdose: pharmacologic rationale and guidelines. J Pediatr 1981;98:825.
17. Spiegel RJ, Cooper PR, Blum RH, et al. Treatment of massive intrathecal methotrexate overdose by ventriculolumbar perfusion. N Engl J Med 1984;311:386.
18. Jakobson AM, Kreuger A, Mortimer O, et al. Cerebrospinal fluid exchange after intrathecal methotrexate overdose. A report of two cases. Acta Paediatr 1992; 81:359.
19. Adamson PC, Balis FM, McCully CL, et al. Rescue of experimental intrathecal methotrexate overdose with carboxypeptidase-G2. J Clin Oncol 1991;9:670.
20. Rudnick SA, Cadman EC, Capizzi RL, et al. High-dose cytosine arabinoside (HDARAC) in refractory acute leukemia. Cancer 1979;44:1189.
21. Dworkin LA, Goldman RD, Zivin LS, et al. Cerebellar toxicity following high-dose cytosine arabinoside. J Clin Oncol 1985;3:613.
22. Herzig RH, Hines JD, Herzig GP, et al. Cerebellar toxicity with high-dose cytosine arabinoside. J Clin Oncol 1987;5:927.
23. Miller L, Link MP, Bologna S, et al. Cerebellar atrophy caused by high-dose cytosine arabinoside: CT and MR findings. AJR Am J Roentgenol 1989;152:343.
24. Winkleman MD, Hines JD. Cerebellar degeneration caused by high-dose cytosine arabinoside. A clinicopathological study. Ann Neurol 1983;14:520.
25. Ritch PS, Hansen RM, Heuer DK. Ocular toxicity from high-dose cytosine arabinoside. Cancer 1983;51:430.
26. Margileth DA, Poplack DG, Pizzo PA, et al. Blindness during remission in two patients with acute lymphoblastic leukemia: a possible complication of multimodality therapy. Cancer 1977;39:58.
27. Ventura GJ, Keating MJ, Castellanos AM, et al. Reversible bilateral lateral rectus muscle palsy associated with high-dose cytosine arabinoside and mitoxantrone therapy. Cancer 1986;58:1633.
28. Malapert D, Degos JD. Painful legs and moving toes. Neuropathy caused by cytarabine. Rev Neurol (Paris) 1989;145:869.
29. Luque FA, Selhorst JB, Petruska P. Parkinsonism induced by high-dose cytosine arabinoside. Mov Disord 1987;2:219.
30. Dunton SF, Nitschke R, Spruce WE, et al. Progressive ascending paralysis following administration of intrathecal and intravenous cytosine arabinoside. A Pediatric Oncology Group study. Cancer 1986;57:1083.
31. Breuer AC, Pitman SW, Dawson DM, et al. Paraparesis following intrathecal cytosine arabinoside: a case report with neuropathologic findings. Cancer 1977;40:2817.
32. Eden OB, Goldie W, Wood T, et al. Seizures following intrathecal cytosine arabinoside in young children with acute lymphoblastic leukemias. Cancer 1978;42:53.
33. Resar LM, Phillips PC, Kastan MD, et al. Acute neurotoxicity after intrathecal cytosine arabinoside in two adolescents with acute lymphoblastic leukemia of B-cell type. Cancer 1993;71:117.
34. Gay CT, Bodensteiner JB, Nitschke R, et al. Reversible treatment-related leukoencephalopathy. J Child Neurol 1989;4:208.
35. Levi J, Wiernik P. A comparative clinical trial of 5-azacytidine and guanazole in previously treated adults with acute nonlymphocytic leukemia. Cancer 1976;38:36.
36. Harris BE, Carpenter JT, Diasio RB. Severe 5-fluorouracil toxicity secondary to dihydropyrimidine dehydrogenase deficiency. A potentially more common pharmacogenetic syndrome. Cancer 1991;68:499.
37. Horton J, Olson KB, Sullivan J, et al. 5-Fluorouracil in cancer: an improved regimen. Ann Intern Med 1970; 73:897.
38. Riehl J-L, Brown WJ. Acute cerebellar syndrome secondary to 5-fluorouracil therapy. Neurology 1965;14:961.
39. MacDonald DR. Neurologic complications of chemotherapy. Neurol Clin 1991;9:955.
40. Greenwald ES. Organic mental changes with flurouracil therapy [letter]. JAMA 1976;235:248.
41. Lynch HT, Droszcz CP, Albano WA, et al. "Organic brain syndrome" secondary to 5-fluorouracil toxicity. Dis Colon Rectum 1981;24:130.
42. Bergevin PR, Patwardhan VC, Weissman J, et al. Neurotoxicity of 5-flurururacil [letter]. Lancet 1975;1:410.
43. Bixenman WW, Nicholls JVV, Warwick OH. Oculomotor disturbances associated with 5-fluorouracil chemotherapy. Am J Ophthalmol 1977;83:789.
44. Doll DD, Yarbro JW. Vascular toxicity associated with chemotherapy and hormonotherapy. Curr Op Oncol 1994;6:345.
45. Campbell TN, Howell SB, Pfeifle C, et al. High-dose allopurinol modulation of 5-FU toxicity: phase I trial of an outpatient dose schedule. Cancer Treat Rep 1982;66:1723.

46. Howell SB, Pfeifle CE, Wung WE. Effect of allopurinol on the toxicity of high-dose 5-fluorouracil administered by intermittent bolus injection. Cancer 1983;51:220.
47. Muggia FM, Camacho FJ, Kaplan BH, et al. Weekly 5-fluorouracil combined with PALA: toxic and therapeutic effects in colorectal cancer. Cancer Treat Rep 1987;71:253.
48. Casper ES, Michaelson RS, Kemeny N, et al. Phase I evaluation of a biochemically designed combination: PALA, thymidine, and 5-FU. Cancer Treat Rep 1984;68:539.
49. Chabner BA, Longo DL (eds). Cancer Chemotherapy and Biotherapy: Principles and Practice (2nd ed). Philadelphia: Lippincott-Raven, 1996.
50. Hook CC, Kimmel DW, Kvols LK, et al. Multifocal inflammatory leukoencephalopathy with 5-fluororuracil and levamisole. Ann Neurol 1992;31:262.
51. Kimmel DW, Schutt AJ. Multifocal leukoencephalopathy: occurrence during 5-fluorouracil and levamisole therapy and resolution after discontinuation of chemotherapy. Mayo Clin Proc 1993;68:363.
52. Heier MS, Fossa SD. Wernicke-Korsakoff-like syndrome in patients with colorectal carcinoma treated with high-dose doxifluridine (5'-dFUrd). Acta Neurol Scand 1986;73:449.
53. Kuzuhara S, Ohkoshi N, Kanemaru K, et al. Subacute leucoencephalopathy induced by carmofur, a 5-fluorouracil derivative. J Neurol 1987;234:365.
54. Suzuki T, Koizumi J, Uchida K, et al. Carmofur-induced organic mental disorders. Jpn J Psychiatry Neurol 1990;44:723.
55. Hochster H, Cassileth P. Fludarabine phosphate therapy of non-Hodgkin's lymphoma. Semin Oncol 1990;17:63.
56. Von Hoff DD. Phase I clinical trials with fludarabine phosphate. Semin Oncol 1990;17(Suppl 8):33.
57. Casper ES, Mittleman A, Kelson J, et al. Phase I clinical trial of fludarabine phosphate (F-ara-AMP). Cancer Chemother Pharmacol 1985;15:233.
58. Grever MR, Kopecky KJ, Coltman CA, et al. Fludarabine monophosphate: a potentially useful agent in chronic lymphocytic leukemia. Nouv Rev Fr Hematol 1988;30:457.
59. Cohen RB, Abdallah JM, Gray JR, et al. Reversible neurologic toxicity in patients treated with standard-dose fludarabine phosphate for mycosis fungoides and chronic lymphocytic leukemia. Ann Intern Med 1993; 118:114.
60. Warrell RP Jr, Berman E. Phase I and II study of fludarabine phosphate in leukemia: therapeutic efficacy with delayed central nervous system toxicity. J Clin Oncol 1986;4:74.
61. Chun HG, Leyland-Jones B, Caryk SM, et al. Central nervous system toxicity of fludarabine phosphate. Cancer Treat Rep 1986;70:1225.
62. Grever M, Leiby J, Kraut E. A comprehensive phase I and II clinical investigation of fludarabine phosphate. Semin Oncol 1990;17(Suppl 8):39.
63. Cheson BD, Vena DA, Foss FM, et al. Neurotoxicity of purine analogs: a review. J Clin Oncol 1994;12:2216.
64. Major PP, Agarwal RP, Kufe DW. Deoxycoformycin: neurological toxicity. Cancer Chemother Pharmacol 1981;5:193.
65. Wiley RG, Gralla RJ, Casper ES, et al. Neurotoxicity of the pyrimidine synthesis inhibitor N-phosphonocetyl-L-aspartate. Ann Neurol 1982;12:175.
66. Holland JF, Scharlau C, Gailani S, et al. Vincrisine treatment of advanced cancer: a cooperative study of 392 cases. Cancer Res 1973;33:1258.
67. Casey EB, Jellife AM, Le Quesne PM, et al. Vincristine neuropathy: clinical and electrophysiological observations. Brain 1973;96:69.
68. McGuire SA, Gospe SM Jr, Dahl G. Acute vincristine neurotoxicity in the presence of hereditary motor and sensory neuropathy type I. Med Pediatr Oncol 1989; 17:520.
69. Perrault DJ, Turley J, Quirt I, et al. A prospective study of vincristine neuropathy [abstract]. Program/Proceedings American Society of Clinical Oncology 1988;7: A1115.
70. Cassady JR, Tonnesen GL, Wolfe LC, et al. Augmentation of vincristine neurotoxicity by irradiation of peripheral nerves. Cancer Treat Rep 1980;64:963.
71. Thant M, Hawley RJ, Smith MT, et al. Possible enhancement of vincristine neuropathy by VP-16. Cancer 1982;49:859.
72. Griffiths JD, Stark RJ, Ding JC, et al. Vincristine neurotoxicity enhanced in combination chemotherapy including both teniposide and vincristine. Cancer Treat Rep 1986;70:519.
73. Weber DM, Dimopoulos MA, Alexanian R. Increased neurotoxicity with VAD-cyclosporin in multiple myeloma [letter]. Lancet 1993;341:558.
74. Carmichael SM, Eagleton L, Ayers CR, et al. Orthostatic hypotension during vincristine therapy. Arch Intern Med 1970;126:290.
75. Gottlieb RJ, Cuttner J. Vincristine-induced bladder atony. Cancer 1971;28:674.
76. Levitt LP, Prager D. Mononeuropathy due to vincristine toxicity. Neurology 1975;25:894.
77. Albert DM, Wong VG, Henderson ES. Ocular complications of vincristine therapy. Arch Ophthalmol (Copenh) 1967;78:709.
78. Mahajan SL, Ikeda Y, Myers TJ, et al. Acute acoustic nerve palsy associated with vincristine therapy. Cancer 1981;47:2404.
79. Delaney P. Vincristine-induced laryngeal nerve paralysis. Neurology 1982;32:1285.
80. Sanderson PA, Kuwabara T, Cogan DG. Optic neuropathy presumably caused by vincristine therapy. Am J Ophthalmol 1976;81:146.
81. Jackson DV Jr, Pope EK, McMahan RA, et al. Clinical trial of pyridoxine to reduce vincristine neurotoxicity. J Neurooncol 1986;4:37.
82. Jackson DV Jr, McMahan RA, Pope EK, et al. Clinical

trial of folinic acid to reduce vincristine neurotoxicity. Cancer Chemother Pharmacol 1986;17:281.
83. Jackson DV, Wells HB, Atkins JN, et al. Amelioration of vincristine neurotoxicity by glutamic acid. Am J Med 1988;84:1016.
84. Le Quesne PM, Fowler CJ, Harding AE. A study of the effects of isaxonine on vincristine-induced peripheral neuropathy in man and regeneration following peripheral nerve crush in the rat. J Neurol Neurosurg Psychiatry 1985;48:933.
85. Van Kooten B, van Diemen HA, Groenhout KM, et al. A pilot study on the influence of a corticotropin (4-9) analogue on *Vinca* alkaloid-induced neuropathy. Arch Neurol 1992;49:1027.
86. Houi K, Mochio S, Kobayashi T. Gangliosides attenuate vincristine neurotoxicity on dorsal root ganglion cells. Muscle Nerve 1993;16:11.
87. Di Gregorio F, Favaro G, Panozzo C, et al. Efficacy of ganglioside treatment in reducing functional alterations induced by vincristine in rabbit peripheral nerves. Cancer Chemother Pharmacol 1990;26:31.
88. Whittaker JA, Parry DH, Bunch C, et al. Coma associated with vincristine therapy. BMJ 1973;4:335.
89. Hurwitz RL, Mahoney DH Jr, Armstrong DL, et al. Reversible encephalopathy and seizures as a result of conventional vincristine administration. Med Pediatr Oncol 1988;16:216.
90. Byrd RL, Rohrbaugh TM, Raney RB Jr, et al. Transient cortical blindness secondary to vincristine therapy in childhood malignancies. Cancer 1981;47:37.
91. Carpentieri U, Lockhart LH. Ataxia and athetosis as side effects of chemotherapy with vincristine in non-Hodgkin's lymphoma. Cancer Treat Rep 1978;62:561.
92. Boranic M, Raci F. A Parkinson-like syndrome as a side effect of chemotherapy with vincristine and adriamycin in a child with acute leukaemia. Biomedicine 1979;31:124.
93. Owens G. Intraarterial chemotherapy of primary brain tumors. Ann NY Acad Sci 1969;159:603.
94. Bleck TP, Jacobsen J. Prolonged survival following the inadvertent intrathecal administration of vincristine: clinical and electrophysiologic analyses. Clin Neuropharmacol 1991;14:457.
95. Dyke RW. Treatment of inadvertent intrathecal injection of vincristine. N Engl J Med 1989;321:1270.
96. Lipton RB, Apfel SC, Dutcher JP, et al. Taxol produces a predominantly sensory neuropathy. Neurology 1989; 39:368.
97. Hilkens PHE, Verweij J, Stoter G, et al. Peripheral neurotoxicity induced by docetaxel. Neurology 1986; 46:104.
98. Rowinsky EK, Eisenhauer EA, Chaudhry V, et al. Clinical toxicities encountered with paclitaxel (TAXOL). Semin Oncol 1993;20(No 4, Suppl 3):1.
99. Kim JH, Khil MS, Kim SH, et al. Clinical and biological studies of estramustine phosphate as a novel radiation sensitizer. Int J Radiat Oncol Biol Phys 1994;29:555.
100. Yoshida D, Piepmeir J, Weinstein M. Estramustine sensitizes human glioblastoma cells to irradiation. Cancer Res 1994;54:1415.
101. Eklov S, Essand M, Carlsson J, et al. Radiation sensitization by estramustine studies on cultured human prostate cancer cells. Prostate 1992;21:287.
102. Calvaletti G, Marzorati L, Bogliun G, et al. Cisplatin-induced peripheral neurotoxicity is dependent on total-dose intensity and single-dose intensity. Cancer 1992;69:203.
103. Siegal T, Haim N. Cisplatin-induced peripheral neuropathy. Frequent off-therapy deterioration, demyelinating syndromes, and muscle cramps. Cancer 1990; 66:1117.
104. Rosenfeld CS, Broder LE. Cisplatin-induced autonomic neuropathy. Cancer Treat Rep 1984;68:659.
105. Boogerd W, ten Bokkel Huinink WW, Dalesio O, et al. Cisplatin induced neuropathy: central, peripheral and autonomic nerve involvement. J Neurooncol 1990; 9:255.
106. Mollman JE, Hogan WM, Glover DJ, et al. Unusual presentation of cis-platinum neuropathy. Neurology 1988;38:488.
107. Grunberg SM, Sonka S, Stevenson LL, et al. Progressive paresthesias after cessation of therapy with very high-dose cisplatin. Cancer Chemother Pharmacol 1989;25:62.
108. Riggs JE, Ashraf M, Snyder RD, et al. Prospective nerve conduction studies in cisplatin therapy. Ann Neurol 1988;23:92.
109. Thompson SW, Davis LE, Kornfeld M, et al. Cisplatin neuropathy. Clinical, electrophysiologic, morphologic, and toxicologic studies. Cancer 1984;54:1269.
110. Gregg RW, Molepo JM, Monpetit VJ, et al. Cisplatin neurotoxicity: the relationship between dosage, time, and platinum concentration in neuologic tissues, and morphologic evidence of toxicity. J Clin Oncol 1992; 10:795.
111. Montpetit VJA, Stewart D, Dancea S, et al. Pathology of dorsal root ganglia (DRG) in cis-platinum therapy [abstract 34]. J Neuropathol Exp Neurol 1988;47:312.
112. Apfel SC, Arezzo JC, Lipson L, et al. Nerve growth factor prevents experimental cisplatin neuropathy. Ann Neurol 1992;31:76.
113. Anderson ME, Naganuma A, Meister A. Protection against cisplatin toxicity by administration of glutathione ester. FASEB J 1990;4:3251.
114. Gao WQ, Dybdal N, Shinsky N, et al. Neurotrophin-3 reverses experimental cisplatinum induced peripheral sensory neuropathy. Ann Neurol 1995;38:30.
115. Van der Hoop RG, Vecht CJ, van der Burg ME, et al. Prevention of cisplatin neurotoxicity with an ACTH (4-9) analogue in patients with ovarian cancer. N Engl J Med 1990;322:89.
116. Moroso MJ, Blair RL. A review of cis-platinum ototoxicity. J Otolaryngol 1983;12:365.
117. Reddel RR, Kefford RF, Grant JM, et al. Ototoxicity in

patients receiving cisplatin: importance of dose and method of drug administration. Cancer Treat Rep 1982;66:19.
118. Schell MJ, McHaney VA, Green AA, et al. Hearing loss in children and young adults receiving cisplatin with or without prior cranial irradiation. J Clin Oncol 1989; 7:754.
119. Meyer WH, Ayers D, McHaney VA, et al. Ifosfamide and exacerbation of cisplatin-induced hearing loss [letter]. Lancet 1993;341:754.
120. Ostrow S, Hahn D, Wiernik PH, et al. Ophthalmologic toxicity after cis-dichlorodiammine-platinum (II) therapy. Cancer Treat Rep 1978;62:1591.
121. Walsh TJ, Clark AW, Parhad IM, et al. Neurotoxic effects of cisplatin therapy. Arch Neurol 1982;39:719.
122. List AF, Kummet TD. Spinal cord toxicity complicating treatment with cisplatin and etoposide. Am J Clin Oncol 1990;13:256.
123. Bruck W, Heise E, Friede RL. Leukoencephalopathy after cisplatin therapy. Clin Neuropathol 1989;8:263.
124. Cattaneo MT, Filipazzi V, Piazza E, et al. Transient blindness and seizure associated with cisplatin therapy. J Cancer Res Clin Oncol 1988;114:528.
125. Highley M, Meller ST, Pinkerton CR. Seizures and cortical dysfunction following high-dose cisplatin administration in children. Med Pediatr Oncol 1992;20:143.
126. Mead GM, Arnold AM, Green JA, et al. Epileptic seizures associated with cisplatin administration. Cancer Treat Rep 1982;66:1719.
127. Berman IJ, Mann MP. Seizures and transient cortical blindness associated with cis-platinum (II) diamminedichloride (PDD) therapy in a thirty-year-old man. Cancer 1980;45:764.
128. Cohen RJ, Cuneo RA, Cruciger MP, et al. Transient left homonymous hemianopsia and encephalopathy following treatment of testicular carcinoma with cisplatinum, vinblastine, and bleomycin. J Clin Oncol 1983;1:392.
129. Walker RW, Cairncross JG, Posner JB. Cerebral herniation in patients receiving cisplatin. J Neurooncol 1988;6:61.
130. Ritch PS. Cis-dichlorodiammineplatinum II-induced syndrome of inappropriate secretion of antidiuretic hormone. Cancer 1988;61:448.
131. Doll DC, List AF, Greco FA, et al. Acute vascular ischemic events after cisplatin-based combination chemotherapy for germ-cell tumors of the testis. Ann Intern Med 1986;105:48.
132. Doll DC, Ringenberg QS, Yarbro JW. Vascular toxicity associated with antineoplastic agents. J Clin Oncol 1986;4:1405.
133. Icli F, Karaoguz H, Dincol D, et al. Severe vascular toxicity associated with cisplatin-based chemotherapy. Cancer 72;1993:587.
134. Frustaci S, Barzan L, Comoretto R, et al. Local neurotoxicty after intra-arterial cisplatin in head and neck cancer. Cancer Treat Rep 1987;71:257.
135. Feun LG, Wallace S, Stewart DJ, et al. Intracarotid infusion of cis-diamminedichloroplatinum in the treatment of recurrent malignant brain tumors. Cancer 1984;54:794.
136. Shimamura Y, Chikama M, Tanimoto T, et al. Optic nerve degeneration caused by supraophthalmic carotid artery infusion with cisplatin and ACNU. Case report. J Neurosurg 1990;72:285.
137. Kupersmith MJ, Frohman LP, Choi IS, et al. Visual system toxicity following intra-arterial chemotherapy. Neurology 1988;38:284.
138. Castellanos AM, Glass JP, Yung WKA. Regional nerve injury after intra-arterial chemotherapy. Neurology 1987;39:834.
139. O'Brien MER, Tonge K, Blake P, et al. Blindness associated with high-dose carboplatin [letter]. Lancet 1992;339:558.
140. Walker RW, Rosenblum MK, Kempin SJ, et al. Carboplatin-associated thrombotic microangiopathic hemolytic anemia. Cancer 1989;64:1017.
141. Burger PC, Kamenar E, Schold SC, et al. Encephalomyelopathy following high-dose BCNU therapy. Cancer 1981;48:1318.
142. Shingleton BJ, Bienfang DC, Albert DM, et al. Ocular toxicity associated with high-dose carmustine. Arch Ophthalmol 1982;100:1766.
143. Wilson WB, Perez GM, Kleinschmidt-DeMasters BK. Sudden onset of blindess in patients treated with oral CCNU and low-dose cranial irradiation. Cancer 1987;59:901.
144. Rosenblum MK, Delattre J-Y, Walker RW, et al. Fatal necrotizing encephalopathy complicating treatment of malignant gliomas with intra-arterial BCNU and irradiation: a pathological study. J Neurooncol 1989; 7:269.
145. Mahaley MS Jr, Whaley RA, Blue M, et al. Central neurotoxicity following intracarotid BCNU chemotherapy for malignant gliomas. J Neurooncol 1986;3:297.
146. Hochberg FH, Pruitt AA, Beck DO, et al. The rationale and methodology for intra-arterial chemotherapy with BCNU as treatment for glioblastoma. J Neurosurg 1985;63:876.
147. Tonn JC, Roosen K, Schachenmayer W. Brain necrosis after intraarterial chemotherapy and irradiation of malignant gliomas—a complication of both ACNU and BCNU? J Neurooncol 1991;11:241.
148. Stewart DJ, Grahovac Z, Russell NA, et al. Phase I study of intracarotid PCNU. J Neurooncol 1987;5:245.
149. Bethlenfalvay NC, Bergin JJ. Severe cerebral toxicity after intravenous nitrogen mustard therapy. Cancer 1972;29:366.
150. Segal GM, Duckert LG. Reversible mechlorethamine-associated hearing loss in a patient with Hodgkin's disease. Cancer 1986;57:1089.
151. Kende G, Sirkin SR, Thomas PR, et al. Blurring of vision: a previously undescribed complication of cyclophosphamide therapy. Cancer 1979;44:69.
152. Tashima CK. Immediate cerebral symptoms during

rapid intravenous administration of cyclophosphamide (NSC-26271). Cancer Chemother Rep 1975;59:441.
153. Goren MP, Wright RK, Pratt CB, et al. Dechlorethylation of ifosfamide and neurotoxicity [letter]. Lancet 1986;2:1219.
154. Pratt CB, Green AA, Horowitz ME, et al. Central nervous system toxicity following the treatment of pediatric patients with ifosfamide/mesna. J Clin Oncol 1986;4:1253.
155. Pratt CB, Goren MP, Meyer WH, et al. Ifosfamide neurotoxicity is related to previous cisplatin treatment for pediatric solid tumors. J Clin Oncol 1990;8:1399.
156. DiMaggio JR, Brown R, Baile WF, et al. Hallucinations and ifosfamide-induced neurotoxicity. Cancer 1994; 73:1509.
157. Cerny T, Kupfer A. The enigma of ifosfamide encephalopathy [editorial]. Ann Oncol 1992;3:679.
158. Kupfer A, Aeschlimann C, Wermuth B, et al. Prophylaxis and reversal of ifosfamide encephalopathy with methylene-blue. Lancet 1994;343:763.
159. Patel SR, Forman AD, Benjamin RS. High-dose ifosfamide-induced exacerbation of peripheral neuropathy. J Natl Cancer Inst 1994;86:305.
160. Heideman RL, Cole DE, Balis F, et al. Phase I and pharmacokinetic evaluation of thiotepa in the cerebrospinal fluid and plasma of pediatric patients: evidence for dose-dependent plasma clearance of thiotepa. Cancer Res 1989;49:736.
161. Woff SN, Herzig RH, Fay JW, et al. High-dose N,N', N''-triethylenethiophospharamide (thiotepa) with autologous bone marrow transplantation: phase I studies. Semin Oncol 1990;17(Suppl 3):2.
162. Gutin PH, Levi JA, Wiernik PH. Treatment of malignant meningeal disease with intrathecal thioTEPA: a phase II study. Cancer Treat Rep 1977;61:885.
163. Vassal G, Deroussent A, Hartmann O, et al. Dose-dependent neurotoxicity of high-dose busulfan in children: a clinical and pharmacological study. Cancer Res 1990;50:6203.
164. Sureda A, de Oteyza P, Garcia Larana J, et al. High-dose busulfan and seizures. Ann Intern Med 1989;111:543.
165. Grigg AP, Shepherd JD, Phillips GL. Busulphan and phenytoin [letter]. Ann Intern Med 1989;111:1049.
166. Martell RW, Sher C, Jacobs P, et al. High-dose busulfan and myoclonic epilepsy. Ann Intern Med 1987;106:173.
167. Djaldetti M, Pinkhas J, Vries AD, et al. Myasthenia gravis in a patient with chronic myeloid leukemia treated by busulfan. Blood 1968;32:336.
168. Gams RA, Carpenter JT. Central nervous system complications after combination treatment with adriamycin (NSC-123127) and 5-(3,3-dimethyl-1-triazeno)imidazole-4-carboxamide (NSC-45388). Cancer Chemother Rep 1974;58:753.
169. Gerner RE, Moore GE, Didolkar MS. Chemotherapy of disseminated malignant melanoma with dimethyl triazeno imidazole carboxamide and dactinomycin. Cancer 1973;32:756.
170. Paterson AHG, McPherson TA. A possible neurologic complication of DTIC [letter]. Cancer Treat Rep 1978;61:105.
171. Lanser JB, van Seters AP, Moolenaar AJ, et al. Neuropsychologic and neurologic side effects of mitotane and reversibility of symptoms [letter]. J Clin Oncol 1992;10:1504
172. Spivack SD. Drugs five years later: procarbazine. Ann Intern Med 1974;81:795.
173. Samuels ML, Leary WV, Alexanian R, et al. Clinical trials with N-isopropyl-alpha-(2-methylhydrazino)-p-tolnamide hydrochloride in malignant lymphoma and other disseminated neoplasia. Cancer 1967;20:1187.
174. Foster BJ, Harding BJ, Leyland-Jones B, et al. Hexamethylmelamine: a critical review of an active drug. Cancer Treat Rev 1986;13:197.
175. Schachter S, Freeman R. Transient ischemic attack and adriamycin cardiomyopathy. Neurology 1982;32:1380.
176. Barbui T, Rambaldi A, Parenzan L, et al. Neurological symptoms and coma associated with doxorubicin administration during chronic cyclosporin therapy [letter]. Lancet 1992;339:1421.
177. Beck WT, Kuttesch JF. Neurological symptoms associated with cyclosporin plus doxorubicin [letter]. Lancet 1992;340:496.
178. Cordon-Cardo C, O'Brien JP, Casals D, et al. Multidrug-resistance gene (P-glycoprotein) is expressed by endothelial cells at blood-brain barrier sites. Proc Natl Acad Sci U S A 1989;86:695.
179. Arico M, Nespoli L, Porta F, et al. Severe acute encephalopathy following inadvertent intrathecal doxorubicin administration. Med Pediatr Oncol 1990; 18:261.
180. Mortensen ME, Cecalupo AJ, Lo WD, et al. Inadvertent intrathecal injection of daunorubicin with fatal outcome. Med Pediatr Oncol 1992;20:249.
181. Neuwelt EA, Pagel M, Barnett P, et al. Pharmacology and toxicity of intracarotid Adriamycin administration following osmotic blood-brain barrier modification. Cancer Res 1981;41:4466.
182. Man A, Brock PG. Intrathecal mitozantrone [letter]. Lancet 1987;1:327.
183. Hall C, Dougherty WG, Lebish IJ, et al. Warning against use of intrathecal mitoxantrone [letter]. Lancet 1989;1:734.
184. Lakhani AK, Zuiable AG, Pollard CM, et al. Paraplegia after intrathecal mitozantrone. Lancet 1986;2:1393.
185. Doll DC, Yarbro JW. Vascular toxicity associated with antineoplastic agents. Semin Oncol 1992;19:580.
186. Leff RS, Thompson JM, Daly MD, et al. Acute neurologic dysfunction after high-dose etoposide therapy for malignant glioma. Cancer 1988;62:32.
187. Van Echo DA, Chiuten DF, Gormley PE, et al. Phase I clinical and pharmacological study of 4'-(9-acridinylamino)-methanesulfon-m-anisidide using an intermittent biweekly schedule. Cancer Res 1979;39:3881.
188. Legha SS, Brodey GP, Keating MJ, et al. Early clinical

evaluation of acridinylaminomethanesulfon-m-anisidide (AMSA) in patients with advanced breast cancer and acute leukemia [abstract C-518]. Proceedings American Association for Cancer Research 1979;20:416.
189. La Rocca RV, Meer J, Gilliatt RW, et al. Suramin-induced polyneuropathy. Neurology 1990;40:954.
190. Russell JW, Windebank AJ, Podratz JL. Role of nerve growth factor in suramin neurotoxicity studies in vitro. Ann Neurol 1994;36:221.
191. Leonard JV, Kay JD. Acute encephalopathy and hyperammonaemia complicating treatment of acute lymphoblastic leukemia with asparaginase. Lancet 1986; 1:162.
192. Ohnuma T, Holland JF, Sinks LF. Biochemical and pharmacological studies with L-asparaginase in man. Cancer Res 1970;30:2297.
193. Feinberg WM, Swenson MR. Cerebrovascular complications of L-asparaginase therapy. Neurology 1988; 38:127.
194. Priest JR, Ramsay NK, Steinherz PG, et al. A syndrome of thrombosis and hemorrhage complicating L-asparaginase therapy for childhood acute lymphoblastic leukemia. J Pediatr 1982;100:984.
195. Taylor LP, Posner JB. Steroid myopathy in cancer patients treated with dexamethasone [abstract]. Neurology 1989;39(Suppl 1):129.
196. Lacomis D, Smith TW, Chad DA. Acute myopathy and neuropathy in status asthmaticus: case report and literature review. Muscle Nerve 1993;16:84.
197. Hirano M, Ott BR, Raps EC, et al. Acute quadriplegic myopathy: a complication of treatment with steroids, nondepolarizing blocking agents, or both. Neurology 1992;42:2082.
198. Khaleeli AA, Edwards RHT, Gohil K, et al. Corticosteroid myopathy: a clinical and pathological study. Clin Endocrinol 1983;18:155.
199. Coomes EN. The rate of recovery of reversible myopathies and the effects of anabolic agents in steroid myopathy. Neurology 1965;15:523.
200. Stiefel FC, Breitbart WS, Holland JC. Corticosteroids in cancer: neuropsychiatric complications. Cancer Invest 1989;7:479.
201. Hu D-S, Silberfarb PM. Management of sleep problems in cancer patients. Oncology (Huntingt) 1991;5:23.
202. Baethge BA, Lidsky MD. Intractable hiccups associated with high-dose intravenous methyl-prednisolone therapy. Ann Intern Med 1986;104:58.
203. Ron IG, Inbar MJ, Barak Y, et al. Organic delusional syndrome associated with tamoxifen treatment. Cancer 1992;69:1415.
204. Pluss JL, DiBella NJ. Reversible central nervous system dysfunction due to tamoxifen in a patient with breast cancer. Ann Intern Med 1984;101:652.
205. Saphner T, Tormey DC, Gray R. Venous and arterial thrombosis in patients who received adjuvant therapy for breast cancer. J Clin Oncol 1991;9:286.
206. Grunberg SM, Weiss MH, Spitz IM, et al. Treatment of unresectable meningiomas with the antiprogesterone agent mifepristone. J Neurosurg 1991;74:861.
207. Adams F, Fernandez F, Mavligit G. Interferon-induced organic mental disorders associated with unsuspected pre-existing neurologic abnormalities. J Neurooncol 1988;6:355.
208. Adams F, Quesada JR, Gutterman JU. Neuropsychiatric manifestations of human leukocyte interferon therapy in patients with cancer. JAMA 1984;252:938.
209. Meyers CA, Scheibel RS, Forman AD. Persistent neurotoxicity of systemically administered interferon-alpha. Neurology 1991;41:672.
210. Bernsen PL, Wong Chung RE, Vingerhoets HM, et al. Bilateral neuralgic amyotrophy induced by interferon treatment. Arch Neurol 1988;45:449.
211. Bauherz G, Soeur M, Lustman F. Oculomotor nerve paralysis induced by alpha II-interferon. Acta Neurol Belg 1990;90:111.
212. Kanda Y, Shigeno K, Kinoshita N, et al. Sudden hearing loss associated with interferon. Lancet 1994;343:1134.
213. Siegel JP, Puri RK. Interleukin-2 toxicity. J Clin Oncol 1991;9:694.
214. Saris SC, Patronas NJ, Rosenberg SA, et al. The effect of intravenous interleukin-2 on brain water content. J Neurosurg 1989;71:169.
215. Bernard JT, Ameriso S, Kempf RA, et al. Transient focal neurologic deficits complicating interleukin-2 therapy. Neurology 1990;40:154.
216. Illowsky Karp B, Yang JC, Khorsand M, et al. Multiple cerebral lesions complicating therapy with interleukin-2. Neurology 1996;47:417.
217. Philip T, Mercatello A, Negrier S, et al. Interleukin-2 with and without LAK cells in metastatic renal cell carcinoma; the Lyon first-year experience in 20 patients. Cancer Treat Rev 1989;16(Suppl A):91.
218. Somers SS, Reynolds JV, Guillou PJ. Multifocal neurotoxicity during interleukin-2 therapy for malignant melanoma. Clin Oncol (R Coll Radiol) 1992;4:135.
219. Vecht CJ, Keohane C, Menon RS, et al. Acute fatal leukoencephalopathy after interleukin-2 therapy. N Engl J Med 1990;323:1146.
220. Meyers CA, Yung WKA. Delayed neurotoxicity of intraventricular interleukin-2: a case report. J Neurooncol 1993;15:265.
221. Loh FL, Herskovitz S, Berger AR, et al. Brachial plexopathy associated with interleukin-2 therapy. Neurology 1992;42:462.
222. Heys SD, Mills KLG, Evemin O. Bilateral carpal tunnel syndrome associated with interleukin-2 therapy. Postgrad Med J 1992;68:587.
223. Neta R, Oppenheim JJ. IL-1. Can we exploit Jekyll and subjugate Hyde? Biological Therapy Cancer Updates 1992;2:1.
224. Forman AD. Neurologic complications of cytokine therapy. Oncology 1994;8:105.
225. Sherman ML, Spriggs DR, Arthur KA, et al. Recombinant humor tumor necrosis factor administered as a

five-day continuous infusion in cancer patients: phase I toxicity and effect on lipid metabolism. J Clin Oncol 1988;6:344.
226. Blick M, Sherwin SA, Rosenblum M, et al. Phase I study of recombinant tumor necrosis in cancer patients. Cancer Res 1987;47:2986.
227. Parkinson DR, Cano PO, Jerry LM, et al. Complications of cancer immunotherapy with Levamisole. Lancet 1977;1:1129.
228. MacDonald JS, Schnall SF. The role of 5-FU plus levamisole in the therapy of colon cancer. Princip Pract Oncol 1991;5:1.
229. Melgaard B, Kohler O, Sand Hansen H, et al. Misonidazole neuropathy. A prospective study. J Neurooncol 1988;6:227.
230. Frytak S, Moertel CH, Childs DS. Neurologic toxicity associated with high-dose metronidazole therapy. Ann Intern Med 1978;88:361.
231. Coleman CN, Halsey J, Cox RS, et al. Relationship between the neurotoxicity of the hypoxic cell radiosensitizer SR2508 and the pharmacokinetic profile. Cancer Res 1987;47:319.
232. Foster BJ, Clagetl-Carr K, Hoth D, et al. Pentamethylmelamine: a review of an aqueous analogue of hexamethylmelamine. Cancer Treat Rep 1986;70:383.
233. Williams MG, Earhart RH, Bailey H, et al. Prevention of central nervous system toxicity of the antitumor antibiotic acivicin by concomitant infusion of an amino acid mixture. Cancer Res 1990;50:5475.
234. Taylor SA, Crowley J, Pollock TW, et al. Objective antitumor activity of Acivicin in patients with recurrent CNS malignacies: a Southwest Oncology Group trial. J Clin Oncol 1991;9:1476.
235. Smith MA, Adamson PC, Balis FM, et al. Phase I and pharmacokinetic evaluation of all-trans-retinoic acid in pediatric patients with cancer. J Clin Oncol 1992;10:1666.
236. Natale R, Waterhouse D, Grove W, et al. Phase I clinical and pharmacokinetic trial of CI-980, a novel mitotic inhibitor. Proc Am Soc Clin Oncol 1992;11:292a.
237. Cheung NV, Lazarus H, Miraldi FD, et al. Ganglioside GD2 specific monoclonal antibody 3F8: a phase I study in patients with neuroblastoma and malignant melanoma. J Clin Oncol 1987;5:1430.
238. Gould BJ, Borowitz MJ, Groves ES, et al. Phase I study of an anti-breast cancer immunotoxin by continuous infusion: report of a targeted toxic effect not predicted by animal studies. J Natl Cancer Inst 1989;81:775.
239. Pai LH, Bookman MA, Ozols RF, et al. Clinical evaluation of intraperitoneal *Pseudomonas* exotoxin immunoconjugate OVB3-PE in patients with ovarian cancer. J Clin Oncol 1991;9:2095.
240. Rougier P, Bugat R. CPT-II in the treatment of colorectal cancer: clinical efficacy and safety profile. Semin Oncol 1996;23(No 1, Suppl 3):34.

Chapter 25

Neurologic Complications of Radiation Therapy

Edward J. Dropcho

Objectives

- To recognize the acute reversible effects of radiotherapy on the brain and spinal cord
- To understand the pathophysiology, clinical diagnosis, and management of radiation-induced focal cerebral necrosis and delayed radiation myelopathy
- To increase familiarity with the spectrum of diffuse cerebral injury induced by irradiation, including in adults and children with primary and metastatic brain tumors
- To appreciate the current concepts regarding toxicity of prophylactic cranial irradiation for adults with small cell lung carcinoma and for children with acute lymphoblastic leukemia
- To become familiar with injury to the optic nerve and other cranial nerves caused by irradiation
- To recognize the cerebrovascular disorders induced by cranial irradiation
- To appreciate the increasingly recognized ability of therapeutic irradiation to induce neoplasms of the central and peripheral nervous systems

The central and peripheral nervous systems are often considered to be relatively resistant to high-energy radiation, although the introduction of megavoltage radiation therapy (RT) in the 1940s was soon followed by reports of neurotoxicity. The neurotoxicity of RT manifests as a spectrum of clinical syndromes, ranging from transient and benign symptoms to disabling and even fatal necrosis of the brain or spinal cord. Over the past 20 years more sensitive neuroimaging techniques and methods of clinical testing have shown that the limits of tolerance of the central nervous system (CNS), especially of the brain, need to be revised downward. In addition to directly injuring the brain, spinal cord, or peripheral nervous system, therapeutic irradiation can induce cerebrovascular disease and is being increasingly recognized as a cause of second neoplasms.

Cerebral Injury

Acute Encephalopathy

Brain injury by therapeutic irradiation has traditionally been classified according to its time of onset into acute, early delayed, and late forms.[1] The acute reaction to cranial irradiation usually occurs during the first several days of RT and consists of headache, nausea, fever, somnolence, and worsening of preexisting focal symptoms. Fatal cerebral herniation has been reported but is rare. Acute RT encephalopathy tends to occur more frequently and to be more severe among patients with a large intracranial mass(es) and in patients who receive large (more than 300 cGy) daily dose fractions of whole-brain irradiation.[2, 3] Increased cerebral edema is the most likely cause of symptoms, but this may not be apparent in neuroimaging studies.[4] Acute toxicity generally responds well to increased doses of dexamethasone.[1] Pretreatment with dexamethasone for 24–72 hours before initiating cranial RT reduces the risk of acute encephalopathy for patients with large or multiple brain tumors.

Early Delayed Encephalopathy

Early delayed encephalopathy typically consists of headache, somnolence, and deterioration in preexisting deficits occurring 1–4 months after the completion of cranial RT.[1] Corticosteroids usually produce symptomatic improvement, but the syndrome resolves after several weeks with or without corticosteroids. Neuropsychological testing shows reversible memory dysfunction in some patients.[5] Early delayed encephalopathy is of particular clinical importance among patients with primary brain tumors because its clinical and neuroimaging features are indistinguishable from those of tumor recurrence or progression. During the 2–4 months after completing standard external beam RT, computed tomographic (CT) or magnetic resonance (MR) scans in as many as 25% of patients with gliomas show worsening edema and mass effect, with or without new contrast enhancement. Complete resolution of the clinical and radiographic changes occurs over the subsequent several months.[6–10] Transient clinical deterioration and worsening MR appearance may occur in up to one-half of children who receive hyperfractionated (twice daily) RT for brain stem gliomas.[11] MR scans in up to one-half of patients who receive stereotactic radiosurgery for primary brain tumors show worsening enhancement, mass effect, edema, or all of these signs as long as 12 months after completion of therapy, sometimes symptomatic, with subsequent resolution.[12]

A subset of early delayed RT encephalopathy is the somnolence syndrome that occurs in children irradiated for primary brain tumors and in 40–60% of children with leukemia who receive 1,800–2,400 cGy of prophylactic whole-brain RT.[13, 14] The syndrome occurs 3–8 weeks after completion of RT and consists of drowsiness, nausea, and irritability, and less commonly fever or transient papilledema.[13, 15] Symptoms resolve completely within 3–6 weeks. Corticosteroids hasten recovery and may also prevent the syndrome if given during the course of RT.[16] The somnolence syndrome is probably more frequent and more severe in children younger than 3 years old.[13, 17] Children who develop the somnolence syndrome do not have a higher risk for delayed cognitive impairment.[14]

There are few neuropathologic descriptions of early delayed encephalopathy, which is not surprising in view of its reversible nature. There are several autopsy reports of patients who developed progressive, fatal clinical deterioration 8–12 weeks after RT.[18–20] The cerebral hemispheres or brain stem of these patients showed multiple "punched-out" foci of demyelination, with loss of oligodendrocytes, "bizarre astrocytes," and prominent perivascular mononuclear cell infiltrates, but without vascular changes or frank necrosis. These findings support the theory that early delayed encephalopathy reflects damage (possibly inflammatory or autoimmune) to myelin, glial cells, or both. It is not clear, however, whether patients with the more common reversible early delayed encephalopathy have a less severe form of the same demyelinating process seen in the few autopsied cases.

Focal Cerebral Necrosis

Delayed RT neurotoxicity can occur several months to 10 or more years after cranial RT. This may either take the form of focal necrosis or diffuse cerebral injury. Focal cerebral radiation necrosis can occur after treatment of primary brain tumors[1, 3, 21] or of metastatic tumors,[22] and after incidental irradiation of the brain during treatment of pituitary adenomas or other extraneural tumors of the head and neck.[23–26] The incidence of focal necrosis after 5,000 cGy or more is generally quoted as 3–5%.[3, 8, 27] Many patients with brain tumors, however, die before they are at risk for developing radiation necrosis, and few published series provide actuarial analysis of the occurrence of focal necrosis. In one of few such studies, there was a 2.8% overall incidence of focal radiation necrosis among patients with malignant gliomas, but the incidence was 9% among 12-month survivors.[21]

Focal radiation necrosis in patients with primary brain tumors most often occurs in close proximity to the tumor, even in patients who received a uniform dose of whole-brain RT without a focal tumor "boost."[4, 28, 29] Occasional patients develop focal necrosis contralateral to the tumor.[29, 30] Necrosis affecting both frontal lobes, temporal lobes, brain stem, or all of these sites is prone to occur after RT for pituitary tumors[23, 31–33] or for nasopharyngeal carcinoma.[26]

The histopathology of focal radiation necrosis features predominant involvement of white matter, with relative but not complete sparing of cerebral cortex and deep gray matter structures. In extreme cases there are confluent foci of coagulative necrosis of all parenchymal elements. Demyelination and loss of oligodendrocytes are present in less severely affected areas, with variable axonal loss, axonal swellings, focal calcifications, fibrillary gliosis, and scattered perivascular infiltrates of mononuclear cells. A nearly constant feature of RT necrosis is extensive vascular injury, most commonly seen as fibrinoid necrosis of vessel walls, hyaline thickening of vessel walls, thrombotic occlusion (of varying ages) of small vessels, proliferation of adventitial fibroblasts, hyaline transudates surrounding affected vessels, and formation of telangiectasias.[7, 23, 34, 35] The frequent localization of focal RT necrosis within or close to the primary tumor site suggests that peritumoral cerebral edema potentiates RT injury.[21, 29]

The latent period between completion of cranial RT and the clinical onset of cerebral necrosis ranges from 4 months to 7 years, with a peak onset at approximately 15–18 months.[1] There is no clear relationship between RT dose and the latency period. The clinical presentation of focal RT necrosis is typically that of a subacute space-occupying lesion, which is nonspecific and in brain tumor patients is indistinguishable from tumor recurrence or progression. CT or MR scans show a mass lesion with a combination of edema and patchy or ring enhancement and cannot distinguish RT necrosis from tumor recurrence.[4, 8, 36–38] Definitive diagnosis of RT necrosis requires pathologic confirmation, although in patients with malignant gliomas there is often an intermingling of active tumor with areas of necrosis, so that stereotactic brain biopsies carry a risk of sampling error.

An alternative method of diagnosing RT necrosis is with positron emission tomography (PET) scanning or single photon emission CT (SPECT). Anaplastic gliomas usually show increased uptake of 18F-fluorodeoxyglucose (FDG) on PET scans, in contrast with low uptake in areas of focal necrosis.[38–41] FDG-PET scanning cannot absolutely distinguish progressive glioma from focal necrosis due to limited spatial resolution, the frequent intermingling of tumor cells with small areas of necrosis, and occasional instances of increased FDG uptake by inflammatory or reactive cells in areas of focal RT necrosis.[42] Increased uptake of ^{201}Tl-thallium in SPECT scans is suggestive of recurrent anaplastic glioma. The accuracy of SPECT scanning to distinguish recurrent tumor from RT necrosis is enhanced by dual imaging for both thallium and ^{99m}Tc technetium.[43, 44] As with PET imaging, SPECT scanning is limited by spatial resolution and carries a significant rate of false-positive and false-negative results.[45]

Dexamethasone or other corticosteroids produce clinical and radiographic improvement in a high percentage of patients with focal radiation necrosis.[23, 46, 47] In most cases, this improvement is temporary, or patients become dependent on the corticosteroid; however, there are exceptional instances in which patients maintain their improvement even after the corticosteroids are discontinued.[26] There are anecdotal reports of definite clinical and radiographic improvement in patients anticoagulated with heparin or warfarin,[48, 49] but the actual likelihood of improvement with anticoagulation is unknown. Surgical debulking of necrotic brain tissue is probably worthwhile in patients who do not show adequate response to conservative measures and who have a focal accessible mass lesion.[23, 35, 46, 50] Some patients with focal RT necrosis continue to deteriorate despite surgical debulking because of progressive necrosis adjacent or contralateral to the original site.[24, 51]

There have been numerous and sometimes conflicting attempts to analyze dose relationships and establish dose thresholds for cerebral RT necrosis.[27, 52] There are several formulas for calculating RT dose equivalents based on total dose, daily dose fractions, and treatment duration in order to allow comparison of the radiobiologic effect of different treatment regimens. The first such dose equivalent was the nominal standard dose (NSD) or rad equivalent therapy (ret) devised by Ellis to compare the biologic effect of different treatment regimens on skin and connective tissue [53]:

$$\text{NSD (ret)} = \text{total dose (cGy)} \times N^{-0.24} \times T^{-0.11}$$

where N is the number of dose fractions and T is the total treatment duration in days. The risk of focal cerebral necrosis is probably very low up to doses of 1,600 rets and increases steeply to 10% or more at doses of more than 1,700 rets.[1, 27, 35]

All recent series agree that the daily dose fraction of RT is a more important determinant of the risk of damage to brain or spinal cord than to non-neural tissues. This has led to several modifications of Ellis' original NSD formula in an effort to more accurately relate dose schedules to the risk of neural tissue injury. Studies of the tolerance of rat spinal cord led to the "neuret"[1]:

$$\text{neuret} = \text{total dose (cGy)} \times N^{-0.44} \times T^{-0.06}$$

Focal cerebral necrosis most frequently occurs in patients receiving 1,000 or more neurets. There are, however, documented cases of focal cerebral necrosis occurring at doses as low as 1,300 rets or 750 neurets.[1, 22, 29] A similar dose equivalent formula is the brain tolerance unit (btu)[54]:

$$\text{btu} = \text{total dose (cGy)} \times N^{-0.45} \times T^{-0.03}$$

The risk of focal cerebral necrosis as a function of btu is reported as a sigmoid curve, with a "very low risk" at less than 1,050 btu and a steep increase in the risk of necrosis at more than 1,200 btu.[54] A commonly used regimen for anaplastic gliomas delivers 6,120 cGy in 34 fractions of 180 cGy per day; this is equivalent to 1,720 rets, 1,031 neurets, or 1,120 btu.

These dosimetric analyses of focal cerebral necrosis have led to several general conclusions:

1. The RT dose per daily fraction is an important determinant of the risk of necrosis.
2. In most studies the risk of focal necrosis as a function of the dose equivalent takes the form of a sigmoid curve.
3. Although the exact dose-risk curves differ among different published studies, most agree that above a critical exposure level the curve is steep and that small increments in dose lead to a significantly higher risk of cerebral necrosis.
4. With safe RT regimens the risk of radiation necrosis is very low, but there is probably no absolute therapeutic dose threshold below which it cannot occur.

Diffuse Cerebral Injury

The most frequent neurotoxic effect of cranial RT is not focal necrosis but diffuse cerebral injury.[38, 55, 56] Diffuse injury may be classified according to the age of the patient and the setting in which cranial RT is administered, but in all these groups (except patients with "methotrexate leukoencephalopathy") a common pathophysiology probably applies. There is not a very strong correlation between abnormalities in neuroimaging studies and the presence or severity of clinical neurologic and neuropsychological deficits.

Primary Brain Tumors in Adults

There are several reports of serial neuroimaging studies in this population, but only a few small neuropsychological studies. This is at least partially due to the fact that only a small minority of adults with glioblastoma multiforme or other malignant primary brain tumors survive long enough for delayed diffuse cerebral injury to become an issue. Serial CT or MR scans in at least one-half of long-term survivors (more than 18–24 months) with malignant gliomas show diffuse cortical atrophy, ventricular dilatation, and signal abnormalities in the hemispheric white matter.[37, 57–62] The severity of white matter changes is positively correlated to the volume of brain irradiated, the total RT dose, and patient age.[63, 64] Neuroimaging abnormalities may progressively worsen over time in up to one-half of patients.[65]

Some but not all patients with these radiographic abnormalities develop clinically important cognitive impairment. Up to 30–50% of adults with malignant gliomas are unable to return to their premorbid employment and functional status because of moderate to severe diffuse cortical dysfunction.[62, 66–69] Formal neuropsychological testing in these patients has shown particular difficulties with tasks requiring attention or problem solving.[70–72] The more severely affected patients are disabled by progressive dementia and gait disturbance.[62, 67] Several autopsies of patients with malignant gliomas and symptomatic diffuse cerebral injury have shown marked cerebral atrophy with diffuse demyelination and spongiform changes in the hemispheric white matter, but with relative preservation of axons and blood vessels.[59, 62] Patients older than 50 years of age at diagnosis appear to be more likely to develop significant cognitive impairment than younger patients.[61, 62, 69] Most published reports of performance status of long-term glioma survivors describe patients who received whole-brain RT (usually 4,000–4,500 cGy) plus a focal tumor boost.[67, 72] Patients treated with focal RT ports rather than whole-brain RT probably have a lower risk of symptomatic diffuse cerebral injury.[68, 73] A potentiating effect of nitrosoureas or other chemotherapy on the neurotoxic effect of RT has been postulated but not proven.[57]

A relatively unusual but increasingly recognized sequela to 6,000 cGy or more for gliomas in adults is the development within 8–36 months of multifocal patchy or spotty enhancing lesions on MR scans.[74] The lesions are either asymptomatic or associated with worsening focal deficits. They have a variable course, including spontaneous resolution over several months, stabilization, appearance of new lesions together with resolution of others, or (rarely) progression to frank focal cerebral necrosis.

Brain Metastases

Focal cerebral necrosis is a rare occurrence after whole-brain RT for brain metastases, because patients generally receive 4,000 cGy or less, and few patients survive long enough to be at risk. On the other hand, as many as 50% of patients with brain metastases who survive more than 1 year after whole-brain RT develop evidence of diffuse cerebral injury on serial CT or MR scans, including diffuse cerebral atrophy, ventricular enlargement, and signal abnormalities in the hemispheric white matter.[62, 75–77]

Most patients with evidence for diffuse cerebral injury on neuroimaging studies do not have gross neurologic deficits or cognitive impairment, although there are few detailed studies of serial neurologic and neuropsychological examinations in this population. A small proportion of long-term survivors with brain metastases develops a syndrome of progressive dementia, psychomotor retardation, and gait disturbance appearing 6–18 months after whole-brain RT.[62, 76, 77] The incidence of RT dementia has been estimated at 2–5% among all patients treated for brain metastases, and as high as 19% of patients who survive more than 12 months after whole-brain RT. A disproportionately high percentage of reported patients with RT dementia received unconventional whole-brain RT regimens, with daily dose fractions of more than 300 cGy.[76, 77] Autopsies in a few of these patients have shown diffuse injury to myelin sheaths with relative preservation of axons and blood vessels.[62, 77] Ventriculoperitoneal shunting produces a temporary and partial improvement in some patients, but to date there is no reliable way to predict which patients would benefit from a shunt.[62, 77]

The high incidence of brain metastases in patients with small cell lung carcinoma despite a good systemic response to chemotherapy supports the concept of the brain as a pharmacologic sanctuary and has led to the use of prophylactic whole-brain RT. Numerous studies have shown that in small cell lung cancer patients with a complete response to systemic therapy, prophylactic whole-brain RT (usually 2,400–3,000 cGy) significantly decreases the overall incidence of brain metastases (from an average of 25–30% to approximately 5–10%) and reduces the incidence of brain metastases as a solitary site of relapse, but does not improve overall patient survival.[78–81] Prophylactic RT is not without risk, however, and its use is still controversial.[82–84] Mild to moderate diffuse cerebral atrophy and signal abnormalities in hemispheric white matter are present on CT or MR scans in a majority of small cell lung cancer patients who survive more than 1 year after prophylactic RT.[85–88] These abnormalities often become progressively worse on serial imaging studies.[89] Gross neurologic deficits are uncommon, but a high percentage of patients tested have impairment of memory and cognitive functions. In published series a varied percentage of patients develops progressive dementia with gait disturbance.[76, 87, 89–93] Clinically overt diffuse cerebral injury is probably more likely to occur in patients who receive high daily dose RT fractions, concomitant systemic chemotherapy during prophylactic RT, or both.[80, 81, 89, 90, 92, 94, 95]

Primary Brain Tumors in Children

The dilemma of treating primary brain tumors in children is that many tumors respond well to aggressive therapy, including cranial or craniospinal RT, but there is little doubt that the developing brain is more sensitive to RT that the adult brain. As with adult brain tumor patients, there is only a rough correlation between abnormalities in neuroimaging studies and the findings of neuropsychological evaluations. Serial CT or MR scans show diffuse cerebral atrophy and signal abnormalities in hemispheric white matter in up to one-half of children with primary brain tumors after 2,500–4,000 cGy whole-brain RT.[96–98] A distinctive pattern of calcifications called *mineralizing microangiopathy* (see following discussion) also occurs in up to one-third of these patients. The calcifications appear most commonly in the basal ganglia, dentate nuclei, and cerebral gray-white matter junction, sometimes as early as 3 months after whole-brain RT, and often become progressively larger and more numerous over time.[36, 97] Children who receive hyperfractionated RT for brain stem glioma may develop multiple enhancing lesions and abnormal white matter signal distributed in the RT field.[99]

Several prospective studies of disease-free survivors of childhood primary brain tumors have demonstrated significant declines in mean IQ scores within 2 years after whole-brain RT.[56, 100–104] Neurobehavioral problems and learning disabilities occurring after whole-brain RT are often present in children whose full-scale IQ still lies in the normal range. These abnormalities include short-term memory loss, attention deficit disorders, visual perceptual difficulties, and impaired fine motor coordination, reflected in poor school performance and the need for special education.[101, 102, 104–106]

Cognitive decline is more frequent and more severe in children who undergo whole-brain RT at a younger age.[100, 102, 104, 107–109] These children have average declines of 20–25 points in full-scale IQ[102] and are much more likely to have IQ scores of less than 80 than are older children. The age cutoff for higher risk of cognitive impairment varies from 3 to 7 years old among different series; there is nearly universal agreement that the risk is especially high for children irradiated before 2 years of age.

Decline in full-scale IQ is much less common among children who receive RT to focal ports rather than to the whole brain.[109] An exception to this is a disproportionately high incidence of cognitive impairment and learning disabilities among children with primary hypothalamic or suprasellar tumors,[109, 110] independent of the presence or absence of hydrocephalus.

Childhood Leukemia

Prophylactic whole-brain RT (1,800–2,400 cGy) and intrathecal methotrexate in children with acute lymphoblastic leukemia are highly effective in reducing the incidence of leukemic meningitis but carry a significant risk of producing several types of diffuse cerebral injury.[17] The most common findings on CT or MR scans after CNS prophylaxis are diffuse cerebral "atrophy," white matter changes, or both, present in 40–50% of patients in whom serial neuroimaging studies are done.[111–116] In some of these patients, however, the scan abnormalities are reversible,[111, 117] and CT or MR scan findings generally do not correlate well with the results of neuropsychological testing.[115, 118, 119]

Most but not all neuropsychological studies of childhood leukemia survivors have demonstrated a risk of delayed cognitive impairment after CNS prophylaxis. There is a large body of literature addressing this issue, with sometimes conflicting results. Many of the published studies have methodologic flaws such as small patient numbers, selection bias, nonuniformity and insensitivity of neuropsychological tests, and short follow-up periods.[56, 120] Several consistent trends do emerge:

1. In most studies the mean full-scale IQ scores of survivors of childhood leukemia who received whole-brain RT remain in the average range, but are either less than the IQ of controls or show a decline on serial testing.[121–124] Performance IQ is more likely to be affected than verbal IQ.[17]
2. Significant neuropsychological dysfunction and learning disabilities can be present in children with IQ scores in the average range.[117,122,125–129]
3. The risk of significant cognitive impairment is higher among children given CNS prophylaxis before 3–6 years of age than in older children.[17, 121, 125, 128, 130–132]
4. In most but not all series cognitive impairment is more likely to occur after CNS prophylaxis with a combination of whole-brain RT plus methotrexate than with methotrexate alone.[17, 125, 130, 133]
5. Children who receive treatment for overt meningeal leukemia have a higher risk of cognitive impairment than children who are given prophylactic treatment.

The second most common CT finding in long-term survivors of childhood leukemia is the presence of intracerebral calcifications, which appear within 5 years of RT in 4–30% of patients.[111–113, 132, 134] The pathologic correlate of these calcifications is mineralizing microangiopathy, most frequently located in the putamen and less often in the depths of cerebral cortical sulci and consisting of calcification of the walls of small blood vessels, luminal occlusion, and a variable amount of "mineralized necrotic neural tissue."[135] Mineralizing microangiopathy has not been reported in patients who received intrathecal methotrexate but no cranial RT.[112, 113, 135] The risk of mineralizing microangiopathy appears to be higher in children irradiated when younger than 5 years old and in children treated for overt leukemic meningitis.[135, 136] Some but not all patients with mineralizing microangiopathy have cognitive impairment, perceptual-motor disability, or neurologic deficits such as seizures, motor signs, or gait impairment.[112, 132, 134, 137] On average, leukemia survivors with intracerebral calcifications on CT or MR scans are more likely to have cognitive impairment than individuals with cerebral atrophy or normal scan results.

The most devastating neurologic syndrome occurring in survivors of childhood leukemia is delayed leukoencephalopathy, which generally begins insidiously with personality changes, confusion, or somnolence 4–24 months after CNS prophylaxis or treatment of meningeal leukemia. Some children show neurologic stabilization or improvement after cessation of methotrexate treatments, but many suffer a progressive course that in the most severe cases leads to profound dementia, spastic quadriparesis, seizures, and coma.[138–141] CT or MR scans show roughly symmetric bilateral signal abnormalities of the deep hemispheric white matter, especially near the frontal horns of the lateral ventricles, with occasional patchy areas of contrast enhancement. Later changes include diffuse atrophy, ventricular dilatation, and intracerebral calcifications.[141–144] The same clinical, radiographic, and pathologic features of leukoencephalopathy may also occur in adults after whole-brain RT and intrathecal methotrexate for leptomeningeal metastases from breast carcinoma or other solid tumors.[145, 146]

Leukoencephalopathy is characterized by multiple foci of coagulative necrosis disseminated randomly throughout the hemispheric white matter, generally sparing the cerebral cortex and basal ganglia. In severe cases, the lesions coalesce to produce massive destruction of the entire centrum semiovale. Demyelination, loss of oligodendrocytes, axonal fragmentation, and axonal swellings are present within and around the necrotic foci. There is reactive astrocytosis but little if any inflammatory response. Vascular changes such as fibrinoid necrosis and fibrin extravasation may be present but are not frequent or severe.[138, 141, 147] The pathologic features of leukoencephalopathy not infrequently coexist with mineralizing microangiopathy.[138, 139]

There is little doubt that the neurotoxic effects of cranial RT and methotrexate have a synergistic effect in the pathogenesis of leukoencephalopathy.[140, 142] Leukoencephalopathy occasionally occurs after intrathecal or high-dose intravenous methotrexate without cranial RT, but whole-brain RT clearly increases the likelihood of developing leukoencephalopathy. The risk of developing leukoencephalopathy is increased in several settings: (1) after high cumulative doses (intrathecal plus intravenous) of methotrexate,[139, 147] (2) when the methotrexate is given during or after whole-brain RT,[142] (3) when whole-brain RT and methotrexate are given for therapy of overt leukemic or carcinomatous meningitis rather than for prophylaxis, and (4) in patients with abnormalities of cerebrospinal fluid (CSF) flow that result in delayed clearance of methotrexate from the CNS.

Cerebrovascular Disease

The most common deleterious effect of RT on the cerebral circulation is development of occlusive disease of major extracranial or intracranial vessels.[148, 149] Stenosis or occlusion of the extracranial carotid arteries most commonly occurs after cervical or supraclavicular RT given for lymphomas, carcinomas of the breast or thyroid, or a variety of other head and neck tumors.[100, 149, 150] Amaurosis fugax, transient ischemic attacks, or cerebral infarcts occur at intervals ranging from 6 months to 50 years after RT, with a median latent period of approximately 15–20 years. Arteriography shows disease limited to the RT ports, including such unusual sites as the proximal common carotid artery and the internal carotid artery distal to the common carotid bifurcation. Carotid endarterectomy is often made difficult by a lengthy span of diseased artery, scarring of periarterial tissues, and tight adherence of plaque to the vessel wall, but the reported morbidity is fairly low.[151, 152] It is impossible from the anecdotal reports of this rare complication to make any confident statements about the relative merits of surgery, antiplatelet agents, or anticoagulation with heparin or warfarin.

RT-induced carotid occlusive disease is generally believed to be the result of acceleration of ordinary atherosclerosis. Many of the reported patients have hypercholesterolemia or other hyperlipidemias.[149–151, 153] Diet-induced hyperlipidemia is known to potentiate RT injury to major vessels in animal studies.[148, 149] Endothelium is most likely the primary site of injury, with a possible additional factor of injury to the vasa vasorum.

RT-induced occlusive disease of intracranial vessels resembles extracranial disease in its symptoms, but occurs in a different group of patients.[149, 154, 155] Stenosis or occlusion of the intracranial internal carotid artery and its major branches most often follows RT for optic glioma, pituitary adenoma, or suprasellar tumors. The reported interval between RT and symptoms in these patients ranges from 2 to 20 years, with a median of 5 years. When RT is administered to adolescents or adults, the most common intracranial vasculopathy is narrowing or occlusion of the supraclinoid internal carotid artery. In contrast, vasculopathy occurring after RT during early childhood (usually for optic or hypothalamic gliomas) most often takes the form of a moyamoya pattern.[156–158] Clinical manifestations in these children include multiple strokes, recurrent transient ischemic attacks, headache, seizures, and cognitive impairment. The vascular pathology resembles that of idiopathic or primary moyamoya syndrome and features intimal fibrosis and marked proliferation of endothelial and myointimal cells, without inflammation or much atheroma. There are anecdotal reports of benefit from extracranial-intracranial bypass surgery.[158]

Other unusual cerebrovascular disorders may occur as late effects of RT for primary brain tumors. Intracranial or intraspinal hemorrhages have been reported occurring 2–6 years after craniospinal RT for primary brain tumors[159]; the hemorrhage occurred distant from the primary tumor site, and pathology showed microscopic vascular anomalies but no other features of focal RT necrosis. Other reports include the development of mass lesions composed of fibrin, hemorrhage, and a tangle of abnormal small blood vessels (often hyalinized or calcified) occurring after RT for optic or hypothalamic gliomas.[160] There are anecdotal reports of intracranial aneurysms and intracerebral hemorrhage 3–20 years after irradiation of primary tumors.[161, 162] Another recently described cerebrovascular sequel is the development of complicated migraine with unilateral headache and transient focal deficits in children after whole-brain RT for primary tumors.[163]

Optic Neuropathy

Radiation injury to the optic nerve and chiasm most often occurs in patients treated for tumors of the orbit or paranasal sinuses, pituitary adenomas, or craniopharyngiomas.[164, 165] For many of these patients it is impossible to spare the anterior visual system when irradiating tumors with curative intent. Optic neuropathy less commonly occurs after whole-brain RT for primary or metastatic brain tumors. In most patients, the optic nerve exposure was 5,000 cGy or more, although optic neuropathy may rarely occur after doses as low as 2,400 cGy.[166, 167] RT regimens using a high daily dose fraction probably carry an increased risk of subsequent optic neuropathy. The median latency period from RT to the onset of symptoms is 12–18 months, without a clear relationship between the RT dose and latent interval. The pathology of radiation-induced optic neuropathy is a nonspecific mixture of axonal loss, demyelination, gliosis, and microvascular changes.

Patients with radiation-induced optic neuropathy generally present with painless monocular loss of acuity, visual field constriction, or both.[164, 165] Visual field deficits include central scotoma, altitudinal loss, or quadrantic loss. Funduscopic examination initially shows optic nerve head swelling with hyperemic disks, telangiectasias, hemorrhages, cotton-wool spots, and narrowed retinal arterioles. Fluorescein angiography shows retinal capillary nonperfusion. Less commonly, the fundus may appear relatively normal if the main injury is to the retrobulbar optic nerve. MR scanning shows patchy enhancement of one or both optic nerves and occasionally of the optic chiasm.[168–170] The optic nerves may also be slightly enlarged. Some patients have MR evidence for concurrent injury to the nearby brain parenchyma.[171] Most patients with radiation optic neuropathy deteriorate rapidly over several weeks to severe, often bilateral vision loss and optic atrophy, although approximately one-third of involved eyes show partial improvement. Corticosteroids or hyperbaric oxygen have no demonstrated beneficial effect.[165, 171]

Other Cranial Neuropathies

Other than the optic nerve, hypoglossal palsy is the most frequent RT-induced cranial neuropathy, occurring 2–10 years after treatment of primary head and neck tumors. The probable mechanism is entrapment of the nerve by fibrosis. Less common are unilateral palsy of the vagus nerve or spinal accessory nerve or multiple lower cranial nerve palsies. Some patients with RT-induced bulbar palsy have myokymia and neuromyotonic electromyographic (EMG) discharges in multiple muscles innervated by the lower cranial nerves.[172, 173] Cranial nerves III–VII seem resistant to ordinary external photon beam RT, but may be injured by proton beam irradiation of pituitary tumors. Hearing loss is a common complication of cranial RT but is generally due to a conductive loss or cochlear damage rather than to the auditory nerve itself.

Spinal Cord Injury

Transient Myelopathy

The most common form of radiation-induced spinal cord injury is a transient syndrome occurring after craniospinal axis irradiation for primary CNS tumors or after incidental irradiation of the cord for treatment of lymphoma or extraneural tumors of the head, neck, or thorax. Transient myelopathy occurs in at least 10–15% of patients receiving mantle field RT for Hodgkin's disease.[174, 175] The syndrome is more frequent among patients receiving a total spinal cord dose of 5,000 cGy or more or daily radiation fractions of 200 cGy or more.[176] Transient myelopathy occurs after a latent period of 1–30 months after the completion of radiation, with the peak onset at 4–6 months.[174, 177] The syndrome consists solely of paresthesias or electric shock sensations radiating down the spine (Lhermitte's symptom) and frequently extending down the limbs as well.[178] These symptoms are often precipitated or worsened by neck flexion or physical exertion. Patients rarely report other symptoms and almost never show any objective signs of myelopathy. MR scans are unrevealing. Transient RT myelopathy is generally believed to be caused by demyelination of the posterior columns. This is supported by some animal studies, but because of the self-limited nature of the syndrome, there is no neuropathologic proof of this in humans. The syndrome resolves gradually over 1–9 months[174, 175] and affected patients are not at higher risk for developing severe delayed RT myelopathy.

Delayed Progressive Myelopathy

The majority of patients who develop delayed severe myelopathy received incidental irradiation of the spinal cord as part of treatment for extraneural primary carcinomas of the lung, esophagus, head and neck, or of lymphoid tumors. Less common are patients in whom the spinal cord itself is targeted in the treatment of a glioma or as part of craniospinal axis RT for medulloblastoma. The reported incidence figures for delayed radiation myelopathy range from 1% to 12%,[177, 179–184] but are probably misleading because many patients do not survive long enough to be at risk for developing this complication. There appear to be bimodal incidence peaks after latent intervals of 12–14 months and 24–28 months.[185] Exceptional patients have latent intervals as short as 3 months or as long as 10 years after RT.[179, 186]

Delayed RT myelopathy usually presents with numbness or dysesthesias in the legs, followed by weakness and sphincter dysfunction, with an upper level of cord dysfunction ascending to lie within the irradiated area.[179, 186] A Brown-Séquard's pattern is fairly common early in the course.[186–188] Pain is not a prominent complaint. In most patients the neurologic deficits progress over weeks to months in a steady or (less commonly) stepwise fashion, leading to paraplegia or quadriplegia in at least 50% of patients.[186, 189, 190] The clinical features of RT myelopathy do not reliably distinguish it from recurrent primary spinal cord glioma, intramedullary spinal metastasis, paraneoplastic necrotizing myelopathy, or myelopathy caused by intrathecal chemotherapy.

The CSF in delayed RT myelopathy is usually normal but may contain slightly elevated protein levels or a mild pleocytosis.[189, 191] Myelography results are typically normal, but a few patients have focal or diffuse fusiform spinal cord enlargement that may actually extend beyond the irradiated spinal segment.[179, 191–193] MR scans usually show enlargement of the affected cord and abnormally high signal intensity on T2-weighted images.[194–198] Most patients have abnormal intramedullary contrast enhancement, either in a streaky or less commonly a ring-enhancing pattern. The MR abnormalities often extend beyond the RT ports and generally persist for several months, followed by spinal cord atrophy in long-term survivors. MR scanning cannot absolutely distinguish RT myelopathy from recurrent spinal cord glioma, intramedullary spinal cord metastasis, or paraneoplastic myelopathy.

Treatment options for patients with severe RT myelopathy are very limited. Some patients show stabilization or partial improvement on corticosteroid therapy.[192–194] There is a single reported instance of partial improvement after anticoagulation with heparin and warfarin.[49] There are also reports of stabilization or improvement with hyperbaric oxygen.[199] All of the anecdotal reports of treatment lack a denominator to estimate the likelihood of a meaningful response.

The histopathology of delayed RT myelopathy is somewhat variable, both between patients and in different areas of the spinal cord in the same patient.[179, 188, 200] White matter is characteristically more severely affected than gray matter, with a predilection for the posterior and superficial lateral columns. Coalescing foci of demyelination and axonal degeneration in these areas are accompanied by wallerian degeneration above and below the necrotic zones. In the most severe cases there are areas of total coagulative necrosis. In cases in which gray matter is involved, the neurons may show central chromatolysis but are often remarkably preserved. There is a spectrum of severity of changes in small blood vessels, including fibrinoid necrosis of the vessel walls, hyaline thickening and obliteration of lumens, telangiectasias, extravasation of hyaline material, and occasional perivascular lymphocytic cuffing. In some cases, the severity of vascular changes appears to be mild compared with the degree of demyelination and parenchymal necrosis. The nerve roots and anterior or posterior spinal arteries are not involved, even adjacent to areas of extensive cord necrosis. There is some evidence that direct damage to glia and myelin predominates in patients with relatively short latent intervals, whereas patients with longer latent intervals show more prominent vascular changes, although there is considerable variability and overlap among patients.[201, 202]

As with radiation cerebral necrosis, there have been numerous attempts to retrospectively correlate the risk of RT myelopathy with a radiation "dose equivalent" (see previous discussion).[177] The risk of delayed RT myelopathy has been estimated at 1% at 1,015 rets and 50% at 1,480 rets.[180] The risk of brain or spinal cord injury sharply increases at doses of more than 1,000–1,100 neurets.[1] The daily RT dose fraction is an important determinant of the risk of developing delayed myelopathy.[184] There is probably an inverse correlation between the equivalent dose of RT and the latent period for delayed myelopathy.[185] Few of the published analyses factor in the length of the spinal cord irradiated, although this clearly has an impact on the risk of delayed myelopathy.[203]

Although the exact risk estimates from different series vary somewhat, several generalizations can be made: (1) The risk of severe delayed RT myelopathy is considerably less than 5% after total spinal cord doses of 5,500 cGy or less given in daily fractions of 200 cGy or less. (2) The risk increases with a higher dose per daily fraction, higher total dose, shorter total treatment duration, and longer extent of spinal cord irradiated. (3) Unexplained differences in individual sensitivity to irradiation result in the occurrence of delayed radiation myelopathy in a small percentage of patients who receive a "safe" radiation regimen.[191, 196, 204] A potentiating effect of concomitant chemotherapy on the risk of developing radiation myelopathy has been postulated but not proven.[177] Re-irradiation of the spinal cord for treatment of head and neck tumors up to total doses of 8,000–9,000 cGy clearly causes an increased risk of myelopathy, although reliable incidence figures are not available.[205]

Motor Neuron Syndrome

A rare syndrome of selective damage to lower motor neurons has occurred in patients treated with spinal

RT for medulloblastoma,[206] lymphoma,[207] and testicular germ cell tumors.[208–210] Patients present with subacute, diffuse leg weakness beginning 4–14 months after completion of RT. Examination shows bilateral but asymmetric muscle atrophy, fasciculations, normal or decreased muscle stretch reflexes, flexor plantar responses, and no sensory or sphincter involvement. Weakness is confined to the legs even in patients who received RT to the entire spine.[206] The syndrome progresses slowly over several months and then stabilizes but does not improve. Motor and sensory nerve conduction velocities are normal, and there is EMG evidence of diffuse denervation, including of the lumbar paraspinal muscles.[210] In a few published cases, spine MR scans were normal.[211] Lumbosacral anterior horn cells are believed to be the primary site of damage in these patients, but there is no published neuropathologic proof for this, and it is possible that the syndrome represents selective damage to proximal motor axons or to motor roots.

Brachial Plexopathy

Injury to the brachial plexus is the most frequent peripheral nervous system complication of RT. Breast carcinoma is the tumor most often associated with RT brachial plexopathy, accounting for 40–75% of patients in the literature, followed by bronchogenic carcinoma and then by lymphoma.[212, 213] RT-induced brachial plexopathy can be divided into relatively rare instances occurring during or shortly after completion of RT, and the more common "delayed progressive" cases.

Acute brachial plexopathy may occur during the course of axillary and supraclavicular RT for Hodgkin's disease.[214] Severe unilateral or bilateral shoulder pain is followed by weakness, mainly involving the deltoid and supraspinatus muscles, with partial recovery. The acute onset of symptoms and the distribution of weakness in these patients closely resemble cryptogenic brachial plexopathy or neuralgic amyotrophy. The restricted occurrence of acute brachial plexopathy during RT for Hodgkin's disease but not for other tumors argues against direct radiation damage to the plexus and in favor of an inflammatory or immune process specifically related to the Hodgkin's disease.

A syndrome of "early delayed" RT brachial plexopathy occurs in approximately 1% of women treated for breast carcinoma.[215, 216] Onset of neurologic symptoms occurs within the first 6 months after completion of RT. Paresthesias of the hand and forearm are the presenting symptoms in 90% of patients with neurologic symptoms, with shoulder and axillary pain in some patients; the pain and sensory symptoms improve over several months. During this time some patients develop mild weakness, which again resolves almost completely.

Delayed RT brachial plexopathy occurs after a latent interval varying from several months up to more than 10 years. In most reported series the latent interval is at least 12 months, with a broad peak of onset from 2 to 4 years after the RT.[212, 217, 218] There is no obvious relationship between the latent period and the details of RT, except for shorter latencies in patients who have received a second course of RT to the plexus.

There is a rough correlation between the risk of delayed brachial plexopathy and the total dose of RT administered to the plexus.[212, 217, 218] The tolerance dose or safety threshold for the brachial plexus is estimated to be 1,700–1,900 rets,[219, 220] with the incidence of plexopathy increasing sharply above 1,900 rets. A course of 5,600 cGy given in daily 200-cGy fractions over 38 days is equivalent to 1,700 rets. This safety threshold is clearly not absolute; there are reports of a low incidence of brachial plexopathy even at 1,920 rets.[221] Conversely, there are reports of a higher than expected incidence of plexopathy after doses of less than 1,600 rets.[222, 223] The risk of delayed brachial plexopathy is increased when large irradiation fields are used, when patients receive two separate courses of subthreshold RT, and probably when patients receive concomitant chemotherapy plus RT.[216, 223] It is clear that unexplained differences in individual susceptibility result in occurrence of brachial plexopathy following seemingly safe RT regimens.

The exact pathophysiology of delayed RT injury to the brachial (or lumbosacral) plexus remains unclear. Most experimental animal studies implicate microvascular injury as the key event,[224] although peripheral axons and myelin sheaths are also clearly susceptible to direct damage by irradiation.[220, 225] Extensive fibrosis within and surrounding nerve trunks of the plexus, with demyelination and loss of axons, is consistently present at surgery or autopsy.[217, 226, 227] It is difficult, however, to reconstruct the pathophysiology based on this end-stage appearance. The occasional finding of hyalinized and obliterated vessels supports the hypothesis that vascular damage is an important, if not the primary, cause of plexopathy.

The most common presenting symptoms of delayed RT brachial plexopathy are numbness and paresthesias of the hand and fingers, with weakness tending to develop later in the course.[212, 213, 226, 228] Less than 20% of patients report pain at the outset, and approximately one-third of patients have minimal or no pain throughout their entire course.[212, 226] In approximately two-thirds of patients the motor and sensory deficits gradually worsen over several years to a level of severe neurologic disability. The remainder of patients have a spontaneous cessation of progression after 1–3 years.[212, 213, 218, 226, 229, 230] Spontaneous recovery of neurologic function is highly unusual. In some patients, the dysesthesias and pain diminish concurrently with worsening weakness, whereas other patients suffer from persistent or even increasing pain with progressive motor and sensory loss.

A frequent clinical dilemma is distinguishing RT brachial plexopathy from tumor metastasis to the plexus. Carcinomas of the breast and lung together account for an overwhelming majority of brachial plexus metastases. Brachial plexus metastases may occur as an isolated site of tumor spread, and some patients have no other evidence for metastatic tumor for several years or more after the onset of metastatic plexopathy.[212, 226] There is considerable overlap in the latent intervals between patients with brachial plexus metastases and RT plexopathy.[212, 226, 228, 231]

Radiation-induced skin changes, lymphedema, and soft tissue induration of the axilla and supraclavicular fossa are each present in 30–75% of patients with RT brachial plexopathy.[212, 226, 228, 231] These changes are also present in a lower but still sizable proportion of patients with brachial plexus metastases.

The distribution of neurologic signs and symptoms varies somewhat between patients with metastatic versus radiation brachial plexopathy, but the degree of overlap does not permit an absolute distinction to be made. In some series, patients with plexus metastases had predominant involvement of C8–T1 roots or of the lower trunk.[212, 228] In contrast, patients with RT brachial plexopathy often report early sensory and motor symptoms localized to the C5–C6 segments.[212] In several other series, however, there was a much less clear-cut clinical distinction between RT plexopathy and plexus metastases. Many patients with RT brachial plexopathy in these series had weakness mainly involving the muscles innervated by the C8–T1 roots or lower trunk.[213, 228] Conversely, diffuse involvement of the plexus was equally common among patients with metastases and patients with radiation damage.[226, 232]

Although not infallible, the two most reliable clinical features to distinguish RT brachial plexopathy from plexus metastases are Horner's syndrome and pain. Horner's syndrome, when present, strongly indicates brachial plexus metastases, because it is present in up to one-half of patients with metastatic plexopathy and is virtually never seen in patients with RT brachial plexopathy.[212, 222, 228] Metastatic brachial plexopathy is characterized by early, severe, and unrelenting pain in more than 80% of patients.[212, 213, 226, 228] Pain often precedes numbness or weakness by up to several months.[212] Pain is generally but not always most severe in a C8–T1 dermatomal distribution.[212] Early and severe pain in patients with RT brachial plexopathy is distinctly unusual.[212, 226]

The electrophysiology features of RT brachial plexopathy include diminished amplitude of sensory nerve action potentials (often the earliest finding), prolongation of F-wave latencies, and EMG evidence for chronic partial denervation.[222, 233] Motor nerve conduction block across the plexus can be demonstrated in the majority of patients.[213, 234] In many patients, the EMG abnormalities are more extensive than would have been predicted by the clinical examination. In agreement with the clinical signs and symptoms, EMG evidence of denervation in many patients with RT plexopathy is diffuse or predominantly present in muscles supplied by the upper trunk.[233] In some patients, however, the EMG abnormalities are mainly in the distribution of C8 and T1.[235]

The electrophysiologic abnormality that most reliably differentiates RT brachial plexopathy from plexus metastases is myokymia, defined as spontaneous, semirhythmic bursts of potentials. Myokymia is present in one or more muscles in 50–70% of patients with RT brachial plexopathy.[213, 228, 236, 237] Other abnormal discharges less frequently seen included low-frequency bizarre discharges, grouped discharges, and myoclonic discharges. The number of myokymic discharges may vary considerably among muscles innervated by the same trunks and cords of the plexus. Myokymia is rarely if ever present in patients with brachial plexus metastases.

CT scan results in patients with RT brachial plexopathy are either normal or show an ill-defined loss of normal tissue planes without any identifiable mass.[213, 221, 238] High-quality contrast-enhanced CT scans in up to 90% of patients with brachial plexus metastases show a circumscribed soft tissue mass, diffuse soft tissue infiltration, or both.[238, 239] MR scans provide simultaneous multiplanar images and better resolution of soft tissue structures. MR appears to be somewhat more sensitive than CT in detecting brachial plexus metastases, although the difference between the two techniques is modest.[232] Even with MR scanning, there are occasional patients who have no obvious tumor mass and have changes consistent with RT injury who turn out to have plexus metastases. Surgical exploration of the brachial plexus may be done as a last resort in attempting to differentiate metastases from radiation damage, but surgery carries morbidity and may miss metastatic tumor.[212, 231]

There are numerous anecdotal reports or uncontrolled studies of surgical attempts to improve neurologic function and relieve pain in patients with RT-induced brachial plexopathy. The most common procedure is neurolysis (opening the epineural sheath) and removal of scar tissue, with or without placement of an omental flap to revascularize the plexus.[240] Some reported patients with severe pain obtained significant pain relief after surgery[230, 241, 242]; however, the likelihood of improvement is difficult to glean from the literature, and there are few reports of long-term follow-up of patients. Neurolysis rarely relieves motor or sensory deficits, and it is not clear whether surgery can halt the progression of deficits.[226, 230, 243, 244] In 20–50% of patients, surgery causes a significant deterioration in sensory or motor function.[241, 242] Some patients who undergo neurolysis are found to have previously unsuspected plexus metastases.[242] There are anecdotal reports of long-lasting pain relief in patients with RT brachial plexopathy following dorsal root entry zone lesions.[245] Anticoagulation with intravenous heparin followed by chronic warfarin has been reported to bring about neurologic improvement in a few patients with RT brachial plexopathy.[49] Based on only a few anecdotal reports, the actual likelihood of neurologic improvement in patients treated with anticoagulants is not known.

Lumbosacral Plexopathy

RT injury to the lumbosacral plexus is less common than brachial plexopathy and has clearly been recognized only over the past 15 years. RT lumbosacral plexopathy most often follows irradiation for pelvic tumors such as carcinomas of the bladder, uterus, or cervix, testicular tumors, or lymphoma involving para-aortic lymph nodes.[227, 246–249] Patients may have received external beam photon therapy, interstitial or intracavitary radiation implants, or both.[249, 250] The latent interval between RT and onset of neurologic symptoms in patients with lumbosacral plexopathy varies from 3 months to 30 years, with a median interval of approximately 5 years.[227, 248] There is no clear correlation between the RT dose and the duration of the latent interval.

The relationship between RT dose and the occurrence of lumbosacral plexopathy is more complicated than for brachial plexopathy. With standard once daily external beam RT, lumbosacral plexopathy has occurred after doses ranging from 3,000 to 6,750 cGy.[227, 246] Many patients received two courses of external beam RT[246] or a combination of external beam treatment plus intracavitary radiation implants, delivering total doses of 8,000 cGy or more.[248, 249] Another factor that must be taken into account is that irradiation of the para-aortic region or pelvis exposes the nerves over long distances. RT injury to peripheral nerves becomes more likely as the field size increases, but this factor is difficult to quantify.[220]

RT-induced lumbosacral plexopathy usually presents as asymmetric bilateral leg weakness.[227] The weakness may involve any muscles innervated by L2–S1 but often has an L5–S1 predominance. Atrophy, fasciculations, and loss of muscle stretch reflexes accompany the weakness. Pain eventually occurs in approximately one-half of patients, but is usually not early or severe. Approximately one-third of patients have early and prominent numbness and paresthesias.[246] Bladder or bowel symptoms are unusual, and if present are often attributable to RT-induced proctitis or bladder fibrosis.[227] The most frequent course of RT lumbosacral plexopathy is one of slow progression over months to years.[227] A few patients have a more rapid tempo of progression, and a few show stabilization of neurologic deficits after a period of progression.[249] Exceptional patients have significant resolution of weakness and sensory symptoms.[251] There is an anecdotal report of improvement with anticoagulation.[49]

Analogous to the brachial plexus, RT injury to the lumbosacral plexus must often be differentiated from metastatic tumor. Metastases to the lumbosacral plexus most often arise from colorectal carcinomas, breast carcinoma, gynecologic carcinomas, retroperitoneal or pelvic sarcomas, or lymphoma.[227, 252] At least 75% of patients with lumbosacral plexus metastases present with early, severe, and unrelenting pain affecting the low back, hip, and thigh.[227, 248, 252] Most patients subsequently develop weakness and sensory symptoms after a lag period of weeks to months. Bladder dysfunction is uncommon. The tempo of progression of symptoms is usually faster in patients with metastases than with RT plexopathy.

Electrophysiologic testing in patients with RT lumbosacral plexopathy shows reduced amplitude of compound muscle action potentials, abnormal or absent sural nerve potentials, fibrillations, and chronic motor unit changes.[227] One-half of patients have fibrillations in paraspinal muscles, indicating additional injury to nerve roots. Myokymic discharges are present in approximately 60% of patients, especially in proximal muscles.[227, 237] The discharges may be widely scattered and are often present in muscles not overly weak. Low-frequency periodic discharges have also been reported.[247] Myokymia is rarely if ever present in patients with lumbosacral plexus metastases.

CT scans of the abdomen and pelvis are normal in patients with radiation lumbosacral plexopathy.[227, 248] CT scans of pelvis or abdomen show lymphadenopathy, tumor masses, bone erosion, or all of these in 75% of patients with lumbosacral plexus metastases.[227, 252] Patients may have a normal scan result; repeat scans generally show tumor within 6 months.[252]

Radiation-Induced Tumors

An increasing number of case reports and epidemiologic studies indicate that tumorigenesis can be a sequela not only to therapeutic doses of cranial RT given for brain tumors, but also to much lower doses. In order of decreasing frequency, the most common RT-induced intracranial tumors are meningiomas, gliomas, and sarcomas.[33, 253, 254] The largest reported series of RT-induced meningiomas describe patients who developed meningiomas many years after low-dose RT for fungal scalp infections.[255, 256] The estimated intracranial dose in these patients was 200 cGy or less. The latency between RT and diagnosis of meningioma ranged from 15 to 58 years, with a peak between 35 and 40 years. More than 80% of the meningiomas occurred along the calvarium, coinciding with the area of maximal RT exposure. Among the numerous reported patients who developed meningioma after much higher doses of cranial RT for primary brain tumors, the median latency was approximately 15 years, suggesting an inverse relationship between the dose of cranial RT and the latent period for tumorigenesis.[253, 257, 258] Meningiomas have also been reported to occur after prophylactic whole-brain RT for childhood leukemia.[259, 260] RT-induced meningiomas do not show any unusual distribution of histologic subtypes, but they do have a higher than expected degree of cellular anaplasia and are more likely to recur after surgery as compared with sporadic meningiomas.[261–263]

Low-grade or anaplastic gliomas can occur after cranial RT in a number of settings, including long-term survivors of medulloblastoma, pituitary adenomas, and suprasellar tumors, and patients irradiated for extracranial diseases.[33, 253, 264, 265] The mean latent period to diagnosis of RT-induced gliomas is approximately 10 years, with no clear correlation between the latency and either the RT dose or patient's age when irradiated. Approximately 75% of RT-induced gliomas are glioblastoma multiforme or anaplastic astrocytoma, and 12% of the tumors are multifocal.[254, 265, 266] There are no distinctive histologic features of RT-induced gliomas and no striking differences in clinical behavior as compared with malignant gliomas in general.

Approximately 40% of reported RT-induced gliomas occurred in long-term survivors of childhood leukemia who received prophylactic whole-brain RT.[253, 265, 267–269] Gliomas are the most common nonhematologic tumors to occur as second neoplasms in survivors of childhood leukemia,[270, 271] with an estimated incidence as high as 2.3% among 5-year survivors after CNS prophylaxis.[272] Most tumors are anaplastic astrocytomas or glioblastoma multiforme. The risk of developing glioma may be higher among children with leukemia who receive cranial RT before 5 years of age.[271] There is probably a genetic link between leukemia and glial tumors in addition to the tumorigenic effect of cranial RT, because glioma can occur in leukemia survivors who never received cranial RT,[273] and there is an excess incidence of hematologic malignancies among family members of children with brain tumors.[270, 274]

Osteogenic sarcoma of the skull base or the calvarium is a rare complication of RT for pituitary tumors or primary brain tumors, respectively.[33, 253, 275] Dural-based fibrosarcoma may occur after RT for pituitary adenoma.[33, 253]

Malignant nerve sheath tumors involving the brachial plexus may occur in patients from 2 to 25 years after 2,000–4,250 cGy irradiation to the region for lymphoma or breast cancer.[253, 276–278] Some of these patients have stigmata of type 1 neurofibromatosis.[276] Postirradiation malignant fibrous histiocytoma or other sarcomas in the brachial or lumbosacral plexus have also been reported.[232, 248, 279]

Conclusion

Therapeutic irradiation can have injurious effects on the brain, spinal cord, peripheral nervous system, and cerebral vasculature. The pathophysiologic mechanisms of radiation-induced neurologic complications include direct injury to neural tissue, damage to microvasculature or to large blood vessels, and induction of neoplasia. Whether patients receive RT for neural tumors or the nervous system receives "incidental" irradiation in the treatment of systemic neoplasms, a low risk for nervous system injury is an inherent part of effective therapy. Other than treating patients within broad guidelines of "safe" RT regimens, little can be done to reduce the risk. For the neurologist the task is usually that of being able to recognize the varied ways in which RT can affect the nervous system and to differentiate these syndromes from other neurologic complications of cancer. Unfortunately, the therapeutic options for treating RT-induced neurologic complications are often somewhat limited.

References

1. Sheline GE. Therapeutic irradiation and brain injury. Int J Radiat Oncol Biol Phys 1980;6:1215.
2. Young DF, Posner JB, Chu F, et al. Rapid course radiation therapy of cerebral metastases: results and complications. Cancer 1974;34:1069.
3. Leibel SA, Sheline GE. Radiotherapy in the Treatment of Cerebral Astrocytomas. In DG Thomas (ed), Neuro-Oncology: Primary Malignant Brain Tumours. London: Edward Arnold, 1990;193.
4. Deck MD. Imaging Techniques in the Diagnosis of Radiation Damage to the Central Nervous System. In HA Gilbert, AR Kagan (eds), Radiation Damage to the Nervous System. New York: Raven, 1980;107.
5. Armstrong C, Ruffer J, Corn B, et al. Biphasic patterns of memory deficits following moderate-dose partial-brain irradiation: neuropsychologic outcome and proposed mechanisms. J Clin Oncol 1995;13:2263.
6. Hoffman WF, Levin VA, Wilson CB. Evaluation of malignant glioma patients during the postirradiation period. J Neurosurg 1979;50:624.
7. Groothuis DR, Vick NA. Radionecrosis of the Central Nervous System: The Perspective of the Clinical Neurologist and Neuropathologist. In HA Gilbert, AR Kagan (eds), Radiation Damage to the Nervous System. New York: Raven, 1980;93.
8. Mikhael MA. Dosimetric Considerations in the Diagnosis of Radiation Necrosis of the Brain. In HA Gilbert, AR Kagan (eds), Radiation Damage to the Nervous System. New York: Raven, 1980;59.
9. Yamashita J, Handa H, Yumitori K, et al. Reversible delayed radiation effect on the brain after radiotherapy of malignant astrocytoma. Surg Neurol 1980;13:413.
10. Graeb DA, Steinbok P, Robertson WD. Transient early computed tomographic changes mimicking tumor progression after brain tumor irradiation. Radiology 1982;144:813.
11. Packer RJ, Zimmerman RA, Kaplan A, et al. Early cystic/necrotic changes after hyperfractionated radiation therapy in children with brain stem gliomas. Cancer 1993;71:2666.
12. Bakardijev AI, Barnes PD, Goumnerova LC, et al. Magnetic resonance imaging changes after stereotactic radiation therapy for childhood low grade astrocytoma. Cancer 1995;78:864.
13. Freeman JE, Johnston PG, Voke JM. Somnolence after prophylactic cranial irradiation in children with acute lymphoblastic leukemia. BMJ 1973;4:523.
14. Berg RA, Ch'ien LT, Lancaster W, et al. Neuropsychological sequelae of postradiation somnolence syndrome. Dev Behav Pediatr 1983;4:103.
15. Ch'ien LT, Aur RJ, Stagner S, et al. Long-term neurological implications of somnolence syndrome in children with acute lymphocytic leukemia. Ann Neurol 1980;8:273.
16. Mandell LR, Walker RW, Steinherz P, et al. Reduced

incidence of the somnolence syndrome in leukemic children with steroid coverage during prophylactic cranial radiation therapy. Cancer 1989;63:1975.
17. Bleyer WA. Central nervous system leukemia. Pediatr Clin North Am 1988;35:789.
18. Lampert P, Tom MI, Rider WD. Disseminated demyelination of the brain following cobalt gamma radiation. Arch Pathol (AMA) 1959;68:322.
19. Lampert PW, Davis RL. Delayed effects of radiation on the human central nervous system: "early" and "late" delayed reactions. Neurology 1964;14:912.
20. Monro P, Mair WG. Radiation effects on the human central nervous system 14 weeks after X-radiation. Acta Neuropathol 1968;11:267.
21. Soffietti R, Sciolla R, Giordana MT, et al. Delayed adverse effects after irradiation of gliomas: clinicopathological analysis. J Neurooncol 1985;3:187.
22. Sundaresan N, Galicich JH, Deck MD, et al. Radiation necrosis after treatment of solitary intracranial metastases. Neurosurgery 1981;8:329.
23. Martins AN, Johnston JS, Henry JM, et al. Delayed radiation necrosis of the brain. J Neurosurg 1977;47:336.
24. Glass JP, Hwang TL, Leavens ME, et al. Cerebral radiation necrosis following treatment of extracranial malignancies. Cancer 1984;54:1966.
25. Woo E, Lam K, Yu YL, et al. Cerebral radionecrosis: is surgery necessary? J Neurol Neurosurg Psychiatry 1987;50:1407.
26. Lee AW, Ng SH, Ho JH, et al. Clinical diagnosis of late temporal lobe necrosis following radiation therapy for nasopharyngeal carcinoma. Cancer 1988;61:1535.
27. Marks JE, Wong J. The risk of cerebral radionecrosis in relation to dose, time and fractionation: a follow-up study. Prog Exp Tumor Res 1985;29:210.
28. Burger PC, Mahaley MS, Dudka L, et al. The morphologic effects of radiation administered therapeutically for intracranial gliomas. Cancer 1979;44:1256.
29. Schiffer D, Giordana MT, Soffietti R, et al. Radio- and chemotherapy of malignant gliomas: pathological changes in the normal nervous tissue. Acta Neurochir 1981;58:37.
30. Shewmon DA, Masdeu JC. Delayed radiation necrosis of the brain contralateral to original tumor. Arch Neurol 1980;37:592.
31. Berge G, Brun A, Hakansson CH, et al. Sensitivity to irradiation of the brain stem: irradiation myelitis in the treatment of a nasopharynx carcinoma. Cancer 1974; 33:1263.
32. Brismar J, Roberson GH, Davis KR. Radiation necrosis of the brain: neuroradiological considerations with computed tomography. Neuroradiology 1976;12:109.
33. Al-Mefty O, Kersh JE, Routh A, et al. The long-term side effects of radiation therapy for benign brain tumors in adults. J Neurosurg 1990;73:502.
34. Rubinstein LJ. Tumors of the Central Nervous System. Washington, DC: Armed Forces Institute of Pathology, 1972.
35. Rottenberg DA, Chernik NL, Deck MD, et al. Cerebral necrosis following radiotherapy of extracranial neoplasms. Ann Neurol 1977;1:339.
36. Kingsley DP, Kendall BE. CT of the adverse effects of therapeutic irradiation of the central nervous system. AJNR Am J Neuroradiol 1981;2:453.
37. Dooms GC, Hecht S, Brant-Zawadzki M, et al. Brain radiation lesions: MR imaging. Radiology 1986; 158:149.
38. Valk PE, Dillon WP. Radiation injury of the brain. AJNR Am J Neuroradiol 1991;12:45.
39. Doyle WK, Budinger TF, Valk PE, et al. Differentiation of cerebral radiation necrosis from tumor recurrence by 18-F FDG and 82-Rb positron emission tomography. J Comput Assist Tomogr 1987;11:563.
40. Di Chiro G, Oldfield E, Wright DC, et al. Cerebral necrosis after radiotherapy and/or intra-arterial chemotherapy for brain tumors: PET and neuropathologic studies. AJR Am J Roentgenol 1988;150:189.
41. Glantz MJ, Hoffman JM, Coleman E, et al. Identification of early recurrence of primary central nervous system tumors by fluorodeoxyglucose positron emission tomography. Ann Neurol 1991;29:347.
42. Janus TJ, Kim EE, Tilbury R, et al. Use of 18F-fluorodeoxyglucose positron emission tomography in patients with primary malignant brain tumors. Ann Neurol 1993;33:540.
43. Schwartz RB, Carvalho PA, Alexander E, et al. Radiation necrosis vs high-grade recurrent glioma: differentiation by using dual isotope SPECT with 201Tl and 99mTc-HMPAO. AJNR Am J Neuroradiol 1991;12:1187.
44. Carvalho PA, Schwartz RB, Alexander E, et al. Detection of recurrent gliomas with quantitative thallium-201/technecium-99m HMPAO single-photon emission computerized tomography. J Neurosurg 1992;77:565.
45. Kahn D, Follett KA, Bushnell DL, et al. Diagnosis of recurrent brain tumor: value of 201Tl SPECT vs. 18F-fluorodeoxyglucose PET. AJR Am J Radiol 1994;163:1459.
46. Edwards MS, Wilson CB. Treatment of Radiation Necrosis. In HA Gilbert, AR Kagan (eds), Radiation Damage to the Nervous System. New York: Raven, 1980;129.
47. Shaw PJ, Bates D. Conservative treatment of delayed cerebral radiation necrosis. J Neurol Neurosurg Psychiatry 1984;47:1338.
48. Rizzoli HV, Paganelli DM. Treatment of delayed radiation necrosis of the brain. J Neurosurg 1984;60:589.
49. Glantz MJ, Burger PC, Friedman AH, et al. Treatment of radiation-induced nervous system injury with heparin and warfarin. Neurology 1994;44:2020.
50. Di Lorenzo N, Nolletti A, Palma L. Late cerebral radionecrosis. Surg Neurol 1978;10:281.
51. Rottenberg DA, Horten B, Kim JH, et al. Progressive white matter destruction following irradiation of an extracranial neoplasm. Ann Neurol 1980;8:76.
52. Kramer S. The hazards of therapeutic irradiation of the central nervous system. Clin Neurosurg 1968;15:301.

53. Ellis F. Nominal standard dose and the ret. Br J Radiol 1971;44:101.
54. Pezner RD, Archambeau JO. Brain tolerance unit: a method to estimate risk of radiation brain injury for various dose schedules. Int J Radiat Oncol Biol Phys 1981;7:397.
55. Crossen JR, Garwood D, Glatstein E, et al. Neurobehavioral sequelae of cranial irradiation in adults: a review of radiation-induced encephalopathy. J Clin Oncol 1994;12:627.
56. Roman DD, Sperduto PW. Neuropsychological effects of cranial radiation: current knowledge and future directions. Int J Radiat Oncol Biol Phys 1995;31:983.
57. Seiler RW. Late results of multimodality therapy of high-grade supratentorial astrocytomas. Surg Neurol 1980;15:88.
58. Foo SH, Hiesinger E, Wise A, et al. Quality of long-term survival of treated patients with malignant glioma [Abstract]. Proc Am Soc Clin Oncol 1986;5:136.
59. Curnes JT, Laster DW, Ball MR, et al. Magnetic resonance imaging of radiation injury to the brain. AJNR Am J Neuroradiol 1986;7:389.
60. Curran WJ, Hecht-Leavitt C, Schut L, et al. Magnetic resonance imaging of cranial radiation lesions. Int J Radiat Oncol Biol Phys 1987;13:1093.
61. Stylopoulos LA, George AE, de Leon MJ, et al. Longitudinal study of parenchymal brain changes in glioma survivors. AJNR Am J Neuroradiol 1988;9:517.
62. Asai A, Matsutani M, Kohno T, et al. Subacute brain atrophy after radiation therapy for malignant brain tumor. Cancer 1989;63:1962.
63. Tsuruda JS, Kortman KE, Bradley WG, et al. Radiation effects on cerebral white matter: MR evaluation. AJR Am J Roentgenol 1987;149:165.
64. Corn BW, Yousem DM, Scott CB, et al. White matter changes are correlated significantly with radiation dose: observations from a randomized dose-escalation trial for malignant glioma (Radiation Therapy Oncology Group 83-02). Cancer 1994;74:2828.
65. Constine LS, Konski A, Ekholm S, et al. Adverse effects of brain irradiation correlated with MR and CT imaging. Int J Radiat Oncol Biol Phys 1988;15:319.
66. Lieberman AN, Foo SH, Ransohoff J, et al. Long term survival among patients with malignant brain tumors. Neurosurgery 1982;10:450.
67. Imperato JP, Paleologos NA, Vick NA. Effects of treatment on long-term survivors with malignant astrocytomas. Ann Neurol 1990;28:818.
68. Kleinberg L, Wallner K, Malkin MG. Good performance status of long-term disease-free survivors of intracranial gliomas. Int J Radiat Oncol Biol Phys 1993;26:129.
69. Vigliani MC, Sichez N, Poisson M, et al. A prospective study of cognitive functions following conventional radiotherapy for supratentorial gliomas in young adults: 4-year results. Int J Radiat Oncol Biol Phys 1996; 35:527.
70. Hochberg FH, Slotnick B. Neuropsychologic impairment in astrocytoma survivors. Neurology 1980;30:172.
71. Maire JP, Coudin B, Guerin J, et al. Neuropsychologic impairment in adults with brain tumors. Am J Clin Oncol 1987;10:156.
72. Archibald YM, Lunn D, Ruttan LA, et al. Cognitive functioning in long-term survivors of high-grade glioma. J Neurosurg 1994;80:247.
73. Taphoorn MJ, Schiphorst AK, Snoek FJ, et al. Cognitive functions and quality of life in patients with low-grade gliomas: the impact of radiotherapy. Ann Neurol 1994;36:48.
74. Peterson K, Clark B, Hall WA, et al. Multifocal enhancing magnetic resonance imaging lesions following cranial irradiation. Ann Neurol 1995;38:237.
75. Cairncross JG, Kim JH, Posner JB. Radiation therapy for brain metastases. Ann Neurol 1980;7:529.
76. Frytak S, Earnest F, O'Neill BP, et al. Magnetic resonance imaging for neurotoxicity in long-term survivors of carcinoma. Mayo Clin Proc 1985;60:803.
77. DeAngelis LM, Delattre JY, Posner JB. Radiation-induced dementia in patients cured of brain metastases. Neurology 1989;39:789.
78. Komaki R, Cox JD, Whitson W. Risk of brain metastases from small cell carcinoma of the lung related to the length of survival and prophylactic irradiation. Cancer Treat Rep 1981;65:9.
79. Rosen ST, Makuch RW, Licther AS, et al. Role of prophylactic cranial irradiation in prevention of central nervous system metastases in small cell lung cancer. Am J Med 1983;74:615.
80. Pedersen AG, Kristjansen PE, Hansen HH. Prophylactic cranial irradiation and small cell lung cancer. Cancer Treat Rev 1988;15:85.
81. Arriagada R, Le Chevalier T, Borie F, et al. Prophylactic cranial irradiation for patients with small-cell lung cancer in complete remission. J Natl Cancer Inst 1995;87:183.
82. Turrisi AT. Brain irradiation and systemic chemotherapy for small-cell lung cancer: dangerous liaisons? J Clin Oncol 1990;8:196.
83. Kristjansen PE, Kristensen CA. The role of prophylactic cranial irradiation in the management of small cell lung cancer. Cancer Treat Rev 1993;19:3.
84. Bunn PA, Kelly K. Prophylactic cranial irradiation for patients with small-cell lung cancer. J Natl Cancer Inst 1995;87:161.
85. Catane R, Schwade JG, Yarr I, et al. Follow-up neurological evaluation in patients with small cell lung carcinoma treated with prophylactic cranial irradiation and chemotherapy. Int J Radiat Oncol Biol Phys 1981; 7:105.
86. Craig JB, Jackson DV, Moody D, et al. Prospective evaluation of changes in computed cranial tomography in patients with small cell lung carcinoma treated with chemotherapy and prophylactic cranial irradiation. J Clin Oncol 1984;2:1151.

87. Johnson BE, Becker B, Goff WB, et al. Neurologic, neuropsychologic, and computed cranial tomography scan abnormalities in 2- to 10-year survivors of small cell lung cancer. J Clin Oncol 1985;3:1659.
88. Lee JS, Umsawadi T, Lee YY, et al. Neurotoxicity in long-term survivors of small cell lung cancer. Int J Radiat Oncol Biol Phys 1986;12:313.
89. Johnson BE, Patronas N, Hayes W, et al. Neurologic, computed cranial tomographic, and MRI abnormalities in patients with small-cell lung cancer: further follow-up of 6- to 13-year survivors. J Clin Oncol 1990; 8:48.
90. So NK, O'Neill BP, Frytak S, et al. Delayed leukoencephalopathy in survivors with small cell lung cancer. Neurology 1987;37:1198.
91. Laukkanen E, Klonoff H, Allan B, et al. The role of prophylactic brain irradiation in limited stage small cell lung cancer: clinical, neuropsychologic, and CT sequelae. Int J Radiat Oncol Biol Phys 1988;14:1109.
92. Fleck JF, Einhorn LH, Lauer RC, et al. Is prophylactic cranial irradiation indicated in small-cell lung cancer? J Clin Oncol 1990;8:209.
93. Lishner M, Feld R, Payne DG, et al. Late neurological complications after prophylactic cranial irradiation in patients with small-cell lung cancer: the Toronto experience. J Clin Oncol 1990;8:215.
94. Bleyer WA. Hobson's choice in the CNS radioprophylaxis of small cell lung cancer. Int J Radiat Oncol Biol Phys 1988;15:783.
95. Van Oosterhout AG, Ganzevles PG, Wilmink JT, et al. Sequelae in long-term survivors of small cell lung cancer. Int J Radiat Oncol Biol Phys 1996;34:1037.
96. Lee Y, Glass P, Eys V, et al. Medulloblastoma in infants and children: computed tomographic follow-up after treatment. Radiology 1985;154:677.
97. Davis PC, Hoffman JC, Pearl GS, et al. CT evaluation of effects of cranial radiation therapy in children. AJR Am J Roentgenol 1986;147:587.
98. Packer RJ, Zimmerman RA, Bilaniuk LT. Magnetic resonance imaging in the evaluation of treatment-related central nervous system damage. Cancer 1986;58:635.
99. Freeman CR, Bourgouin PM, Sanford RA, et al. Long term survivors of childhood brain stem gliomas treated with hyperfractionated radiotherapy: clinical characteristics and treatment related toxicities. Cancer 1996;77:555.
100. Ellenberg L, McComb JG, Siegel SE, et al. Factors affecting intellectual outcome in pediatric brain tumor patients. Neurosurgery 1987;21:638.
101. Duffner PK, Cohen ME, Parker MS. Prospective intellectual testing in children with brain tumors. Ann Neurol 1988;23:575.
102. Packer RJ, Sutton LN, Atkins TE, et al. A prospective study of cognitive function in children receiving whole-brain radiotherapy and chemotherapy: 2-year results. J Neurosurg 1989;70:707.
103. Duffner PK, Cohen ME. The long-term effects of central nervous system therapy on children with brain tumors. Neurol Clin 1991;9:479.
104. Radcliffe J, Packer RJ, Atkins TE, et al. Three- and four-year cognitive outcome in children with noncortical brain tumors treated with whole-brain radiotherapy. Ann Neurol 1992;32:551.
105. Kun LE, Mulhern RK. Neuropsychologic function in children with brain tumors: serial studies of intellect and time after treatment. Am J Clin Oncol 1983;6:651.
106. LeBaron S, Zeltzer PM, Zeltzer LK, et al. Assessment of quality of survival in children with medulloblastoma and cerebellar astrocytoma. Cancer 1988;62:1215.
107. Spunberg JJ, Chang CH, Goldman M, et al. Quality of long-term survival following irradiation for intracranial tumors in children under the age of two. Int J Radiat Oncol Biol Phys 1981;7:727.
108. Chin HW, Maruyama Y. Age at treatment and long-term performance results in medulloblastoma. Cancer 1984;53:1952.
109. Jannoun L, Bloom HJ. Long-term psychological effects in children treated for intracranial tumors. Int J Radiat Oncol Biol Phys 1990;18:747.
110. Danoff BF, Cowchock FS, Marquette C, et al. Assessment of the long-term effects of primary radiation therapy for brain tumors in children. Cancer 1982;49:1580.
111. Lund E, Hamborg-Pedersen B. Computed tomography of the brain following prophylactic treatment with irradiation therapy and intraspinal methotrexate in children with acute lymphoblastic leukemia. Neuroradiology 1984;26:351.
112. Riccardi R, Brouwers P, Di Chiro G, et al. Abnormal computed tomography brain scans in children with acute lymphoblastic leukemia: serial long-term follow-up. J Clin Oncol 1985;3:12.
113. Brecher ML, Berger P, Freeman AI, et al. Computerized tomography scan findings in children with acute lymphocytic leukemia treated with three different methods of central nervous system prophylaxis. Cancer 1985;56:2430.
114. Paakko E, Vainionpaa L, Lanning M, et al. White matter changes in children treated for acute lymphoblastic leukemia. Cancer 1992;70:2728.
115. Kingman A, Mooyaart EL, Kamps WA, et al. Magnetic resonance imaging of the brain and neuropsychological evaluation in children treated for acute lymphoblastic leukemia at a young age. Am J Pediatr Hematol Oncol 1993;15:231.
116. Matsumoto K, Takahashi S, Sato A, et al. Leukoencephalopathy in childhood hematopoietic neoplasm caused by moderate-dose methotrexate and prophylactic cranial radiotherapy: an MR analysis. Int J Radiat Oncol Biol Phys 1995;32:913.
117. Ochs J, Mulhern R, Fairclough D, et al. Comparison of neuropsychologic functioning and clinical indicators of neurotoxicity in long-term survivors of childhood leukemia given cranial radiation or parenteral methotrexate: a prospective study. J Clin Oncol 1991;9:145.

118. Poplack DG, Brouwers P. Adverse sequelae of central nervous system therapy. Clin Oncol 1985;4:263.
119. Kramer JH, Norman D, Brant-Zawadzki M, et al. Absence of white matter changes on magnetic resonance imaging in children treated with CNS prophylaxis therapy for leukemia. Cancer 1988;61:928.
120. Williams JM, Dvais KS. Central nervous system prophylactic treatment for childhood leukemia: neuropsychological outcome studies. Cancer Treat Rev 1986; 13:113.
121. Jannoun L. Are cognitive and educational development affected by age at which prophylactic therapy is given in acute lymphoblastic leukemia? Arch Dis Child 1983;58:953.
122. Moss HA, Nannis ED, Poplack DG. The effects of prophylactic treatment of the central nervous system on the intellectual functioning of children with acute lymphocytic leukemia. Am J Med 1981;71:47.
123. Anderson V, Smibert E, Ekert H, et al. Intellectual, educational, and behavioural sequelae after cranial irradiation and chemotherapy. J Neurol Neurosurg Psychiatry 1994;70:476.
124. Jankovic M, Brouwers P, Valsecchi MG, et al. Association of 1800 cGy cranial irradiation with intellectual function in children with acute lymphoblastic leukaemia. Lancet 1994;344:224.
125. Meadows AT, Massari DJ, Fergusson J, et al. Declines in IQ scores and cognitive dysfunction in children with acute lymphocytic leukemia treated with cranial irradiation. Lancet 1981;2:1015.
126. Moore I, Kramer JH, Wara W, et al. Cognitive function in children with leukemia: effect of radiation dose and time since irradiation. Cancer 1991;68:1913.
127. Butler RW, Hill JM, Steinherz PG, et al. Neuropsychologic effects of cranial irradiation, intrathecal methotrexate, and systemic methotrexate in childhood cancer. J Clin Oncol 1994;12:2621.
128. Haupt R, Fears TR, Robison LL, et al. Educational attainment in long-term survivors of childhood acute lymphoblastic leukemia. JAMA 1994;272:1427.
129. Smibert E, Anderson V, Godber T, et al. Risk factors for intellectual and educational sequelae of cranial irradiation in childhood acute lymphoblastic leukaemia. Br J Cancer 1996;73:825.
130. Rowland JH, Glidewell OJ, Sibley RF, et al. Effects of different forms of central nervous system prophylaxis on neuropsychologic function in childhood leukemia. J Clin Oncol 1984;2:1327.
131. Giralt J, Ortega JJ, Olive T, et al. Long-term neuropsychologic sequelae of childhood leukemia: comparison of two CNS prophylactic regimens. Int J Radiat Oncol Biol Phys 1992;24:49.
132. Mulhern RK, Kovnar E, Langston J, et al. Long-term survivors of leukemia treated in infancy: factors associated with neuropsychologic status. J Clin Oncol 1992;10:1095.
133. Mulhern RK, Fairclough D, Ochs J. A prospective comparison of neuropsychologic performance of children surviving leukemia who received 18-Gy, 24-Gy, or no cranial irradiation. J Clin Oncol 1991;9:1348.
134. McIntosh S, Fischer DB, Rothman SG, et al. Intracranial calcification in childhood leukemia: an association with systemic chemotherapy. J Pediatr 1977;91:909.
135. Price RA, Birdwell DA. The central nervous system in childhood leukemia: mineralizing microangiopathy and dystrophic calcification. Cancer 1978;42:717.
136. Carli M, Perilongo G, Laverda AM, et al. Risk factors in long-term sequelae of central nervous system prophylaxis in successfully treated children with acute lymphocytic leukemia. Med Pediatr Oncol 1985; 13:334.
137. Brouwers P, Riccardi R, Fedio P, et al. Long-term neuropsychologic sequelae of childhood leukemia: correlation with CT brain scan abnormalities. J Pediatr 1985;106:723.
138. Rubinstein LJ, Herman MM, Long TF, et al. Disseminated necrotizing leukoencephalopathy: a complication of treated central nervous system leukemia and lymphoma. Cancer 1975;35:291.
139. Ch'ien LT, Aur RJ, Verzosa MS, et al. Progression of methotrexate-induced leukoencephalopathy in children with leukemia. Med Pediatr Oncol 1981;9:133.
140. Phillips PC. Methotrexate Neurotoxicity. In DA Rottenberg (ed), Neurological Complications of Cancer Treatment. Boston: Butterworth–Heinemann, 1991;115.
141. Robain O, Dulac O, Dommergues JP, et al. Necrotizing leukoencephalopathy complicating treatment of childhood leukaemia. J Neurol Neurosurg Psychiatry 1984;47:65.
142. Bleyer WA, Griffin TW. White Matter Necrosis, Mineralizing Microangiopathy, and Intellectual Abilities in Survivors of Childhood Leukemia: Associations with Central Nervous System Irradiation and Methotrexate Therapy. In HA Gilbert, AR Kagan (eds), Radiation Damage to the Nervous System. New York: Raven, 1980;155.
143. Shalen PR, Ostrow PT, Glass PJ. Enhancement of the white matter following prophylactic therapy of the central nervous system for leukemia. Radiology 1981;140:409.
144. Miyatake S, Kikuchi H, Oda Y, et al. A case of treatment-related leukoencephalopathy: sequential MRI, CT and PET findings. J Neurooncol 1992;14:143.
145. Wasserstrom WR, Glass JP, Posner JB. Diagnosis and treatment of leptomeningeal metastases from solid tumors: experience with 90 patients. Cancer 1982; 49:759.
146. Obbens EA, Leavens ME, Beal JW, et al. Ommaya reservoirs in 387 cancer patients: a 15-year experience. Neurology 1985;35:1274.
147. Price RA, Jamieson PA. The central nervous system in childhood leukemia: subacute leukoencephalopathy. Cancer 1975;35:306.
148. McCready RA, Hyde GL, Bivins BA, et al. Radiation-induced arterial injuries. Surgery 1983;93:306.

149. Murros KE, Toole JF. The effect of radiation on carotid arteries: a review article. Arch Neurol 1989;46:449.
150. Silverberg GD, Britt RH, Goffinet DR. Radiation-induced carotid artery disease. Cancer 1978;41:130.
151. Loftus CM, Biller J, Hart MN, et al. Management of radiation-induced accelerated carotid atherosclerosis. Arch Neurol 1987;44:711.
152. Atkinson JL, Sundt TM, Dale AJ, et al. Radiation-induced atheromatous disease of the cervical carotid artery: report of seven cases and review of the literature. Neurosurgery 1989;24:171.
153. Werner MH, Burger PC, Heinz ER, et al. Intracranial atherosclerosis following radiotherapy. Neurology 1988;38:1158.
154. Painter MJ, Chutorian AM, Hilal SK. Cerebrovasculopathy following irradiation in childhood. Neurology 1975;25:189.
155. Mori K, Takeuchi J, Ishikawa M, et al. Occlusive arteriopathy and brain tumor. J Neurosurg 1978;49:22.
156. Beyer RA, Paden P, Sobel DF, et al. Moyamoya pattern of vascular occlusion after radiotherapy for glioma of the optic chiasm. Neurology 1986;36:1173.
157. Kestle JR, Hoffman HJ, Mock AR. Moyamoya phenomenon after radiation for optic glioma. J Neurosurg 1993;79:32.
158. Bitzer M, Topka H. Progressive cerebral occlusive disease after radiation therapy. Stroke 1995;26:131.
159. Allen JC, Miller DC, Budzilovich GN, et al. Brain and spinal cord hemorrhage in long-term survivors of malignant pediatric brain tumors: a possible late effect of therapy. Neurology 1991;41:148.
160. Epstein MA, Packer RJ, Rorke LB, et al. Vascular malformation with radiation vasculopathy after treatment of chiasmatic/hypothalamic glioma. Cancer 1992;70:887.
161. Azzarelli B, Moore J, Gilmor R, et al. Multiple fusiform intracranial aneurysms following curative radiation therapy for suprasellar germinoma. J Neurosurg 1984;61:1141.
162. Casey AT, Marsh HT, Uttley D. Intracranial aneurysm formation following radiotherapy. Br J Neurosurg 1993;7:575.
163. Shuper A, Packer RJ, Vezina LG, et al. Complicated migraine-like episodes in children following cranial irradiation and chemotherapy. Neurology 1995;45:1837.
164. Kline LB, Kim JY, Ceballos R. Radiation optic neuropathy. Ophthalmology 1985;92:1118.
165. Macdonald DR, Rottenberg DA, Schutz JS, et al. Radiation-induced optic neuropathy. In DA Rottenberg (ed), Neurological Complications of Cancer Treatment. Boston: Butterworth–Heinemann, 1991;37.
166. Fishman ML, Bean SC, Cogan DG. Optic atrophy following prophylactic chemotherapy and cranial radiation for acute lymphocytic leukemia. Am J Ophthalmol 1976;82:571.
167. Brown GC, Shields JA, Sandborn G, et al. Radiation optic neuropathy. Ophthalmology 1982;89:1489.
168. Guy J, Mancuso A, Beck R, et al. Radiation-induced optic neuropathy: a magnetic resonance imaging study. J Neurosurg 1991;74:426.
169. Hudgins PA, Newman NJ, Dillon WP, et al. Radiation-induced optic neuropathy: characteristic appearances on gadolinium-enhanced MR. AJNR Am J Neuroradiol 1992;13:235.
170. Young WC, Thornton AF, Gebarski SS, et al. Radiation-induced optic neuropathy: correlation of MR imaging and radiation dosimetry. Radiology 1992;185:904.
171. Roden D, Bosley TM, Fowble B, et al. Delayed radiation injury to the retrobulbar optic nerves and chiasm. Ophthalmology 1990;97:346.
172. Poncelet AN, Auger RG, Silber MH. Myokymic discharges of the tongue after radiation to the head and neck. Neurology 1996;46:259.
173. Shapiro BE, Rordorf G, Schwamm L, et al. Delayed radiation-induced bulbar palsy. Neurology 1996;46:1604.
174. Carmel RJ, Kaplan HS. Mantle irradiation in Hodgkin's disease. Cancer 1976;37:2813.
175. Word JA, Kalokhe UP, Aron BS, et al. Transient radiation myelopathy (Lhermitte's sign) in patients with Hodgkin's disease treated by mantle irradiation. Int J Radiat Oncol Biol Phys 1980;6:1731.
176. Fein DA, Marcus RB, Parsons JT, et al. Lhermitte's sign: incidence and treatment variables influencing risk after irradiation of the cervical spinal cord. Int J Radiat Oncol Biol Phys 1993;27:1029.
177. Goldwein JW. Radiation myelopathy: a review. Med Pediatr Oncol 1987;15:89.
178. Jones A. Transient radiation myelopathy. Br J Radiol 1964;37:727.
179. Palmer JJ. Radiation myelopathy. Brain 1972;95:109.
180. Wara WM, Phillips TL, Sheline GE, et al. Radiation tolerance of the spinal cord. Cancer 1975;35:1558.
181. Lambert PM. Radiation myelopathy of the thoracic spinal cord in long term survivors treated with radical radiotherapy using conventional fractionation. Cancer 1978;41:1751.
182. McCunniff AJ, Liang MJ. Radiation tolerance of the cervical spinal cord. Int J Radiat Oncol Biol Phys 1989;16:675.
183. Marcus RB, Million RR. The incidence of myelitis after irradiation of the cervical spinal cord. Int J Radiat Biol Oncol Phys 1990;19:3.
184. Jeremic B, Djuric L, Mijatovic L. Incidence of radiation myelitis of the cervical spinal cord at doses of 5500 cGy or greater. Cancer 1991;68:2138.
185. Schultheiss TE, Higgins EM, El-Mahdi AM. The latent period in clinical radiation myelopathy. Int J Radiat Oncol Biol Phys 1984;10:1109.
186. Dynes JB, Smedal MI. Radiation myelitis. AJR Am J Roentgenol 1960;83:78.
187. Atkins HL, Tretter P. Time-dose considerations in radiation myelopathy. Acta Radiol Ther Phys Biol 1966;5:79.
188. Jellinger K, Sturm KW. Delayed radiation myelopathy in man: report of twelve necropsy cases. J Neurol Sci 1971;14:389.

189. Pallis CA, Louis S, Morgan RL. Radiation myelopathy. Brain 1961;84:460.
190. Reagan TJ, Thomas JE, Colby MY. Chronic progressive radiation myelopathy. JAMA 1968;203:128.
191. Sundaresan N, Gutierrez FA, Larsen MB. Radiation myelopathy in children. Ann Neurol 1978;4:47.
192. Godwin-Austen RB, Howell DA, Worthington B. Observations on radiation myelopathy. Brain 1975; 98:557.
193. Worthington BS. Diffuse cord enlargement in radiation myelopathy. Clin Radiol 1979;30:117.
194. Michikawa M, Wada Y, Sano M, et al. Radiation myelopathy: significance of gadolinium-DTPA enhancement in the diagnosis. Neuroradiology 1991;33:286.
195. Wang PY, Shen WC, Jan JS. MR imaging in radiation myelopathy. AJNR Am J Neuroradiol 1992;13:1049.
196. Yasui T, Yaura H, Komiyama M, et al. Significance of gadolinium-enhanced magnetic resonance imaging in differentiating spinal cord radiation myelopathy from tumor. J Neurosurg 1992;77:628.
197. Melki PS, Halimi P, Wibault P, et al. MRI in chronic progressive radiation myelopathy. J Comput Assist Tomogr 1994;18:1.
198. Phuphanich S, Jacobs M, Murtagh FR, et al. MRI of spinal cord radiation necrosis simulating recurrent cervical cord astrocytoma and syringomyelia. Surg Neurol 1996;45:362.
199. Angibaud G, Ducasse JL, Baille G, et al. Potential value of hyperbaric oxygenation in the treatment of post-radiation myelopathies. Rev Neurol 1995;151:661.
200. Burns RJ, Jones AN, Robertson JS. Pathology of radiation myelopathy. J Neurol Neurosurg Psychiatry 1972;35:888.
201. Reinhold HS, Van Putten WL, Hopewell JW, et al. The latent period in clinical radiation myelopathy. Int J Radiat Oncol Biol Phys 1984;10:2385.
202. Schultheiss TE, Stephens LC, Maor MH. Analysis of the histopathology of radiation myelopathy. Int J Radiat Oncol Biol Phys 1988;14:27.
203. Cohen L, Creditor M. An iso-effect table for radiation tolerance of the human spinal cord. Int J Radiat Oncol Biol Phys 1981;7:961.
204. Zweig G, Russell EJ. Radiation myelopathy of the cervical spinal cord: MR findings. AJNR Am J Neuroradiol 1990;11:1188.
205. Schultheiss TE. Spinal cord radiation "tolerance": doctrine versus data. Int J Radiat Oncol Biol Phys 1990;19:219.
206. Sadowsky CH, Sachs E, Ochoa J. Postradiation motor neuron syndrome. Arch Neurol 1976;33:786.
207. Gallego J, Delgado G, Tunon T, et al. Delayed postirradiation lower motor neuron syndrome. Ann Neurol 1986;19:308.
208. Greenfield MM, Stark FM. Post-irradiation neuropathy. AJR Am J Roentgen 1948;60:617.
209. Kristensen O, Melgard B, Schiodt AV. Radiation myelopathy of the lumbosacral spinal cord. Acta Neurol Scandinav 1977;56:217.
210. Horowitz SL, Stewart JD. Lower motor neuron syndrome following radiotherapy. Can J Neurol Sci 1983;10:56.
211. De Carolis P, Montagna P, Cipulli M, et al. Isolated lower motoneuron involvement following radiotherapy. J Neurol Neurosurg Psychiatry 1986;49:718.
212. Kori SH, Foley KM, Posner JB. Brachial plexus lesions in patients with cancer: 100 cases. Neurology 1981;31:45.
213. Harper CM, Thomas JE, Cascino TL, et al. Distinction between neoplastic and radiation-induced brachial plexopathy, with emphasis on the role of EMG. Neurology 1989;39:502.
214. Pezzimenti JE, Bruckner HW, DeConti RC. Paralytic brachial neuritis in Hodgkin's disease. Cancer 1973;31:626.
215. Salner AL, Botnick LE, Herzog AG, et al. Reversible brachial plexopathy following primary radiation therapy for breast cancer. Cancer Treat Rep 1981;65:797.
216. Pierce SM, Recht A, Lingos TI, et al. Long-term radiation complications following conservative surgery and radiation therapy in patients with early stage breast cancer. Int J Radiat Oncol Biol Phys 1992;23:915.
217. Stoll BA, Andrews JT. Radiation-induced peripheral neuropathy. BMJ 1966;1:834.
218. Basso-Ricci S, della Costa C, Viganotti G, et al. Report on 42 cases of postirradiation lesions of the brachial plexus and their treatment. Tumori 1980;66:117.
219. Svensson H, Westling P, Larsson LG. Radiation-induced lesions of the brachial plexus correlated to the dose-time-fraction schedule. Acta Radiol Ther 1975; 14:228.
220. Thomas PK, Holdorff B. Neuropathy Due to Physical Agents. In PJ Dyck, PK Thomas, JW Griffin, et al. (eds), Peripheral Neuropathy (3rd ed). Philadelphia: Saunders, 1993;1000.
221. Barr LC, Kissin MW. Radiation-induced brachial plexus neuropathy following breast conservation and radical radiotherapy. Br J Surg 1987;74:855.
222. Mondrup K, Olsen NK, Pfeiffer P, et al. Clinical and electrodiagnostic findings in breast cancer patients with radiation-induced brachial plexus neuropathy. Acta Neurol Scand 1990;81:153.
223. Olsen NK, Pfeiffer P, Johannsen L, et al. Radiation-induced brachial plexopathy: neurological follow-up in 161 recurrence-free breast cancer patients. Int J Radiat Oncol Biol Phys 1993;26:43.
224. Haymaker W, Lindgren M. Nerve Disturbances Following Exposure to Ionizing Radiation. In PJ Vinken, GW Bruyn (eds), Handbook of Clinical Neurology. Amsterdam: Elsevier, 1970;388.
225. Sunderland S. Nerves and Nerve Injuries. New York: Churchill Livingstone, 1978.
226. Thomas JE, Colby MY. Radiation-induced or metastatic brachial plexopathy? A diagnostic dilemma. JAMA 1972;222:1392.
227. Thomas JE, Cascino TL, Earle JD. Differential diagno-

sis between radiation and tumor plexopathy of the pelvis. Neurology 1985;35:1.
228. Lederman RJ, Wilbourn AJ. Brachial plexopathy: recurrent cancer or radiation? Neurology 1984;34:1331.
229. Burns RJ. Delayed radiation-induced damage to the brachial plexus. Clin Exp Neurol 1978;15:221.
230. Killer HE, Hess K. Natural history of radiation-induced brachial plexopathy compared with surgically treated patients. J Neurol 1990;237:247.
231. Bagley FH, Walsh JW, Cady B, et al. Carcinomatous versus radiation-induced brachial plexus neuropathy in breast cancer. Cancer 1978;41:2154.
232. Thyagarajan D, Cascino T, Harms G. Magnetic resonance imaging in brachial plexopathy of cancer. Neurology 1995;45:421.
233. Wilborn AJ. Electrodiagnosis of plexopathies. Neurol Clin 1985;3:511.
234. Esteban A, Traba A. Fasciculation-myokymic activity and prolonged nerve conduction block. A physiological relationship in radiation-induced brachial plexopathy. Electroenceph Clin Neurophysiol 1993;89:382.
235. Fardin P, Lelli S, Negrin P, et al. Radiation-induced brachial plexopathy: clinical and electromyographical considerations in 13 cases. Electromyogr Clin Neurophysiol 1990;30:277.
236. Albers JW, Allen AA, Bastron JA, et al. Limb myokymia. Muscle Nerve 1981;4:494.
237. Stohr M. Special types of spontaneous electrical activity in radiogenic nerve injuries. Muscle Nerve 1982; 5:578.
238. Cascino TL, Kori S, Krol G, et al. CT of the brachial plexus in patients with cancer. Neurology 1983;33:1553.
239. Fishman EK, Campbell JN, Kuhlman JE, et al. Multiplanar CT evaluation of brachial plexopathy in breast cancer. J Comput Assist Tomogr 1991;15:790.
240. LeQuang C. Postirradiation lesions of the brachial plexus: results of surgical treatment. Hand Clin 1989;5:23.
241. Kline DG. Operative management of selected brachial plexus lesions. J Neurosurg 1983;58:631.
242. Dubuisson AS, Kline DG, Weinshel SS. Posterior subscapular approach to the brachial plexus: report of 102 patients. J Neurosurg 1993;79:319.
243. Match RM. Radiation-induced brachial plexus paralysis. Arch Surg 1975;110:384.
244. Lusk MD, Kline DG, Garcia CA. Tumors of the brachial plexus. Neurosurgery 1987;21:439.
245. Zeidman SM, Rossitch EJ, Nashold BS. Dorsal root entry zone lesions in the treatment of pain related to radiation-induced brachial plexopathy. J Spinal Dis 1993;6:44.
246. Ashenhurst EM, Quartey GR, Starreveld A. Lumbosacral radiculopathy induced by radiation. Can J Neurol Sci 1977;4:259.
247. Aho K, Sainio K. Late irradiation-induced lesions of the lumbosacral plexus. Neurology 1983;33:953.
248. Pettigrew LC, Glass JP, Maor M, et al. Diagnosis and treatment of lumbosacral plexopathies in patients with cancer. Arch Neurol 1984;41:1282.
249. Georgiou A, Grigsby PW, Perez CA. Radiation induced lumbosacral plexopathy in gynecologic tumors: clinical findings and dosimetric analysis. Int J Radiat Oncol Biol Phys 1993;26:479.
250. Stryker JA, Sommerville K, Perez R, et al. Sacral plexus injury after radiotherapy for carcinoma of cervix. Cancer 1990;66:1488.
251. Enevoldson TP, Scadding JW, Rustin GJ, et al. Spontaneous resolution of a postirradiation lumbosacral plexopathy. Neurology 1992;42:2224.
252. Jaeckle KA, Young DF, Foley KM. The natural history of lumbosacral plexopathy in cancer. Neurology 1985;35:8.
253. Devinsky O. Radiation-Induced Tumors of the Central and Peripheral Nervous System. In DA Rottenberg (ed), Neurological Complications of Cancer Treatment. Boston: Butterworth–Heinemann, 1991;79.
254. Kaschten B, Flandroy P, Reznik M, et al. Radiation-induced gliosarcoma: case report and review of the literature. J Neurosurg 1995;83:154.
255. Soffer D, Pittaluga S, Feiner M, et al. Intracranial meningiomas following low-dose irradiation to the head. J Neurosurg 1983;59:1048.
256. Rubinstein AB, Shalit MN, Cohen ML, et al. Radiation-induced cerebral meningioma: a recognizable entity. J Neurosurg 1984;61:966.
257. Ghim TT, Seo JJ, O'Brien M, et al. Childhood intracranial meningiomas after high-dose irradiation. Cancer 1993;71:4091.
258. Starshak RJ. Radiation-induced meningioma in children: report of two cases and review of the literature. Pediatr Radiol 1996;26:537.
259. Stein ME, Drumea K, Guilbord JN, et al. Late aggressive meningioma following prophylactic cranial irradiation for acute lymphoblastic leukemia. Br J Radiol 1995;68:1123.
260. Foreman NK, Laitt RD, Chambers EJ, et al. Intracranial large vessel vasculopathy and anaplastic meningioma 19 years after cranial irradiation for acute lymphoblastic leukemia. Med Pediatr Oncol 1995; 24:265.
261. Harrison MJ, Wolfe DE, Lau TS, et al. Radiation-induced meningiomas: experience at the Mount Sinai Hospital and review of the literature. J Neurosurg 1991;75:564.
262. Mack EE, Wilson CB. Meningiomas induced by high-dose cranial irradiation. J Neurosurg 1993;79:28.
263. Musa BS, Pople IK, Cummins BH. Intracranial meningiomas following irradiation: a growing problem? Br J Neurosurg 1995;9:629.
264. Kitanaka C, Shitara N, Nakagomi T, et al. Postirradiation astrocytoma: report of two cases. J Neurosurg 1989;70:469.
265. Salvati M, Artico M, Caruso R, et al. A report on radiation-induced gliomas. Cancer 1991;67:392.

266. Cavin LW, Dalrymple GV, McGuire EL, et al. CNS tumor induction by radiotherapy: a report of four new cases and estimate of dose required. Int J Radiat Oncol Biol Phys 1990;18:399.
267. Dropcho EJ, Wisoff JH, Walker RW, et al. Supratentorial malignant gliomas in childhood: a review of fifty cases. Ann Neurol 1987;22:355.
268. Fontana M, Stanton C, Pompili A, et al. Late multifocal gliomas in adolescents previously treated for acute lymphoblastic leukemia. Cancer 1987;60:1510.
269. Shapiro S, Mealey J, Sartorius C. Radiation-induced intracranial malignant gliomas. J Neurosurg 1989; 71:77.
270. Meadows AT, Baum E, Fossati-Bellani F, et al. Second malignant neoplasms in children: an update from the Late Effects Study Group. J Clin Oncol 1985;3:532.
271. Neglia JP, Meadows AT, Robison LL, et al. Second neoplasms after acute lymphoblastic leukemia in childhood. N Engl J Med 1991;325:1330.
272. Albo V, Miller D, Leiken S, et al. Nine brain tumors as a late effect in children "cured" of acute lymphoblastic leukemia from a single protocol study [Abstract]. Proc Am Soc Clin Oncol 1985;4:172.
273. Malone M, Lumley H, Erdohazi M. Astrocytoma as a second malignancy in patients with acute lymphoblastic leukemia. Cancer 1986;57:1979.
274. Farwell JR, Flannery JT. Cancer in children with central nervous system neoplasms. N Engl J Med 1984; 311:749.
275. Dodick DW, Mokri B, Shaw EG, et al. Sarcomas of calvarial bones: rare remote effect of radiation therapy for brain tumors. Neurology 1994;44:908.
276. Foley KM, Woodruff JM, Ellis FT, et al. Radiation-induced malignant and atypical peripheral nerve sheath tumors. Ann Neurol 1980;7:311.
277. Trojanowski JQ, Kelinman GM, Proppe KH. Malignant tumors of nerve sheath origin. Cancer 1980;46:1202.
278. Ducatman BS, Scheithauer BW. Postirradiation neurofibrosarcoma. Cancer 1983;51:1028.
279. Gorson KC, Musaphir S, Lathi ES, et al. Radiation-induced malignant fibrous histiocytoma of the brachial plexus. J Neurooncol 1995;26:73.

Chapter 26

Complications of Immunization

Hema Patel and Bhuwan P. Garg

Objectives

- To know the recommended immunization schedule
- To recognize the importance of immunization
- To recognize the various complications associated with immunizations
- To understand the clinical manifestations of complications associated with immunizations
- To understand the relative risk of immunization
- To understand that the risk of complications following immunization is minimal and that the incidence of these complications still remains lower than that following natural infection

Immunoprophylaxis has markedly reduced the incidence, morbidity, and mortality of many infectious diseases. The global eradication of small pox was achieved in 1980, mainly due to an effective immunization program. In the United States, immunization has practically eradicated diphtheria, measles, mumps, pertussis, poliomyelitis, congenital and acquired rubella, tetanus, and *Haemophilus influenzae* type B disease. The current schedule for childhood immunization recommended by the Advisory Committee on Immunization Practices (ACIP) and the American Academy of Pediatrics (AAP) is outlined in Table 26.1.[1]

Immunization may be associated with complications, many of these being neurologic in nature. The frequency and severity of immunization-related complications is difficult to judge because most reports are anecdotal, although an effort has recently been made to collect data in a more systematic fashion. The Monitoring System for Adverse Events Following Immunization (MSAEFI) of the Centers for Disease Control and Prevention (CDC) and the more recent Vaccine Adverse Event Reporting System (VAERS) are passive surveillance systems for collecting data on illnesses temporally associated with immunization. Because of the method of data collection, these systems are not very accurate in ascertaining the frequency of these complications.

Measles, Mumps, and Rubella Immunization

Immunization against measles, mumps, and rubella (MMR) has been administered in a combined vaccine in the United States since 1975.[2]

Measles Vaccine

Measles is a viral infection caused by a member of the paramyxovirus group. A live, highly attenuated measles virus (Enders strain) vaccine is available for general use.[3, 4] By 1982, 97% of all children entering school in the United States had been vaccinated against measles. The incidence of measles had fallen from almost 500 per 100,000 population in 1950 to 0.5 per 100,000 population in 1982. During that period, the reported annual

Table 26.1. Childhood Immunization Schedule

Recommended Age	Immunizations
Birth	Hepatitis B
2 mos	DTaP or DTP, OPV, Hib, hepatitis B
4 mos	DTaP or DTP, OPV, Hib
6 mos	DTaP or DTP, Hib, hepatitis B
6–18 mos	OPV
12–18 mos	Varicella
15–18 mos	DTaP or DTP
12–15 mos	MMR, Hib
4–6 yrs	DTaP or DTP, OPV
11–12 yrs	Hepatitis B and varicella (if not administered during infancy), MMR (may also be given at 4–6 yrs), Td

DTaP = diphtheria, tetanus, acellular pertussis; DTP = diphtheria, tetanus, whole cell pertussis; OPV = trivalent oral polio vaccine; Hib = *Haemophilus influenzae* type B; MMR = measles, mumps, rubella; Td = tetanus and diphtheria toxoid. Source: Adapted from Immunization of adolescents. Recommendations of the Advisory Committee on Immunization Practices, the American Academy of Pediatrics, the American Academy of Family Physicians and the American Medical Association. Pediatrics 1997;99:479.

deaths from measles declined from 700 to 2, and reports of measles encephalitis declined from 300 to 1. It is estimated that during the first 20 years of the measles vaccine program the vaccine resulted in 52 million fewer cases of measles and prevented 5,200 deaths and 17,400 cases of mental retardation.[2]

Local and Systemic Reactions

Mild measles-like symptoms such as fever, rash, cough, and rhinorrhea may occur 1–2 weeks after immunization.[3]

Neurologic Complications

Encephalopathy and Encephalitis. The terms *encephalopathy* and *encephalitis* have been used interchangeably in the literature. Encephalopathy refers to any acute or chronic disturbance of brain function characterized by altered level of consciousness, convulsions, headache, or focal neurologic deficits. Encephalitis refers to an encephalopathy associated with an inflammatory response in the brain.

Many uncontrolled observational studies describe encephalopathy after the administration of measles vaccine.[5–7] From 1963 to 1971, 51 million doses of measles vaccine were distributed, and 59 patients with new-onset neurologic disease after vaccination without evidence of other causes were reported to the CDC. The onset of symptoms was clustered around 6–15 days after immunization. Diagnoses included encephalopathy (60%), encephalomyelitis, aseptic meningitis, and transverse myelitis. Although there was no way to prove that these complications were vaccine related, the clustering of cases 6–15 days after immunization, which is also the time of maximal viral replication, appears significant. The incidence of encephalopathy was 1.16 cases per 1,000,000 distributed doses, compared with a background incidence of encephalitis of 2–3 per 1,000,000 children of similar age.[6] The incidence of encephalitis after natural measles infection is 1 per 1,000 cases.[8]

Therefore, although a cause-and-effect relationship between measles immunization and encephalopathy has not been conclusively established, the clustering of cases in the second week after immunization is worrisome. Even if all these cases were caused by measles vaccination, the incidence still remains much lower than that following natural infection, and comparable with that in healthy controls.

Subacute Sclerosing Panencephalitis. Subacute sclerosing panencephalitis (SSPE) is a devastating form of measles panencephalitis that follows natural measles infection in 5–10 out of every 1,000,000 cases of measles.[9] Development of SSPE after administration of the live attenuated vaccine and a negative history of natural measles was first reported in 1968.[10] Thereafter, several additional reports of SSPE in individuals vaccinated against measles appeared,[6, 9, 11] with the latency ranging from 3 weeks[6] to 5 years[11] between vaccination and onset of SSPE. The National Registry for SSPE, founded in 1969, reported a decline in SSPE from 48.6 new cases per year between 1967 and 1971 to 4.2 new cases per year from 1982–1986.[12] Though there was a decline in the absolute number of cases of SSPE, there was an increase in the proportion of cases that occurred after measles vaccination from 13% of all cases of SSPE in 1967–1970 to 38.5% in 1974.[9] It is thought that the live attenuated measles virus vaccine may be capable of contributing to the pathogenesis of SSPE with a shorter incubation period for SSPE after vaccination than after natural (wild) measles infection.[12] The risk of SSPE after vaccination is lower than after natural measles; the incidence of SSPE with natural measles infection was 8.5 per million compared with 0.7 per million vaccine recipients who had not had measles. It is therefore not a contraindication to routine immunization against measles.[13]

Immunosuppressive Encephalopathy. Immunosuppressive encephalopathy is distinct from acute measles encephalitis and SSPE. It has been documented in two immunocompromised children.[14, 15] Measles virus of the vaccine strain was isolated from the cerebrospinal fluid (CSF) of a 7-year-old girl with acute lymphoblastic leukemia 10 weeks after she had received MMR.[14] Another case occurred in a leukemic child involving the Schwarz strain of measles vaccine.[15] Therefore, measles immunization should be administered with caution in immunosuppressed individuals.

Seizures. Febrile and afebrile seizures may occur 7–14 days after measles immunization.[16–18] Normal children who experience febrile or afebrile seizures after measles vaccination usually recover completely without neurologic sequelae, although some children may have further simple febrile seizures.

Ophthalmologic Complications

Two children have been reported with transitory oculomotor palsy associated with systemic symptoms of measles infection following immunization. One patient had ptosis; the other had a complete third nerve palsy.[19, 20] One case of optic neuritis complicating MMR immunization has also been reported.[21] Bilateral measles retinitis associated with symptoms of systemic measles infection was reported in a 16-month-old girl after immunization. She presented with total blindness and had incomplete recovery of vision.[22]

Mumps Vaccine

Mumps vaccine is a live attenuated virus vaccine introduced in 1967.[23] The Jeryl Lynn strain is used in the United States, and the Urabe strain is used in Japan. Neutralizing antibody response is usually detected within 2 weeks after the vaccination, although this may be delayed up to 6 weeks in some recipients.[24] Immunity is assumed to be long-lasting, but this has not been proved. Because mumps vaccine is administered with measles and rubella in a combined vaccine as MMR, it is difficult to distinguish the adverse effects of the individual antigens.

Neurologic Complications

Mumps is associated with aseptic meningitis. Mumps virus (both wild-type and vaccine strains) has been isolated from the CSF in patients with aseptic meningitis. This relation is firmly established for the Urabe strain, with an incidence of 1.1 cases per 1,000 vaccine recipients. The aseptic meningitis occurs within 2 months of vaccination. There have been no reports of severe illness or long-term sequelae.[25] Data concerning aseptic meningitis in association with the Jeryl Lynn strain are scarce. Eleven cases of meningitis occurring after MMR vaccination were reported in the United States to the VAERS from 1990 to 1992. In none of these was the strain identified or the virus isolated, however, so there is inadequate evidence to implicate the Jeryl Lynn strain.

Otologic Complications

Sensorineural deafness has been reported to occur in 4% of patients after natural mumps infection[26–28] and has also been reported after MMR vaccination. A 7-year-old girl developed total deafness in the left ear 11 days after an injection of MMR without subsequent recovery,[26] and a 3-year-old girl who had received MMR vaccination at 15 months of age developed moderate to severe bilateral unremitting sensorineural deafness.[27]

Rubella (German Measles) Vaccine

Rubella is caused by a virus of the Togavirus group. The original rubella vaccines containing live attenuated virus were licensed for use in the United States in 1969 and were produced using three different cell cultures—viz duck embryo, dog kidney, and rabbit kidney cells. In January 1979, all of these vaccines were replaced by the current strain, which is Wistar RA 27/3 prepared in human diploid cell culture. This new vaccine produces an immune response that closely parallels the natural infection.[29]

Systemic Reactions

Up to 40% of people (adults more often than children) receiving the current rubella vaccine may develop transitory arthralgias and paresthesias beginning 3–25 days after immunization and lasting 1–11 days. Symptoms are mild after vaccination with RA27/3 when compared with the more severe neuritis caused by the original vaccines.[30]

Neurologic Complications

Peripheral Neuropathy. During the mass immunization program of children that began in 1969 and continued for several years thereafter, two fairly well-defined syndromes of peripheral neuropathy were recognized after immunization with all three of the original rubella vaccines: brachial radiculoneuritis (arm syndrome) and lumbosacral radiculoneuritis (leg syndrome).[31–34] The arm syndrome occurred 10–62 days after immunization and was characterized by nocturnal episodes of pain involving the wrists and hands, associated with paresthesias lasting up to 5 weeks. The leg syndrome occurred 29–70 days after immunization and was characterized by asymmetric popliteal pain and inability to straighten the legs or bear weight, with worsening of symptoms at night. The leg pain lasted for 2–14 days with periodic recurrences during 2.5 years of follow-up.[31] These complications have not been described after vaccination with the current (RA 27/3) vaccine.

Demyelinating Diseases. There are isolated case reports of young women who developed transverse myelitis, sometimes associated with optic neuritis, after rubella immunization.[35, 36] This complication is not seen in children and may represent the first manifestation of multiple sclerosis. The relationship between immunization and symptoms may be coincidental, or the immunization-induced fever may have triggered the first attack of multiple sclerosis.[36]

Congenital Rubella Syndrome

Congenital rubella syndrome is caused by infection of the fetus via the maternal blood stream. One of the most important reasons for rubella immunization is to protect the unborn child from acquiring congenital rubella syndrome.[37] The older vaccines (not RA 27/3) may cross the placenta and infect the fetus.[37–39]

The CDC surveillance of rubella vaccination during gestation included 555 women. Of these, 119 were susceptible at the time of vaccination and carried the infant to term. One-third of these women had been vaccinated with RA 27/3 vaccine from 1 week before to 4 weeks after conception, during the highest risk period for viremia and fetal infection. No infant had evidence of congenital rubella syndrome.[40] Although no cases of congenital rubella syndrome were noted in the CDC study, others have reported isolation of rubella virus in the products of conception from abortions after inadvertent immunization.[38] Approximately 1–2% of infants born to susceptible vaccinated mothers had serologic evidence of subclinical infection, with the rate of rubella virus isolation being much higher with the older vaccines. Data indicate that the risk of placental or fetal infection from the RA 27/3 vaccine is present, although minimal.[41]

Even though the risk of congenital rubella syndrome after vaccination appears to be minimal, this small risk should be avoided by vaccinating susceptible women only if not pregnant and advising them not to become pregnant for at least 3 months after vaccination.[41] Physicians should determine the immune status of all women of child-bearing age in their care and vaccinate those who are inadequately immunized.

Poliomyelitis Vaccine

Poliomyelitis is caused by an enterovirus. There are three types of poliovirus (types 1, 2, and 3) with no cross-immunity. Two forms of polio vaccine are available. The original Salk vaccine, an inactivated poliovirus vaccine (IPV) administered by the parenteral route, was developed in 1953 by Jonas Salk and licensed for use in 1959. This was replaced by the oral polio vaccine (OPV), developed by Albert Sabin and licensed for use in 1963. Both IPV and

OPV are trivalent and effective; however, the OPV, a live attenuated virus vaccine, is preferred because it produces secretory mucosal immunity within the gastrointestinal tract as well as serum humoral immunity. The live attenuated virus is shed from the gastrointestinal tract and spreads to unvaccinated individuals, leading to herd immunity. Also, being an oral preparation, it is better tolerated than the injectable form.[42] OPV was recommended for general use by the AAP in 1964. If IPV is used, it should be given according to the same schedule as OPV. The relative value of using the Salk or Sabin vaccine has been reexamined.[43–46] The live attenuated OPV preparation remains the preferred vaccine except for individuals who are immunocompromised or have immunocompromised contacts, because of the risk of developing acute paralytic poliomyelitis as mentioned in the following discussion.

Systemic Reactions

IPV has an excellent safety record, producing only low-grade fever for the first 2 days in 5% of recipients and restlessness in 15%.[46, 47]

Neurologic Complications of Oral Polio Vaccine

Acute Paralytic Poliomyelitis

There are two types of vaccine-related poliomyelitis: that occurring in vaccine recipients, and that in the contacts of vaccinated individuals, especially those with impaired immunity.[48] Acute paralytic poliomyelitis is a major complication seen only after OPV. It has a low incidence, occurring approximately once in every 3.22 million doses of OPV distributed.[49] Most cases of paralytic poliomyelitis in the United States are now vaccine related. Approximately 35% of cases occur in healthy vaccine recipients, usually after the first immunization. Fifteen percent occur in recipients or contacts with immune deficiency states, and the remainder occur in healthy close contacts of vaccine recipients. The interval between vaccine administration and onset of illness may be from 11 to 58 days. In healthy individuals, the onset of symptoms is generally 1 month after exposure to the virus, whereas the latent period may be longer in immunosuppressed individuals. The incidence is greater with the first dose of vaccine. The CDC has estimated that the overall dose-related incidence is 1 in 520,000 first doses distributed versus 1 per 12.3 million subsequent doses distributed. This is still a much lower risk than that after naturally occurring poliomyelitis.[50] Only one of several reports made to the VAERS between November 1990 and July 1992 provided sufficient information to be a well-documented case of vaccine-associated poliomyelitis. With the increasingly younger age of entry into daycare, there is a growing group of non-immunized infants who may be exposed to infants recently immunized with OPV.[51, 52] Administration of a single dose of IPV before beginning OPV immunization to prevent OPV paralytic disease has been suggested.[53]

Guillain-Barré Syndrome

After a nationwide immunization campaign with OPV for children and adults in Finland during a 5-week period between February 10 and March 15, 1985, 10 patients with Guillain-Barré syndrome (GBS) were reported. Six patients were diagnosed within the first 6 weeks of vaccination, and all of the cases of GBS occurred within 10 weeks after vaccination. The crude annual incidence rate was estimated at 1 case per 100,000 population.[54] This evidence favors a causal relation between OPV and GBS. If GBS occurs within 5 days to 6 weeks of a vaccination, subsequent vaccinations with OPV may be associated with an increased risk of repeat GBS.[55]

Diphtheria, Tetanus, and Pertussis Vaccines

Routine immunization against diphtheria, tetanus, and pertussis in infancy and early childhood since the 1940s has played a major role in reducing the incidence of cases and deaths from each of these diseases.

Diphtheria and Tetanus Vaccines

Tetanus is caused by the gram-positive, spore-forming anaerobic bacillus *Clostridium tetani*. In the United States, tetanus has decreased dramatically from 560 reported cases in 1947 to an average of 57 cases reported annually from 1985 to 1994.[56] Although rare in the United States, tetanus occurs exclusively among unvaccinated or inadequately vaccinated individuals and neonates.

Diphtheria is an acute respiratory infection caused by *Corynebacterium diphtheriae*. In the United States, the incidence of diphtheria has decreased because of immunization, from more than 200,000 cases in 1921 to only 15 cases reported from 1990 to 1994.[56]

Diphtheria and tetanus toxoid are generally administered together as tetanus and diphtheria toxoid (Td) in adults and diphtheria and tetanus toxoid (DT) or DTP (a combination that includes pertussis vaccine) in children. DT should be used in children younger than 7 years of age in whom pertussis vaccine is contraindicated. Td should be used in individuals older than 7 years. Td has a lower concentration of diphtheria toxoid than DT. Monovalent tetanus toxoids are also available. Protective antibody levels are achieved in most children and adults after two doses given 4 or more weeks apart, although children younger 1 year of age may require a third dose. These protective levels may be short-lived in infants and older adults, requiring a reinforcing booster dose 6–12 months after the primary series.[57] To maintain protective levels of antitoxin antibody, recall immunization is suggested at 10-year intervals. The accepted protective antibody level is 0.01 antitoxin units per ml or greater. Because of a possibility of developing serious neuropathy due to overimmunization with tetanus toxoid, a careful history of prior immunization should be taken before administrating routine booster injections.[58–60] Clean minor wounds require no booster in a fully immunized person (last booster within 10 years). Persons with contaminated wounds should receive a booster if more than 5 years have elapsed since the last dose. The only contraindication to the use of the toxoids is history of a neurologic or severe hypersensitivity reaction following a previous dose.[61]

Diphtheria and tetanus toxoids are administered together so frequently that it is difficult to analyze the adverse reactions of each separately. There are no known serious adverse reactions to diphtheria toxoid, though data are limited.

Local and Systemic Reactions

Minor reactions, including local pain, erythema, and swelling, may occur within 48 hours after immunization with tetanus toxoid.[58, 62, 63] Severe local reactions associated with systemic manifestations such as fever and malaise are infrequent. These are classified as an Arthus reaction in which immune complexes form locally in the walls of small arteries. They are usually seen with larger doses of toxoid and high antibody levels before immunization.[58, 64]

Anaphylaxis

Anaphylactoid reactions can occur within 2 hours of immunization with tetanus toxoid. Symptoms include urticaria, angioedema, shortness of breath, pruritus, and hypotension.[62] No cases of anaphylaxis associated with the administration of diphtheria toxoid alone have been reported.

Neurologic Complications

Demyelinating Diseases. Several case reports of acute disseminated encephalomyelitis have been described in association with tetanus toxoid administration.[65, 66] Transverse myelitis[67, 68] and optic neuritis have also been reported.[69] However, the evidence to date is inadequate to establish a causal relation between tetanus toxoid, DT, or Td and demyelinating diseases of the central nervous system.

Guillain-Barré Syndrome. The most common neurologic complication to occur after tetanus toxoid administration is polyradiculoneuritis, or GBS. Most reported cases have occurred in adults who received either tetanus toxoid alone or a combination of tetanus toxoid and antitetanus toxin serum.[65, 70–72] These case reports do not demonstrate a definite cause-and-effect relationship between tetanus toxoid and polyradiculoneuritis. The most convincing exception is the case of a patient who received tetanus toxoid on three separate occasions over a period of 13 years and developed a well-documented polyneuropathy of the GBS type after each administration with latencies of 21, 14, and 10 days. He had minimal residual neurologic signs after the second episode and made full functional recovery after the third.[73] A few cases of GBS occurring after vaccination with DT have also been reported. The MSAEFI lists four cases between 1979 and 1990 in relation to DT. The VAERS lists two patients with GBS between 1990 and 1992 with Td, both of whom simultaneously received MMR as well.

Thus, there appears to be a causal relation between tetanus toxoid, alone or as part of a vaccine (DT and Td), and GBS. If GBS occurs 5 days to 6 weeks after vaccination, subsequent vaccinations could be associated with a greater risk of GBS. A previous history of GBS unrelated to vaccination should be of concern but has not been established as a risk factor.

Other Neuropathies. Administration of tetanus and diphtheria toxoids alone or in combination has also been linked to the occurrence of mononeuropathy due to nerve damage from injection of the vaccine directly into the nerve rather than due to the vaccine itself.[59] Cranial mononeuropathies and brachial neuritis have also been reported.[74–76] The latter is thought to be a result of an allergic or hypersensitivity reaction.[74]

Encephalopathy. Tetanus and diphtheria toxoids have not been associated with increased risk of encephalopathy or seizures.

Pertussis Vaccine

Pertussis is caused by a gram-negative coccobacillus *Bordetella pertussis*. Pertussis was first described in 1579 and became a nationally reportable disease in 1922. Encephalopathy occurring after pertussis is associated with significant neurologic sequelae. Reports of pertussis in the United States reached a peak of 265,269 cases and 7,518 deaths in 1934. After widespread immunization against pertussis in the United States since 1947, the number of reported cases and associated mortality declined.[77] Since the 1980s, however, the incidence has gradually been increasing.[56, 78, 79] There were 27,826 cases of pertussis reported to the CDC from 1980 to 1989, for an average annual incidence of 1.2 cases per 100,000 population, with the increase being disproportionately large among adolescents and adults. Infants younger than 2 months of age were at highest risk (average annual incidence 62.8 per 100,000). These infants had the highest rates of hospitalizations (82%), seizures (4%), encephalopathy (1%), and death (1%). This may reflect poor rates of immunization as 64% of children 3 months to 4 years of age who were reported to have pertussis had not been appropriately immunized.[78] Whooping cough can occur in vaccinated individuals but is less severe.[80, 81] Also, immunization prevents the disease but not the infection, so immunized children may carry the organism and infect other children or adults.[82]

Complications

Local and Systemic Reactions. Local reactions are more frequently seen after the use of combined DTP vaccine than with DT alone. These include local erythema, swelling, and pain. Systemic reactions such as fever, drowsiness, anorexia, vomiting, and persistent crying may also be seen.[83]

Hypotonic-Hyporesponsive Episodes. Hypotonic-hyporesponsive episodes may occur within 4 hours of immunization and are characterized by pallor, hypotonia, and unresponsiveness for a period ranging from 10 minutes to 36 hours. The pathogenesis of hypotonic-hyporesponsive episodes is poorly understood.[83] They are not associated with permanent sequelae.[84]

Neurologic Complications

SEIZURES. The incidence of seizures after pertussis vaccination has been estimated at 1 in 1,750–10,000 injections.[83, 85] Febrile convulsions are the most common adverse neurologic reaction to pertussis vaccination[16, 86] and are not associated with permanent neurologic sequelae.[84] They usually occur within 48 hours of the third immunization, which is usually given at 6 months of age, an age when simple febrile convulsions are common.[18, 87] More than one-half of children with postimmunization febrile convulsions have a personal or family history of febrile convulsions. Postimmunization afebrile convulsions occur less frequently, and these children may have a personal, but not a family history of convulsions.[86] Because it is extremely difficult to differentiate a simple febrile seizure from one that is due to a reaction to pertussis vaccine, any seizure closely following pertussis vaccination should be considered a contraindication to further pertussis immunization.

INFANTILE SPASMS. Because the age at which DTP is administered is also the peak age of onset of infantile spasms, a cause-and-effect association has been suspected. Independent surveys from Denmark, Japan, and the United Kingdom have examined this association.

In Denmark, the national immunization program was changed in 1970. Before 1970, children were immunized with DTP at 5, 6, and 15 months of age. After 1970, DTP was abandoned, and only pertussis vaccine was given at 5 weeks, 9 weeks, and 10 months of age. However, the peak age of onset of infantile spasms remained constant at 5 months before and after 1970. This study concluded that a causal relationship between pertussis immunization and infantile spasms was unlikely.[88] In Japan, 200 consecutive patients with infantile spasms were examined, and one child had pertussis identified as the only risk factor before the onset of infantile spasms. A rate of 1 per 200 is no different from that in the general population.[89] In the United Kingdom, The National Childhood Encephalopathy Study (NCES), received reports on 269 patients with infantile spasms. An excess risk of infantile spasms in the 28 days after immunization could not be demonstrated. However, there was an excess risk in the first 7 days after either DTP or DT immunization that was later offset by a decreased risk in the 21 days that followed. This suggests that vaccination may trigger the onset of infantile spasms and bring them to attention more quickly. Subsequent neurologic outcome is no different in children whose spasms are immunization triggered from those in whom they began spontaneously.[90]

ENCEPHALOPATHY. Postpertussis vaccination encephalopathy is characterized by seizures, alterations in mental status, and other signs of cerebral involvement beginning hours to days after immunization.[83, 91] The diagnosis is primarily based on the temporal relationship between immunization and the onset of symptoms.

In the United Kingdom, 50 children were evaluated in 1974 for neurologic illness that may have been related to DPT immunization. Thirty-two suffered convulsions, and 22 were subsequently mentally retarded. The authors concluded that "the clustering of cases in the first 24 hours after inoculation suggested a causal rather than a coincidental relation" and recommended a prospective study.[92] Unfortunately, due to media sensationalism of this report, the vaccination rate in the United Kingdom decreased to 31%, leading to the pertussis epidemic of 1977–1979.[93]

An NCES in 1976 assessed the risk of neurologic complications of immunization. The study identified all children ages 2 months to 3 years admitted during a 3-year period with encephalitis or encephalopathy, unexplained coma, convulsions lasting more than 30 minutes or followed by persistent neurologic complications, infantile spasms, or Reye's syndrome. A total of 1,182 children were registered. Two controls matched for sex, age, and area of residence were selected for each child with encephalopathy. A rate of 3.5% of encephalopathies were temporally related to pertussis immunization. The attributable risk (difference between the incidence of encephalopathy in immunized versus nonimmunized children) was approximately 1 case per 110,000 injections. The difference between the encephalopathic and control group was greatest during the first 72 hours after immunization. The NCES also estimated the risk of permanent brain damage in previously normal children to be 1 case per 310,000 injections. Of 11 such children reported, possible alternative explanations were present in six. Two patients had encephalitis, one due to coxsackie B5 and the other due to rhinovirus; three had infantile spasms; one had Reye's syndrome.[93] Because no attempt has been made to provide a precise definition of the clinical syndrome or to exclude other causes of encephalopathy, predicted incidences may be overestimates.[94]

Data from the CDC for the years 1978 through 1981 suggest a rate for severe reactions of 1 per 230,000 doses of vaccine, but provide no information on long-term sequelae.[95] By comparison, 5 of 1,277 children with natural pertussis infection during 1979 through 1981 had acute encephalopathy as a result of pertussis infection.[96] This suggests a much higher risk of encephalopathy due to natural infection than due to pertussis vaccine.

Contraindications

Absolute contraindications to pertussis vaccination are given in Table 26.2.[61, 97, 98] Pertussis vaccination should also be deferred in children with progressive neurologic disorders, personal history of convulsions, and suspected neurologic conditions that predispose to seizures. Some authors recommend that a previous history of seizure or positive family history of seizures is a contraindication to pertussis immunization.[86, 99]

Table 26.2. Absolute Contraindications to Pertussis Vaccine

Allergic hypersensitivity to the vaccine components
Development of fever of 40.5°C or higher within 48 hours after vaccination
Collapse or shock-like state (hypotensive-hyporesponsive episode) within 48 hours after vaccination
Persistent screaming lasting 3 hours or longer within 48 hours after vaccination
Encephalopathy within 7 days of vaccination
Convulsions with or without fever occurring within 3 days of vaccination
Evolving neurologic disorders

Sources: Adapted from Acel-Imune package insert. Pearl River, NY: Lederle Laboratories, Division American Cyanamid Co., January 3, 1997; American Academy of Pediatrics, Report of the Committee on Infectious Diseases. Pertussis vaccine. Pediatrics 1984;74:303; and Recommendations of the Immunization Practices Advisory Committee (ACIP). Supplementary statement of contraindications to receipt of pertussis vaccine. MMWR Morb Mortal Wkly Rep 1984;33:169.

The ACIP has concluded that a family history of convulsions in parents and siblings is not a contraindication to pertussis vaccination and that children with such family histories should receive pertussis vaccination according to the recommended schedule. DTP vaccination may be postponed in the presence of ongoing febrile illness that is moderate or severe. Minor illness such as a mild upper respiratory infection with or without low-grade fever is not a contraindication. Pertussis vaccine should be given to all children unless absolute contraindications exist.[61]

The Child Neurology Society issued the following conclusions in a consensus statement[100]:

1. Administration of pertussis vaccine is associated with a short-term increased risk of seizures, mostly febrile seizures, and complete recovery is expected.
2. The association between pertussis vaccine and progressive or chronic neurologic disorder raised by case reports has not been conclusively proven by controlled studies.
3. At present there is no means by which the diagnosis of pertussis vaccine encephalopathy can be established in an individual case.

In addition, there is a causal relationship between pertussis vaccine and an unusual shock-like state referred to as a *hypotonic-hyporesponsive episode*, as well as inconsolable crying, probably caused by pain at the injection site.

Acellular Pertussis Vaccine

Acellular pertussis vaccines (DTaP) were developed with the aim of achieving adequate protection against pertussis with fewer side effects. Acellular vaccines contain purified, inactivated *B. pertussis* antigens, including pertussis toxoid, filamentous hemagglutinin, 69-kDa outer membrane proteins (pertactin), and agglutinogens (fimbriae). Acellular pertussis vaccines contain two or more of these denatured elements of *B. pertussis* required for immunity.

Until now, DTaP had been approved for use as booster dose for the fourth and fifth doses in children who had received the first three doses of whole cell vaccine.[101] Toward the end of 1996, DTaP was licensed for use in all five doses of the immunization series, including completion of the series in children who received one or more doses of the whole cell DTP. Approximately 15% of pertussis cases in the United States occur in adolescents and adults. Use of acellular vaccines in those 7 years or older, although currently not recommended, should be considered in the future to reduce the reservoir and circulation of *B. pertussis,* thereby reducing the incidence of pertussis in infants too young to benefit from immunization.

Acellular vaccines are as effective as whole cell DTP. The major advantage of the acellular or component vaccines is that they contain little or no endotoxin, and therefore there is reduction in both the local injection site reactions as well as in the systemic reactions. The incidence of crying, hypotonic-hyporesponsive episodes, and seizures is also reduced in comparison to the whole cell vaccine.[61, 102]

The ACIP and AAP contraindications for whole cell pertussis vaccine should also be considered as contraindications for the use of acellular vaccine.

Haemophilus influenzae Type b Vaccine

Before the introduction of *H. influenzae* type b (Hib) vaccines, the cumulative incidence of invasive Hib disease in the first 5 years of life in the United States was estimated to be approximately 1 in 200 children. Nearly 75% of cases occurred in children younger than 2 years of age. This susceptibility correlates with their lack of antibody to the type b capsular polysaccharide, polyribosylribitol phosphate (PRP). The mortality for children with meningitis was 3–6%, and 19–45% of survivors have permanent sequelae, including hearing loss, mental retardation, and seizures.[103]

In the 1970s, a plain polysaccharide vaccine composed of purified PRP was prepared; however, it is without protective efficacy in children younger than 18 months of age. In addition, a possible increased incidence of disease in the postimmunization period (7 days) has been noted.[104] Therefore, in the late 1980s, a series of vaccines using PRP conjugated with other compounds to increase vaccine efficacy were developed. These vaccines differ in the molecular size of the Hib polysaccharide, the protein used as the carrier, and in the methods used to link the polysaccharide to the protein. Variations in the type or frequency of adverse effects may occur because of differences in the polysaccharide or protein content of these vaccines. Conjugated preparations include PRP-D (diphtheria toxoid), HbOC (*C. diphtheriae* protein), PRP-OMP (*Neisseria meningitidis* outer membrane protein complex), and PRP-T (tetanus toxoid).

The plain PRP vaccines do not provide protective amounts of antibody until after the age of 2 years, whereas the conjugate vaccines stimulate anti-PRP antibody responses in young infants and also induce production of larger amounts of these antibodies. In addition, they induce an anti-PRP antibody response in many individuals who do not respond well to natural infection with Hib or to the plain PRP vaccine, including patients with Hib disease before the age of 2 years and those with splenectomy, sickle cell disease, and malignancy.[105, 106] Protective levels of antibody to Hib vaccine are seen within 1 month of immunization with the conjugate vaccines.[107] The AAP and the ACIP recommend routine immunization of infants with a Hib conjugate vaccine, and this practice has resulted in a marked decrease in the incidence of Hib disease in the United States.[108]

Local and Systemic Reactions

Local reactions, including pain, tenderness, swelling, and erythema at the injection site, and systemic reactions, including low-grade fever and irritability, may occur within 24–72 hours of vaccination with Hib. These reactions are mild and transient. They are seen in approximately 5–25% of vaccine recipients, with overall reaction rates being lower after plain PRP vaccine than after conjugate vaccines.[109]

Neurologic Complications

Guillain-Barré Syndrome

Seven cases of GBS were reported after immunization with three different Hib conjugate vaccines during a period when several million doses of the vaccines were distributed[110, 111] (VAERS November 1990 to July 1992). Five of these cases fit criteria for vaccine-related GBS, though Hib conjugate vaccine was the only potential predisposing factor in three.[110, 111] These data with only 5 cases per several million doses are therefore insufficient to support a definite causal link between GBS and Hib vaccine.

Transverse Myelitis

There is inadequate evidence to support an association between Hib vaccines and transverse myelitis.

Early Susceptibility to **Haemophilus influenzae** *Type b*

Early-onset Hib disease after immunization is defined as a case of serious systemic infection caused by Hib that occurs within the 7-day interval after immunization for Hib. There is evidence to suggest that immunization of children older than 18 months of age with unconjugated PRP vaccine is associated with an increased risk of disease for 7 days thereafter.[104, 112] Because PRP vaccine contains purified capsular polysaccharide only, the early onset cases of Hib infection could not have been caused by infectious material in the vaccine itself. Increased susceptibility to infection in the immediate postimmunization period might be related to a transient decrease in preexisting antibody level caused by formation of antigen-antibody complexes, although other mechanisms have also been postulated.[113–115] Early-onset Hib disease developing within 72 hours after immunization is more likely to be manifested by cellulitis and epiglottitis, rather than meningitis.[116] There is no evidence to suggest a causal relation between immunization with conjugate Hib vaccines and an increased risk of disease in the early postvaccination interval.[117]

Hepatitis B Vaccine

Hepatitis B virus infection may result in acute massive hepatic necrosis or chronic active hepatitis and cirrhosis of the liver. It has been estimated that more than 170 million people in the world today are infected with hepatitis B virus. In the United States, 60–80% of neonates and 6–10% of adults infected with the hepatitis B virus are estimated to become carriers.[118] The risk of becoming a carrier decreases with age.

A plasma-derived hepatitis B vaccine, licensed for use in the United States from 1981 to 1988, is no longer produced. The first vaccine using recombinant DNA technology was licensed in the United States in 1986. Hepatitis vaccine is indicated in people of all ages, especially those who will be at increased risk for exposure to hepatitis B virus infection. These include health care personnel, patients on hemodialysis or requiring frequent transfusions of blood or blood products, institutionalized patients and their close contacts, adolescents, as well as infants born to mothers who have positive results for hepatitis B surface antigen.[118]

Hepatitis B recombinant vaccines are given in a three-dose series. The sequence consists of two priming doses given 1 month apart, followed by a third dose given 6 months after the first. Those who have not been vaccinated against hepatitis B during infancy should complete the series during any childhood visit. The maximal immune response is in children 2–19 years old, with diminished response in older adults and persons with immunosuppressive illnesses.[118]

Local and Systemic Reactions

Local reactions, including soreness, erythema, and local induration are seen in approximately one-third of recipients of both the plasma-derived and recombinant vaccines[119, 120]; 10–15% may experience systemic reactions such as fatigue, headache, or fever.[120]

Anaphylaxis

Hepatitis B vaccines may rarely cause anaphylaxis (VAERS November 1990 to July 1992).

Neurologic Complications

Although there have been some reports of GBS following hepatitis B vaccination, the evidence is insufficient to support an association.[121] Other uncommon side effects include transverse myelitis,[121] optic neuritis,[121] and multiple sclerosis.[122]

Influenza Vaccine

Influenza is characterized by an abrupt onset of fever, myalgia, sore throat, cough, malaise, and in severe cases, pneumonia. It is estimated that more than 20,000 influenza-associated deaths occurred during each of the 10 different U.S. epidemics from 1972 to 1973 and from 1990 to 1991.[123]

The efficacy of influenza vaccine depends on the age and immunocompetence of the recipient as well as the degree of similarity between the vaccine virus strains and those that circulate during the influenza season. The vaccine has been shown to prevent illness in approximately 70% of healthy individuals younger than 65 years and in 30–70% of the uninstitutionalized elderly. Among elderly nursing home residents, the vaccine can be 50–60% effective in preventing complications such as pneumonia and 80% effective in preventing death.[123]

The vaccine is recommended especially for those 65 years of age or older; residents of chronic care facilities that care for people with chronic medical conditions; patients with chronic cardiopulmonary disorders; patients with diabetes, renal dysfunction, or immunosuppression; and children on chronic aspirin therapy who are at risk for developing Reye's syndrome after influenza. Health care workers and close contacts of individuals in chronic care facilities should also be vaccinated. In addition, influenza vaccine may be administered to any person who wishes to reduce the chance of becoming infected with influenza.[123] Each year, the influenza vaccine contains strains representing the viruses that are likely to circulate in the United States that winter. Yearly vaccination of those at high risk before the influenza season is currently the most effective method of reducing the impact of influenza.

Local and Systemic Reactions

The most frequent side effect, reported by fewer than one-third of patients, is soreness at the vaccination site lasting up to 2 days. Systemic reactions including fever, malaise, and myalgias are infrequent and may last for 1 or 2 days.[123]

Allergic Reactions

Immediate allergic reactions, including hives, angioedema, and anaphylaxis, may result from hypersensitivity to a vaccine component, most commonly residual egg protein. Therefore, those with egg allergy should consult a physician for appropriate evaluation to determine if the vaccine should be administered.[123]

Neurologic Complications

Neurologic complications of influenza immunization were rarely reported before 1976. In that year, a national immunization program was established against the "swine flu" (A/New Jersey) strain of influenza virus. Over the next 2 months, an increase in cases of GBS was documented. The risk of GBS attributable to influenza immunization was estimated at 1 per 100,000 immunizations, with onset usually occurring 5–10 weeks after the immunization.[124] Subsequent vaccines prepared from other virus strains have not clearly been associated with GBS. Therefore, vaccination should be avoided in a person known to have developed GBS within 6 weeks of a previous influenza vaccination.

Neurologic disorders temporally associated with influenza vaccination such as encephalopathy,[125–127] brachial plexus neuropathy or neuralgic amyotrophy,[128] acute transverse myelitis,[129] and isolated cranial neuropathies[130] have been reported. However, these complications are too infrequent to establish a causal relationship.

Varicella Vaccine

Varicella is a highly communicable disease caused by varicella zoster virus. In the United States, approximately 3.5 million cases of varicella occurred annually from 1980 to 1994, with a peak incidence in those between 5 and 9 years of age.[131] The attack rate of varicella after household exposure among healthy susceptible children is 87%.[132]

The varicella vaccine (OKA strain) is a live attenuated virus vaccine that was licensed for use in the United States in March 1995. Vaccination is indicated in individuals 12 months of age and older who have not had varicella. Children between 12 months to 12 years of age should receive a single dose. When given after 13 years of age, a second dose should be administered 4–8 weeks later because natural varicella is more severe and complications more frequent in older individuals. The duration of protection after vaccination is not known, and the need for booster doses has not been defined. Severity of varicella after vaccination is much milder than in unvaccinated children.[133, 134]

Contraindications and Precautions

Varicella vaccine is contraindicated in patients with history of hypersensitivity to any component of the vaccine or anaphylactoid reaction to neomycin. Other contraindications include immunodeficiency, family history of congenital or hereditary immunodeficiency, tuberculosis, active febrile illness, and pregnancy. Vaccination should be deferred for at least 5 months after blood or plasma transfusions or administration of immune globulin including varicella zoster immune globulin. Immune globulin should not be administered for 2 months after immunization. Salicylates should be avoided for 6 weeks after vaccination because Reye's syndrome occurring after the use of salicylates during natural varicella infection has been reported. Vaccine recipients should avoid close contact with susceptible high-risk individuals for up to 6 weeks—for example, newborns, pregnant women, and immunocompromised individuals. Pregnancy should be avoided for 3 months after vaccination.[133, 134]

Complications

Varicella vaccine is generally well tolerated. A mild maculopapular or varicelliform rash at the injection site or elsewhere may occur in 7–8% of individuals and local pain and redness in 25–35%. Other reported adverse reactions include fever, headache, irritability, fatigue, cough, diarrhea, anorexia, lymphadenopathy, myalgia, arthralgia, pneumonitis, and febrile seizures, but a causal link has not been established. Anaphylaxis, encephalitis, ataxia, and erythema multiforme have also been reported.[133, 134]

Conclusion

Routine immunization has been instrumental in reducing the morbidity and mortality due to infectious diseases in all age groups. The risks associated with the use of vaccines vary from trivial and inconvenient to severe and life threatening; however, it is important to recognize that the benefits of immunization far outweigh the risks and complications associated with both immunization and the natural illness.

References

1. Immunization of adolescents: recommendations of the Advisory Committee on Immunization Practices, the American Academy of Pediatrics, the American Academy of Family Physicians and the American Medical Association. Pediatrics 1997;99:479.
2. Bloch AB, Orenstein WA, Stetler HC, et al. Health impact of measles vaccination in the United States. Pediatrics 1985;76:524.
3. Meyer HM Jr, Hopps HE, Parkman PD, et al. Control of measles and rubella through use of attenuated vaccines. Am J Clin Pathol 1978;70:128.
4. Hilleman MR, Buynak EB, Weibel RE, et al. Development and evaluation of the Moraten measles virus vaccine. JAMA 1968;206:587.
5. Nader PR, Warren RJ. Reported neurologic disorders following live measles vaccine. Pediatrics 1968;41:997.
6. Landrigan PJ, Witte JJ. Neurologic disorders following live measles-virus vaccination. JAMA 1973;223:1459.
7. Alderslade R, Bellman MH, Ross EM, et al. The National Childhood Encephalopathy Study: a report on 1,000 cases of serious neurological disorders in infants and young children from the NCES research team. In Department of Health and Social Security. Whooping Cough: Reports from the Committee on the Safety of Medicines and the Joint Committee on the Vaccination and Immunization. London: Her Majesty's Stationary Office, 1981.
8. Miller DL. Frequency of complications of measles, 1963: report on a National Inquiry by the Public Health Laboratory Service in collaboration with the Society of Medical Officers of Health. BMJ 1964;2:75.
9. Modlin JF, Jabbour JT, Witte JJ, et al. Epidemiologic studies of measles, measles vacine and subacute sclerosing panencephalitis. Pediatrics 1977;59:505.
10. Schneck SA. Vaccination with measles and central nervous system disease. Neurology 1968;18(Part II):79.
11. Cho CT, Lansky LJ, D'Souza BJ. Panencephalitis following measles vaccination [letter]. JAMA 1973; 224:1299.
12. Dyken PR, Cunningham SC, Ward LC. Changing character of subacute sclerosing panencephalitis in the United States. Pediatr Neurol 1989;5:339.
13. Subacute sclerosing panencephalitis Surveillance: United States. MMWR Morb Mortal Wkly Rep 1982;31:585.
14. Valmari P, Lanning M, Tuokko H, et al. Measles virus in the cerebrospinal fluid in postvaccination immunosuppressive measles encephalopathy. Pediatr Infect Dis J 1987;6:59.
15. Mitus A, Holloway A, Evans AE, et al. Attenuated measles vaccine in children with acute leukemia. Am J Dis Child 1962;103:243.
16. Hirtz DG, Nelson KB, Ellenberg JH. Seizures following childhood immunizations. J Pediatr 1983;102:14.
17. Griffin MR, Ray WA, Mortimer EA, et al. Risk of seizures after measles-mumps-rubella immunization. Pediatrics 1991;88:881.
18. Pollock TM, Morris J. A 7-year survey of disorders attributed to vaccination in northwest Thames region. Lancet 1983;1:753.
19. Pampiglione G, Griffith AH, Bramwell EC. Transient cerebral changes after vaccination against measles. Lancet 1971;2:5.
20. Chan CC, Sogg RL, Steinman L. Isolated oculomotor palsy after measles immunization. Am J Ophthalmol 1980;89:446.
21. Kazarian EL, Gager WE. Optic neuritis complicating measles, mumps and rubella vaccination. Am J Ophthalmol 1978;86:544.
22. Marshall GS, Wright PF, Fenichel GM, et al. Diffuse retinopathy following measles, mumps and rubella vaccination. Pediatrics 1985;76:989.
23. Buynak ZB, Hilleman MR. Live attenuated mumps virus vaccine. I. Vaccine development. Proc Soc Exp Biol Med 1966;123:768.
24. Hilleman MR, Buynak EB, Weibel RE, et al. Live

attenuated mumps-virus vaccine. N Engl J Med 1968;278:227.
25. Fujinaga T, Motegi Y, Tamura H, et al. A prefecture-wide survey of mumps meningitis associated with measles, mumps and rubella vacccine. Pediatr Infect Dis J 1991;10:204.
26. Nabe-Nielsen J, Walter B. Unilateral deafness as a complication of the mumps, measles and rubella vaccination. BMJ 1988;297:489.
27. Brodsky L, Stanievich J. Sensorineural hearing loss following live measles virus vaccination. Int J Pediatr Otorhinolaryngol 1985;10:159.
28. Healy CE. Mumps vaccine and nerve deafness [letter]. Am J Dis Child 1972;123:612.
29. Orenstein WA, Bart KJ, Hinman AR, et al. The opportunity and obligation to eliminate rubella from the United States. JAMA 1984;251:1988.
30. Preblud SR. Some current issues relating to rubella vaccine. JAMA 1985;254:253.
31. Kilroy AW, Schaffner W, Fleet WF, et al. Two syndromes following rubella immunizations: clinical observations and epidemiological studies. JAMA 1970;214:2287.
32. Gilmartin RC, Jabbour JT, Duenas DA. Rubella vaccine myeloradiculoneuritis. J Pediatr 1972;80:406.
33. Speier JE. Complications of Rubella vaccination [letter]. JAMA 1970;213:2272.
34. Schaffner W, Fleet WF, Kilroy AW, et al. Polyneuropathy following rubella immunization. A follow-up study and review of the problem. Am J Dis Child 1974;127:684.
35. Holt S, Hudgins D, Krishnan KR, et al. Diffuse myelitis associated with rubella vaccination. BMJ 1976;2:1037.
36. Kline LB, Margulies SL, Oh SJ. Optic neuritis and myelitis following rubella vaccination. Arch Neurol 1982;39:443.
37. Modlin JF, Brandling-Bennet D, Witte JJ, et al. A review of five years experience with rubella vaccine in the United States. Pediatrics 1975;55:20.
38. Wyll SA, Herrmann KL. Inadvertent rubella vaccination of pregnant women. Fetal risk in 215 cases. JAMA 1973;225:1472.
39. Vaheri A, Vesikari T, Oker-Blom N, et al. Isolation of attenuated rubella-vaccine virus from human products of conception and uterine cervix. N Engl J Med 1972;286:1071.
40. Rubella vaccination during pregnancy: United States 1971–1983. MMWR Morb Mortal Wkly Rep 1984;33:365.
41. Preblud SR, Stetler HC, Frank JA Jr, et al. Fetal risk associated with rubella vaccine. JAMA 1981;246:1413.
42. Nightingale EO. Recommendations for a national policy on poliomyelitis vaccination. N Engl J Med 1977;297:249.
43. Salk D. Eradication of poliomyelitis in the United States: I. Live virus vaccine-associated and wild poliovirus disease. Rev Infect Dis 1980;2:228.
44. Salk D. Eradication of poliomyelitis in the United States: II. Live virus vaccine-associated and wild poliovirus disease. Rev Infect Dis 1980;2:243.
45. Salk D. Eradication of poliomyelitis in the United States: III. Live virus vaccine-associated and wild poliovirus disease. Rev Infect Dis 1980;2:258.
46. Fox JP. Eradication of poliomyelitis in the United States: a commentary on the Salk reviews. Rev Infect Dis 1980;2:277.
47. Ruuskanen O, Salmi TT, Stenvik M, et al. Inactivated poliovaccine: adverse reactions and antibody responses. Acta Paediatr Scand 1980;69:397.
48. Henderson DA, Witte JJ, Morris L, et al. Paralytic disease associated with oral polio vaccines. JAMA 1964;190:41.
49. Centers for Disease Control. Poliomyelitis—United States, 1975–1984. MMWR Morb Mortal Wkly Rep 1986;35:180.
50. Nkowane BM, Wassilak SG, Orenstein WA, et al. Vaccine-associated paralytic poliomyelitis, United States: 1973 through1984. JAMA 1987;257:1335.
51. Bergeisen GH, Bauman RJ, Gilmore RL. Neonatal paralytic poliomyelitis: a case report. Arch Neurol 1986; 43:192.
52. Wilson J, Robinson R. Poliomyelitis after contact with recently vaccinated infant [letter]. BMJ 1974;2:53.
53. Fenichel GM. Neurological Complications of Immunization. In KF Swaiman (ed), Pediatric Neurology: Principles and Practice. St. Louis: Mosby, 1993;1189.
54. Kinnunen E, Farkkila M, Hovi T, et al. Incidence of Guillain-Barré syndrome during a nationwide oral polio virus vaccine campaign. Neurology 1989;39:1034.
55. Institute of Medicine. Polio Vaccines. In KR Stratton, CJ Howe, RB Johnston (eds), Adverse Events Associated with Childhood Vaccines: Evidence Bearing on Causality. Institute of Medicine. Washington DC: National Academy Press, 1994;187.
56. Centers for Disease Control. Summary of Notifiable Diseases, United States, 1994. MMWR Morb Mortal Wkly Rep 1995;43:70.
57. Peebles TC, Levine L, Eldred MC, et al. Tetanus toxoid emergency boosters: a reappraisal. N Engl J Med 1969;280:575.
58. Collier LH, Polakoff S, Mortimer J. Reactions and antibody responses to reinforcing doses of adsorbed and plain tetanus vaccines. Lancet 1979;1:1364.
59. Blumstein GI, Kreithin H. Peripheral neuropathy following tetanus toxoid administration. JAMA 1966;198:1030.
60. Centers for Disease Control. Diphtheria, tetanus, and pertussis: guidelines for vaccine prophylaxis and other preventive measures. JAMA 1985;254:895.
61. Acel-Imune package insert. Pearl River, NY: Lederle Laboratories, Division American Cyanamid Co., January 3, 1997.
62. Jacobs RL, Lowe RS, Lanier BQ. Adverse reactions to tetanus toxoid. JAMA 1982;247:40.
63. Jones AE, Melville-Smith M, Watkins J. Adverse reactions in adolescents to reinforcing doses of plain and adsorbed tetanus vaccines. Community Med 1985;7:99.
64. Facktor MA, Bernstein RA, Fireman P. Hypersensitivity to tetanus toxoid. J Allergy Clin Immunol 1973;52:1.

65. Schlenska GK. Unusual neurological complications following tetanus toxoid administration. J Neurol 1977;215:299.
66. Schwarz G, Lanzer G, List WF. Acute midbrain syndrome as an adverse reaction to tetanus immunization. Intensive Care Med 1988;15:53.
67. Whittle E, Roberton NRC. Transverse myelitis after diphtheria, tetanus and polio immunization. BMJ 1977;1:1450.
68. Read SJ, Schapel GJ, Pender MP. Acute transverse myelitis after tetanus toxoid vaccination [letter]. Lancet 1992;339:1111.
69. Topaloglu H, Berker M, Kansu T, et al. Optic neuritis and myelitis after booster tetanus toxoid vaccination [letter]. Lancet 1992;339:178.
70. Quast U, Hennessen W, Widmark RM. Mono- and polyneuritis after tetanus vaccination (1970–1977). Dev Biol Stand 1979;43:25.
71. Reinstein L, Pargament JM, Goodman JS. Peripheral neuropathy after multiple tetanus toxoid injections. Arch Phys Med Rehabil 1982;63:332.
72. Holliday PL, Bauer RB. Polyradiculoneuritis secondary to immunization with tetanus and diphtheria toxoids. Arch Neurol 1983;40:56.
73. Pollard JD, Selby G. Relapsing neuropathy due to tetanus toxoid: report of a case. J Neurol Sci 1978;37:113.
74. Tsairis P, Dyck PH, Mulder DW. Natural history of brachial plexus neuropathy: report on 99 patients. Arch Neurol 1972;27:109.
75. Baust W, Meyer D, Wachsmuth W. Peripheral neuropathy after administration of tetanus toxoid. J Neurol 1979;222:131.
76. Kiwit JC. Neurologic amyotrophy after administration of tetanus toxoid [letter]. J Neurol Neurosurg Psychiatry 1984;47:320.
77. Recommendations of the Immunization Practices Advisory Committee (ACIP). Diphtheria, tetanus and pertussis: recommendations for vaccine use and other preventive measures. MMWR Morb Mortal Wkly Rep 1991;40:RR-10.
78. Farizo KM, Cochi SL, Zell ER, et al. Epidemiological features of pertusssis in the United States, 1980–1989. Clin Infect Dis 1992;14:708.
79. Pertussis Surveillance—United States, January 1992–June 1995. MMWR Morb Mortal Wkly Rep 1995;44:525.
80. Miller CL, Fletcher WB. Severity of notified whooping cough. BMJ 1976;1:117.
81. Church MA. Evidence of whooping-cough-vaccine efficacy from the 1978 whooping-cough epidemic in Hertfordshire. Lancet 1979;2:188.
82. Cherry JD, Brunell PA, Golden GS, et al. Report of the Task Force on Pertussis and Pertussis Immunization—1988. Pediatrics 1988;81:939.
83. Cody CL, Baraff LJ, Cherry JD, et al. Nature and rates of adverse reactions associated with DTP and DT immunizations in infants and children. Pediatrics 1981;68:650.
84. Baraff LJ, Shields D, Beckwith L, et al. Infants and children with convulsions and hypotonic-hyporesponsive episodes following diphtheria-tetanus-pertussis immunization: follow-up evaluation. Pediatrics 1988;81:789.
85. Ouvrier RA. Whooping cough immunizations: a neurologist's viewpoint. Med J Aust 1978;2:300.
86. Stetler HC, Orenstein WA, Bart KJ, et al. History of convulsions and use of pertussis vaccine. J Pediatr 1985;107:175.
87. Harker P. Primary immunization in febrile convulsions in Oxford in 1972–1975. BMJ 1977;2:490.
88. Melchior JC. Infantile spasms and early immunization against whooping cough. Arch Dis Child 1977;52:134.
89. Matsumoto A, Watanabe K, Negoro T, et al. Infantile spasms: etiological factors, clinical aspects and long term prognosis in 200 cases. Eur J Pediatr 1981; 135:239.
90. Bellman MH, Ross EM, Miller DL. Infantile spasms and pertussis immunization. Lancet 1983;1:1031.
91. Berg JM. Neurological complications of pertussis immunization. BMJ 1958;2:24.
92. Kulenkampff M, Schwartzman JS, Wilson J. Neurological complications of pertussis inoculation. Arch Dis Child 1974;49:46.
93. Miller DL, Ross EM, Alderslade R, et al. Pertussis immunization and serious acute neurological illness in children. BMJ 1981;282:1595.
94. Fenichel GM. Neurologic Complications of Immunization. In KF Swaiman (ed), Pediatric Neurology: Principles and Practice. St. Louis: Mosby, 1989;925.
95. Cherry JD. The epidemiology of pertussis and pertussis immunization in the United Kingdom and the United States: a comparative study. Curr Probl Pediatr 1984; 14:53.
96. Pertussis Surveillance 1979–1981. MMWR Morb Mortal Wkly Rep 1982; 31:333.
97. American Academy of Pediatrics. Report of the Committee on Infectious Diseases: pertussis vaccine. Pediatrics 1984;74:303.
98. Recommendations of the Immunization Practices Advisory Committee (ACIP): supplementary statement of contraindications to receipt of pertussis vaccine. MMWR Morb Mortal Wkly Rep 1984;33:169.
99. Toomey JA. Reactions to pertussis vaccine. JAMA 1949;139:448.
100. Child Neurology Society Consensus Statement. Pertussis immunization and the central nervous system. Ann Neurol 1991;29:458.
101. Centers for Disease Control. Pertussis vaccination: acellular pertussis vaccine for reinforcing and booster use—supplementary ACIP statement: recommendations of the Immunizations Practice Advisory Committee (ACIP). MMWR Morb Mortal Wkly Rep 1992;41:RR-1.
102. Feldman S, Perry S, Andrew M, et al. Comparison of acellular (B type) and whole-cell pertusis-component diphtheria-tetanus-pertussis vaccines as the first booster

immunization in 15 to 24 month old children. J Pediatr 1992;121:857.
103. Cochi SL, Broome CV, Hightower AW. Immunization of US children with *Hemophilus influenzae* type b polysaccharide vaccine: a cost effectiveness model of strategy assessment. JAMA 1985;253:521.
104. Shapiro ED, Murphy TV, Wald ER, et al. The protective efficacy of *Hemophilus* b polysaccharide vaccine. JAMA 1988;260:1419.
105. Frank AL, Labotka RJ, Rao S, et al. *Haemophilus influenzae* type b immunization of children with sickle cell diseases. Pediatrics 1988;82:571.
106. Feldman S, Gigliotti F, Shenep JL, et al. Risk of *Hemophilus influenzae* type b disease in children with cancer and response of immunocompromised leukemic children to a conjugate vaccine. J Infect Dis 1990;161:926.
107. Kayhty H, Peltola H, Eskola J, et al. Immunogenicity of *Haemophilus influenzae* oligosaccharide-protein and polysaccharide-protein conjugate vaccination of children at 4, 6, and 14 months of age. Pediatrics 1989;84:995.
108. Adams WG, Deaver KA, Cochi SL, et al. Decline of childhood *Hemophilus influenza* type b (Hib) disease in the Hib vaccine era. JAMA 1993;269:221.
109. Ahonkhai VI, Lukacs LJ, Jonas LC, et al. *Haemophilus influenzae* type b conjugate vaccine (meningococcal protein conjugate) (PedvaxHIB): clinical evaluation. Pediatrics 1990;85:676.
110. D'Cruz OF, Shapiro ED, Spiegelman KN, et al. Acute inflammatory demyelinating polyradiculoneuropathy (Guillain-Barré syndrome) after immunization with *Hemophilus influenzae* type b conjugate vaccine. J Pediatr 1989;115:743.
111. Gervaix A, Caflisch M, Suter S, et al. Guillain-Barré syndrome following immunization with *Haemophilus influenzae* type b conjugate vaccine. Eur J Pediatr 1993;152:613.
112. Black SB, Shinefield HR, Hiatt RA, et al. Kaiser Permanente Pediatric vaccine study group. Efficacy of *Hemophilus influenzae* type b capsular polysaccharide vaccine. Pediatr Infect Dis J 1988;7:149.
113. Sood SK, Daum RS. Disease caused by *Haemophilus influenzae* type b in the immediate period after homologous immunization: immunologic investigation. Pediatrics 1990;85:698.
114. Marchant CD, Band E, Froeschle JE, et al. Depression of anticapsular antibody after immunization with *Hemophilus influenzae* type b polysaccarhide-diptheria conjugate vaccine. Pediatr Infect Dis J 1989;8:508.
115. Patel H, Garg BP. Neurological Complications of Immunization. In K Roos (ed), CNS Infectious Diseases and Therapy. New York: Marcel Dekker, 1997;79.
116. Hiner EE, Frasch CE. Spectrum of disease due to *Hemophilus influenzae* type b occurring in immunized children. J Infect Dis 1988;158:343.
117. Santosham M, Wolff M, Reid R, et al. The efficacy in Navajo infants of a conjugate vaccine consisting of *Hemophilus influenzae* type b polysaccharide and *Neisseria meningitidis* outer-membrane protein complex. N Engl J Med 1991;324:1767.
118. Centers for Disease Control. Protection against viral hepatitis: recommendations of the Immunization Practices Advisory Committee (ACIP). MMWR Morb Mortal Wkly Rep 1990;39:RR-2.
119. Szmuness W, Stevens CE, Harley EJ, et al. Hepatitis B vaccine: demonstration of efficacy in a controlled trial in a high risk population in the United States. N Engl J Med 1980;303:833.
120. Andre FE. Summary of safety and efficacy data on a yeast-derived hepatitis B vaccine. Am J Med 1989; 87:14S.
121. Shaw FE, Graham DJ, Guess HA, et al. Postmarketing surveillance for neurologic adverse events reported after hepatitis B vaccination: experience of the first three years. Am J Epidemiol 1988;127:337.
122. Herroelen L, De Keyser J, Ebinger G. Central-nervous-system demyelination after immunization with recombinant hepatitis B vaccine. Lancet 1991;338:1174.
123. Recommendations of the Advisory Committee on Immunization Practices (ACIP). Prevention and control of Influenza. MMWR Morb Mortal Wkly Rep 1996;45:RR-5.
124. Schonberger LB, Bregman DJ, Sullivan-Bolyal JZ, et al. Guillain-Barré syndrome following vaccination in the national influenza immunization program, United States 1976–1977. Am J Epidemiol 1979;110:105.
125. Cherington M. Locked-in syndrome after "swine-flu" inoculation [letter]. Arch Neurol 1977;34:258.
126. Gens RD, Beecham HJ. Meningoencephalitis after influenza inoculation [letter]. N Engl J Med 1978; 299:721.
127. Yahr MD, Lobo-Antunes J. Relapsing encephalomyelitis following the use of influenza vaccine. Arch Neurol 1972;27:182.
128. Weintraub MI, Chia DTS. Paralytic brachial neuritis after swine flu vaccination [letter]. Arch Neurol 1977;34:518.
129. Wells CEC. A neurological note on vaccination against influenza. BMJ 1971;3:755.
130. Felix JK, Schwartz RH, Myers GJ. Isolated hypoglossal nerve paralysis following influenza vaccination. Am J Dis Child 1976;130:82.
131. Preblud SR. Varicella: complications and costs. Pediatrics 1986;78:728.
132. Ross AH. Modification of chickenpox in family contacts by administration of gamma globulin. N Engl J Med 1962;267:369.
133. American Academy of Pediatrics, Committee on Infectious Diseases. Recommendations for the use of live attenuated varicella vaccine. Pediatrics 1995;95:791.
134. Varivax package insert. West Point, PA: Merck and Co., May 1996.

Index